TRAUMA MANAGEMENT
Volumes I and II, Second Edition

Series Editors

F. William Blaisdell, M.D.
Professor and Chairman
Department of Surgery
University of California, Davis
Sacramento, California

Donald D. Trunkey, M.D.
Professor and Chairman
Department of Surgery
The Oregon Health Sciences University
Portland, Oregon

ABDOMINAL TRAUMA

SECOND EDITION

With additional revised chapters from Urogenital Trauma, Volume II

F. William Blaisdell, M.D.
Professor and Chairman
Department of Surgery
University of California, Davis
Sacramento, California

Donald D. Trunkey, M.D.
Professor and Chairman
Department of Surgery
The Oregon Health Sciences University
Portland, Oregon

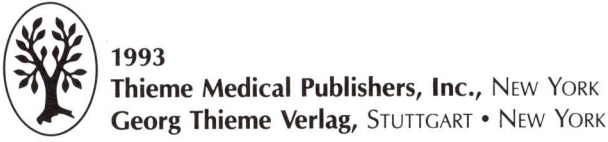

1993
Thieme Medical Publishers, Inc., NEW YORK
Georg Thieme Verlag, STUTTGART • NEW YORK

Thieme Medical Publishers, Inc.
381 Park Avenue South
New York, New York 10016

ABDOMINAL TRAUMA, SECOND EDITION
F. William Blaisdell
Donald D. Trunkey

Library of Congress Cataloging-in-Publication Data

Abdominal trauma, second edition : with additional revised chapters from Urogenital trauma,
 volume II / [edited by]F. William Blaisdell, Donald D. Trunkey.— 2nd ed.
   p.   cm.—(Trauma management ; v. 1–2)
  Includes bibliographical references and index.
  ISBN 0-86577-453-6 (Thieme Medical Publishers).—ISBN
3-13-598902-X (Georg Thieme Verlag)
  1. Abdomen—Wounds and injuries. I. Blaisdell, F. William (Frank
William), 1927–   . II. Trunkey, Donald D. III. Urogenital trauma.
III. Series.
  [DNLM: 1. Abdominal Injuries—surgery. 2. Urogenital System—
injuries. WO 700 T776 1982 v. 1–2]
RD540.A2 1992
617.5'5044—dc20
DNLM/DLC
for Library of Congress   92-49807
                                                                                         CIP

Copyright © 1993 by Thieme Medical Publishers, Inc. This book, including all parts thereof, is legally protected by copyright. Any use, exploitation or commercialization outside the narrow limits set by copyright legislation, without the publisher's consent, is illegal and liable to prosecution. This applies in particular to photostat reproduction, copying, mimeographing or duplication of any kind, translating, preparation of microfilms, and electronic data processing and storage.

Important note: Medicine is an ever-changing science. Research and clinical experience are continually broadening our knowledge, in particular our knowledge of proper treatment and drug therapy. Insofar as this book mentions any dosage or applications, readers may rest assured that the authors, editors, and publishers have made every effort to ensure that such references are strictly in accordance with the state of knowledge at the time of production of the book. Nevertheless, every user is requested to carefully examine the manufacturers' leaflets accompanying each drug to check on his own responsibility whether the dosage schedules recommended therein or the contraindications stated by the manufacturers differ from the statements made in the present book. Such examination is particularly important with drugs that are either rarely used or have been newly released on the market.

Some of the product names, patents, and registered designs referred to in this book are in fact registered trademarks or proprietary names even though specific reference to this fact is not always made in the text. Therefore, the appearance of a name without designation as proprietary is not to be construed as a representation by the publisher that it is in the public domain.

Printed in the United States of America.

5   4   3   2   1

TMP ISBN 0-86577-453-6
GTV ISBN 3-13-598902-X

Contents

	Contributors	v
	Foreword	vii
	Preface	ix
1.	General Assessment of Penetrating and Blunt Abdominal Trauma *David H. Wisner, M.D.*	1
2.	Resuscitation *Lee Halvorsen, M.D., and James W. Holcroft, M.D.*	13
3.	Peritoneal Lavage, Computerized Tomography, Angiography, Ultrasound, and Magnetic Resonance Imaging *David H. Wisner, M.D., and Lawrence A. Danto, M.D.*	32
4.	Indications for and General Conduct of the Operation *David H. Wisner, M.D.*	57
5.	Chest and Abdominal Wall Injuries *F. William Blaisdell, M.D.*	72
6.	Diaphragm Rupture *Sandra L. Beal, M.D.*	83
7.	Pelvic Fractures *Felix Battistella, M.D.*	94
8.	Esophageal, Gastric, and Omental Injuries *Richard A. Crass, M.D., and Richard J. Mullins, M.D.*	110
9.	Trauma to the Pancreas and Duodenum *Charles Frey, M.D., and Tatsuo Araida, M.D.*	118
10.	Injuries to the Liver and Extrahepatic Ducts *John Ragsdale, M.D., and Donald D. Trunkey, M.D.*	160
11.	Small Bowel and Mesentery *Michael Smith, M.D., and Norman Christensen, M.D.*	190
12.	Trauma to the Colon and Rectum *E. John Harris, Jr., M.D., and Donald D. Trunkey, M.D.*	209

13. **Splenic Injury** 230
    Sandra L. Beal, M.D., and Donald D. Trunkey, M.D.

14. **The Management of Renal and Ureteral Trauma** 250
    Peter R. Carroll, M.D., Christopher M. Dixon, M.D., and Jack W. McAninch, M.D.

15. **Urethral and Bladder Injuries** 277
    Christopher M. Dixon, M.D., Jack W. McAninch, M.D., and Peter R. Carroll, M.D.

16. **Genital Injuries** 293
    Jack W. McAninch, M.D., Christopher M. Dixon, M.D., and Peter R. Carroll, M.D.

17. **Female Genital Trauma and Sexual Assault** 311
    M. Margaret Knudson, M.D., and William R. Crombleholme, M.D.

18. **Trauma in Pregnancy** 324
    M. Margaret Knudson, M.D.

19. **Abdominal Arterial Trauma** 341
    William R. Fry, M.D.

20. **Abdominal Venous Trauma** 371
    F. William Blaisdell, M.D.

21. **Retroperitoneal Hematoma** 398
    Anthony A. Meyer, M.D., Kenneth A. Kudsk, M.D., and George F. Sheldon, M.D.

    Index 414

Contributors

Tatsuo Araida, M.D.
Visiting Fellow in Gastrointestinal Surgery
University of California, Davis
Sacramento, California

Felix Battistella, M.D.
Assistant Professor of Surgery
University of California, Davis
Sacramento, California

Sandra L. Beal, M.D.
Assistant Professor of Surgery
University of California, Davis
Sacramento, California

F. William Blaisdell, M.D.
Professor and Chairman
Department of Surgery
University of California, Davis
Sacramento, California

Peter R. Carroll, M.D.
Assistant Professor of Urology
University of California School of Medicine
and San Francisco General Hospital
San Francisco, California

Norman Christensen, M.D.
Associate Clinical Professor of Surgery
University of California, San Francisco
San Francisco, California

Richard A. Crass, M.D.
Professor of Surgery
The Oregon Health Sciences University
Portland, Oregon

William R. Crombleholme, M.D.
Associate Professor of Obstetrics and
  Gynecology
University of California, San Francisco
San Francisco, California

Lawrence A. Danto, M.D.
Associate Clinical Professor of Surgery
University of California, Davis
Sacramento, California

Christopher M. Dixon, M.D.
Assistant Professor of Urology
University of California School of Medicine
and San Francisco General Hospital
San Francisco, California

Charles Frey, M.D.
Professor of Surgery
University of California, Davis
Sacramento, California

William R. Fry, M.D.
Assistant Professor of Surgery
University of California, Davis
Sacramento, California

Lee Halvorsen, M.D.
Assistant Professor of Surgery
University of California, Davis
Sacramento, California

E. John Harris, Jr., M.D.
Instructor in Surgery
The Oregon Health Sciences University
Portland, Oregon

James W. Holcroft, M.D.
Professor and Vice Chairman
Department of Surgery
University of California, Davis
Sacramento, California

M. Margaret Knudson, M.D.
Assistant Professor of Surgery
University of California, San Francisco
San Francisco, California

Kenneth A. Kudsk, M.D.
Associate Professor of Surgery
University of Tennessee
Memphis, Tennessee

Jack W. McAninch, M.D.
Professor of Urology
University of California School of Medicine
and San Francisco General Hospital
San Francisco, California

Anthony A. Meyer, M.D.
Professor of Surgery
University of North Carolina
Chapel Hill, North Carolina

Richard J. Mullins, M.D.
Professor of Surgery
The Oregon Health Sciences University
Portland, Oregon

John Ragsdale, M.D.
Professor of Surgery
The Oregon Health Sciences University
Portland, Oregon

George F. Sheldon, M.D.
Professor and Chairman
Department of Surgery
University of North Carolina
Chapel Hill, North Carolina

Michael Smith, M.D.
Assistant Clinical Professor of Surgery
University of California, Davis
Sacramento, California

Donald D. Trunkey, M.D.
Professor and Chairman
Department of Surgery
The Oregon Health Sciences University
Portland, Oregon

David H. Wisner, M.D.
Associate Professor of Surgery
University of California, Davis
Sacramento, California

Foreword

As academic surgeons, our interest in trauma developed for multiple reasons. Our discipline, surgery, through the act of operation itself, inflicts trauma. Thus, the study of trauma provides insight into surgical illness and recovery from operation. The pursuit of trauma involves the need to investigate basic mechanisms of wound healing, immunology, biochemistry, and physiology. Trauma is the oldest, and will remain the most secure, of all surgical disciplines since the treatment of injury can not be resolved by medical measures, as is potentially true of cardiovascular disease, cancer, and biliary and gastrointestinal disorders. Finally, despite increasing specialization, the trauma surgeon must remain a generalist since under emergency circumstances he must be prepared to deal with unexpected problems in any area, involving any body cavity.

In the process of developing trauma surgery as a distinct discipline in our university settings, we have acquired colleagues with similar interests. Thus, we have accumulated a large clinical experience and a uniform approach to trauma that seems to merit collection in a treatise on trauma rather than remain as a large number of articles scattered throughout the medical literature in journals and book chapters. We are bringing together clinicians from the respective staffs of four institutions—the University of California, San Francisco, at San Francisco General Hospital; the University of California, Davis, at our Sacramento Medical Center and Highland General Hospital, Oakland; The Oregon Health Sciences University; and the University of North Carolina. We feel this is a coordinated and united approach to trauma.

To make the material more manageable and to permit subsequent revision and expansion of particular areas in which changes are the most rapid, we have elected to organize our work into a series of monographs rather than to incorporate it into a single volume. Our first, *Abdominal Trauma*, has been of the widest general interest and has set the tone for the subsequent monographs on *Urogenital Trauma* (incorporated into this second edition), *Cervicothoracic Trauma*, *Burn Trauma*, *Craniospinal Trauma*, and *Extremity Trauma*.

The orientation of our trauma monographs is toward the senior surgical resident and general surgeons who treat trauma in their private practice. We believe our orientation will be both practical and conservative, aimed toward saving the maximum number of lives with minimum morbidity.

F. William Blaisdell, M.D.
Donald D. Trunkey, M.D.

Preface

Abdominal Trauma, the first monograph in the series, was completed ten years ago. Since that date, there have been many advances in trauma management. The current edition of *Abdominal Trauma* presents a complete update of all the previous chapters and includes revised chapters from *Urogenital Trauma*, previously Vol. II in this series. As is true of all of the previous volumes, the contributions to this new edition have come from our colleagues with whom we work and as such, we believe, represents a unified and consistent approach to the management of abdominal trauma.

This second edition of *Abdominal Trauma* was designed to be our primary treatise on trauma. It is fitting that *Abdominal Trauma* be the first volume in our series and the first to be updated since the abdomen is the focal point of the evaluation of injury in the multiply-injured patient. Abdominal injury is the most subtle of all the injuries to the body, and is the most likely to tax the diagnostic skills of the trauma surgeon. Autopsy studies repeatedly confirm that abdominal injury is the most frequent cause of readily preventable death. Our philosophic approach to trauma, which may seem conservative to some, is to recommend exploratory laparotomy if there is doubt concerning the presence of abdominal injury. There are no statistics available that support the contention that patients die from complications secondary to exploratory laparotomy, whereas it is relatively easy to prove that patients die of delays in the diagnosis of abdominal trauma. It is a fact that many patients die in sophisticated hospitals of readily treatable injuries as a result of having their injury recognized late or not at all. We remain surprised at the reluctance of surgeons to explore the abdomen of a traumatized patient and at the same time readily accept a negative exploration rate of 20% to 30% for appendicitis as representing good practice.

Although new diagnostic techniques such as peritoneal lavage and computed tomographic scanning have provided valuable assistance in making a prompt diagnosis of abdominal injury, there is no substitute for clinical judgment since all ancillary diagnostic methods have inherent false negative rates. For peritoneal lavage, for example, the false negative rate varies from 1% to 5%, but most likely is closer to the higher figure in medical centers that see and treat trauma only occasionally. The tragedy of one preventable death in a previously healthy young person may have permanent impact on the unfortunate surgeon responsible for treatment, or lack thereof.

The contributions to this and successive volumes come from our colleagues with whom we work or have worked, as we believe the value of this series is that it provides a uniform approach to trauma. This experience we describe represents an optimal approach for us as we deal with thousands of trauma victims each year in our combined environments. We believe the guidelines for patient management that we have laid down should be of assistance to those who deal with trauma less frequently as well.

We, the editors, are grateful to our secretaries who have assisted us with the manuscript preparation by turning out draft after draft. Our special thanks goes to Ms. Shirley Cable, who has assisted in editing all of the current chapters to ensure consistent grammatical style. We are indebted to our surgery residents, many of whom have initiated or assisted us with statistical evaluation of our results that have led to numerous papers and manuscripts. Moreover, their suggestions regarding patient management have led to new concepts of patient care and operative management. We congratulate our new artist, Kathy Hirsh, who has updated and added to the illustrative material provided by Marsha Dohrmann in the first edition. In particular, we are indebted to our long-suffering wives and children, who have tolerated our emergency commitments so well and in so doing have helped our surgical careers.

F. William Blaisdell, M.D.
Donald D. Trunkey, M.D.

1
General Assessment of Penetrating and Blunt Abdominal Trauma

DAVID H. WISNER, M.D.

HISTORY: Definitive surgical treatment for abdominal injuries for all practical purposes has developed in only this century. Previously, survival depended more on the individual's inherent ability to recuperate than on the medical care he received.

King William, the Conquerer of England, was a famous early victim of abdominal trauma. In 1087, he was faced with a revolt led by his son Robert, treason by his half-brother Odo, and war with King Philip of France. William crossed the channel to engage the French and fell on them at the town of Mantes in a surprise attack. The city was taken and burned and the destruction was so complete that today it is hard to find traces of 11th-century buildings in the town. As William rode through the streets of the devastated city, his horse, frightened by burning embers, threw the corpulent king against the high pommel of his saddle with such force that he was lethally ruptured. He died 3 weeks later after great suffering from abdominal sepsis. The body was removed to Caen where the final insult occurred. As the bloated corpse was being forced into a too-small stone coffin, the abdomen burst, filling the church with an incredible stench. The tomb was subsequently destroyed in 1562 by Calvinists. A single femur was all that survived of William's remains and even this was subsequently lost during the revolutionary riots of 1793. Today a simple stone is all that marks the grave of William the Conquerer.

During the 19th century, several surgeons attempted laparotomy for gunshot wounds of the abdomen and met with mixed results. Mortality for abdominal wounds was very high, approaching 98% during the American Civil War. During the Boer war near the turn of the century, there were isolated reports of successful surgical treatment of major abdominal trauma but more patients died after operative intervention than survived, seemingly confirming the prevailing notion that the best course of action in patients with penetrating abdominal wounds was observation and expectant management.

> *World War I brought improvements in surgical techniques and perioperative care such that operative intervention was increasingly used and mortality after gunshot wounds to the abdomen dropped to 45%. This was further reduced to 25% during World War II, to 12% during the Korean conflict, and to 8.5% in Vietnam. During the same period since World War I, civilian mortality from abdominal gunshot wounds dropped from 55% to less than 5% today. Many of the improvements in care and mortality rate have resulted from putting into practice lessons learned during the management of wartime injuries.*[3,4,10,11,13,16,18,21,22,24]

Autopsy studies show that head and chest trauma are the primary killers after injury in industrialized societies (Table 1–1). Abdominal injuries are nonetheless responsible for approximately 10% of deaths from blunt and penetrating trauma. Fatal isolated blunt abdominal trauma is relatively rare since associated head, chest, or pelvic injuries are usually present. Isolated penetrating abdominal trauma more often leads to death, usually secondary to exsanguination from major vascular injury or from septic complications of bowel injury.[14,15,19,21,26]

PATHOPHYSIOLOGY AND ETIOLOGY

The likelihood of injury to different viscera after penetrating abdominal trauma is related to the amount of space they occupy. As a consequence, hollow viscera such as the small and large intestine are most commonly injured. The mechanism of injury for blunt trauma is completely different and solid organs such as the liver and spleen are most vulnerable. This is of more than epidemiologic significance, as the index of suspicion for different injuries and their associated complications is different for the two different mechanisms.

Table 1–1 Cause of Death in 425 Trauma Cases (San Francisco General Autopsy Study)

TYPE OF INJURY	PERCENTAGE
Head injury	45
Burns	11
Heart injury	10.5
Lung injury	8
Liver injury	6.5
Aortic injury	4
Hemorrhage	4
Pelvic fracture	2.5
Miscellaneous	3.0
Hospital related*	6.5

*Primarily sepsis and respiratory failure.

Penetrating Trauma

Stab wounds are relatively benign injuries unless a major blood vessel has been lacerated. A recent review of 200 stab wounds suffered in the Folsom prison population in which there was almost universal intent to kill the victim disclosed a mortality rate of only 3%.[28] Most of the deaths were due to exsanguination from vascular injury. Many stab wounds of the abdominal wall fail to penetrate the peritoneal cavity and even if the peritoneal cavity is violated, there is often minimal or no injury to intraperitoneal viscera. Gunshot wounds, on the other hand, result in significant intraperitoneal injury more than 90% of the time.[7] The devastation caused by bullet and shotgun wounds depends not only on the organs struck by the projectile but also on the nature of wounding weapon and bullet and the range from which the shooting took place.

Terminal ballistics, the amount of energy imparted to tissues by a projectile, largely determines the resultant injury and killing power. A first approximation of the terminal ballistics of a given projectile is related to its kinetic energy (KE), which is determined by multiplying the mass of the projectile by the square of its velocity and dividing by a constant:

$$KE = mV^2/2g,$$

where KE = kinetic energy
      m = mass of the projectile
      V = velocity of the projectile
      g = the force of gravity

It follows that kinetic energy of a bullet is linearly related to the weight but increases markedly with even small increases in its velocity. Table 1–2 gives the muzzle velocity of a number of different weapons. Because of the importance of velocity in determining kinetic energy and killing power, weapons capable of generating a muzzle velocity of greater than 2000 feet per sec are termed "high velocity" weapons and the remainder classified as "low velocity" weapons.[29]

Kinetic energy determined by the muzzle velocity of a weapon gives only a first approximation of the injuring power of a projectile because the real determinant of injury is the amount of kinetic energy deposited in the tissue, or the kinetic energy upon entrance minus the kinetic energy upon exit. Thus, the wounding power of a low velocity projectile that does not exit and imparts all of its kinetic energy to the tissue can be greater than that

Table 1–2 Examples of Muzzle Velocity

WEAPON	VELOCITY (FT/SEC)
.22 Long rifle	1335
.22 Magnum	2000
.220 Swift	2800
.270 Winchester	3580
.357 Magnum	1550
.38 Colt	730
.44 Magnum	1850
.45 ACP	850

of a high velocity projectile that enters and exits the tissue without losing much of its kinetic energy. In this respect, bullet design is also important. For maximal injury potential, a bullet should dissipate all of its energy to the tissue. This has led to the development of missiles such as soft point or hollow nose bullets that deform or disintegrate on impact. If a bullet disintegrates, the damage produced is increased by secondary missiles or fragments of bone and other tissue.[5,6,25]

Close-range shotgun blasts, although they are low velocity injuries, cause the most devastating injuries of any weapon to which civilians are exposed because of the number and shape of the projectiles and because all of the kinetic energy is imparted to the tissue (Fig. 1–1). Sherman and Parrish have classified shotgun wounds into three categories based on range: Type I, sustained at long range (greater than 7 yards); Type II, sustained at short range (3–7 yards); and Type III, sustained at very short range (less than 3 yards).[23] An example of a Type III injury is seen in Figure 1–1. Type I injuries usually produce a widely scattered pattern of injury and may not even penetrate visceral cavities from distances of greater than 40 yards. Expectant management in the absence of clinical findings suggestive of visceral injury is often appropriate. At a range of 20 yards, penetration becomes increasingly likely and expectant management becomes increasingly less advisable. Type II injuries usually involve damage to deep structures and require aggressive treatment. Type III wounds produce massive tissue injury and carry a very high mortality rate (85–90%). Trying to determine range based on the pattern of the shot scatter is not always reliable as the presence of a choke on the shotgun barrel can significantly narrow the pattern of even long-range wounds. The type of shot used is also important in determining how deeply the shot has penetrated at a given range.[20,27]

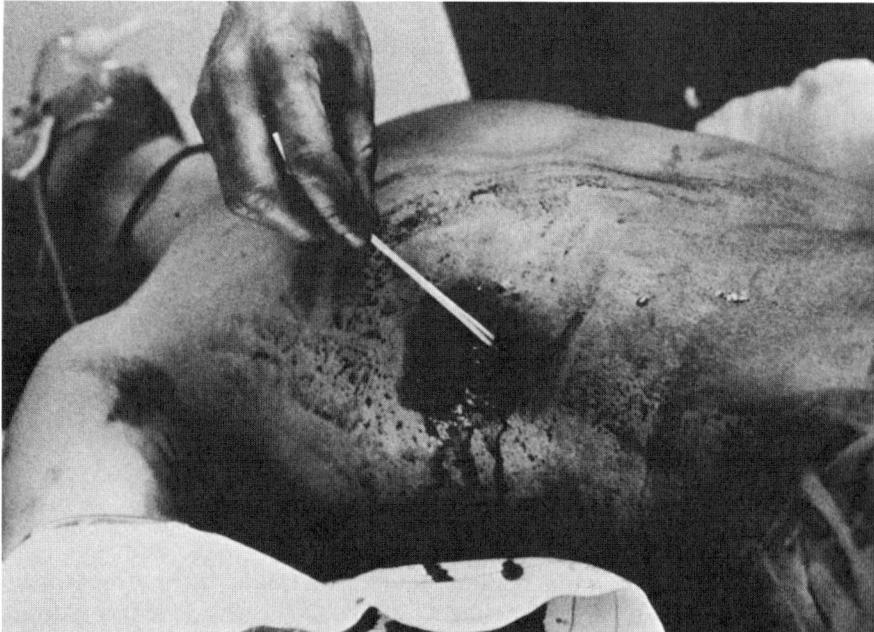

Figure 1–1. Close-range shotgun injury of the lower chest and right upper quadrant of the abdomen.

Blunt Injury

Blunt injury can be caused by direct impact, deceleration, rotary forces, and shear forces. Direct impact may cause significant injury and the severity can be estimated by knowing the force and duration of impact as well as the mass of the patient contact area. Determinants of injury are the speed of a motor vehicle at impact, whether the patient was a driver or passenger, and the degree of deformity of the vehicle. Table 1–3 lists the most common sites of injury from motor vehicle accidents, which are the most frequent mechanism for blunt trauma. Ejection, steering assembly impact, windshield or instrument panel impact, and rear collision account for most of these injuries.

Deceleration injuries are most often associated with high speed motor vehicle accidents and falls from heights. As the body impacts, the organs continue to move forward at the terminal velocity, tearing vessels and tissues from points of attachment. Rotary forces also tend to cause tearing injuries from a tumbling type of movement.

Shear forces produce degloving of injuries such as are apt to occur when a patient is run over by a large vehicle. As the vehicle passes over the body the skin and subcutaneous tissues are pushed ahead, tearing nutrient blood supply from its muscular sources below and separating subcutaneous fat from underlying fascia. This mechanism can also be caused by shear forces from a seatbelt in a high speed motor vehicle accident. Soft tissue necrosis and loss is common after shear injuries.

ASSESSMENT

Primary Survey

The initial evaluation of blunt and penetrating trauma is essentially the same (Table 1–4).[1] The first priority should be airway maintenance. If the patient is unconscious or *in extremis*, there should be a low threshold for endotracheal intubation. This ensures maximal oxygenation if the patient is perfusing poorly and decreases the risk of aspiration. Similarly, if the patient is tachypneic or complains of dyspnea, the intubation threshold should be low as these are signs of impending respiratory arrest. Except for instances of brain stem injury (which is almost universally fatal) or the ingestion of depressant drugs, all serious

Table 1–3 Frequency of Injuries in Traffic Accident Victims

	57 PEDESTRIANS	64 AUTO OCCUPANTS	6 MOTORCYCLE OR BICYCLE
Head	35 (22)*	43 (30)	6 (6)
Chest	17 (4)	31 (12)	3
Abdomen	14 (2)	24 (10)	—
Spine	4 (2)	4 (1)	—
Upper extremity	14 (0)	17 (0)	1
Pelvis and lower extremity	40 (16)	27 (2)	2
Genitourinary	5 (0)	4 (1)	—

*The number of times that each injury was the primary cause of death is indicated in parentheses.
From Perry and McClellan.[21] Reprinted with permission.

Table 1–4 Primary Survey

A–Airway maintenance
B–Breathing and ventilation
C–Circulation/hemorrhage control
D–Disability/neurologic status
E–Exposure

types of respiratory dysfunction are associated with an increased respiratory rate (Table 1–5). A respiratory rate of more than 25 per min means that something is wrong and should lower the threshold for intubation and prompt arterial blood gas analysis. A respiratory rate of more than 35 per min is an absolute indication for intubation. If the patient is conscious, he should be asked to take a deep breath. The ability to take a deep inspiratory effort without discomfort rules out most thoracic injuries. If the patient is unable to take a deep breath or if he splints with respiratory effort, chest wall injury should be assumed. The location of pain with inspiration is an indicator of the location of the chest wall injury. This is helpful in the evaluation of possible abdominal injury because injuries to the lower six ribs raise the possibility of intraabdominal injury.

The second priority after airway maintenance is breathing, or ensuring that the patient is adequately oxygenated and ventilated. If the patient's spontaneous ventilatory efforts are inadequate, ventilation should be assisted with positive pressure ventilation either by bagging or with a mechanical ventilator. The adequacy of ventilation is assessed both clinically and with frequent determinations of arterial blood gas values. The vast majority of trauma patients who require intubation also require positive pressure ventilation. Vigorous ventilation also reduces intracranial pressure in patients at risk for intracranial hypertension and helps to maximize oxygenation.

The third priority of management is circulation. The blood pressure should be noted but it should be borne in mind that young patients, by vasoconstricting, can maintain a relatively good blood pressure even though considerable volume has been lost. The pulse rate is not helpful in the acutely injured patient. Rapid pulse rates can be caused by anxiety, pain, or illicit drugs. Slow pulse rates are also misleading and are seen in up to 50% of seriously injured patients who are seriously hypovolemic. Assessment of peripheral perfusion and cerebral function are useful in defining the level of shock (Fig. 1–2). Urine output is not helpful initially because of residual urine in the bladder, but it can be a useful indicator of perfusion if the patient is followed for a number of hours. Warm extremities, good peripheral perfusion, and good urinary output often provide the best assurance that the blood volume is not seriously depleted.

In addition to assessment of the circulatory status in the patient with abdominal injury,

Table 1–5 Respiratory Rate/Min

< 10:	Central nervous system depression or injury
10–25:	Probably adequate
25–35:	Pathology likely
> 35:	Intubate and investigate urgently

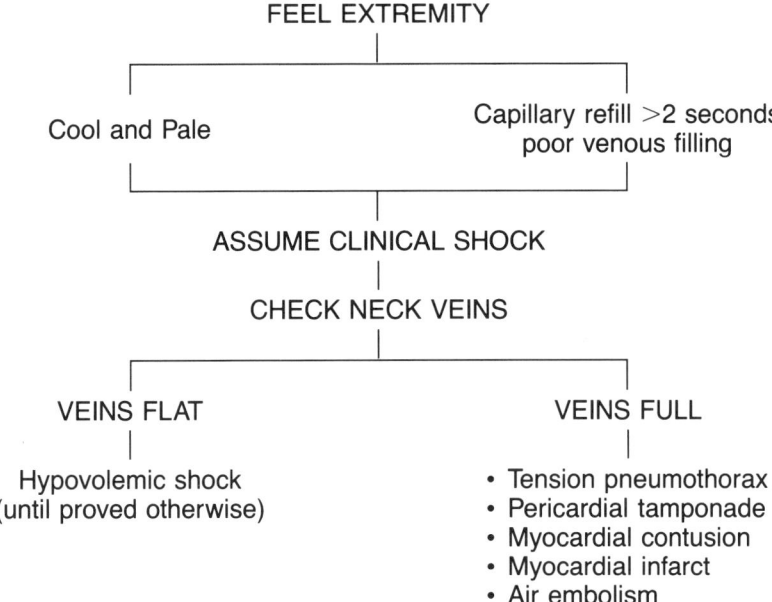

Figure 1–2. Quick assessment of shock.

measures should be taken to provide access to the intravascular space and to replete intravascular volume. Large-bore intravenous lines should be placed in at least two sites and an infusion with isotonic crystalloid solution begun. We favor avoiding the neck veins in such situations because of the simultaneous priority of airway management, the collapsed state of the neck veins, and the risk of pneumothorax. Instead, cutdowns are placed in the saphenous vein at the ankle. These veins will often admit the cut end of the intravenous tubing, a large-bore line that allows for the rapid infusion of large volumes of fluid if necessary.[12]

Another aspect of the circulatory priority of the primary survey is the control of obvious external bleeding. Overt hemorrhage should be treated with immediate tamponade with a finger, fist, gauze sponge, or pressure dressing. Scalp and facial bleeding can be massive and occasionally result in exsanguination while other occult bleeding is being ruled out. These wounds should be controlled initially with pressure. Rapid closure of scalp wounds is sometimes necessary for temporary control while further evaluation is carried out. If this is done, it should be remembered that the rationale for the closure is rapid hemorrhage control. Speed is of the essence and minimal attention should be paid to cosmesis. After the patient has been completely evaluated and all other sources of hemorrhage controlled, the laceration can be reapproximated with cosmesis in mind.

The fourth priority of the primary survey is determination of any neurologic disability. This includes a brief assessment of state of consciousness and a determination of the size, reactivity, and equality of the pupils. The states of consciousness are classified as alert, responsive to voice, responsive to pain, or unresponsive and provide a baseline exam of the level of consciousness. A progressive fall in the level of consciousness can be a manifestation of increasing intracranial pressure requiring decompression. An awake, conscious patient obviously has a good margin for safety. More elaborate determinations of the level of consciousness such as the Glasgow Coma Scale are reserved for the secondary survey.

The fifth and final priority of the primary survey is exposure. The patient should be completely disrobed to facilitate the elements of the secondary survey and further therapy and monitoring.

Secondary Survey

The secondary survey is a head-to-toe evaluation. Each region of the body should be examined individually.

The head should be inspected for scalp lacerations and the possibility of depressed skull fractures. The ears should be checked for hemotympanum. The face should be palpated for the presence of fractures and extraocular motions tested if possible. The neck should be examined for step-offs, which might indicate an underlying fracture, and if the patient can cooperate with a physical examination, the cervical spine should be checked for tenderness. If the patient is conscious, is nontender in the cervical spine, and moves his head without discomfort, the probability of an unstable cervical spine fracture is minimal.[2,17] If he is unconscious or reports cervical discomfort either on questioning or palpation, the head and neck should remain immobilized until fractures can be ruled out radiographically.[8] The neck veins should be examined for distention but they can look normal even in the face of tamponade, if the patient is also severely hypovolemic.

The chest should be inspected for flail segments with spontaneous ventilation and the location of any penetrating wounds noted. The chest should also be palpated for the presence of subcutaneous air or crepitus and to detect pain associated with rib fractures or sternal trauma. The screening maneuver of asking the patient to take a deep breath is a reliable way of ruling out chest wall injury. It will also help to localize rib fractures and allow the physician to avoid excessive palpation in areas known to be painful. If the comatose patient responds to stimuli, gentle pressure over the lower ribs can establish whether rib fractures are present. Auscultation should also be carried out. Absent breath sounds may indicate hemothorax or pneumothorax. Bowel sounds may indicate a ruptured diaphragm and distant heart sounds may be associated with cardiac tamponade. Although auscultation is sometimes rewarded by the rapid diagnosis of intrathoracic pathology, the stethoscope is notoriously unreliable in a noisy emergency department setting and auscultation should always be followed in the later stages of the evaluation with a chest x-ray (Fig. 1–3).

One of the areas that is often neglected in the physical examination is the back side of the patient. The patient should be log-rolled with someone supporting his head and neck while the back, flank, buttocks, and posterior aspects of the thighs are inspected. This is sometimes most easily accomplished upon the patient's arrival in the emergency room during transfer from the ambulance stretcher to the emergency room gurney. Even if the back has been inspected before the secondary survey, the thoracic and lumbar spine should be palpated at this time for deformity and tenderness.

Blunt injuries to the lower six ribs or penetrating trauma through the sixth interspace or below implies the possibility of abdominal injury. Depending on the phase of respiration, the intraabdominal viscera can rise as high as the level of the fifth intercostal space. This

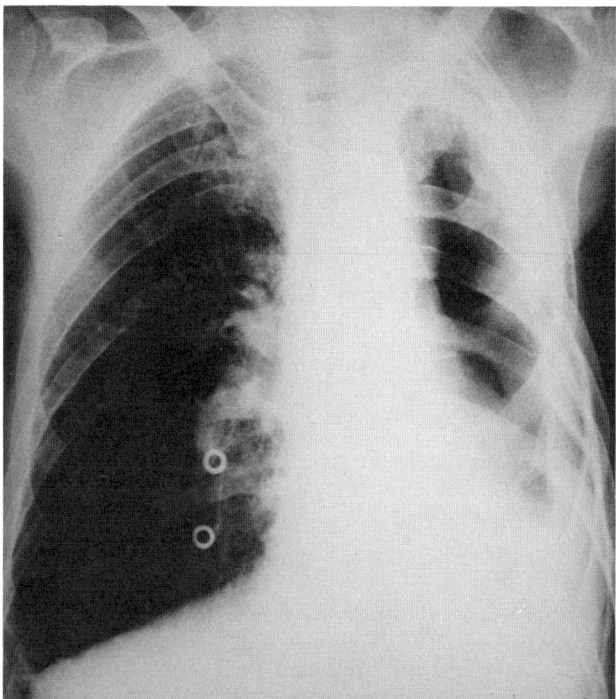

Figure 1–3. Right tension pneumothorax. The mediastinum is shifted to the left with compromise of function of the good lung.

is an important consideration in the evaluation of penetrating thoracic trauma when considering the possibility of underlying abdominal injury (Fig. 1–4).

The contour of the abdomen should be noted. The normal fasting abdomen is scaphoid. The abdomen may be relatively full after a large meal and of course the contour of the abdomen in an obese patient may be convex rather than scaphoid. Auscultation of the abdomen is neither sensitive nor specific for underlying injury and is not helpful. Gentle palpation of the abdomen should be carried out initially by laying a hand on the abdominal wall. This permits assessment of local areas of increased tone, which may suggest underlying injury. The location of any penetrating wounds should be noted. An attempt should be made to match the number of bullet holes with any information about the number of shots fired. Two holes may mean either two bullets or a through-and-through injury. An odd number of holes implies the presence of a foreign body inside the patient and it is important to locate the bullet on x-ray so that its path can be reconstructed. Deeper palpation should be carried out to elicit guarding, tenderness, and rebound. The flanks should be palpated and the iliac crests and symphysis pubis compressed to look for an unstable pelvic fracture. The reliability of physical exam to detect even major pelvic fractures is poor, however, and the pelvis should also undergo subsequent radiographic evaluation in patients who have suffered major blunt trauma.[9]

A rectal examination is also part of the secondary survey. Fullness in the pelvis is diagnostic of retroperitoneal hematoma and pelvic fracture. Blood on the examining finger

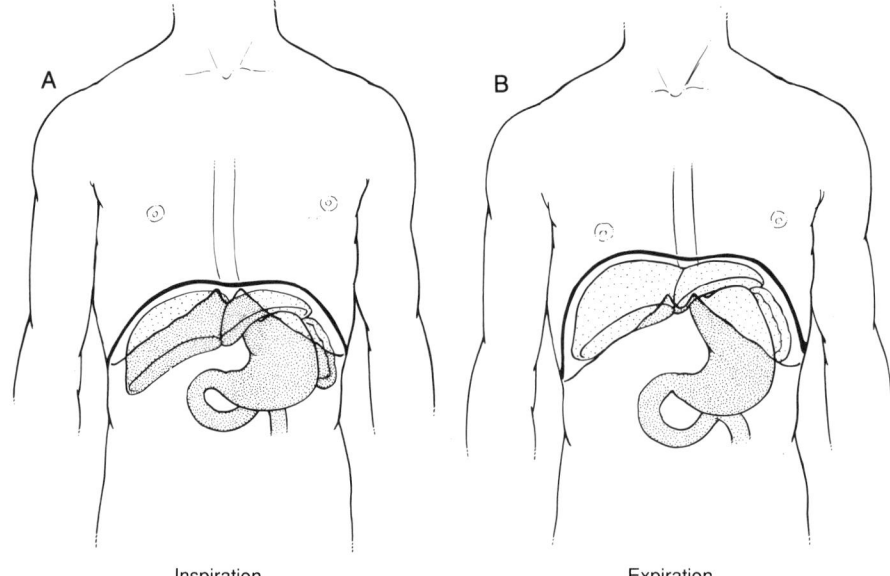

Figure 1–4. **A:** The average location of the diaphragm. **B:** With expiration the diaphragm moves upward as far as the fifth intercostal interspace.

suggests lower gastrointestinal injury. A high-riding prostate gland or perineal laceration may be associated with pelvic fractures. A rectal exam also gives some indication of the degree of rectal tone.

The genitalia should be inspected. Blood at the urethral meatus should be taken as a sign of urethral injury until proven otherwise.

The secondary survey should also include a more detailed neurological exam, including a determination of the level of consciousness as measured by the Glasgow Coma Scale as well as testing of motor function, sensation, and deep tendon reflexes.

Finally, the extremities should be examined for tenderness, deformity, swelling, lacerations, and vascularity. If the patient is awake and can move both lower extremities without discomfort, the probability of fracture is low. Passive motion of the extremities should also be done. If the patient is unable to cooperate but responds to pain, pain on passive motion points to a site of probable injury. Instability, of course, is diagnostic of fracture or dislocation. The upper extremities should be examined in a similar fashion, and all four extremities palpated for pulses, evidence of hematomas, and sites of tenderness, which may be associated with fracture or ligamentous injury.

HISTORY

Although the history is important, preoccupation with history taking should not interfere with the rapid conduct of the primary survey. Often, history can be obtained from the patient, family, or prehospital emergency personnel at the same time that the primary and secondary surveys are being carried out. A useful mnemonic for remembering appropriate information that should be obtained during the initial history taking is AMPLE.[1]

    A—Allergies
    M—Medications
    P—Past illnesses
    L—Last meal
    E—Events/Environment related to the injury

LABORATORY AND X-RAY EXAMINATIONS

After completion of the primary survey and simultaneous with history taking and the secondary survey, appropriate laboratory and roentgenographic studies should be obtained. Top laboratory priorities are hematocrit and arterial blood gas determinations as well as sending a sample of blood for typing and crossmatching and a sample of urine for urinalysis. A normal value for the hematocrit shortly after the time of injury does not rule out significant blood loss but a low value can be a sign of hemorrhage. A baseline value is important for comparison if the patient is to be followed subsequently with serial abdominal examinations and hematocrit determinations. A mean corpuscular volume (MCV) determination, measured either at the time of admission or subsequently, occasionally provides clues about a preexisting iron deficiency, nutritional, or thallasemic anemia. Lower priorities are determinations of serum electrolytes, serum amylase, and white blood cell count as well as a toxicology screen and a blood alcohol determination.

    The highest priority with respect to x-ray examinations is a chest x-ray. A chest x-ray should be obtained in all patients with blunt trauma, penetrating injury in proximity to the thoracic cavity, or a decreased level of consciousness (looking for signs of aspiration). In blunt trauma patients or patients with penetrating trauma to the neck, particularly if there is a depressed level of consciousness, the second x-ray priority is a lateral x-ray of the cervical spine. Demonstration of the lower cervical spine is enhanced by inferior traction on the upper extremities during the taking of the film. The final initial radiologic priority in patients with blunt trauma is an anteroposterior x-ray of the pelvis to look for pelvic fracture. All of these films (the chest x-ray, lateral cervical spine view, and anteroposterior view of the pelvis) should be obtained in the resuscitation area of the emergency department in seriously injured patients rather than in the x-ray suite. Routine views of the abdomen in blunt trauma patients and in patients without penetrating injury in proximity to the abdomen are of minimal value and should not be obtained. In patients with penetrating trauma, especially gunshot wounds, x-rays should also be taken of the injured areas to locate retained bullets. Whenever any x-rays are taken after penetrating trauma, entrance wounds should be marked with a staple or a paper clip taped to the skin at the site so that the location of the wounds can be seen on the film.

    After these initial x-rays have been taken, subsequent studies are determined by the stability of the patient and the nature of the patient's injuries (see subsequent chapters). The need for further radiologic evaluation is common in blunt trauma patients, with the most common x-rays required being computerized tomography of the head in patients with a depressed level of consciousness, a complete cervical spine series to rule out vertebral column injury, and x-rays of suspected fractures of the extremities.

The relative merits of further diagnostic measures such as peritoneal lavage, computerized tomography of the abdomen, intravenous pyelography, and angiography will be discussed in later chapters.

REFERENCES

1. American College of Surgeons. Advanced Trauma Life Support Course; 1989.
2. Bachulis BL, Long WB, Hynes GD, et al. Clinical indications for cervical spine radiographs in the traumatized patient. *Cerv Spine Radiogr Trauma*. 1987; 153:473–477.
3. Bailey H. *Surgery in Modern Warfare*. 3rd ed. Baltimore: Williams & Wilkins; 1944:II.
4. DiVincenti FC. Blunt abdominal trauma. *J Trauma*. 1968; 8:1004.
5. Fackler ML, Bellamy RF, Malinowski JA. The wound profile: illustration of the missile-tissue interaction. *J Trauma*. 1988; S21–S32.
6. Fackler ML. Wound ballistics: a review of common misconceptions. *JAMA*. 1988; 259:2730–2736.
7. Feliciano DV, Burch JM, Spjut-Patrinely V, et al. Abdominal gunshot wounds. *Ann Surg*. 1988; 208:362–370.
8. Fisher RP. Cervical radiographic evaluation of alert patients following blunt trauma. *Ann Emerg Med*. 1984; 13:905–907.
9. Gillott A, Rhodes M, Lucke J. Utility of routine pelvic x-ray during blunt trauma resuscitation. *J Trauma*. 1988; 28:1570–1574.
10. Griswald RA, Cellier HS. Blunt abdominal trauma. *Abst Surg*. 1961; 112:209.
11. Heaton LD, et al. Military surgical practices in the US Army in Vietnam. *Curr Probl Surg*. Nov. 1966.
12. Holcroft JW, Blaisdell FW. Trauma to the torso. In: Wilmore DW, Brennan MF, Harken AH, Holcroft JW, Meakins JL, eds. *American College of Surgeons Care of the Surgical Patient*. New York: Scientific American; 1989:1–56.
13. Hopsen WB, et al. Stab wounds of the abdomen. *Am Surg*. 1966; 32:213.
14. Hossack DW. The pattern of injuries received by 500 drivers and passengers killed in road accidents. *Med J Aust*. 1972; 2:193–195.
15. Hossack DW. Investigation of 400 people killed in road accidents with special reference to blood alcohol levels. *Med J Aust*. 1972; 2:225–258.
16. Kazarian KK, et al. Stab wounds of the abdomen, an analysis of 500 patients. *Arch Surg*. 1971; 102:465.
17. Kreipke DL, Gillespie KR, McCarthy MC, et al. Reliability of indications for cervical spine films in trauma patients. *J Trauma*. 1989; 29:1438–1439.
18. Loria FL. *Historical Aspects of Abdominal Injuries*. Springfield, Ill: Charles C Thomas; 1968.
19. Mucha P, Daly R, Farnell M. Selective management of blunt splenic trauma. *J Trauma*. 1986; 26:970.
20. Ordog GJ, Wasserberger J, Balasubramaniam S. Shotgun wound ballistics. *J Trauma*. 1988; 28:624–631.
21. Perry JF Jr, McClellan RJ. Autopsy findings in 127 patients following fatal traffic accidents. *Surg Gynecol Obstet*. 1964; 119:586–590.
22. Pridgen JE, et al. Penetrating wounds of the abdomen: analysis of 776 operative cases. *Ann Surg*. 1967; 165:901.
23. Sherman RT, Parrish RA. Management of shotgun injuries. *J Trauma*. 1963; 3:76.
24. Surgery in World War II, General Surgery, Office of the Surgeon General, Department of the Army, Washington, DC, 1955.
25. Sykes LN Jr, Champion HW, Fouty WJ. Dum-dums, hollow-points, and devastators: techniques designed to increase wounding potential of bullets. *J Trauma*. 1988; 28:618–623.
26. Trunkey DD, Lim RC Jr. Analysis of 425 consecutive trauma fatalities: an autopsy study. *J Am Coll Emerg Phys*. 1974; 368.
27. Walker ML, Poindexter JM Jr, Stovall I. Principles of management of shotgun wounds. *Surg Gynecol Obstet*. 1990; 170:97–105.
28. Walton CB, Blaisdell FW, Jordan RG, Bodai BI. The injury potential and lethality of stab wounds: a Folsom Prison study. *J Trauma*. 1989; 29:99–101.
29. Wilson JM. Shotgun ballistics and shotgun injuries. *West J Med*. 1978; 129:149–155.

2
Resuscitation

LEE HALVORSEN, M.D.
JAMES W. HOLCROFT, M.D.

HISTORY: Resuscitation of the trauma victim involves ensuring adequate ventilation and circulation. The former was less complex and has been easier to understand historically. The factors leading to the breakdown of the circulation, however, were not as easily recognized. Many of the clinical observations of shock initially took place as a result of human conflict. Although it was accepted early that soldiers could die as a result of severe blood loss, late deaths in soldiers who had survived their initial insult remained a mystery.[59] Therapeutic bleedings were frequently undertaken in the 1700s to remove toxins from the blood that were thought to be responsible for morbidity. Although this therapy was not successful, the concept of shock plasma and toxic hematologic factors continued to be a prevalent theme in trauma research.[13] By the time of the American Civil War, amputation had replaced phlebotomy as the principal form of therapy for severe trauma, thus ridding the body of the "toxic injured tissue." Surgeons were able to salvage some patients using this treatment, but mortality from simple extremity wounds remained high, especially if extensive time and difficult transport were involved.[1,21]

During World War I, a major step in the treatment of extremity injuries was made when Sir Robert Jones brought the Thomas splint to the British trenches. This device reduced the immediate mortality of femoral fractures from 70% to 10%. Although we now know that these splinting devices limit the compartmental volume of the thigh and thus limit bleeding into soft tissue, internal losses of blood and fluid were not appreciated as an important factor in shock until the hind limb injury studies of Blalock in 1929.[14]

The cardiovascular changes associated with hemorrhagic shock were first investigated at the end of the 19th century by Crile. In animal studies, Crile noted that central venous pressure fell during hemorrhage and that restoration of central pressures by saline infusion improved overall survival.[24] Henderson expanded on this work in 1910, noting the important relationship between central venous pressure, cardiac output, and arterial blood pressure.[38] Front-line field studies performed during World War II by Beecher and his associates correlated this earlier laboratory work in the human clinical setting and provided some of the first hard evidence that a decreased blood volume was the principal cause of shock and death in soldiers.[9,48] In the civilian setting, the cardiac catheterization studies of Cournard demonstrated that the severity of plasma volume depletion measured during hemorrhagic shock closely paralleled the low cardiac outputs of of these patients.[23] This key study also contrasted the hemodynamic derangements in patients with burn shock and severe head injury from those with a pure hemorrhagic mechanism. Finally, the introduction of blood banking and blood transfusion lent further support to the hypovolemic theory and resulted in a significant improvement in overall survival of military casualties.

INTRODUCTION

The term "shock" has been used loosely to describe the body's generalized response to traumatic injury.[83] However, in the stricter sense, shock should be thought of as the clinical manifestation of a series of derangements in the cardiovascular system that result in the inadequate delivery of oxygen and other nutrients to tissues. These derangements, if severe, lead to a vicious cycle of ischemia, acidemia, and cellular death and to extensive morbidity and mortality. Prevention and prompt correction of shock form the mainstays of trauma resuscitation.

The immediate aspects in both the evaluation and treatment of the traumatized patient are to ensure an adequate airway for ventilation and to control external exigent hemorrhage. If this is not accomplished, the patient will rapidly suffer further circulatory collapse, diffuse tissue and organ damage, and eventual cardiac arrest. In this regard, our priorities are slightly modified from those of the American College of Surgeons and consist of airway, bleeding, and circulation. The final immediate priority is the central nervous system (Table 2–1).

THE AIRWAY

When thoracic penetration is present or when there have been rib fractures, there is always the probability that associated lung laceration may be present. When positive pressure ventilation is initiated as part of resuscitation or when anesthesia is induced for the surgical treatment of other injuries, a minor lung laceration can produce lethal tension pneumothorax as air is forced out of the laceration because of increased atmospheric pressure in the airway. For this reason, chest tubes are used liberally as part of initial resuscitation,

Table 2–1 Priorities and Goals of Resuscitation

VENTILATORY SYSTEM	CARDIOVASCULAR SYSTEM	CENTRAL NERVOUS SYSTEM
Establish stable unobstructed airway	Restore plasma volume	Correct hypoxemia
Correct alveolar hypoxemia	Control hemorrhage	Lower pCO_2 to 25–30 mm Hg
Compensate for metabolic acidemia	Maximize cardiac output	Increase serum osmolality
Normalize blood pH and artery O_2 saturation	Reestablish flow to vital organs and distal tissues	Lower intracranial pressure
	Minimize reperfusion injury	Minimize cerebral edema
	Turn off systemic "pressor" response	

particularly if the unstable condition of the patient contraindicates immediate chest x-ray. In the stable patient, chest tube insertion can await indications based on chest x-ray. However, if the patient with thoracic penetration is going to require immediate abdominal surgery, prophylactic chest tube insertion may be judicious when there has been thoracic penetration or evidence of rib fractures despite the absence of hemothorax or pneumothorax.

Although it is clear that not all trauma patients will require mechanical ventilation, a liberal approach toward endotracheal intubation should be adopted and should include such broad categories of patients as those with evidence of a major head injury, chest wall injury, or laryngeal injury, those with labored respirations or a respiratory rate greater than 25 per min, and those with evidence of CO_2 retention or hypoxemia.[4]

A respiratory rate under 10 per min results from hypothermia, ingestion of sedative drugs, or brain stem injury. The former two causes are best treated temporarily with ventilator support. In almost all other instances, ventilation compromise will result in an abnormal increase in respiratory rate. A respiratory rate that exceeds 30 per min demands that the cause be found and treated promptly and serial blood gases followed; that over 35 per min is an indication for intubation and mechanical ventilation unless immediately reversible.

Early intervention is the key, and the surgeon's visual impression of the patient is the essential data for making the decision to intubate, not the results of arterial blood gases. Although many authors have pointed out that small endotracheal cannulas can provide adequate oxygenation on a temporary basis, whenever possible, a larger size 8.5 to 9.5 F soft cuff endotracheal tube should be used in the adult.[17] This decreases airway resistance, enhances suctioning and later bronchoscopic capabilities, and makes the patient more comfortable during the weaning period.

Another indication for endotracheal intubation is altered consciousness with loss of gag, cough, and swallowing reflexes so that the patient is at risk for aspiration; major maxillofacial injury that produces bleeding into the upper airway is another. Thus, whenever the patient has altered ventilation as manifested by tachypnea or altered consciousness, the airway must be protected and ensured.

The early postintubation period is often a key time in resuscitation triage, a time when rapid movement to the operating room may be needed in response to deterioration in the patient's vital signs. Immediately after intubation, the surgeon should bag ventilate the patient, anticipating a right mainstem intubation; if the tube appears to be in the right position but the patient is still difficult to ventilate with the AMBU bag, there may be an unrecognized pneumothorax. The abrupt rise in central venous pressure associated with positive pressure ventilation may also precipitate the sudden decompression of a major vena caval or hepatic venous injury, in which case the patient's blood pressure may plummet. It can also cause the sudden worsening of pericardial tamponade. Finally, if a major bronchial disruption has occurred, positive airway pressure can cause air to embolize into the coronary circulation and result in sudden cardiac arrest.

When the patient has stabilized, mechanical ventilation should be set up such that the initial tidal volumes are kept low at 8 to 9 ml/kg, ventilation is rapid at 20 to 26 breaths per minute, FiO_2 is 0.1 (100%), and positive end expiratory pressure (PEEP) is zero. These deviations from the standard intensive care unit (ICU) settings minimize cardiac compressive forces, rapidly compensate for metabolic acidemia, and provide maximum inspired oxygen concentration[45,65,68] (Table 2–2).

Table 2–2   Ventilator Settings in the Emergency Room

Large endotracheal tube: suctioning, bronchoscopy, weaning
Initiate bag ventilation: hard to bag—pneumothorax or R main stem intubation
Vital sign recheck for sudden decompensation: pericardial tamponade, hepatic venous injury, coronary air embolism?
Suction the airway: clear airway of aspirate
Institute mechanical ventilation with following settings:
  FiO_2 1.0 (100%): maximize cardiac compressive forces
  Initial rate of 25.0: assume metabolic acidemia
  No PEEP: minimize cardiac compression, enhance ventricular filling, lower intracranial pressure
  If a head injury is present, adjust ventilation rate to keep pCO_2 at 25–30: use cerebral vasoconstriction to shift cerebral volume pressure curve down
  If there is no head injury, adjust rate to maintain pH of 7.35–7.40: slight acidemia is safe and may enhance the distal unloading of oxygen from hemoglobin

THE CIRCULATION

Once the airway has been secured, the surgeon should begin a secondary appraisal of the patient's injuries so that the principal cause of any decreased perfusion can be identified (Fig. 2–1). Three types of shock are commonly seen in the emergency room trauma patient: hemorrhagic shock, cardiac compressive shock, and neurogenic shock. Thus, the priorities in the secondary survey should be the relief of tamponade, the identification of internal hemorrhage, and the better definition of intracranial and extracranial neurologic injury. Each of these will be discussed in detail in other sections.

Septic shock and sepsis syndrome are uncommon during the initial presentation of the traumatized patient and usually require 3 to 10 days to develop after massive injury.[85] They will not be discussed in this chapter. Cardiogenic shock can be a primary etiology for trauma under unusual circumstances, e.g., when an elderly patient suffers a myocardial infarction with syncope and collapses behind the wheel of a moving vehicle. These patients

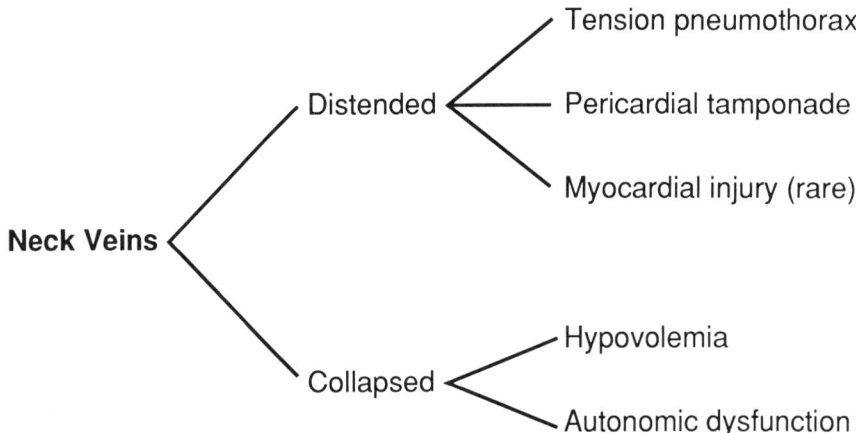

Figure 2–1.   Utilization of the status of neck veins for initial shock triage.

present a special challenge to the trauma surgeon because of their poor tolerance of fluid administration, anesthesia, and surgery.

Pathophysiology

During the post–War World II period, Wiggers and his associates performed a series of important shock studies on anesthetized dogs in which they bled animals into a fluid reservoir elevated at a set height above the animals' right atrium in order to produce a desired level of hypotension. It was noted that during the later phases of hemorrhagic shock the animals would begin to take blood back up from the reservoir even though the arterial pressure would remain the same.[93] At this point in the experiment, simple replacement of shed blood would not insure the dog's survival. Wiggers considered this the phase of decompensated or irreversible shock, and it was commonly assumed that injuries severe enough to produce this level of shock were not compatible with survival.

During the early phases of the Korean conflict, the concept of decompensated shock was used clinically to explain late death after what initially seemed to be successful resuscitation. Severely traumatized patients frequently developed renal failure as a pre-terminal event and, during the later phases of the Korean war, physicians used infusions of large quantities of fluid in an effort to prevent this renal failure.[53] Although many patients responded, it was unclear as to why volumes greater than 3 to 4 times the estimated blood loss were often necessary. These large volume requirements were investigated by Shires and Trunkey in the 1970s with a series of intracellular studies using micropuncture technique. Their work suggested that sodium and water moved into the intracellular space during the later stages of hemorrhagic shock.[79] They postulated that this intracellular fluid shift led to the progressive contraction of the patient's interstitial and intravascular spaces, to decreased cardiac filling, and ultimately to insufficient cardiac output. Large volumes seemed logical because of the need to resuscitate both the interstitial and intravascular spaces. Clinical studies supported Shires' findings and advocated isotonic solutions of sodium chloride as the most effective solution for the correction of this interstitial defect.[20]

When these concepts were applied during the Vietnam conflict, large volume isotonic resuscitation resulted in decreased morbidity from renal failure. And yet, as with the other conflicts, a new syndrome consisting of refractory hypoxemia, decreased lung compliance, and interstitial lung edema, otherwise known as the respiratory distress syndrome (RDS) of shock and trauma, emerged as a cause of late mortality due to respiratory failure.[11] Investigators initially had difficulty weighing the relative contributions of the severity of tissue trauma, the duration of shock, and the volume of fluid administered during resuscitation in the etiology of this clinical entity. With the advent of the Swan-Ganz catheter, it became apparent that many of the RDS patients actually had low atrial pressures, making overzealous fluid administration an unlikely etiology. Furthermore, clinical experience suggested that fluid restriction in RDS patients actually contributed to mortality.[19,54]

Experimental studies of lower extremity ischemia and crush injury in several species now indicate that massive tissue trauma and peripheral ischemia can result in a diffuse activation of the inflammatory and coagulation cascades.[12] Subsequent work by Beal and Klausner confirmed evidence of platelet microembolization and polymorphonuclear leukocyte trapping in the lung with local inflammation in the pulmonary microvasculature.[5,49] Increases in pulmonary microvascular permeability follow this local inflammation and allow leakage of proteinaceous fluid from the intravascular space into the pulmonary interstitium and the alveoli, which results in the formation of noncardiogenic pulmonary edema.

The unraveling of the RDS mystery helped to emphasize that the microvascular endothelial membrane is a target organ of severe shock and that the ultimate goal of resuscitation should be to restore circulatory function before microvascular permeability syndromes develop. With this in mind, trauma resuscitation today should emphasize the rapid correction of hypovolemia and an aggressive attitude toward the diagnosis and treatment of internal hemorrhage.[32] Although restoration of blood pressure and cardiac output in the field would be ideal, the prehospital administration of intravenous fluids has come under serious criticism. Retrospective analysis suggests that the volumes of isotonic crystalloid solution given to the average trauma patient during prehospital transport are well under those required for adequate resuscitation.[51] The delays associated with failures in obtaining vascular access further compound this problem.[47,62] Although many institutions have been forced to adopt a "scoop and run policy" regarding prehospital resuscitative therapy, recent laboratory and clinical studies suggest that infusion of small volumes of hyperosmolar hyperoncotic fluids may allow prehospital rescuers to restore plasma volume rapidly and correct shock in the field or during transport.[42] These hypertonic saline dextran solutions promote the rapid movement of water from the intracellular to the extracellular space, thus using the patient's own intracellular fluid reservoir to restore intravascular volume temporarily.[57] Hypertonic saline formulations are still experimental and comprise only one of a number of new therapies aimed at providing prompt resuscitation, immune modulation, and prevention of late end-organ failure.[89]

Hemorrhagic Shock

Hemorrhagic shock is by far the most common type of shock encountered in both military and civilian trauma.[81] The severity of hemorrhagic shock can be broken down into three clinical categories—mild, moderate, or severe—based on the magnitude of blood lost (Table 2–3). The signs and symptoms at each level of severity are a function of the body's progressive attempt to compensate for the decreased blood volume by limiting perfusion to

Table 2–3 Clinical Classification of Hemorrhagic Shock

Mild shock: (up to 20% blood volume loss)	
Pathophysiology:	Decreased perfusion of nonvital organs and tissues (skin, fat, skeletal muscle, and bone)
Manifestations:	Pale, cool skin, patient complains of feeling cold, hypotension if intoxicated with alcohol
Moderate shock: (20–40% blood volume loss)	
Pathophysiology:	Decreased perfusion of splanchnic organs and kidneys
Manifestations:	Oliguria, postural hypotension, mild agitation; pregnant patient shows signs of mild shock and fetal distress
Severe shock: (40% blood volume loss or greater)	
Pathophysiology:	Decreased perfusion of the heart and brain
Manifestations:	Restlessness, agitation, coma, cardiac ischemic changes, cardiac arrest

ischemia-tolerant tissues and thereby preserving blood flow to vital organs.[88] Compensation begins with stimulation of the sympathetic adrenergic nerves. In mild shock (20% blood loss or less), the peripheral veins and venules go into spasm, displacing the blood back to the right atrium. Concurrently, the arterioles in the skin, skeletal muscle, and fat constrict.[29,58,60] The patient may complain of feeling thirsty and cold and may shiver. The skin will be cool, pale, and moist and the subcutaneous veins will be collapsed. Blood flow to the coronary, cerebral, renal, and splanchnic arteries is preserved, and the blood pressure, heart rate, and mental status may be normal.[77]

As the level of shock deepens to a moderate level (20–40% blood loss), blood flow to the renal arteries decreases, leading to the release of renin from the juxtaglomerular apparatus. Vasopressin is released from the posterior pituitary gland, promoting further arterial vasoconstriction in the peripheral and splanchnic vascular beds.[39,66,74] The renin–angiotensin interaction and aldosterone enhance absorption of sodium and water at the level of the renal tubule. This causes the patient to develop a low volume (<0.5 ml/kg/hr in the adult and <2 ml/kg/hr in the infant) of concentrated urine. The insertion of a Foley catheter is frequently necessary to monitor this evolving condition. Later, shunts in the medullary area of the kidney result in underperfusion of the renal cortex.[18,96] If the renal cortex is bypassed for 24 or more hours, renal cortical necrosis will develop. As one progresses into moderate hemorrhagic shock, blood flow to the coronary arteries and cerebral arteries begins to decrease and cardiac output is depressed 30% to 40%. Blood pressure may be normal in the supine position, but it will fall if the head of the bed is elevated (i.e., postural hypotension).[78]

In severe shock, (>40% blood loss) cardiac output is severely depressed, vasoconstriction is no longer effective, and the vital perfusion of the brain and heart is obviously compromised. The patient often becomes agitated, combative, or obtunded and the electrocardiogram may show signs of ischemia in the form of S-T segment depression or new Q waves. Heart rate may increase, but this is not a reliable indication of the level of hypovolemia, and a bradycardiac rhythm may be seen in the preterminal state.[52] Laboratory data will demonstrate a progressive metabolic acidemia as cellular function deteriorates; the patient will be at high risk for the development of increased microvascular permeability.[64]

In addition to the physical examination assessment of hypovolemia, serial monitoring of the whole blood hematocrit in the emergency room is essential so that the surgeon can anticipate the patient's clinical course and assess the rate of ongoing bleeding. Hematocrit values should be obtained at least hourly in the emergency room and as frequently as every 20 min if the patient has suffered a concurrent pelvic or severe long bone fracture. As a general rule, the hematocrit will fall 3% to 4% for each unit (500 ml) of whole blood lost.[23] Because the initial packed cell volume of the patient is not known, several serial values will be necessary to calculate the slope, e.g., the rate of ongoing bleeding. An initial hematocrit of under 30% or a progressive fall suggesting greater than a 500-ml blood loss should prompt consideration of unrecognized intraabdominal hemorrhage.

Acute ethanol intoxication masks some of the cutaneous and renal signs of hemorrhagic shock. Ethanol in moderate concentration can override the effects of the adrenergic nervous system.[61] In addition, ethanol inhibits the release of vasopressin from the pituitary gland, promotes an osmotic diuresis, and produces a warm, seemingly well perfused patient.[63,84] Hemorrhagic shock can be recognized in the intoxicated patient by frequent measurements of the arterial blood pressure and the blood hematocrit. Mean arterial blood pressure will fall early in the intoxicated patient because of a disabled peripheral vasoconstrictive mechanism and because ethanol appears to decrease myocardial contractility.[30,43,56] The hematocrit may be lowered initially by the increase in serum osmolarity associated with alcohol ingestion, but the serial changes in hematocrit will still be valid. Combative or obtunded behavior may be the result of intoxication or shock and for this reason all inebriated individuals should be followed closely for hemodynamic changes.[91]

The administration of hypertonic saline dextran solutions in the prehospital setting may also alter the initial presentation of a patient who has suffered a significant blood loss. These hyperosmolar solutions cause cutaneous vasodilation and a subjective feeling of warmth much like ethanol.[40] Additionally, hypertonic sodium chloride solutions promote an increase in the renal excretion of sodium and an increased urine output.[50] Unlike the intoxicated patient, however, the patient resuscitated with hypertonic saline has an expanded plasma volume and should maintain a normal blood pressure in the emergency room if hemorrhage has stopped. A history of a severe mechanism of injury or hypotension in the field, a low hematocrit on initial presentation, or a delayed fall in blood pressure may be clinical clues suggesting significant blood loss.

Shock Resuscitation

In all cases of hemorrhagic shock, once the patient has entered the emergency room, intravenous (IV) access should be obtained immediately with an IV line large enough to infuse fluid faster than the rate of ongoing bleeding.[51] In the case of mild shock with minimal associated injury, a single percutaneous catheter may be all that is necessary. However, if the clinical history suggests violent injury, multiple large-bore IV catheters should be placed. Effective vascular access can be achieved rapidly in the emergency room via the direct insertion of sterile IV tubing (12 gauge or greater) into a venotomy in the greater saphenous vein as it crosses the medial malleolus of the ankle (Fig. 2–2). This vein can be palpated directly and has no important nervous structures near it.[71] Access using this site also avoids the risk of arterial injury and pulmonary laceration associated with subclavian venous punctures in hypovolemic patients. Alternative large-bore IVs can be established through the conversion of an existing percutaneous 16-gauge IV catheter to a 8.5 F introducer sheath. This is performed by disconnecting the IV at the hub and passing a 0.032-mm guide wire through the existing catheter. The IV cannula is then removed, and a small skin incision is made to facilitate the dilator–sheath complex, which is then slid over the wire into the cephalic or median cubital vein. This technique may be especially useful in the case of bilateral lower extremity fractures when veins are not accessible or when caval occlusion may be required, although fluids given through saphenous cutdowns in the latter instance will find their way back to the right atrium through collateral venous channels in the retroperitoneum.

After venous access has been obtained, fluid resuscitation should begin with the rapid infusion of 2 to 3 liters of isotonic crystalloid solution. This volume of fluid will resuscitate patients in mild shock with arrested hemorrhage. Ringer's lactate, Ringer's acetate, and normal saline are all examples of appropriate isotonic solutions.[28,34] Because a metabolic acidemia is associated with hypoperfusion, we prefer crystalloids with a mild buffering capacity and, if normal saline is to be used, 1 to 2 ampules of bicarbonate can be added to each liter to compensate for the hyperchloremic nature of this solution. One may wish to avoid lactated solutions in patients with liver disease because of the possibility of impaired hepatic conversion of lactate to bicarbonate. Fluids containing dextrose should also be

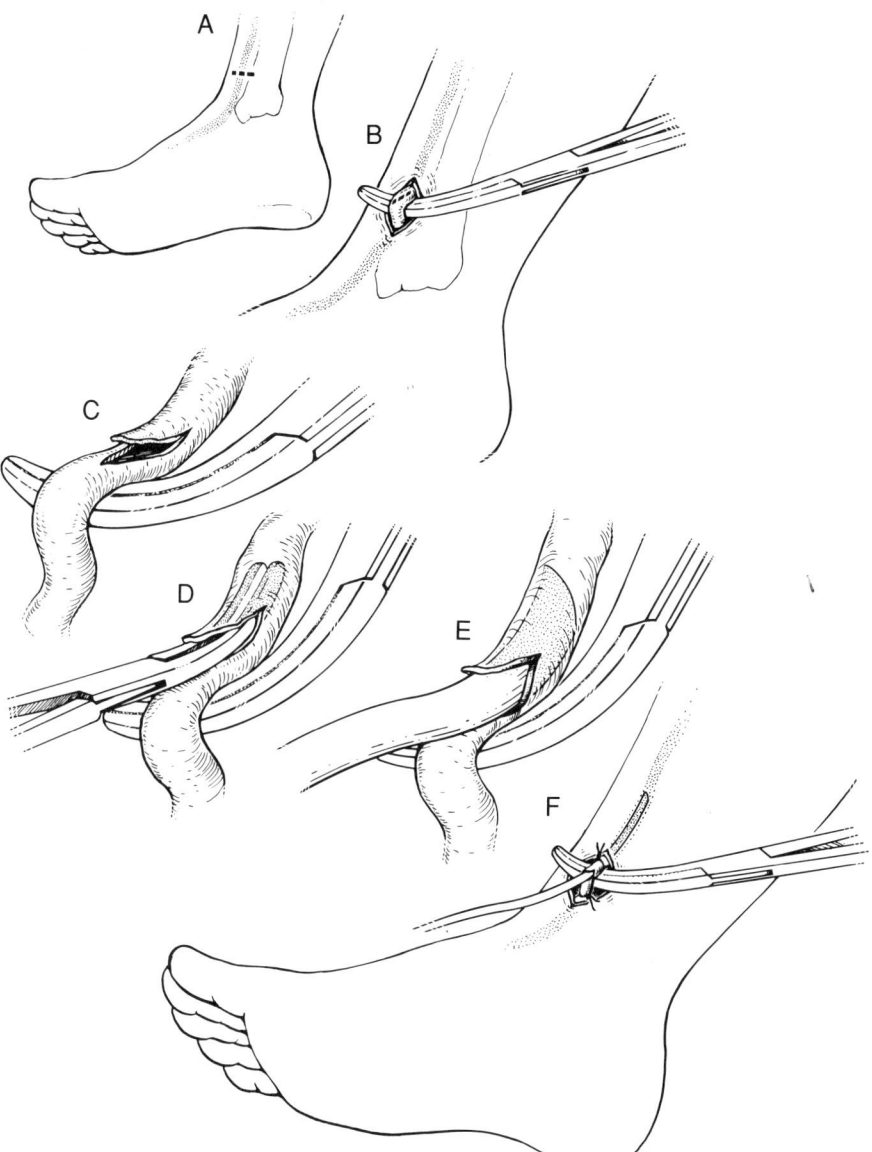

Figure 2–2. Saphenous vein cutdown. **A,B:** A generous transverse incision should be made centering on the groove anterior to the medial malleolus; the vein will lie on the fascia and can be picked up by thrusting a curved hemostat under it. **C,D:** The point of a #11 blade should be thrust transversely through the center of the vein, which then slashes outward to give a "fishmouthed" transverse opening that is then dilated with the tips of a small hemostat. **E,F:** An obliquely cut section of IV tubing is then advanced into the vein and the vein tied proximally and distally after the catheter is proven functional.

avoided in the initial resuscitation of hemorrhagic shock, as these solutions can exacerbate shock-generated hyperglycemia and induce an inappropriate osmotic diuresis.

The administration of fluid is both diagnostic and therapeutic. If the patient remains hypotensive after the first 2 to 3 liters of fluid, this should raise the suspicion of unrecognized internal hemorrhage. Isotonic crystalloid solutions distribute throughout the entire extracellular fluid, and volumes equaling 2 to 3 times the presumed blood loss may be necessary to restore adequate ventricular preload.[40] However, the total volume of isotonic fluid ultimately required for complete resuscitation will depend on many factors that take into account the severity of the microvascular permeability defect and the degree of cellular swelling in addition to the absolute volume of blood lost. The endpoint of initial resuscitation is the restoration of normal (and in some cases supranormal) cardiac output, not on the absolute quantity of fluid given, as this can easily exceed 20 liters by the time the patient leaves the operating room. Once hemorrhage has been controlled, further fluid requirements within the first 24 hr after initial resuscitation function as an index of the degree of cellular ischemic damage, reperfusion injury, and as a predictor of late morbidity and mortality.[87]

Colloidal solutions such as plasma, dextran, albumin, or hetastarch are also effective volume expanders under conditions of simple injury and theoretically could be used for the correction of hemorrhagic hypovolemia.[90] However, in the severely shocked state, diffuse increases in microvascular permeability can occur.[26,40,46] The result is a loss of endothelial integrity that alters the normal forces governing transcapillary fluid flux.[82] Once this syndrome develops, proteins and synthetic colloids can move more freely into the interstitial space.[70] Under these circumstances the administration of colloidal solutions may be no more effective in increasing or maintaining plasma volume than crystalloid solutions.[41] The colloidal solutions carry with them the theoretical risks of transmission of viral diseases, antigenicity, and anaphylaxis. They are also much more expensive, and although we prefer crystalloid for initial resuscitation, late supplementation of plasma and interstitial oncotic pressure with albumin or plasma may be beneficial in the elderly or nutritionally debilitated patient during the recovery period once the patient's capillary "leak" has sealed and may speed Phase III fluid mobilization.[15] This issue is currently under study.

Patients suffering from hemorrhagic shock may also require the transfusion of whole blood or packed red blood cells for the restoration of oxygen-carrying capacity. But the administration of blood products is no longer a simple issue, and when contemplating transfusion, the short-term side effects of anemia must be weighed against the potential risks of long-term morbidity due to the transmission of hepatitis and human immunodeficiency virus infection (see Chapter 13, Table 13–3).[6,10,31,55,69]

With these risks in mind, many patients can avoid transfusion if hemorrhage is promptly and definitively controlled and injuries are simple.[37] Clinical observation of young, anemic trauma patients suggest that hematocrits of 20% or more are well tolerated and that hematocrits as low as 12% to 15% may be tolerated temporarily. Elderly patients with atherosclerotic coronary artery disease and patients with closed head injuries, on the other hand, will not tolerate significant anemia and should be transfused to a hematocrit approaching 30% to 36%.[40,94,95] We prefer to restrict transfusion in the emergency room whenever possible and advocate the use of red cell reclamation systems if there has not been frank contamination of the shed blood with bowel contents.

One notable exception to this anti–emergency room transfusion philosophy is the specific case of the severely displaced Malgaigne pelvic fracture. Patients with this injury should be viewed with the same degree of urgency as the patient with a rupturing aortic aneurysm, because, if untreated, they will exsanguinate before definitive orthopedic stabilization can take place. Transfusion in these patients should be initiated in the emergency room with O negative or type-specific blood if necessary to maintain a margin of safety. The hematocrit also should be checked much more frequently (every 20 min or less) than usual.

Cardiac Compressive Shock

Compression of the inferior or superior vena cava or of the ventricular chambers themselves will lead to shock based on a restriction of ventricular filling and inadequate cardiac output.[68] In the setting of trauma, this condition often results from the presence of a tension pneumothorax with mediastinal shift, a hemopericardium, or a diaphragmatic rupture. The patient typically presents with signs and symptoms similar to hypovolemic shock but has findings suggesting an elevated right atrial pressure. These features include the classic jugular–venous distention (Fig. 2–3) as well as two more subtle signs, namely the pulsus paradoxus and Kussmaul's sign. A pulsus paradoxus is a drop of greater than 10 mm Hg in systolic blood pressure with spontaneous inspiration. Kussmaul's sign is said to be present when there is an elevation in central venous pressure with spontaneous inspiration.[40] Rapid

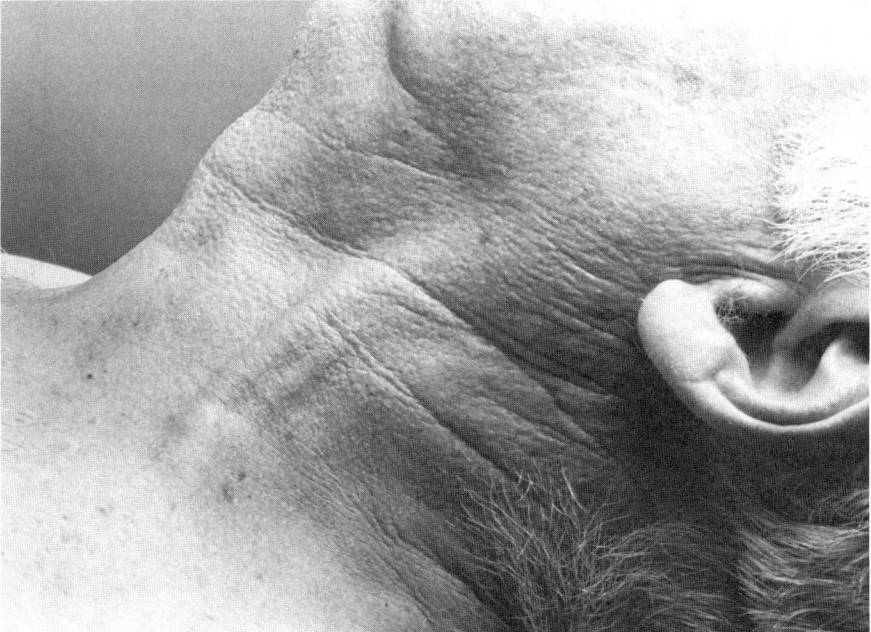

Figure 2–3. If the patient is not responding to fluid resuscitation, the x-ray does not show a tension pneumothorax, and the neck veins are distended, the patient is in cardiogenic shock.

bedside assessment of these signs can be performed by palpating the radial pulse or blowing up a blood pressure cuff and observing the jugular venous wave after asking the patient to take a deep breath. The physician should be aware, however, that these signs may be masked by hypovolemia and may only be present after an initial 2 to 3 liters of intravenous fluid have been administered. Cardiac compressive shock should also be suspected any time a previously stable patient rapidly deteriorates in the emergency room or during surgery. Effective therapy for cardiac compressive shock hinges on correction of any intravascular volume deficit that may exist and the rapid diagnosis and relief of the compressing force.

The most common cause of cardiac compressive shock, tension pneumothorax, is suggested by labored respirations, crepitance or obviously broken ribs on palpation of the chest wall, the presence of unequal breath sounds on auscultation, contralateral shift of the midline trachea, or difficulty in bag ventilation of an intubated patient. Treatment in the context of trauma consists of tube thoracostomy in the fourth intercostal space midaxillary line. A large, 36 F tube should be placed straight into the chest and directly posteriorly after an intrathoracic finger sweep to break up any adhesions that might be present. We believe that time should not be sacrificed for the creation of a subcutaneous tunnel as the chest wall exit site will usually seal rapidly after the tube is removed. Moreover, attempts at oblique placement in emergency circumstances may result in the tube encircling rather than penetrating the chest wall. Prevention in many ways is the best "treatment" for this form of shock and to avoid confusion, it is often wise to place prophylactic chest tubes in patients with severe chest wall injuries before surgery.[35]

Hemopericardium is suggested by the history of a rapid deceleration of the sternum, palpable sternal fracture, a penetrating injury to the chest, or a widened mediastinum on chest x-ray. The type and location of treatment depends on the stability of the patient. Unconscious patients with frank hypotension in suspected tamponade should be treated in the emergency room by needle pericardiocentesis with removal of 50 ml of blood or left anterolateral thoracotomy depending on the acuteness of the situation. The patient should then be moved immediately to the operating room for definitive repair of the tamponading lesion rather than attempting repair in the resuscitation area. The stable, conscious patient with tamponade can be brought urgently to the operating room, where he should be prepped and draped before the application of positive pressure ventilation. This precaution is taken because positive ventilatory pressures enhance cardiac compression and may result in sudden cardiac arrest.[86]

Diaphragmatic rupture is suggested by signs of respiratory distress with the additional finding of bowel sounds in the chest on physical examination and a gastric bubble or large bowel in the thorax on chest x-ray.[76] Emergency room treatment consists of volume expansion and the placement of a nasogastric tube for drainage of intragastric contents. This may help relieve cardiac compression if the stomach is one of the herniated organs. We believe that operative repair of the diaphragmatic injury is often best accomplished through an abdomen approach as this allows for inspection of the viability of the herniated viscera in addition to repair of the actual diaphragmatic defect.

Neurogenic Shock

Neurogenic shock in the trauma patient usually results from a compression, hemorrhagic contusion, or laceration of the spinal cord. The pathogenesis of the hypotension associated with this form of shock is a loss of sympathetic adrenergic tone in the peripheral vasculature below the level of the injury. High spinal cord lesions are the most profound in this regard, often involving loss of the sympathetic cardiac nerves that arise at the level of T4. When vasomotor tone is lost, blood pools in the veins and venules below the level of injury, thereby decreasing venous return and ultimately decreasing cardiac output.[73] Impairment of the cardiac adrenergic nerves may cause the vagal parasympathetic fibers to predominate, with the result being a relative bradycardia. Compensatory arterial tone is lost in severe neurogenic shock and this compounds the patient's hypotension. At the level of the microvasculature, peripheral arterial vasodilation may cause both a physiological as well as an anatomical shunt of oxygen away from the stromal cells.[25,92]

The patient in neurogenic shock may initially appear warm and well perfused, and the urine output may temporarily be normal depending on the integrity of the adrenergic nerves to the kidney. The diagnosis should be obvious based on the mechanism of injury and the patient's abnormal neurological examination. Diving accidents, unhelmeted motorcycle accidents, and motor vehicle accidents with ejection should always raise the suspicion of spinal cord injury.[36]

Treatment should be aimed at definitive stabilization of the spine and the restoration of ventricular filling. In the case of mild neurogenic shock, venous return may be increased by expanding the patient's plasma volume by giving intravenous fluid and by placing the patient in the Trendelenburg position (if this is compatible with the remainder of his or her evaluation).[78,80] With severe involvement, intravenous fluids will be less effective and the administration of systemic alpha-adrenergic agents such as phenylephrine may be necessary to restore a normal degree of venous and arterial tone. Pressor drugs should be started at a low dose (0.5 µg/kg/min in the case of phenylephrine) and may be titrated up and down rapidly so as to improve venous return while avoiding systemic arterial vasospasm. Renal ischemia functions as the hallmark of pressor overdose. This can be detected by careful quantification of the urine output. Pressor agents may be used in the patient with isolated neurogenic shock at low doses for a short period of time (≤24 hr) without the use of a Swan-Ganz catheter. Concurrent hemorrhagic shock, complex insensible losses, and the presence of a microvascular permeability syndrome are all indications for more detailed cardiac monitoring; most patients with a combined shock lesion should have their cardiac outputs directly measured as part of the postoperative ICU care. Finally, patients in neurogenic shock can lose a tremendous amount of heat because of their vasodilated state. Active external or internal warming techniques may be necessary to prevent further heat loss and restore normothermia in these patients.

RESUSCITATION OF PATIENTS WITH A CONCURRENT HEAD INJURY

The presence of a closed head injury in the face of hemorrhagic shock can pose a special challenge to the resuscitative skills of the trauma team. Whereas the goals of cerebral and peripheral resuscitation are similar regarding reestablishment of oxygen delivery, they differ in that injured brain tissue has a fixed volume in which to expand in response to local inflammation or intracranial hemorrhage. Functionally, this means that the trauma surgeon must correct hypoxemia and hypovolemia without overexpanding the patient's extracellular fluid volume to avoid unnecessary iatrogenic exacerbations of intracranial pressure. On the other hand, uncorrected shock greatly exacerbates head injury and elevates intracranial pressure, and the development of a microvascular permeability syndrome in this setting is the worst possible scenario.

On admission, many trauma patients have evidence of both a closed head injury and mild to moderate hemorrhagic shock. In addition to the usual signs of hypovolemia, e.g., cool skin, venospasm, and oliguria, the head-injured patient may manifest bradycardia, tachypnea, and hypertension, otherwise known as the Cushing reflex. Teleologically, this can be thought of as the body's attempt to maintain cerebral perfusion against a mounting intracranial pressure. The neurological examination may suggest a mass lesion via a blown pupil (typically on the side of the lesion) or the presence of a hemiparesis. The Glasgow Coma Scale will generally be under 6 (Table 2–4). Because delays in diagnosis are associated with a much worse prognosis, the patient with signs of head trauma should be definitively evaluated for a neurosurgically correctable mass lesion before exploratory laparotomy by obtaining a base computed tomography (CT) scan of the head without contrast. This provides the neurosurgeons with diagnostic information and can ultimately expedite care by allowing a two-team approach in the operating room.

We do not advocate a blanket policy of set-volume fluid restriction in our head-injured patients. It is important to remember that hypotension in a polytrauma setting is a feature of either mild to moderate hypovolemic shock or severe terminal brain injury with tentorial herniation. Patients with signs of herniation on admission are frequently unsalvageable, whereas hemorrhagic hypotension with low cerebral perfusion pressure will almost always improve with intravascular volume expansion. Thus, a diagnostic IV fluid bolus should never be withheld from the polytrauma patient for the sake of preventing cerebral edema. The optimal fluid to use for that bolus is a subject of considerable controversy, however, and the latest trends suggest that hyperosmolar resuscitation with either mannitol or hypertonic saline may restore effective circulation using smaller fluid volumes and without exacerbating cerebral edema.[97,99] Mannitol is usually given in a dose of 0.7 to 1.0 g/kg, which works out to a 50- to 70-g initial dose in the average adult.[8] The use of hypertonic saline solutions in head injury is still experimental, although the animal data appear quite promising.[98] Diuretics, which may be beneficial in the isolated head injury, should not be given in a polytrauma setting as they may cause contraction of the intravascular volume and exacerbate hypovolemic shock.

In terms of ventilatory management, hyperventilation is almost always beneficial and is compatible with both resuscitation of hypovolemia and head injury. Although the natural

Table 2–4 Glasgow Coma Scale

EYE OPENING	MOTOR RESPONSE	VERBAL RESPONSE
4 Spontaneous	6 Follows commands	5 Oriented
3 To sound	5 Localizes stimulus	4 Confused
2 To pain	4 Withdraws	3 Words
1 None	3 Flexion posturing	2 Sounds
	2 Extension posturing	1 None
	1 No movement	

tendency of the patient will be to breath rapidly, endotracheal intubation and mechanical ventilation gives the physician much tighter control over the patient's pCO_2. Lowering the arterial pCO_2 causes cerebral vasoconstriction and shifts the cerebral volume pressure curve back toward normal range.[33] The recommended pCO_2 is 25 to 30.

PATIENT *IN EXTREMIS* MANAGEMENT

Controversy exists regarding the treatment of trauma patients who present to the emergency room *in extremis* or with apparent cardiac arrest. Although little debate exists concerning the need for immediate intubation and ventilation in these patients, somewhat conflicting data have been presented regarding the role of emergency thoracotomy and operating room resuscitation.[16] Resuscitative thoracotomy theoretically allows the surgeon to vent a tension pneumothorax, relieve pericardial tamponade, control bleeding rapidly from small cardiac and pulmonary hilar lacerations, and perform more effective open cardiac massage in the emergency room. Operating room resuscitation theoretically allows rapid laparotomy and media sternotomy concurrent with resuscitation. We propose a somewhat selective use of these maneuvers based on the mechanism of injury and signs of life on physical examination, realizing that these are desperate measures. This selective approach seems justified because the survival figures in blunt trauma cardiopulmonary resuscitation cases have been poor, as have been those cases of patients in full cardiac arrest before arrival in the emergency room with a penetrating mechanism, and because these procedures place a tremendous drain on a trauma center's resources.[2,22,75]

In our algorithm, the patient who presents to the emergency department in apparent cardiac arrest should be intubated immediately and checked for "signs of life" (Fig. 2–4). These signs include the presence of a pulse; spontaneous respirations; a history of life in the field with loss of vital signs in the ambulance; or any rhythm, other than agonal, when the patient is connected to the cardiac monitor. Patients without any of these signs are declared "dead on arrival." If a sign of life is present, however, one may elect to perform anterolateral thoracotomy if the injury appears to be in the thorax or take the patient directly to the operating room for resuscitation if the exsanguinating lesion appears to be in the abdomen.

Emergency room thoracotomy is performed by creating a bold curved incision in the fifth intercostal space starting 1 cm lateral to the sternum, proceeding under the pectoralis major muscle in the pectoral or submammary groove, and ending at the posterior axillary line. The incision should go down to the parietal pleura with the first stroke, followed by blunt disruption of the pleura by the surgeon's finger, which avoids pulmonary laceration. A finger is then thrust across the inferior aspect of the middle mediastinum to relieve a potential tension pneumothorax on the other side. The pericardium is incised in a longitudinal manner to avoid the phrenic nerve. Blood is evacuated from the pericardium and the heart is cradled in the surgeon's hand with the second through fifth fingers resting against the left ventricle and the thumb positioned anteriorly against the right ventricle or on top of the sternum. Any cardiac laceration should be controlled with finger pressure while open cardiac massage is performed. The patient should then be taken immediately to the operating room. Saphenous cutdowns are extremely beneficial in these patients and may be placed by other members of the resuscitation team while thoracotomy is being per-

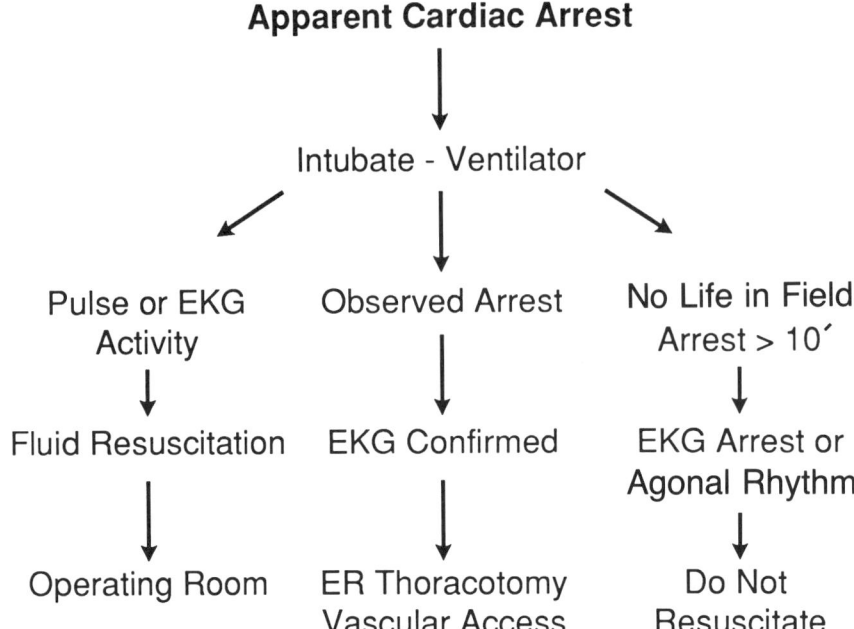

Figure 2–4. Triage of the trauma patient who is in apparent cardiac arrest. In the case of observed arrest in the victim of blunt trauma, the salvage rate is so low that it may be appropriate not to carry out thoracotomy except in infants and children.

formed. They should not delay transport to the operating room, however, because once the patient is in the operating room fluids can usually be given much more rapidly.

Operating room resuscitation has been proposed as the most rapid means of controlling exsanguination hemorrhage from intraabdominal or thoracoabdominal lesions without the time delays associated with stopping in the emergency room to intubate and place lines.[44] If one elects to perform so-called resuscitation laparotomy, the abdomen should be rapidly opened in the midline and packed. Manual pressure can be placed on the abdominal aorta to increase coronary artery diastolic filling pressure, but this must be released periodically to prevent renal and splanchnic ischemia. Once the abdomen is packed, the surgeon should then stop and let anesthesia catch up with fluid administration to reestablish preload. Only after adequate cardiac filling and circulation has been restored should the operation proceed.

The results of emergency thoracotomy have been generally disappointing.[16,22,45] Mortality appears to be higher in the blunt trauma population who receive emergency room thoracotomy than in patients with a penetrating mechanism; when the "signs of life" criteria are strictly applied, fewer blunt trauma patients will be true candidates for thoracotomy. Massive injuries to the cardiac chambers and great vessels, prolonged cardiac ischemia, and low diastolic coronary artery filling pressures in these trauma patients may explain the low salvage rates. Although preliminary data suggest similar statistical outcomes in the pediatric population, heroic efforts may be more appropriate in young children because of the child's general resiliency in tolerating ischemia and overall enhanced recovery powers.[7,67]

REFERENCES

1. Archibald EW, McLean WS. Observations upon shock with particular relevance to the condition as seen in war surgery. *Ann Surg.* 1917; 66:281.
2. Baker CC, Thomas AN, Trunkey DD. The role of emergency room thoracotomy in trauma. *J Trauma.* 1980; 20:848–854.
3. Baker DP. Trauma in the pregnant patient. *Surg Clin North Am.* 1982; 62:275–289.
4. Barone JE, Pizzi WF, Nealon TF Jr, Richman H. Indications for intubation in blunt chest trauma. *J Trauma.* 1986; 26:334–338.
5. Beal SL, Reed RL, Heimbach D, Chi E, Reynolds L. Pulmonary microembolism: a cause of lung injury. *J Surg Res.* 1987; 43:303–310.
6. Beal SL, Spisso JM. The risk of splenorrhaphy. *Arch Surg.* 1988; 123:1158–1163.
7. Beaver BC, Columlani PH, Bush JR, Dudgeon DL, Bohrer SL, Haller JA. Efficacy of emergency room thoracotomy in pediatric trauma. *J Pediatr Surg.* 1987; 22:19–23.
8. Becker DP, Gade GF, Young HF, Feureman TF. Diagnosis and treatment of head injury in adults. In: Youmans JR, ed. *Neurological Surgery.* 3rd ed. Philadelphia: WB Saunders; 1982:2017–2149.
9. Beecher HK. The physiologic effects of wounds. Medical Department, U.S. Army, Washington, DC, 1952.
10. Berkman SA. Infectious complications of blood transfusion. *Blood Rev.* 1988; 2:206–210.
11. Blaisdell FW, Lewis FR Jr. *Respiratory Distress Syndrome of Shock and Trauma.* Philadelphia: WB Saunders; 1977.
12. Blaisdell FW, Lim RC, Amberg JR, Choy SH, Hall AD, Thomas AN. Pulmonary microembolism. *Arch Surg.* 1966: 93:776.
13. Blaisdell FW. Traumatic shock: the search for a toxic factor. *Bull Am Coll Surg.* 1983; 68:1.
14. Blalock A. Experimental shock: the cause of low blood pressure produced by muscle injury. *Arch Surg.* 1930; 20:959.
15. Bock JC, Barker BC, Clinton AG, Wilson MB, Lewis FR. Post-traumatic changes in, and effect of colloid osmotic pressure on the distribution of body water. *Ann Surg.* 1989; 210:395.
16. Bodai BI, Smith JP, Blaisdell FW. The role of emergency thoracotomy in blunt trauma. *J Trauma.* 1982; 22: 487–491.
17. Boyce JR, Peters G. Vessel dilator cricothyrotomy for transtracheal jet ventilation. *Can J Anesth.* 1989; 36: 350–353.
18. Burke TJ, Burnier M, Langberg H, Shanley P, Schrier RW. Renal response to shock. *Ann Emerg Med.* 1986; 15:1397–1400.
19. Cafferata HT, Aggeler PM, Robinson AJ, Blaisdell FW. Intravascular coagulation in the surgical patient: its significance and diagnosis. *Am J Surg.* 1969; 118:281.
20. Canizaro PC, Prager MD, Shires GT. The infusion of Ringer's lactate solution during shock. *Am J Surg.* 1971; 122:494.
21. Cannon WB. *Traumatic Shock.* New York: Appleton and Co; 1923.
22. Cogbill TN, Moore EE, Millikan JS, et al. Rationale for selective application of emergency department thoracotomy in trauma. *J Trauma.* 1983; 23:452–460.
23. Cournand A, Riley RL, Bradley SE, et al. Studies of the circulation in clinical shock. *Surgery.* 1943; 13:964.
24. Crile GW. *Experimental Research into Surgical Shock.* Philadelphia: JB Lippincott; 1899.
25. Cryer HM, Garrison RN, Harris PD. Role of muscle microvasculature during hyperdynamic and hypodynamic phases of endotoxic shock in decelerate rats. *J Trauma.* 1988; 28:312–318.
26. Demling RH. Effect of plasma and interstitial protein content on tissue edema formation. *Curr Stud Hematol Blood Transfusion.* 1986; 53:36–52.
27. Dilts PV, Brinkman CR, Kirschbaum TH, Assali NS. Uterine and systemic hemodynamic interrelationships and their response to hypoxia. *Curr Dev Eval.* 1969; 103:138–157.
28. Drucker WR, Chadwick CDJ, Gann DS. Transcapillary refill in hemorrhage and shock. *Arch Surg.* 1983; 116:1344–1353.
29. Eckstein JW, Wendling MG, Abboud FM. Forearm venous responses to stimulation of adrenergic receptors. *J Clin Invest.* 1965; 44:1151–1159.
30. Eisenhofer G, Lombia DG, Johnson RH. Effects of ethanol ingestion on α-adrenoceptor–mediated circulating response in man. *Br J Clin Pharmacol.* 1989; 18:581–586.
31. Federal Drug Administration Drug Bulletin: use of blood components. *FDA Drug Bull.* 1989; 19:14.
32. Finch CA, Lenfant C. Oxygen transport in man. *N Engl J Med.* 1972; 286:407–414.
33. Gade GF, Becker DP, Miller JD, Dwan PS. Pathology and pathophysiology of head injury. In: Youmans JR, ed. *Neurological Surgery.* 3rd ed. Philadelphia: WB Saunders; 1982:1965–2016.
34. Gann DS, Carlson DE, Byrnes GJ, Pirkle JC Jr, Allen-Rowlands CF. Role of solute in the early restitution of blood volume after hemorrhage. *Surgery.* 1983; 94:439.
35. Glinz W. Priorities in diagnosis and treatment of blunt chest injuries. *Surgery.* 1986; 17:318–321.

36. Green BA, Eismont FJ, O'Heir JT. Spinal cord injury—a system's approach: Prevention, emergency medical services and emergency room management. *Crit Care Clin.* 1987; 3:471–493.
37. Greenburg AG. Indications for transfusion. In: Wilmore DW, Brennan MF, Harken AH, Holcroft JW, Meakins JL, eds. *American College of Surgeons: Care of the Surgical Patient, Vol. 1, Critical Care.* A Publication of the Committee on Pre and Postoperative Care. New York: Scientific American; 1989.
38. Henderson Y. Acapnea in shock, the failure of the circulation. *Am J Physiol.* 1910; 27:152.
39. Hock CE, Su J-Y, Lefer AM. Role of AVP in maintenance of circulatory homeostasis during hemorrhagic shock. *Am J Physiol.* 1984; 246:H174.
40. Holcroft JW. Shock. In: Wilmore DW, Brennan MF, Harken AH, Holcroft JW, Meakins JL, eds. *American College of Surgeons: Care of the Surgical Patient, Vol. 1, Critical Care.* A Publication of the Committee on Pre and Postoperative Care. New York: Scientific American; 1989.
41. Holcroft JW, Trunkey DD. Extravascular lung water following hemorrhagic shock in the baboon: comparison between resuscitation with lactated Ringer's and plasmanate. *Ann Surg.* 1974; 180:408–417.
42. Holcroft JW, Vassar MJ, Turner JE, Derlet RW, Kramer GC. 3% NaCl and 7.5% NaCl/Dextran 70 in the resuscitation of severely injured patients. *Ann Surg.* 1987; 206:279.
43. Horton JW. Hemorrhagic shock complicated by chronic ethanolism. *Am J Physiol.* 1989; 257:H198–208.
44. Hoyt DB, Shackford SR, Davis JW, MacKersie RC, Hollingsworth-Fredlund P. Thoracotomy during trauma resuscitation—an appraisal by board-certified general surgeons. *J Trauma.* 1989; 29:1318–1321.
45. Hoyt DB, Shackford SR, McGill T, MacKersie R, Davis J, Hansbrough J. The impact of in-house surgeons and operating room resuscitation on outcome of traumatic injuries. *Arch Surg.* 1989; 124:906–910.
46. Jin LJ, Lalonde C, Demling RH. Lung dysfunction after thermal injury in relation to prostanoid and oxygen radical release. *J Appl Physiol.* 1986; 61:103–112.
47. Jones SE, Nesper TP, Alcoulou E. Prehospital intravenous line placement: a prospective study. *Ann Emerg Med.* 1989; 18:244–246.
48. Keith NM. *Blood Volume in Wound Shock.* London: Medical Research Committee Special Report; Series 26, 1919.
49. Klausner JM, Asner H, Paterson IS, et al. Lower torso ischemia-induced lung injury is leukocyte dependent. *Ann Surg.* 1988; 208:761–767.
50. Kramer GC, Perron PR, Lindsey DC, et al. Small-volume resuscitation with hypertonic saline dextran solution. *Surgery.* 1986; 100:239–247.
51. Lewis FR Jr. Prehospital intravenous fluid therapy: physiologic computer modelling. *J Trauma.* 1986; 26: 804–811.
52. Little RA. 1988 Fitts lecture: heart rate changes after haemorrhage and injury—A reappraisal. *J Trauma.* 1989; 29:903.
53. Lordon RE, Burton JR. Post-traumatic renal failure in military personnel in southeast Asia: experience at Clark USAF Hospital, Republic of the Phillipines. *Am J Surg.* 1972; 53:137–147.
54. Lowe RJ, Moss GS, Jilek J, Levine HD. Crystalloid vs colloid in the etiology of pulmonary failure after trauma: a randomized trial in man. *Surgery.* 1977; 81:676.
55. Luna GK, Dellinger EP. Nonoperative observation therapy for splenic injuries: a safe therapeutic option? *Am J Surg.* 1987; 153:462–468.
56. Malt SH, Baue AE. The effects of ethanol as related to trauma in the awake dog. *J Trauma.* 1971; 11: 76–78.
57. Mazzoni MC, Borgstrom P, Arfors KE, Intaglietta M. Dynamic fluid redistribution in hyperosmotic resuscitation of hypovolemic hemorrhage. *Am J Physiol.* 1988; 255:H629–637.
58. Mellander S, Johansson B. Control of resistance, exchange, and capacitance functions in the peripheral circulation. *Pharmacol Rev.* 1968; 20:117.
59. Morris EA. *A Practical Treatise on Shock After Operations and Injuries.* London: Hartwicke Publishers; 1867.
60. Motulsky HJ, Insel PA. Adrenergic receptors in man: direct identification, physiologic regulation, and clinical alterations. *N Engl J Med.* 1982; 307:18–29.
61. Newsome HH Jr. Ethanol modulation of plasma norepinephrine response to trauma and hemorrhage. *J Trauma.* 1988; 28:1–9.
62. O'Gorman M, Trabulsey P, Pilcher DB. Zerotime prehospital I.V. *J Trauma.* 1989; 29:84–86.
63. Pang CCY. Effect of vasopressin antagonist and saralasin on regional blood flow following hemorrhage. *Am J Physiol.* 1983; 245:H749.
64. Pepe PE. The clinical entity of adult respiratory distress syndrome. Definition, prediction, and prognosis. *Crit Care Clin.* 1986; 2:377–403.
65. Piene H. Pulmonary arterial impedance and right ventricular function. *Physiol Rev.* 1986; 66:606.
66. Pirkle JC, Gann DS. Restitution of blood volume after hemorrhage: role of the adrenal cortex. *J Physiol* 1976; 230:1683–1687.
67. Powell RW, Gill EA, **Jurkovich GJ, Ramenofsky** ML. *Resuscitative thoracotomy in children and adolescents.* Presented in the 55th Annual Assembly of the Southeastern Surgical Congress; March 16–18, 1987.

68. Rankin JS, Olsen CO, Arentzen CE, et al. The effects of airway pressure on cardiac function in intact dogs and man. *Circulation.* 1982; 66:108.
69. Reesink HW, Van der Poll CL. Blood transfusion and hepatitis: still a threat? *Blut.* 1989; 58:1–6.
70. Renkin EM. Some consequences of capillary permeability to macromolecules: Starling's hypothesis reconsidered. *Am J Physiol.* 1986; 250:706–710.
71. Rhee KJ, Derlet RW, Beal SL. Rapid venous access using saphenous vein cutdown at the ankle. *Am J Emerg Med.* 1989; 7:263–266.
72. Romney SL, Gabel PV, Takeda Y. Experimental hemorrhage in late pregnancy: effects on maternal and fetal hemodynamics. *Am J Obstet Gynecol.* 1963; 87:636–649.
73. Rothe CF. Venous system: physiology of the capacitance vessels. In: Shepherd JT, Abboud FM, Geiger SR, eds. *Handbook of Physiology, Section 2. The Cardiovascular System, Vol. III. Peripheral Circulation and Organ Blood Flow, Part 1.* Bethesda, Md: American Physiological Society; 1984:397–452.
74. Schmid PG, Abboud FM, Wendling MG, et al. Regional vascular effects of vasopressin: Plasma levels and circulatory responses. *Am J Physiol.* 1974; 227:998–1004.
75. Schwab CW, Adcock OT, Max MH. Emergency department thoracotomy (EDT); a 26 month experience using an "agonal" protocol. *Am Surg.* 1986; 52:20–29.
76. Sharma OP. Traumatic diaphragmatic rupture: not an uncommon entity—personal experience with collective review of the 1980's. *J Trauma.* 1989; 29:678–682.
77. Shenkin HA, Cheney RH, Govons SR, Hardy JD, Fletcher AG, Starr I. On the diagnosis of hemorrhage in man: a study of volunteers bled large amounts. *Am J Med Sci.* 1944; 208:421–436.
78. Shepherd JT, Vanhoutte PM. Role of the venous system in circulatory control. *Mayo Clin Proc.* 1978; 53: 247–255.
79. Shires GT, Cunningham JN, Baker CRF, et al. Alterations in cellular membrane function during hemorrhagic shock in primates. *Ann Surg.* 1972; 176:288.
80. Sibbald WJ, Paterson NAM, Holliday RL, Baskerville J. The Trendelenburg position: hemodynamic effects in hypotensive and normotensive patients. *Crit Care Med.* 1979; 7:218.
81. Simeone FA. Shock, trauma, and the surgeon. *Ann Surg.* 1963; 158:759.
82. Starling DH. On the absorption of fluids from connective tissue spaces. *J Physiol Lond.* 1896; 19:312–326.
83. Thal AP. *Shock: A Physiologic Basis for Treatment.* Chicago: Year Book Medical Publishers; 1971.
84. Thiagarajan AB, Mifford IN, Estay RL. Acute effect of intragastric ethanol administration on plasma levels of stress hormones. *Adv Alcohol Substance Abuse.* 1988; 7:227–230.
85. Trunkey DD, Illner H, Wagner IY, Shires GT. The effect of septic shock on skeletal muscle action potentials in the primate. *Surgery.* 1979; 85:638.
86. Tyson GS, Maier GW, Olsen CO, Davis JW, Rankin JS. Pericardial influences on ventricular filling in the conscious dog. *Circ Res.* 1984; 54:173–184.
87. Vassar MJ, Moore J, Perry CA, Spisso J, Holcroft JW. Early fluid requirements in trauma patients. A predictor of pulmonary failure and mortality. *Arch Surg.* 1988; 123:1149–1157.
88. Vatner SF. Effects of hemorrhage on regional blood flow distribution in dogs and primates. *J Clin Invest.* 1974; 54:225.
89. Vedder NB, Fouty BW, Winn RK, Harlan JM, Rice CL. Role of neutrophils in generalized reperfusion injury associated with resuscitation from shock. *Surgery.* 1989; 106:509–516.
90. Virgilio RW, Rice CL, Smith DE, et al. Crystalloid vs colloid resuscitation: is one better? *Surgery.* 1979; 85:129.
91. Ward RE, Flynn TC, Miller PW, et al. Effects of ethanol ingestion on the severity and outcome of trauma. *Am J Surg.* 1982; 144:153–157.
92. Wiegman DL, Miller FN, Harris PD. Modification of α-adrenergic responses of small arteries by altered PCO_2 and pH. *Eur J Pharm.* 1979; 57:307–315.
93. Wiggers CJ. *Physiology of Shock.* New York: The Commonwealth Fund Publications; 1950.
94. Wilkerson DK, Rosen AL, Sehgal LR, Gould SA, Sehgal HL, Moss GS. Limits of cardiac compensation in anemic baboons. *Surgery.* 1988; 103:665.
95. Wilmore DW, Brennan MF, Harken AH, Holcroft JW, Meakins JL, eds. *American College of Surgeons: Care of the Surgical Patient, Vol. 1, Critical Care, A Publication of the Committee on Pre and Postoperative Care.* New York: Scientific American; 1989.
96. Wilson DR, Honrath V. Inner medullary collecting duct function in ischemic acute renal failure. *Clin Invest Med.* 1988; 11:157–166.
97. Wisner D, Busche F, Sturm J, Gaob M, Meyer H. Traumatic shock and head injury: Effect of fluid resuscitation on the brain. *J Surg Res.* 1989; 46:49–59.
98. Wisner D, Schuster L, Quinn C. Hypertonic saline resuscitation of head injury; Effects on cerebral water content. *J Trauma.* 1990; 30:75–78.
99. Zornow, MH, Scheller MS, Shackford SR. Effect of a hypertonic lactated Ringer's solution on intracranial pressure and cerebral water content in a model of traumatic brain injury. *J Trauma.* 1989; 29:484–488.

3
Peritoneal Lavage, Computerized Tomography, Angiography, Ultrasound, and Magnetic Resonance Imaging

DAVID H. WISNER, M.D.
LAWRENCE A. DANTO, M.D.

HISTORY: The diagnosis of traumatic injuries to the abdomen before this century relied largely on the history and physical exam. Paré, in his book The Methods of Treating Wounds Made by Arquebueses and Other Firearms, *described how he would have the patient assume the position he was in at the time of injury to determine the course of a projectile through the body. Simple diagnostic tests and procedures have been developed only during the last 100 years. We take for granted such routine diagnostic studies as the hematocrit and chest x-ray in the setting of trauma, but hematocrit determinations began only in the 1890s[1] and the use of x-rays began only after the publication of Roentgen's* A New Kind of Ray *in 1895. Paracentesis and peritoneal lavage in the diagnosis of trauma date back only to the 1960s and the use of more sophisticated diagnostic tests such as computerized tomography, ultrasonography, and angiography is only about 15 years old. Magnetic resonance imaging, widely available for only the last 5 years, is the most recent development in the diagnostic sphere. In trauma, as in many other areas, a role for this new test is currently being defined.*

The use of paracentesis is a relatively old idea, first advanced for the diagnosis of intraperitoneal disease by Saloman in 1906.[2] Paracentesis was advocated for use in the diagnosis of trauma, pancreatitis, and peritonitis by Neuhof and Cohen in 1926.[3]

Williams and Zollinger systematically studied the use of paracentesis in the trauma patient in the 1950s and reported a 79% accuracy in the diagnosis of intraabdominal injury.[4] Others showed that the ability of paracentesis to diagnosis intraabdominal injury was critically dependent on the amount of blood in the abdomen.[5] This severely limited the use of the test in certain types of injury and hampered its widespread acceptance despite its simplicity and rapidity.

The ingenious addition of lavage to paracentesis by Root et al. in 1965 markedly increased the sensitivity of the procedure in trauma patients and led to its increased use.[6] Lavage of the peritoneal cavity allowed for sampling of fluid in dependent areas such as the pericolonic gutters and the pelvis. This markedly increased sensitivity and negative results of the procedure approached the same reliability as positive results.

Increased use of paracentesis and peritoneal lavage in trauma, however, raised new problems. If the lavage is negative but the patient manifests a continued fall in hematocrit or elevation in white blood cell count, at what point should the results be ignored and laparotomy carried out? Gross blood on paracentesis obviously constituted a positive study, but how should the lavage results be interpreted? What was the relationship between cell counts and other findings in the lavage fluid and the presence of intraperitoneal injury? Guidelines to increase the specificity of peritoneal lavage were developed in the decade after Root's description of the technique.[7–13] Not surprisingly, peritoneal lavage was also applied to the diagnosis of penetrating abdominal injury.[14–18]

PERITONEAL LAVAGE

Most patients with immediately life-threatening injuries will declare themselves shortly after arrival in the emergency department. Prolonged and sophisticated diagnostic procedures are not appropriate in such patients and should not delay needed operative intervention. Most patients, however, will be stable enough to undergo the initial laboratory and radiologic tests described in the previous chapter. More elaborate diagnostic tests are warranted based on the presenting complaint and the patient's status. Technological advances have been applied increasingly to the early diagnosis of trauma patients and are appropriate in many circumstances. It should be emphasized, however, that these tests are often time-consuming and should be done only in hemodynamically stable patients. Prolonged delays to obtain further diagnostic information are self-defeating if they lead to increased morbidity or mortality.

Rationale and Indications

Diagnosis of intraabdominal injury by physical exam can be very difficult, especially after blunt trauma.[9,11,13,19,20] Clinical signs of visceral injury are notoriously nonspecific and the overall inaccuracy of the initial physical exam in detecting intraabdominal injury has been

Table 3–1 Indications for Peritoneal Lavage

Triage of multiple casualties
Altered mental status/unreliable abdominal exam
Need for prolonged anesthesia for associated injuries
Multiply injured patient

reported to be between 16% and 45%.[4,7,9,10,12,21–29] Since delays in diagnosis are associated with increased morbidity, a more objective means of diagnosis is important.[9,10,29–32]

Patients with obvious peritoneal signs should have expeditious abdominal exploration (Table 3–1). Patients with reliable abdominal exams without peritoneal signs should be observed with serial blood counts and abdominal exams. Lavage in such patients is invasive, uncomfortable, and technically difficult if the patient is obese or has had previous abdominal operations. Observation and serial examination is preferred in such situations. A falling hematocrit during the observation period should prompt either abdominal exploration or computerized tomography (CT) of the abdomen. Exploratory laparotomy should be done if increasing abdominal tenderness or peritoneal signs develop.

One of the major virtues of peritoneal lavage is its rapidity. It can be done in the emergency department in a matter of minutes, lends itself to early diagnosis and triage, and the patient remains under continuous observation. There are several situations in which lavage is particularly valuable. It allows for rapid triage when multiple patients arrive simultaneously in the emergency department. Patients with positive paracentesis or lavage are triaged to the operation room; those with negative lavage can be triaged to further diagnostic studies of associated injuries. Patients with altered mental status are also ideal candidates. Alcohol or drug intoxication and closed head injury with altered mental status make physical examination of the abdomen difficult and unreliable. When rapid evaluation of such patients is necessary to plan diagnostic studies of associated injuries, peritoneal lavage can rapidly rule intraabdominal injury either in or out. In the multiply injured patient such as one with extensive extremity injuries and minimal to moderate evidence of torso trauma, evaluation of the abdomen may be difficult. Moreover, the hematocrit cannot be relied on to monitor intraabdominal bleeding. Peritoneal lavage is of great value in such circumstances (Table 3–2).

Imminent need for surgery to treat associated injuries is another indication for peritoneal lavage. Patients operated on for orthopedic or other injuries will often be anesthetized for prolonged periods of time. These operations can lead to extensive blood loss and hemodynamic instability. Peritoneal lavage done at the beginning of the anesthetic provides some assurance that intraoperative hemodynamic instability and postoperative decreases in hematocrit are not due to occult intraperitoneal injury.

Peritoneal lavage in awake and alert patients should rarely be done. In triage situations when multiple casualties present simultaneously, peritoneal lavage may be appropriate. In most other situations, however, serial hematocrits and abdominal exams or abdominal CT should be done instead (Table 3–2). Patients with obvious peritoneal signs should have expeditious abdominal exploration.

Lavage can also be useful in the diagnosis of intraabdominal injury after penetrating trauma. Gunshot wounds to the abdomen are associated with an 80% to 90% incidence of

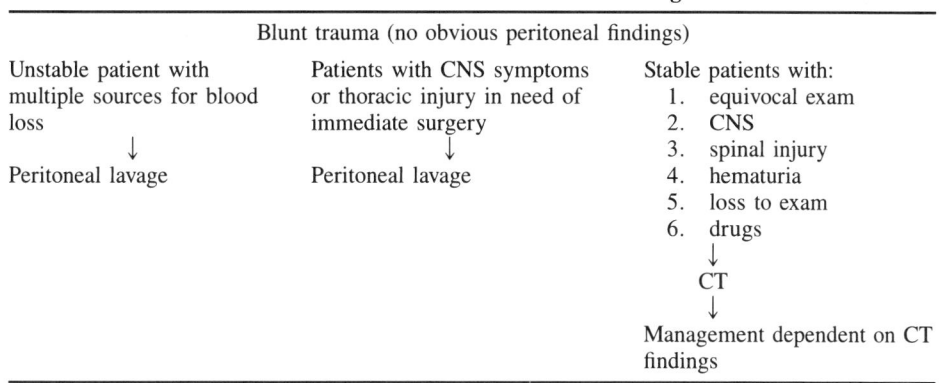

Table 3-2 Blunt Abdominal Trauma—Management

intraperitoneal injury and should be explored. Stab wounds to the anterior abdomen, on the other hand, can be explored in all instances, examined serially, and operated on selectively or triaged with peritoneal lavage. Guidelines for the interpretation of lavage results are different for blunt and penetrating trauma in some series, however, and this must be borne in mind when interpreting cell counts obtained from the lavage of stab wound patients.[15] The sensitivity of peritoneal lavage in such a setting has proven to be very good and the use of peritoneal lavage leads to a decreased number of negative and nontherapeutic laparotomies (Table 3-3).

Contraindications

The most important contraindications to the use of lavage are peritoneal signs on abdominal exam or the persistence of hemodynamic instability despite vigorous fluid resuscitation. Such patients are candidates for abdominal exploration and time should not be wasted confirming the presence of hemoperitoneum. Multiple previous abdominal incisions are a relative contraindication. Adhesions lead to compartmentalization of the abdomen and can result in false negative results. There is also increased danger of iatrogenic injury to loops of bowel adherent to the anterior abdominal wall. Pelvic fractures can result in false positive

Table 3-3 Penetrating Abdominal Trauma—Management

	Penetrating wound	
Unstable		Stable
↓	Gunshot wound	Peritoneal lavage
Operation	↓	or
	Operation	Operation

lavage results for several reasons. Retroperitoneal blood dissecting up the anterior abdominal wall in the preperitoneal space can lead to false positive results if the catheter goes through or into this layer. This problem can largely be circumvented by doing the lavage above rather than below the umbilicus. Diapedesis of red blood cells across the peritoneum from retroperitoneal hematomas associated with a pelvic fracture can also result in false positive lavage results, especially if a number of hours elapse between the time of injury and the lavage.

Pregnancy is not a contraindication to lavage if the lavage is done by careful open technique in a supraumbilical location.[26] With appropriately sized catheters, children can be lavaged with much the same technique used in adults.[33,34] We have a bias against performing lavage in stable patients who are awake and alert and can cooperate with a physical exam of the abdomen. Lavage in such patients is uncomfortable, can be technically difficult, and is invasive. Fortunately, for many of the situations in which there are relative contraindications to the performance of peritoneal lavage, CT of the abdomen can be used as an alternative.

Technique

A quiet patient is of great benefit in the performance of peritoneal lavage. When the patient is alert and cooperative, it is helpful to explain in advance how the lavage will be done. Intubation and paralysis facilitate both lavage and the evaluation of associated injuries in uncooperative patients with altered mental status, most of whom will also need to undergo CT of the head. When there is an indication for anesthesia to treat associated injuries such as fractures, lavage can be carried out after induction. Short-term intubation with the performance of lavage in a quiet, controlled setting is safer, will decrease the complication rate, and provides more reliable results.

Once a quiet field is assured, the bladder should be decompressed with a urinary catheter. A nasogastric or orogastric tube should be passed and placed to suction if the abdomen is distended or supraumbilical rather than infraumbilical lavage is to be carried out.

The lavage should usually be done in an infraumbilical position. We use an open technique in which the peritoneum is opened under direct vision. Although such an approach results in an increased incidence of minor wound complications compared to puncture and needle lavage techniques, we feel that the incidence of serious complications is reduced.[6,10,12,20,22,35–37] One exception to this approach is in obese patients, where closed techniques may be advantageous (Fig. 3–1). The skin is cleaned with an iodinated solution and infiltrated with lidocaine containing epinephrine. The epinephrine is important in minimizing contamination of the lavage specimen by blood from the incision and infiltration should therefore be done even in unconscious patients. A longitudinal midline incision is then made, generally approximately 2 to 3 cm in length (Fig. 3–2). A longer incision may be necessary in obese patients to retract the subcutaneous fat and visualize fascia adequately. After the skin incision has been made, the subcutaneous tissue is bluntly retracted and the linea alba incised for a short distance. As with the skin incision, this fascial incision must be long enough to allow for retraction of the preperitoneal fat and visualization of the peritoneum. After retraction of the preperitoneal fat, the peritoneum is located and elevated into the wound. This can be done either with forceps or by pulling up on the fascia with

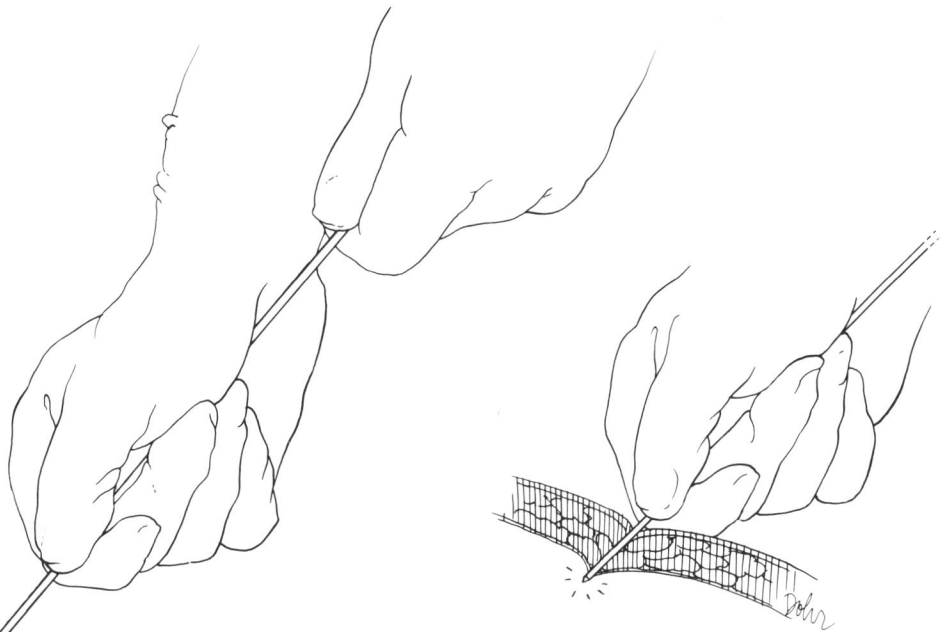

Figure 3–1. Peritoneal lavage using a closed technique is occasionally indicated. The obturator should be grasped as shown to preclude uncontrolled or excessively deep penetration. One hand acts as the guard while the other applies the force necessary to push the trocar through the abdominal wall.

towel clips. A small hole is made in the peritoneum and the lavage catheter inserted (Fig. 3–2). The ideal catheter is a peritoneal dialysis catheter, which is fairly stiff and has multiple side holes (Fig. 3–3). The catheter should slide easily into the peritoneal cavity. If it does not, it may be in the preperitoneal space and the hole through which the catheter has been placed should be reexamined to ensure that it is indeed a hole in the peritoneum and not a hole in a layer of preperitoneal fat. The catheter should be directed toward the pelvis because in the supine position this is the most dependent portion of the peritoneal cavity and is where intraperitoneal blood is most likely to collect (Fig. 3–4).

When the catheter is in satisfactory position, its proximal end should be attached by way of an extension tubing to a fitting that allows for aspiration with a 10-ml syringe. If aspiration results in the return of 10 or more ml of gross blood, the study is positive, the procedure is over, and the catheter can be removed. If the aspiration is negative for gross blood, lavage should be done. This is done by running isotonic fluid (either lactated Ringer's solution or normal saline) by gravity into the peritoneal cavity. A liter of lavage fluid should be used in adults and approximately 20 ml/kg in children. The lavage fluid is then removed by placing the empty fluid container on the floor below the level of the patient and allowing it to siphon out of the abdomen. Distribution and mixing of the lavage fluid in the peritoneal cavity is facilitated by pushing lightly on the anterior abdominal wall and shifting the patient gently from side to side. Return of the fluid is sometimes slow and may require manipulation of the catheter. It is also important to avoid running all of the fluid from the lavage container into the peritoneal cavity. When this is done, no fluid

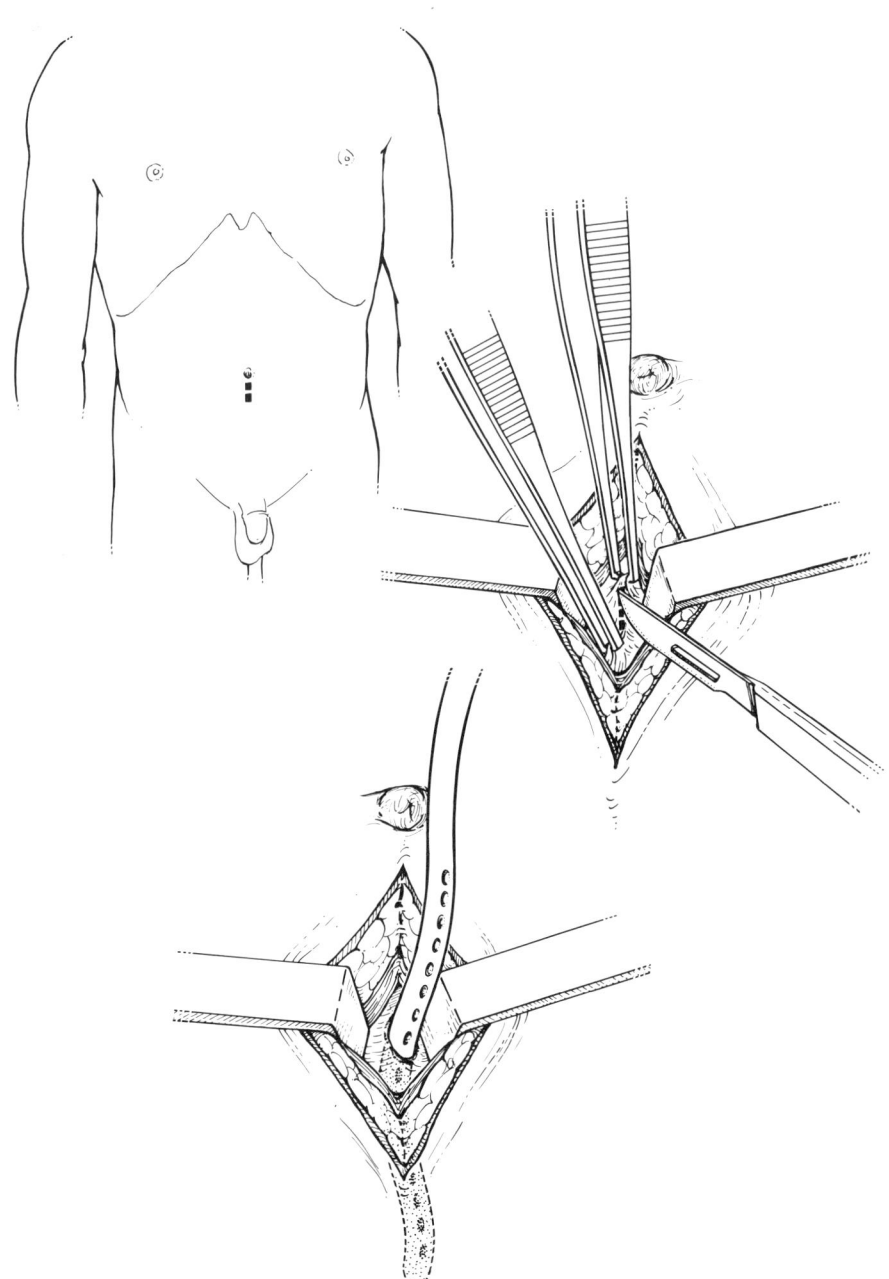

Figure 3–2. Peritoneal lavage using the open or "minilap" technique. After opening of the fascia, the preperitoneal fat is cleared from the underlying peritoneum and the peritoneum tented with forceps or hemostats. A hole is made in the peritoneum and the catheter inserted under direct vision.

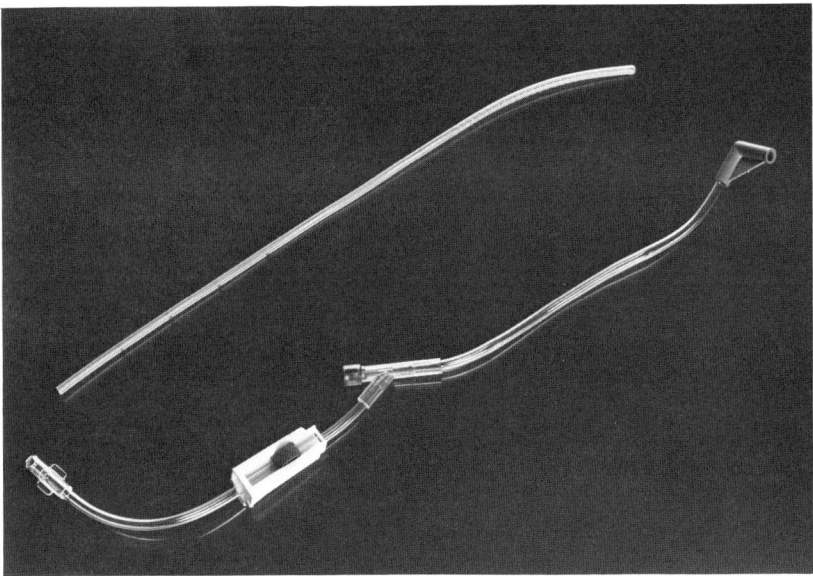

Figure 3–3. A peritoneal dialysis catheter with multiple side holes at one end is ideal for use in paracentesis and peritoneal lavage

remains in the tubing connecting the peritoneal fluid with the lavage container. This inhibits the siphon effect necessary for adequate fluid return.

After siphon removal has begun, a subjective observation of the color of the fluid can be made and an aliquot sent for microscopic analysis. Counting the number of red blood cells per milliliter is the most important component of the lavage fluid analysis (Table 3–2) but analysis for white blood cell count, amylase concentration, bilirubin, vegetable matter,

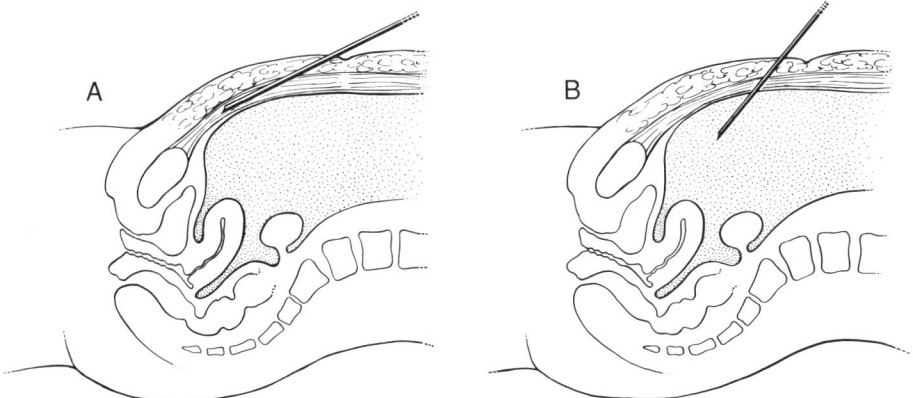

Figure 3–4. **A:** Avoid preperitoneal placement. **B:** The lavage catheter should be placed through the hole in the peritoneum and directed into the pelvis, where fluid is most likely to accumulate in the supine position.

and gram stain can also be done. The aliquot for analysis should not be taken from the initial return of fluid, as this fluid does not adequately sample the contents of the pelvis.

Siphon removal should be continued until there is no more return. As mentioned above, this is facilitated by manipulation of the catheter during siphoning. It is not necessary to remove all of the infused fluid before discontinuing the lavage, as long as enough has been returned to allow for adequate subjective evaluation of color and aliquot sampling (at least 300–400 ml).

After the return of lavage fluid has stopped, the catheter is removed and the fluid discarded. It is not necessary to close the peritoneum. The hole in the midline fascia is closed with interrupted or running absorbable suture; we usually use a #1 polyglycolic acid suture for this purpose because the needle is a good size and the suture ties easily. No subcutaneous sutures or drains are necessary and the skin can be closed with either suture or skin staples. If the aspiration or lavage is obviously positive, we prefer to leave the lavage incision open; closure is done in the operating room.

Interpretation

As mentioned above, the most important parameter used in determining whether the procedure is positive or negative is the presence of gross blood or large numbers of red blood cells (Table 3–4). Gross blood on aspiration obviates the need for instillation of lavage fluid. Subjective evaluation of the color of the lavage fluid has been proposed as a reliable means of determining the presence of intraperitoneal injury but we have found this to be misleading. A little bit of blood goes a long way toward coloring the lavage fluid pink and there is a tendency to overestimate the red blood cell count when this is done subjectively. It has also been suggested that inability to read newsprint through the lavage tubing is a sensitive sign of intraperitoneal bleeding.[11] We have been disappointed with the use of this "poor man's cell count" and have found that it leads, like subjective evaluation of the lavage fluid, to large numbers of false positive interpretations. Although the turnaround time for cell analysis results from the laboratory may be as long as 1 to 2 hr in some hospitals, the vast majority of patients with bleeding slow enough to require microscopic proof of a positive lavage will tolerate the delay.

Table 3–4 Paracentesis/Peritoneal Lavage Interpretation

Indeterminate
  Small amount gross blood
  50,000–100,000 RBC/ml
  100–500 WBC/ml
  75–175 U/100 ml amylase
Positive
  Free aspiration of 10 ml blood
  > 100,000 RBC/ml
  > 500 WBC/ml
  > 175 U/100 ml amylase
  Bilirubin
  Vegetable matter

A red blood cell count of greater than 100,000/ml in blunt trauma patients is considered positive and mandates laparotomy. Counts below 50,000/ml are negative and stable patients without peritoneal signs may be observed. Intermediate counts of 50,000 to 100,000/ml are indeterminate and the decision to explore the patient cannot be made on the basis of the lavage results alone. In order of decreasing importance, lavage values for white blood cells, vegetable matter, amylase, and bilirubin are of much less value than the red blood cell count in the diagnosis of blunt intraabdominal injury. White blood cell values above 500/ml are sometimes the only clue to the presence of bowel rupture. Values between 100 and 500/ml, like red blood cell counts between 50,000 and 100,000/ml, are indeterminate. Elevated amylase levels above 175 units/100 ml are also occasionally indicative of bowel rupture, pancreatic injury, or duodenal injury. The retroperitoneal location of the pancreas and duodenum, however, limits the sensitivity of this measurement.[38-41] Vegetable matter is also a sign of bowel injury but is rarely present in isolation without associated large numbers of red or white blood cells. Testing for bilirubin, which should not normally be present in the peritoneal cavity, can also be done but positive results will be present in isolation only in the rare instances in which blunt rupture of the gall bladder is the only intraabdominal injury.

Peritoneal lavage interpretation after stab wounds is different from that after blunt trauma. Because serious penetrating injuries such as bowel perforation are less often associated with hemorrhage, the red blood cell count required for positivity should be reduced to 10,000/ml to increase sensitivity.[15] In these circumstances the white blood cell count and the presence of bile, amylase, or particulate matter assumes greater importance.

Results

Results of paracentesis and peritoneal lavage have generally been excellent. False positive rates of large series are approximately 3% and false negative rates around 1.5%.[4,6,7,9,11-13,20,22,26,28,29,33,34,41-49] False positive tests can be due to bleeding from the lavage site or injury of the omentum or mesentery by the lavage catheter. Passage of the catheter into the preperitoneal space in patients with large retroperitoneal hematomas associated with a pelvic fracture can also lead to false positive results.

False negative results are most often due to faulty catheter placement, usually in the preperitoneal space, but can also be due to compartmentalization of the abdomen by adhesions from previous abdominal operations. Lavage can also be negative if done immediately after injury if bleeding is slow or contamination from a hollow viscous injury is minimal. Traumatic rupture of the diaphragm, because of a tendency for collection of blood and lavage fluid in the pleural cavity, can also lead to false negative results.[40,49-51] Intraperitoneal bladder ruptures, because they are not always associated with a great deal of bleeding and because of dilution of the lavage fluid by urine, can also be missed by peritoneal lavage. Penetrating injuries of the bowel can be missed, particularly if the lavage is done very early after injury and the criteria of positivity for blunt trauma are used.[14,15,28] If a red blood cell criteria for positivity of 10,000/ml is used after penetrating trauma, 100% sensitivity rates have been reported.[15] A small percentage of bowel and other injuries will be missed if the standard criteria of peritoneal lavage for blunt trauma to the abdomen are used.[14,20]

Although reported false negative rates for peritoneal lavage are impressively low for both blunt and penetrating injuries, these rates can be somewhat misleading. False negative rates give an indication of how many missed injuries there were in *all* patients undergoing peritoneal lavage. Perhaps more important is the positive predictive value, or the number of negative lavages in patients with intraabdominal injury. If the reliability of peritoneal lavage is described in this way, a much higher incidence of injuries, 4% to 5%, are missed.

Complications

Complications after paracentesis and peritoneal lavage can be classified as either major or minor. Minor complications include wound infections, hematomas, and breakdown of the fascial closure with subsequent hernia formation. These complications are most common after the open technique described above. Although a nuisance, none are life-threatening or cause serious morbidity. Review of collected series of peritoneal lavage reveals a minor complication rate of approximately 1%.[6,7,9,11–13,20,22,24,26,28,33,34,41–46,48,52]

Major complications reported with paracentesis and peritoneal lavage include iatrogenic perforation of the stomach, small bowel, colon, mesentery, and pelvic vasculature. The rate of such complications in the large collected series described above was 0.5% and they were more often associated with closed paracentesis techniques. Many required operative intervention for repair; rarely, they resulted in serious morbidity.

COMPUTERIZED TOMOGRAPHY

History

CT is a relatively recent development that has enjoyed major clinical application only since the 1970s and its use in the diagnosis of intraabdominal injuries is an even more recent phenomenon. First suggested for widespread use in trauma patients by Federle and Trunkey in the late 1970s and early 1980s, CT, particularly after blunt injury, has enjoyed increasing popularity.[53–55] The initial blush of enthusiasm for this noninvasive means of examining the peritoneal cavity and retroperitoneum has been tempered by a number of subsequent analyses of the reliability of CT and by the realization that sending a freshly injured patient to the scanner removes the patient from direct observation and can lead to difficulties with monitoring.[56–59] Increasing experience has pointed to these limitations and emphasized the critical importance of patient selection. Nonetheless, there is no question that CT plays an important role in the initial evaluation of many patients and when used properly complements rather than competes with other diagnostic procedures.

Rationale and Indications/Contraindications

CT is best suited to the hemodynamically stable blunt trauma patient with possible intraperitoneal or retroperitoneal injury. Patients presenting to the emergency department with stable vital signs and equivocal abdominal exams are also good candidates for scanning, as are patients with negative or equivocal abdominal exams in whom serial hematocrits show an unexpected drop. CT is also helpful when there are relative contraindications to peritoneal lavage, such as in patients with multiple previous abdominal procedures. Scanning can be done to evaluate injuries to the kidneys and other retroperitoneal organs or when patients require CT scanning of other body regions. CT of the head after closed head injury has become the standard of care and CT scanning is also being used for an increasing number of other extraabdominal injuries. Examples of extraabdominal injuries in which CT scanning is being employed with increasing frequency are facial fractures, spinal trauma, mediastinal widening, and complex pelvic and acetabular fractures. Adding an abdominal scan in stable patients being evaluated for these injuries is usually a relatively simple matter.

Many patients with blunt trauma are admitted for serial abdominal exams and hematocrit determinations. Some of these patients will manifest a fall in their hematocrit over the course of their first 12 to 24 hr in the hospital. The dilemma for the surgeon caring for such patients is to determine whether the drop in hematocrit is due to bleeding from associated injuries, hydration with intravenous fluids, or occult intraabdominal or retroperitoneal bleeding. CT scanning, highly sensitive for intraperitoneal fluid, is an ideal test in such circumstances.

As with paracentesis and peritoneal lavage, patients unstable despite vigorous fluid resuscitation are best treated with laparotomy rather than a CT scan. CT scanning can be dangerous in patients with marginal hemodynamic stability. Although the scan time itself may be short, especially with the most recent generation of scanners, the total time needed for a scan is at least 30 to 60 min in even the best centers when transport and interpretation times are taken into account. This delay can have serious consequences in patients with ongoing intraabdominal hemorrhage. Performance of a scan also places some distance between the patient and the physician, as the patient is in a separate room during the scan. Although automatic blood pressure cuffs and pulse oximeters allow for some monitoring, the ability to follow the patient closely is compromised to a degree.

CT, although very good at detecting free intraperitoneal blood, is less sensitive for the diagnosis of pancreatic injury and blunt rupture of the bowel (Fig. 3–5), particularly if the scan is done shortly after injury.[58–60] For this reason, we rarely scan even stable patients if they have peritoneal signs on physical exam. The reliability of the scan increases with the passage of time in bowel and retroperitoneal injuries so that follow-up scans done the day after trauma can be of value in detecting previously unsuspected problems.

Because CT scanning frequently misses injuries to hollow viscera in the early posttraumatic period, it is less useful for stab wounds to the abdomen. Abdominal gunshot wounds, because of the high incidence of visceral injuries, should be routinely explored and CT scanning plays no role in the work-up of these patients.

Technique

Abdominal CT scanning requires a quiet and cooperative patient to minimize motion artifact. There is also some advantage to having the patient hold his breath during the performance of each cut of the scan. When patients are intoxicated, uncooperative, or have an altered mental status from head injury, intubation and paralysis may be necessary. Optimally, both oral and intravenous contrast should be given. If the patient cannot take the oral contrast by mouth, it can be instilled via a nasogastric or orogastric tube. Typically, 1-cm coronal cuts are taken between the xiphoid and the lower margin of the kidneys. One

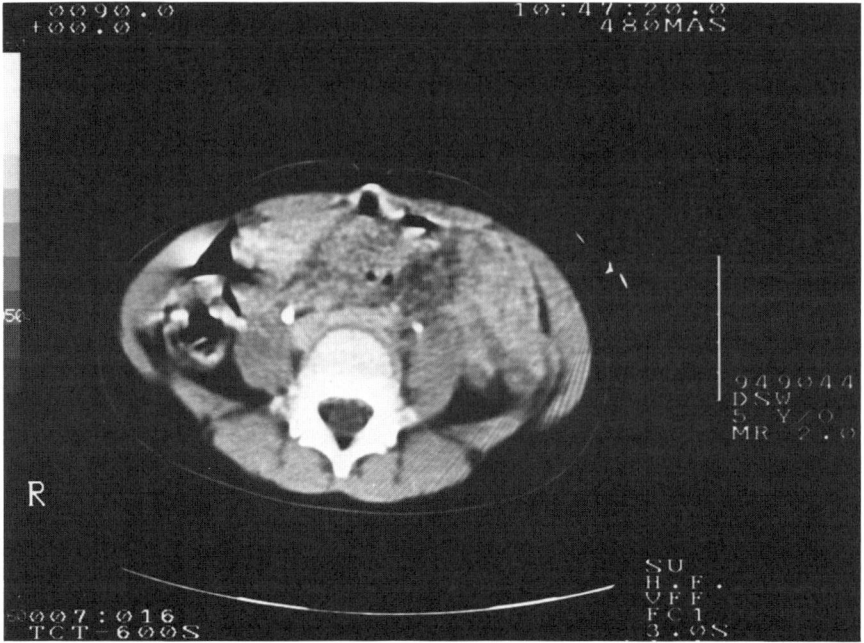

Figure 3–5. An abdominal CT scan obtained 1 hr after admission in a 5-year-old boy involved in a motor vehicle accident. The scan was normal. Because of increasing abdominal pain and peritoneal signs exploratory laparotomy was performed 24 hr after admission. A perforation of the jejunum was found.

and a half–centimeter cuts are then taken for the remainder of the scan through the pelvis. Scanning time varies with the type of scanner but ranges between 40 min for older scanners and 15 to 20 min for the newest generation of machines. The cuts can be read directly from a monitor for rapidity or from a hard copy of the scan.

Free blood or other fluid tends to collect in dependent areas of the peritoneal cavity. In the supine position, these are the pelvis (Fig. 3–6), the right and left pericolic gutters, the subhepatic space, and the posterior aspects of the subphrenic spaces (Fig. 3–7). CT scanning is sensitive for as little as 100 to 200 ml of free fluid in the adult peritoneal cavity.[61] Fluid in the subphrenic spaces is particularly easy to detect because it is immediately adjacent to the spleen or liver (Fig. 3–7).

CT scanning can also pick up parenchymal injuries to the liver (Fig. 3–8), spleen (Fig. 3–9), pancreas (Fig. 3–10), and kidney (Fig. 3–11). Intrahepatic hematomas without associated intraperitoneal blood are detected in instances in which peritoneal lavage would be negative. Retroperitoneal hematomas can be diagnosed and differentiated from intraperitoneal blood (Fig. 3–11).

Associated injuries to the chest and bony pelvis are also sometimes first picked up by CT scanning of the abdomen. Scanning is very sensitive for small amounts of blood in the pleural cavity and can make the diagnosis of hemothorax when the chest x-ray is

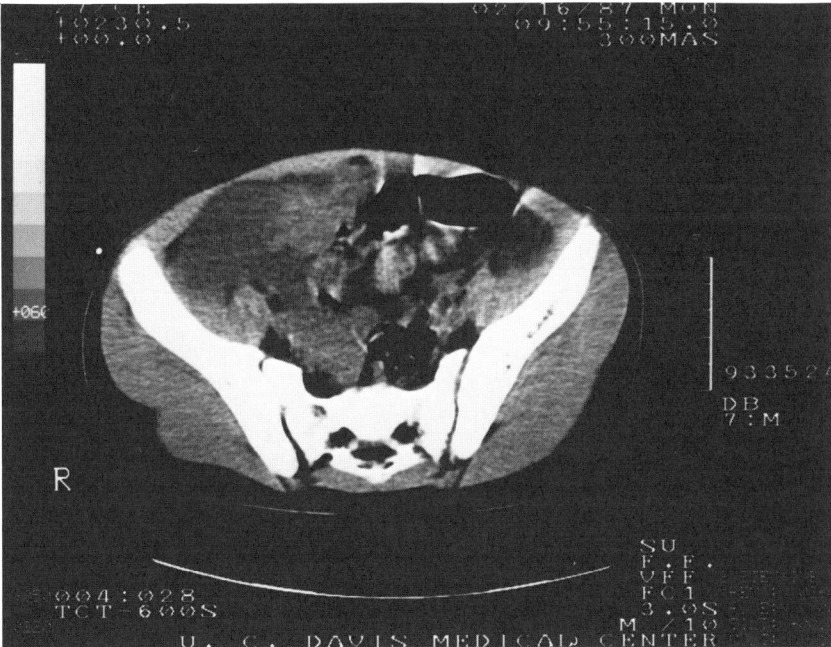

Figure 3–6. A CT scan obtained approximately 24 hr after admission in a 7-year-old boy involved in a pedestrian versus motor vehicle accident. There is a large amount of blood in the pelvis on this cut of the scan. CT scanning also revealed a ruptured spleen and a perinephric hematoma. A hemisplenectomy was performed at laparotomy.

negative or equivocal (Fig. 3–12). Pelvic and acetabular fractures not always obvious on standard x-ray views will sometimes show up on CT (Fig. 3–13).

Results

As with any radiographic examination, interpretation of abdominal CT scans after trauma is critically dependent on the level of expertise of the interpreter. False negative rates as low as 1.6% and false positive rates as low as 3.2% have been reported at centers where expert interpretation is available around the clock.[62] At centers where afterhours interpretation falls to less experienced radiologic personnel and surgeons, accuracy of interpretation decreases appreciably.[58,59] Certain injuries, such as ruptured bowel and isolated pancreatic injuries, can be difficult to diagnose with CT scanning even for experienced readers, particularly when the scan is done shortly after the time of injury. Bowel rupture is manifested on CT by the presence of intraperitoneal fluid and scanning done before significant amounts of fluid have leaked out into the peritoneal cavity will be negative (Fig. 3–5). Similarly, fractures across the body of the pancreas due to compression against the vertebral column may be associated with minimal bleeding and may be difficult to diagnose until a vigorous inflammatory response to leaking pancreatic fluid has occurred.

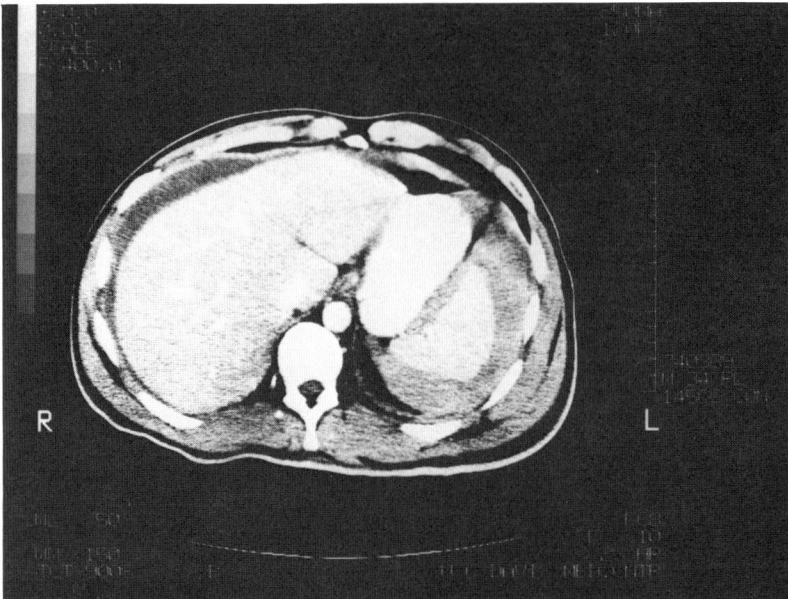

Figure 3–7. Ruptured spleen diagnosed by CT in 34-year-old man after a fall down some stairs. The patient was hemodynamically stable and the scan was performed several hours after admission. Note the perihepatic and perisplenic blood collections. The patient underwent splenectomy.

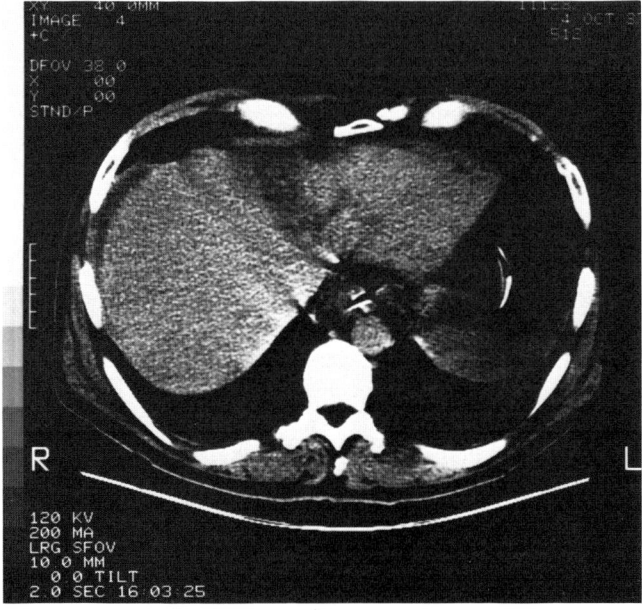

Figure 3–8. A CT scan demonstrating a large liver laceration and hemoperitoneum in a 55-year-old man after a motor vehicle accident. The scan also demonstrates pneumoperitoneum. The patient was found to have perforations of both the large and small bowel on exploration in addition to the liver laceration.

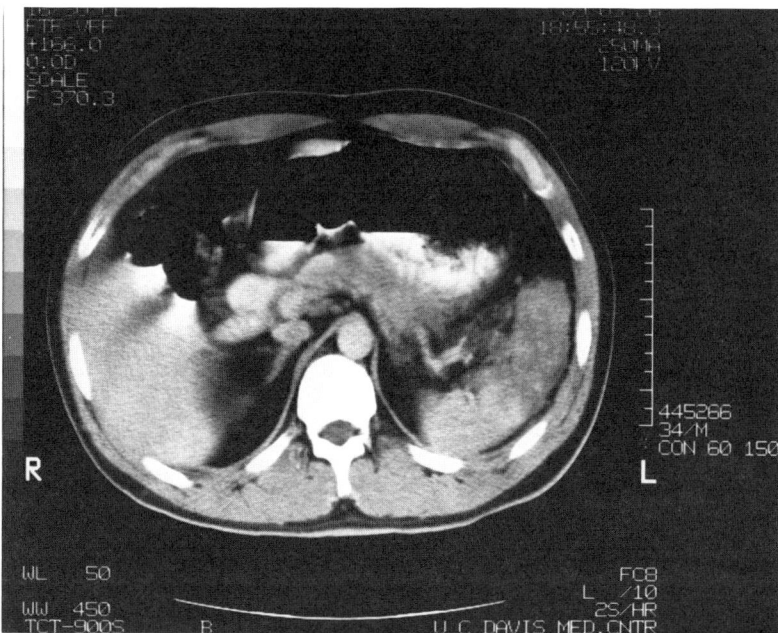

Figure 3–9. This scan demonstrates a ruptured spleen in a 34-year-old man sustained after a fall. The patient was explored and required splenectomy.

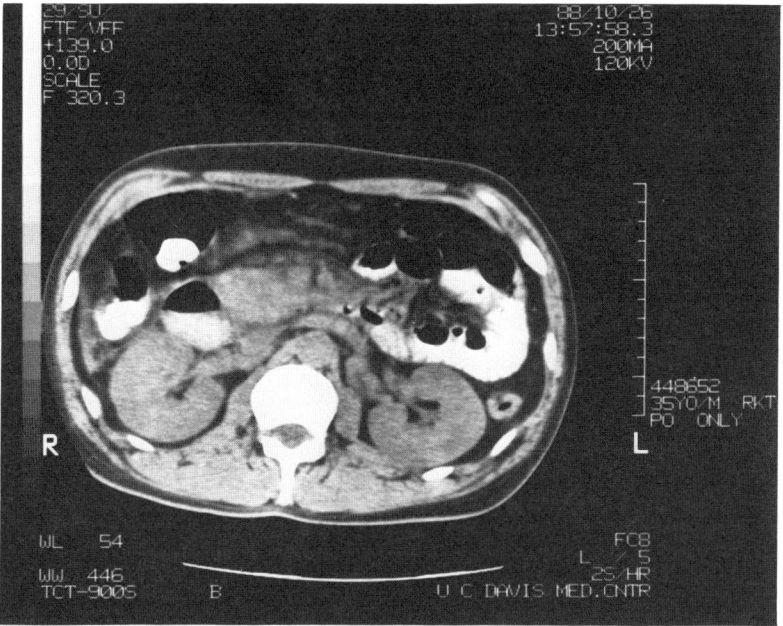

Figure 3–10. A contusion of the head of the pancreas in a 34-year-old man involved in a motor vehicle accident. The head of the pancreas is enlarged and indistinct in this scan done 7 hr after admission. The patient was explored and the head of the pancreas drained.

48 Abdominal Trauma

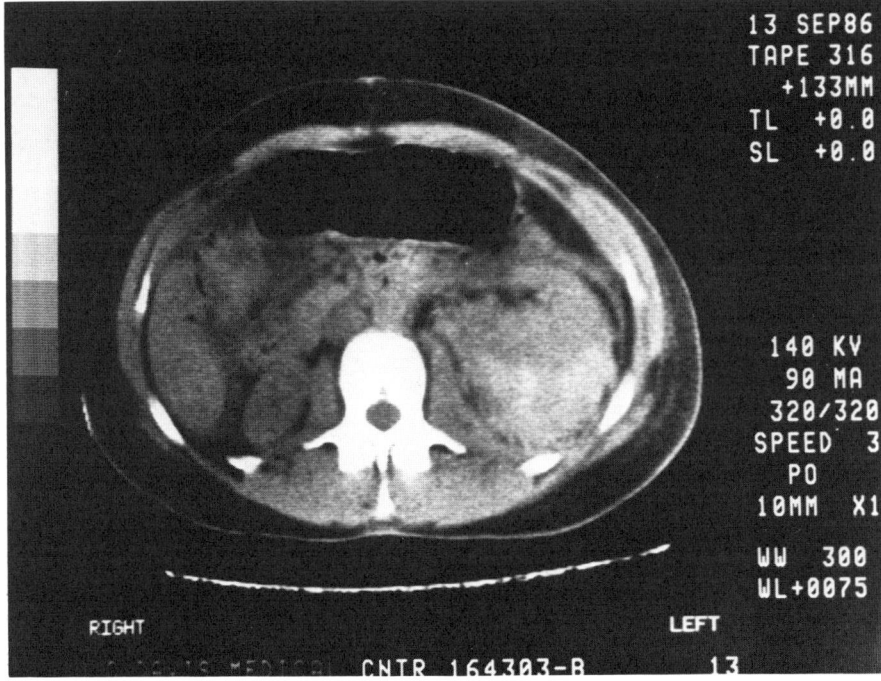

Figure 3–11. The left kidney is fractured in this scan of a 40-year-old woman injured in a motor vehicle accident. There is a large associated perinephric hematoma. The injury was treated conservatively.

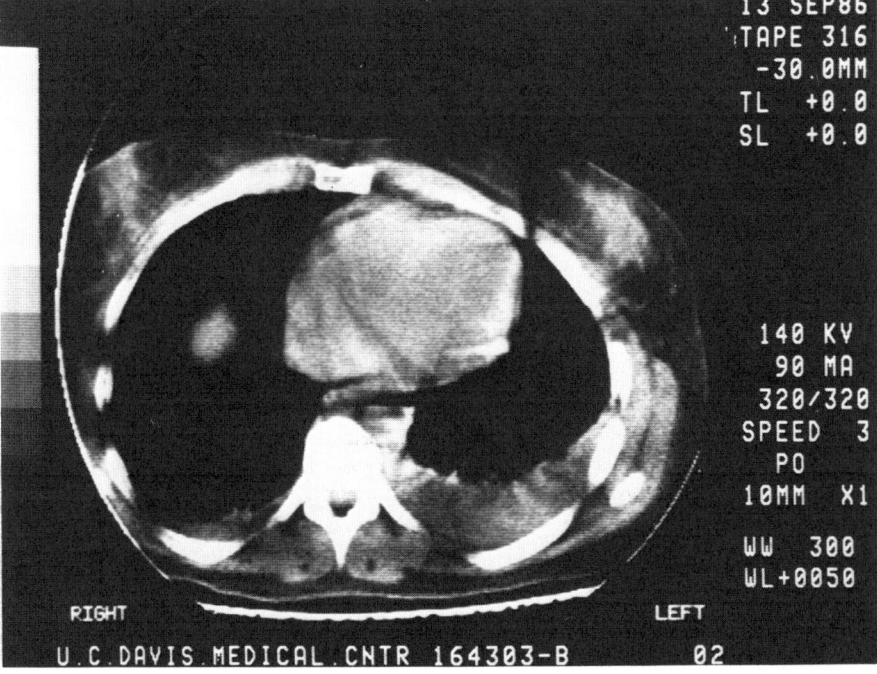

Figure 3–12. This scan revealed bilateral hemothoraces in a patient whose chest x-ray showed minimal evidence of intrathoracic fluid.

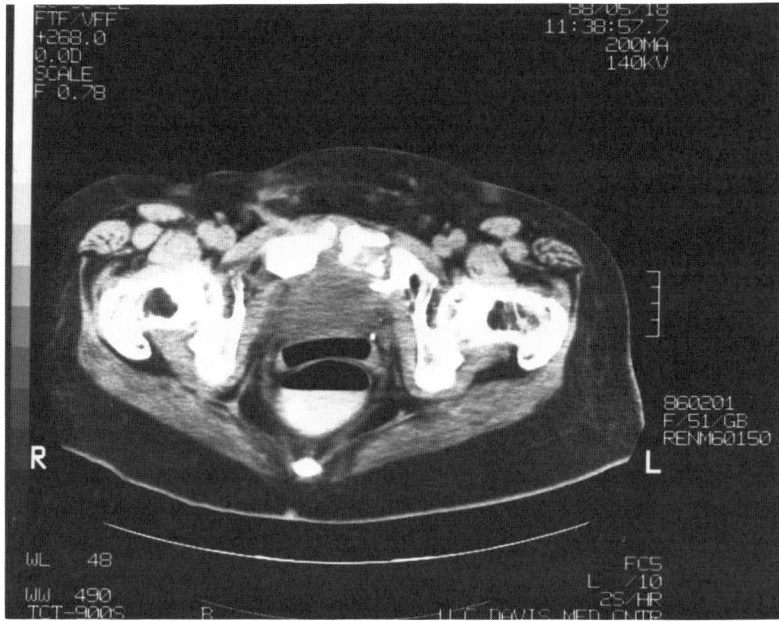

Figure 3–13. This 50-year-old woman was hit by a car. She complained of pelvic pain. An anteroposterior x-ray of the pelvis suggested a pelvic fracture. This was better delineated by a CT scan of the pelvis, which demonstrates bilateral pubic ramus fractures.

Peritoneal Lavage Versus Computerized Tomography

The relative roles of peritoneal lavage and CT in patients with blunt trauma are controversial. We believe the two tests are complementary and each is appropriate in certain circumstances. Peritoneal lavage can be performed rapidly in an emergency department setting and allows for quick triage of patients. This is particularly important in the setting of multiple simultaneous casualties and when hemodynamic stability is uncertain. It is also of great value in the determination of the sequence of tests to be used in patients with multiple blunt trauma. A common clinical scenario is the patient with closed head injury, associated orthopedic trauma, and a possible intraabdominal injury that cannot be ruled out by physical exam. A quick decision must be made as to whether the patient should undergo abdominal exploration or can safely be sent for CT of the head for the diagnosis of surgical intracranial lesions such as subdural, epidural, or intracerebral hematoma. Peritoneal lavage is useful in such instances to rule out gross hemoperitoneum before scanning of the head. If the patient demonstrates focal or lateralizing neurologic signs and the index of suspicion about an intracranial mass lesion is high, paracentesis alone will suffice. If paracentesis is negative for gross blood, the lavage catheter can be left in place and the lavage fluid run into the peritoneal cavity while the patient is being transported. Siphon removal and sampling of the fluid can be done at a convenient juncture during or after the head CT scan. Peritoneal lavage is also of value in patients being taken to the operating room for treatment of extraabdominal injuries. A negative lavage result at the beginning of surgery is reassuring during a prolonged anesthetic with significant intraoperative blood loss and puts the postoperative hematocrit into perspective.

CT is useful in hemodynamically stable patients in whom the index of suspicion for rapid intraabdominal bleeding is low. It is particularly useful when there are relative contraindications to peritoneal lavage such as multiple abdominal incisions or when scanning is required for associated injuries. CT is also of value in the work-up of patients being followed in the hospital in whom the hematocrit falls or there have been other changes in the clinical course that suggest the possibility of injury. Finally, CT is helpful for the diagnosis of intraabdominal abscess in the posttraumatic and postoperative periods (Fig. 3–14).

Both peritoneal lavage and CT are appropriate in certain circumstances. It should be emphasized again, however, that neither of these tests is a substitute for exploratory laparatomy in patients with hemodynamic instability or peritoneal signs on initial abdominal exam.

ANGIOGRAPHY

History

The idea of injecting contrast into blood vessels followed rapidly on the heels of the discovery of the diagnostic possibilities of x-rays. By 1910 Frank and Alwens had

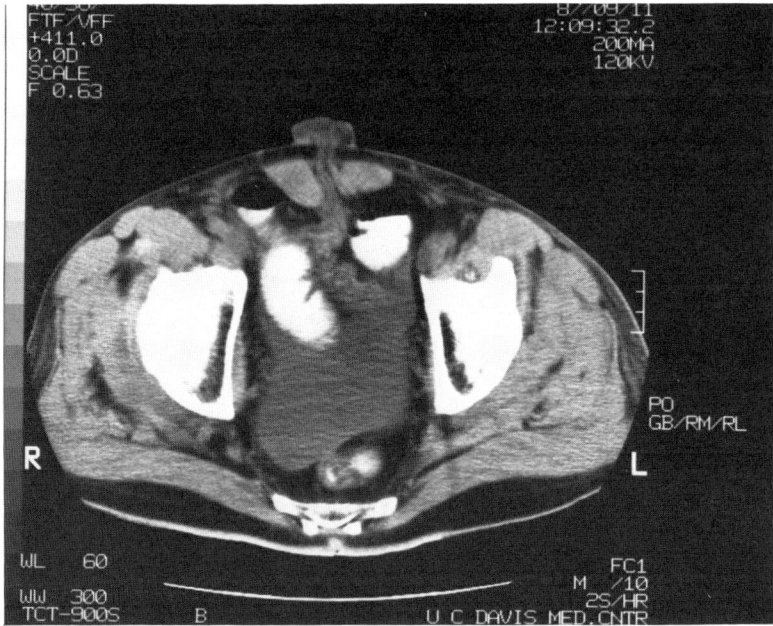

Figure 3–14. A large pelvic abscess demonstrated by CT in a 22-year-old man who had sustained a close-range gunshot wound of the abdomen 10 days earlier with multiple perforations of both the large and small bowel. The abscess was drained operatively.

successfully injected contrast into live animals.[63] These early attempts at angiography were hampered by the lack of a contrast agent with minimal toxicity when injected intraarterially. In the late 1920s, an organic, water-soluble, iodinated contrast agent synthesized originally as a therapeutic agent in the treatment of staphylococcal infections of the gall bladder was gradually modified for use in angiography.[64] A second and then a third iodine atom were added to the original contrast compound to improve radiodensity. Other modifications between 1930 and the 1950s further decreased toxicity.[65]

The development of improved angiographic techniques was coincident with improvements in contrast agents. Early angiography was generally done by direct injection of the vessel of interest, including injections of the carotid arteries and thoracic aorta.[66,67] More sophisticated angiographic equipment led to the increased use of catheter techniques for angiography culminating in the description of the Seldinger method of transfemoral catheter angiography in the early 1950s.[68] Not surprisingly, angiography was found to be of great usefulness in trauma and was applied increasingly to the work-up of injured patients. The advent and increased use of CT have led to a decreasing role for angiography after abdominal trauma but it is still useful in selected circumstances.

Indications

Angiography helps to characterize vascular anatomy in patients with known injuries to the liver or mesentery and defines anatomy before intervention. Suspected renovascular injuries suggested by a nonvisualizing or poorly visualizing kidney on intravenous pyelography may require angiography to rule out a renal pedicle injury (Fig. 3–15). CT is an alternative to angiography in such patients and provides information about the presence and function of the kidneys but does not give any detailed information about the renal vasculature.

Angiography plays a therapeutic role in the treatment of severe pelvic fractures with

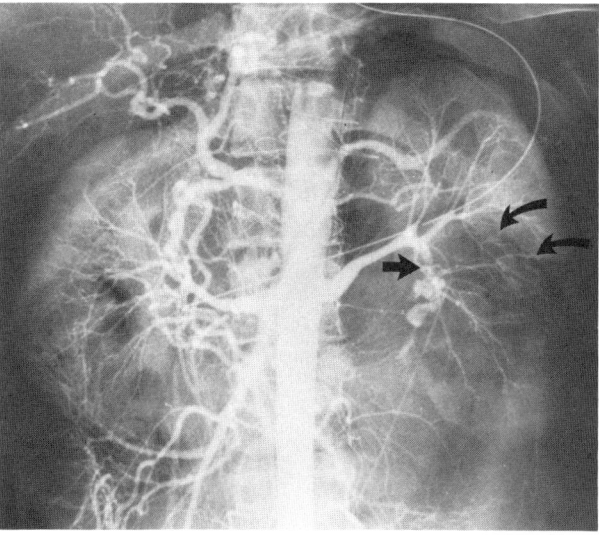

Figure 3–15. Renal fracture arteriogram. Lower pole of kidney fails to opacify (*curved arrows*). Artery to lower pole is avulsed and extravasates contrast material (*straight arrow*).

retroperitoneal bleeding.[69–72] In the vast majority of pelvic fractures, the retroperitoneal hematoma is self-limited and does not require angiographic intervention, particularly if early attention is paid to stabilization of the fracture fragments. In a very small minority, however, angiographic localization and embolization of arterial bleeding sites in the pelvis can be life-saving. Angiographic localization and embolization can also be used in the later posttraumatic period for the diagnosis and treatment of hemobilia. If there is suspicion about a tear or occlusion of the aorta or one of its major branches after blunt injury, angiography is indicated. Diagnosis of suspected aortic or visceral arterial injuries in stable patients with penetrating injuries to the back can be made angiographically. The delay and monitoring limitations outlined above for CT are also important in patients sent for an angiogram and angiography should not be done in patients with unstable hemodynamics or obvious peritoneal signs. In the occasional instance when a stable but potentially complex vascular injury is recognized at operation, (e.g., mesenteric or periaortic anteriovenous fistula) arteriography, either in the operating room or angiography suite, may facilitate identification of the anatomy of the injury.

ULTRASOUND

The use of ultrasonography in the initial diagnosis of patients with blunt abdominal trauma has been used most widely in Europe and its use to date has been limited in the United States, where CT has become the noninvasive diagnostic procedure of choice.[73–76] The

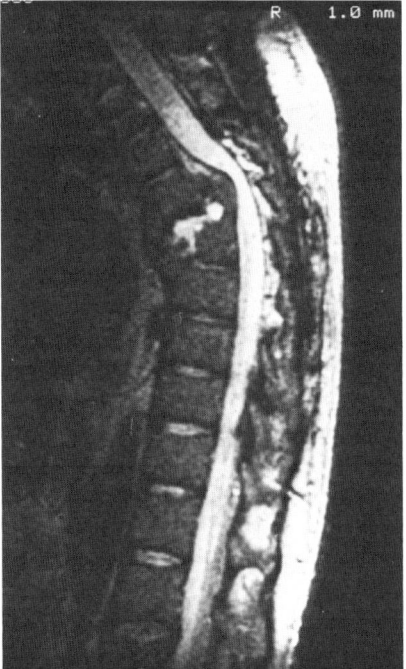

Figure 3–16. A magnetic resonance image of a severe thoracic spine fracture with angulation and loss of integrity of the vertebral column as well as compression of the spinal cord. MRI demonstrates the course of the spinal cord nicely without the use of any contrast agents.

advantages of ultrasound relative to paracentesis and peritoneal lavage are that it is noninvasive and provides at least a limited look at the intraabdominal anatomy. Advantages relative to CT are decreased cost and the ability to perform the test at the bedside in the emergency department.

Disadvantages of ultrasonography are its lack of sensitivity for subtle injuries or those not resulting in intraperitoneal fluid and its dependence on experienced personnel both for performance and interpretation. Standard sagittal and transverse views of the abdomen are obtained and can be interpreted either from the video screen or from a hard-copy image. Sensitivity rates for intraperitoneal fluid approach 90% in the largest series and it appears as though bedside examiners can achieve such rates with practice.[77-79] Parenchymal injuries to intraperitoneal organs are more difficult to diagnose and examination of the retroperitoneum is even more limited. Despite these limitations, ultrasonography in the emergency room is an attractive idea that merits more investigation and comparisons with the sensitivity and specificity rates for peritoneal lavage and CT. In addition, ultrasound may play a role in the future in the intraoperative evaluation of complex injuries to the liver and pancreas. Ultrasound techniques might also be applicable to the detection of subtle injuries of the vasculature before vessel thrombosis.

Ultrasonography can also be useful in the care of trauma patients in the intensive care phase of their hospital course. Ultrasonography is helpful in the diagnosis of both calculous and acalculous cholecystitis in critically ill patients and can also be used for a directed bedside search for intraabdominal abscess in unstable and ventilated patients in whom a trip to the CT scanner might prove dangerous.

MAGNETIC RESONANCE IMAGING

The use of magnetic resonance imaging (MRI) techniques is the latest application of new technology to the diagnosis of abdominal trauma. Its use to date in trauma patients has largely been limited to the diagnosis of neurologic and orthopedic injuries in stable patients (Fig. 3-16). Use in trauma, for the reasons outlined above for CT of the abdomen, should be limited to hemodynamically stable patients. A further logistical problem with MRI in acutely injured patients is the fact that metallic objects cannot be placed in the vicinity of the MRI machine because of the powerful magnetic field needed to create nuclear magnetic resonance. This complicates the study of ventilated patients, those with complex monitoring devices, and those with external fixator devices. Motion artifacts also make application of MRI to the study of torso trauma difficult. Although not yet widely applied to the study of patients with abdominal trauma, the increasing availability of MRI and increasing familiarity with its interpretation will almost certainly lead to its increasing use. It remains to be seen, however, if the images obtained with MRI will be sufficiently superior to those obtained with CT to justify its increased expense and the development of solutions to the logistical problems described above.

REFERENCES

1. Garrison FH. *History of Medicine*. Philadelphia: WB Saunders; 1929.
2. Saloman H. Diagnostiche puncktion des bauches. *Berl Klin Wchnschr*. 1906; 43:45.

3. Neuhof H, Cohen I. Abdominal puncture in the diagnosis of acute intraperitoneal disease. *Ann Surg.* 1926; 83:454–462.
4. Parvin S, Smith DE, Asher WM, Virgilio RW. Effectiveness of peritoneal lavage in blunt abdominal trauma. *Ann Surg.* 1972; 181:255–261.
5. Ciacobine JW, Siler VE. Evaluation of diagnostic abdominal paracentesis with experimental and clinical studies. *Surg Gynecol Obstet.* 1960; 110:676–686.
6. Root HD, Hauser CW, McKinely CR, LaFave JW, Mendiola RP. Diagnostic peritoneal lavage. *Surgery.* 1965; 57:633–637.
7. Bivins BA, Jona JZ, Belin RP. Diagnostic peritoneal lavage in pediatric trauma. *J Trauma* 1976; 16:739–742.
8. Caffee HH, Benfield JR. Is peritoneal lavage for the diagnosis of hemoperitoneum safe? *Arch Surg.* 1971; 103:4–7.
9. Engrav LH, Benjamin CI, Strate RG, Perry JF Jr. Diagnostic peritoneal lavage in blunt abdominal trauma. *J Trauma.* 1975; 15:854–859.
10. Olsen WR, Hildreth DH. Abdominal paracentesis and peritoneal lavage in blunt abdominal trauma. *J Trauma.* 1971; 11:824–829.
11. Olsen WR, Redman HC, Hildreth DH. Quantitative peritoneal lavage in blunt abdominal trauma. *Arch Surg.* 1972; 104:536–543.
12. Pacey J, Forward AD, Preto AF. Peritoneal tap and lavage in patients with blunt abdominal trauma: their contribution to surgical decisions. *CMAJ.* 1971; 105:365–370.
13. Perry JF Jr, Strate RG. Diagnostic peritoneal lavage in blunt abdominal trauma: indications and results. *Surgery.* 1972; 71:898–901.
14. Feliciano DV, Bitondo CG, Steed G, Mattox KL, Burch JM, Jordan GL Jr. Five hundred open taps or lavages in patients with abdominal stab wounds. *Am J Surg.* 1984; 148:772–777.
15. Oreskovich MR, Carrico CJ. Stab wounds of the anterior abdomen: analysis of a management plan using local wound exploration and quantitative peritoneal lavage. *Ann Surg.* 1983; 198(4):411–419.
16. Alyono D, Perry JF Jr. Significance of repeating diagnostic peritoneal lavage. *Surgery.* 1982; 91:656–659.
17. Shaftan GW. How we handle penetrating wounds of the abdomen. *Med Times.* 1976; 104:60–64.
18. Thompson JS, Moore EE, Van Duzer-Moore S, Moore JB, Galloway AC. The evolution of abdominal stab wound management. *J Trauma.* 1980; 20:178–184.
19. Jones TJ, Walsh JW, Maull KI. Diagnostic imaging in blunt trauma of the abdomen. *Surg Gynecol Obstet.* 1983; 157:389–398.
20. Ahmad W, Polk HC. Blunt abdominal trauma: a study of the relation between diagnosis and outcome. *South Med J.* 1973; 66:1127–1131.
21. Baker RJ. Newer techniques in evaluation of injured patients. *Surg Clin North Am.* 1975; 55:31–42.
22. Danto LA, Thomas CW, Gornbein S, Wolfman EF Jr. Penetrating torso injuries: the role of paracentesis and lavage. *Am Surg.* 1977; 43:164–170.
23. Davis JJ, Cohn I Jr, Nance FC. Diagnosis and management of blunt abdominal trauma. *Ann Surg.* 1976; 183: 672–678.
24. Fischer RP, Beverlin BC, Engrav LH, Benjamin CI, Perry JF Jr. Diagnostic peritoneal lavage: fourteen years and 2586 patients later. *Am J Surg.* 1978; 136:701–704.
25. Rothenberger DA, Quattlebaum FW, Zabel J, Fischer RP. Diagnostic peritoneal lavage for blunt trauma in pregnant women. *Am J Obstet.* 1977; 129:479–481.
26. Perry JF Jr. A five-year survey of 152 acute abdominal injuries. *J Trauma.* 1965; 5:53–61.
27. Shaftan GW. Indications for operation in abdominal trauma. *Am J Surg.* 1960; 99:657–664.
28. Thal ER. Evaluations of peritoneal lavage and local exploration in lower chest and abdominal stab wounds. *J Trauma.* 1977; 17:642–648.
29. Williams RD, Zollinger RM. Diagnosis and prognostic factors in abdominal trauma. *Am J Surg.* 1959; 97: 575–581.
30. Perry JF. A five-year survey of 152 acute abdominal injuries. *J Trauma.* 1965; 5:53–61.
31. Foley RW, Harris LS, Pilcher DB. Abdominal injuries in automobile accidents; review of care of fatally injured patients. *J Trauma.* 1977; 17:611–615.
32. Ben-Menachem Y, Fisher RG, Ward RE. Are "occult" intra-abdominal and extraperitoneal injuries really occult? *Radiol Clin North Am.* 1981; 19:125–140.
33. Drew R, Perry JF Jr, Fischer RP. The expediency of peritoneal lavage for blunt abdominal trauma in children. *Surg Gynecol Obstet.* 1977; 145;855–888.
34. Powell RW, Smith DE, Zarins CK, Parvin S, Virgilio RW. Peritoneal lavage in children with blunt abdominal trauma. *J Pediatr Surg.* 1976; 11:973–977.
35. Sachatello CR, Bivins B. Technic for peritoneal dialysis and diagnostic peritoneal lavage. *Am J Surg.* 1976; 131:637–640.
36. Stephens GL, Amis RE. Polyethylene tube technique of diagnostic paracentesis. *J Trauma.* 1965; 5:805–811.
37. Veith FJ, Webber WB, Karl RC, Deysine M. Peritoneal lavage in acute abdominal disease: normal findings and evaluation in 100 patients. *Am Surg.* 1967; 166:290–295.

38. Olsen WR. The serum amylase in blunt abdominal trauma. *J Trauma.* 1973; 13(3):200–204.
39. Gomez GA, Alvarez R, Plasencia G, et al. Diagnostic peritoneal lavage in the management of blunt abdominal trauma: a reassessment. *J Trauma.* 1987; 27(1):1–5.
40. Soderstrom CA, DuPriest RW, Cowley RA. Pitfalls of peritoneal lavage in blunt abdominal trauma. *Surg Gynecol Obstet.* 1980; 151:513–518.
41. Thal ER, Shires GT. Peritoneal lavage in blunt abdominal trauma. *Am J Surg.* 1973; 125:64–69.
42. Bivins BA, Sachatello CR, Daugherty ME, Ernst CB, Griffin WO Jr. Diagnostic peritoneal lavage is superior to clinical evaluation in blunt abdominal trauma. *Am Surg.* 1978; 44:637–641.
43. DuPriest RW Jr, Rodriguez A, Khaneja SC, et al. Open diagnostic peritoneal lavage in blunt trauma victims. *Surg Gynecol Obstet.* 1979; 148:890–894.
44. Gumbert JL, Froderman SE, Mercho JP. Diagnostic peritoneal lavage in blunt abdominal trauma. *Ann Surg.* 1967; 165:70–72.
45. Jacob ET, Cantor E. Discriminate diagnostic peritoneal lavage in blunt abdominal injuries: accuracy and hazards. *Am Surg.* 1979; 45:11–14.
46. Jahadi MR. Diagnostic peritoneal lavage. *J Trauma.* 1972; 12:936–938.
47. McAlvanah MJ, Shaftan GW. Selective conservatism in penetrating abdominal wounds: a continuing reappraisal. *J Trauma.* 1978; 18:206–212.
48. Sloop RD. The dominant role of paracentesis technics in the early diagnosis of blunt abdominal trauma. *Am J Surg.* 1978; 136:145–150.
49. Brotman S, Clayton HS, Cowley RA. False negative peritoneal lavage. *Am Surg.* 1981; 47:309–310.
50. Freeman T, Fischer RP. The inadequacy of peritoneal in diagnosing acute diaphragmatic rupture. *J Trauma.* 1976; 16:538–542.
51. Beal SL, McKennan M. Blunt diaphragm rupture: a morbid injury. *Arch Surg.* 1988; 123:828–832.
52. Hornyak SW, Shaftan GW. Value of "inconclusive lavage" in abdominal trauma management. *J Trauma.* 1979; 19:329–333.
53. Federle MP, Goldberg HI, Kaiser JA, et al. Evaluation of abdominal trauma by computed tomography. *Radiology.* 1981; 138:637.
54. Federle MP. Computed tomography of blunt abdominal trauma. *Radiol Clin North Am.* 1983; 21:461.
55. Federle MP, Crass RA, Jeffrey RB, Trunkey DD. Computed tomography in blunt abdominal trauma. *Arch Surg.* 1982; 117:745.
56. Fabian TC, Mangiante EC, White TJ, Patterson CR, Boldreghini S, Britt LG. A prospective study of 91 patients undergoing both computed tomography and peritoneal lavage following blunt abdominal trauma. *J Trauma.* 1986; 26:602–608.
57. Marx J, Moore EE, Jorden RC, Eule JE Jr. Limitations of computed tomography in the evaluation of acute abdominal trauma: a prospective comparison with diagnostic peritoneal lavage. *J Trauma.* 1985; 25:933–937.
58. Pagliarello G, Hanna SS, Gregory WD, et al. Abdominopelvic computerized tomography and open peritoneal lavage in patients with blunt abdominal trauma: a prospective study. *Can J Surg.* 1987; 30:10–13.
59. Frame SB, Browder IW, Lang EK, McSwain NE. Computed tomography versus diagnostic peritoneal lavage: usefulness in immediate diagnosis of blunt abdominal trauma. *Ann Emerg Med.* 1989; 18:513–516.
60. Davis RA, Shayne JP, Max MH, Woolfitt RA, Schwab W. The use of computerized axial tomography versus peritoneal lavage in the evaluation of blunt trauma: a prospective study. *Surgery.* 1985; 98:845–849.
61. Federle MP, Jeffrey RB. Body computed tomography: hemoperitoneum studied by computed tomography. *Radiology.* 1983; 148:187–192.
62. Wing VW, Federle MP, Morris JA Jr, Jeffrey RB, Bluth R. The clinical impact of CT for blunt abdominal trauma. *Am J Roentgen Ray.* 1985; 145:1191–1194.
63. Franck O, Alwens W. Kreislaufstudien am Röntgenschirm. *Münch Med Wochenschr.* 1910; 57:1950.
64. Binz A, Räth C, von Lichtenberg A. Die Wiedergabe von Nieren und Harnwegen in Röntgenbilde durch Jodpyridonderivate. *Angewandte Chem.* 1930; 43:452.
65. McAfee J. A survey of complications of abdominal aortography. *Radiology.* 1957; 68:825.
66. Moniz E. L'encéphalographic artérielle, son importance dans la localisation des tumeurs cérébrales. *Rev Neurol.* 1927; 2:72.
67. Nuvoli L. Arteriografia dell'aorta toracica mediante punture dell'aorta ascendente o del ventriculos. *Policlinico (Prat.).* 1936; 43:227.
68. Seldinger S. Catheter replacement of the needle in percutaneous arteriography. *Acta Radiol.* 1953: 39:368.
69. Ward RE, Miller P, Clark DG, Benmenachem Y, Duke JH. Angiography and peritoneal lavage in blunt abdominal trauma. *J Trauma.* 1981; 21:848–853.
70. Mucha P Jr, Welch TJ. Hemorrhage in major pelvic fracturees. *Surg Clin North Am.* 1988; 68:757–773.
71. Ward RE, Clark DG. Management of pelvic fractures. *Radiol Clin North Am.* 1981; 19:167–170.
72. Casarella WJ, Martin EC. Angiography in the management of abdominal trauma. *Semin Roentgenol.* 1984; 19:321–327.

73. Weill F. Real-time ultrasonography in emergencies. In: *Real-time Ultrasonography. Clinics in Diagnostic Ultrasound*. New York: Churchill Livingstone; 1982; 10:95–116.
74. Ferrucci JT. Body ultrasonography (second of two parts). *N Engl J Med*. 1979; 300:590–602.
75. Asher WM, Parvin S, Virgilio RW, Haber K. Echographic evaluation of splenic injury after blunt trauma. *Radiology*. 1975; 118:411–415.
76. Viscomi GN, Gonzalez R, Taylor KJ, Crade M. Ultrasonic evaluation of hepatic and splenic trauma. *Arch Surg*. 1980; 115:320–321.
77. Vallon AG, Lees WR, Cotton PB. Grey-scale ultrasonography and endoscopic pancreatography after pancreatic trauma. *Br J Surg*. 1979; 66:169–172.
78. Tiling T, Bouillon B, Schweins M, Steffens H. Ultrasound in blunt abdominal trauma—10 years' experience from a prospective trial. *J Trauma*. In press.
79. Jarowenko DG, Hess RM, Herr RM, Herr MS, Young WW, Beyer FC. Use of ultrasonography in the evaluation of blunt abdominal trauma. *J Trauma*. In press.

4
Indications for and General Conduct of the Operation

DAVID H. WISNER, M.D.

HISTORY: Interest in abdominal trauma, like the treatment of a number of different types of injuries, centered initially around the treatment of battlefield wounds. Matthaeus Gottfried Purman, a surgeon of the Brandenburg Army in 1675, acquired great skill and courage in performing operations in the field and is credited with first suturing wounds of the intestine.[16] His aggressive treatment of abdominal wounds was exceptional for his time, however, and most cases were treated with expectant management. The rationale for this approach was that aggressive operative intervention was associated with a high morbidity and mortality. During the American Civil War (1861–1865), treatment of wounds to the abdomen was generally expectant unless injured bowel had eviscerated and was thus easily available for repair.[3] In 1881, the great American surgeon James Marion Sims published "The Careful Aseptic Invasion of the Peritoneal Cavity for the Arrest of Hemorrhage, the Suture of Intestinal Wounds and the Cleansing of the Peritoneal Cavity" in which he espoused exploration of the abdomen in some cases of abdominal trauma.[39] It is an indication of how little had changed between the time of Purman and the time of Sims that the merits of expectant versus operative intervention were still the subject of lively debate. James Garfield, who had been inaugurated as President only months earlier, was shot in the abdomen in an assassination attempt while entering a railroad station in Washington, D.C., in July 1881, a year after the publication of Sims' book. Garfield was treated nonoperatively and died several months later of abdominal sepsis.

By the late 1880s and early 1890s there was increasing sentiment for operative management of abdominal trauma. At the 1899 meeting of the Southern Surgical Association, H.H. Grant of Louisville made a strong case for operative intervention and chided the timidity of those of his colleagues who still advocated expectant management: ". . . it is clear that to delay, in a delusive hope, until peritonitis shows its folly is almost a crime. The practical [operative] management of a suspected penetrating wound is as plain a duty as the tying of a bleeding artery."[17]

A sometimes polemic and vituperative debate over operative versus expectant management continued through the first World War, although the weight of opinion gradually swung toward operative intervention.[2,22,29] It is of interest that this gradual swing in opinion toward more aggressive management was led by civilian surgeons and was made over the strenuous objections of the military surgeons of the day, many of the most famous of whom still favored expectant management. Perhaps this was because wartime injuries were more serious in nature and generally not amenable to operative treatment given the anesthetic, surgical, and postoperative capabilities available at the time, particularly in a wartime setting. This contrasted with the less severe injuries and superior facilities seen in a civilian practice.

By World War II the general principles of the treatment of abdominal injury had evolved essentially to those of the present.[42] Blood transfusion became available, principles of management of colonic injuries developed, and small bowel injuries underwent primary repair. Antibiotics became available by the end of the conflict. Progress in abdominal injury management came as a result of more rapid transport, better resuscitation from shock, and earlier definitive care.[18]

Although the weight of opinion since the early part of this century has favored operative intervention in abdominal trauma, there is still controversy about the management of certain kinds of injury. This controversy is most vigorous with respect to stab wounds to the abdomen and the management of blunt abdominal trauma.[29,30] Controversies also exist with respect to the management of colonic injuries, the management of injuries to major blood vessels in the abdomen, and the merits of splenic salvage.

INDICATIONS FOR OPERATION

Penetrating Trauma

Decisions regarding management of penetrating trauma of the chest and abdomen are easier than those for blunt trauma. The injury is often obvious and it is easier to predict possible underlying visceral injuries with penetrating than with blunt trauma.

Because the major volume of the abdominal cavity is filled with hollow viscera, penetrating trauma is statistically most likely to produce an injury to these organs (Table 4–1). Assessment of the possibility of hollow viscus injury involves an evaluation for peritoneal or retroperitoneal contamination. The full bowel, when injured, readily evacuates into the peritoneal cavity and signs of injury are usually obvious. When the bowel is empty, however, or when the site of penetration is in the retroperitoneum, early egress of bowel contents may be negligible. Initial findings may therefore be minimal. These injuries will manifest themselves with increasing abdominal tenderness and this finding therefore demands exploration. An elevated white blood cell count or fever appearing several hours after the injury are also clues to the presence of injury. These findings take on added significance in penetrating abdominal trauma patients with altered mental status or associated head injury because of the inability to assess the presence and degree of abdominal tenderness.

Table 4–1 Penetrating Trauma (Relative Incidence of Organ Injury) Collected Series

ORGAN	PERCENTAGE
Small bowel	30
Mesentery and omentum	18
Liver	16
Colon	9
Diaphragm	8
Stomach	7
Spleen	6
Kidney	5
Major vascular	4
Pancreas	3
Duodenum	2
Bladder	1
Ureter	1
Biliary	1

The likelihood of a major vascular injury is far higher with penetrating as opposed to blunt abdominal injury in those patients who survive to reach the hospital. If a patient presents in shock a short time after the injury, the probability of a major vascular injury should be assumed and appropriate resuscitation initiated. Unless an obvious extraabdominal source of blood loss exists, immediate abdominal exploration is indicated.

Although there is controversy regarding treatment of penetrating injuries to the abdomen, we believe in the general principle that most penetrating trauma should be explored immediately.[6,32,41] When a hollow viscus has been injured, delay in treatment results in progression of intraperitoneal or retroperitoneal contamination to the point of invasive infection and a high incidence of septic complications.[6,14] When compared to the minimal risks of morbidity associated with abdominal exploration done through an upper midline incision, the risks of delayed diagnosis and missed injuries take on increased importance.[32,43]

All gunshot wounds that penetrate the lower chest or the abdominal wall should be explored without inordinate delay. The incidence of major intraabdominal injury exceeds 90% in almost all series.[13]

Patients with abdominal stab wounds or stab wounds of the chest wall at or below the level of the sixth intercostal space should undergo immediate laparotomy if there is any clinical evidence of intraabdominal injury such as otherwise unexplained hypotension or peritonitis. In the absence of such findings, we advocate a policy of "selective mandatory exploration" for stab wounds. The abdominal wall is divided into anterior and posterior portions, with the dividing line located in the posterior axillary line. We have found that 90% of stab wounds to the abdomen anterior to the posterior axillary line that have penetrated fascia have also violated the peritoneal cavity.[6,32] If there is any question of the depth of the injury, the wound should be explored under local anesthesia in the emergency room. Demonstrated fascial penetration or an inability to determine definitively the absence of fascial penetration are, in general, indications for abdominal exploration. It can be particularly difficult to determine whether or not the fascia has been penetrated in obese patients and those with large hematomas of the abdominal wall. Certain stiletto type wounds and other wounds of minimal width in the absence of any physical findings may be observed. Since we have found that wounds posterior to the posterior axillary line have a lower incidence of peritoneal penetration, injuries to the back and flank may be observed expectantly if no physical, laboratory, or x-ray findings are present that might suggest intraabdominal injury. The abdominal wall and lower intercostal spaces between the anterior axillary line and the posterior axillary line constitute a "gray zone" between the anterior abdominal wall and the back, and stab wounds to this area can be selectively managed. However, because retroperitoneal colonic injury is possible, laparotomy is used liberally in such injuries in the presence of abdominal findings. The use of serial determinations of the white blood cell count is also of importance in these patients.

This policy of abdominal trauma management was subjected to review.[6] Of 757 patients who underwent exploratory laparotomy for blunt and penetrating abdominal trauma, only 12 of 159 patients with gunshot wounds of the abdomen did not have a major visceral injury. The bullet did not penetrate the peritoneal cavity in most of these patients because penetration of the peritoneal cavity by a gunshot wound necessitated repair or drainage of an abdominal viscus in 99.3% of cases. This reconfirmed our belief that all patients with gunshot wounds suspected of entering the peritoneal cavity should be treated by mandatory laparotomy; this agrees with other large series.[13,14,45]

Of the 367 patients with stab wounds of the abdomen, 106 (30%) had insignificant or absent intraabdominal injury.[6] The main determinant of the need for laparotomy in the patients with negative findings at exploration had been possible peritoneal penetration. Signs of peritoneal irritation were present in 38 patients or 40% of those who had a negative exploration. However, in 21 of these there had been no peritoneal penetration. Eighteen patients in this group with negative findings had laparotomy based on clinical suspicion of penetration alone in the absence of clinical, laboratory, or x-ray abnormalities.

Nineteen complications occurred in the 118 patients whose laparotomy was negative after penetrating trauma from gunshot wounds and stab wounds.[32] Most of the complications were minor and did not prolong hospitalization; the mean hospital stay was 6 days. Hospitalization was prolonged in two patients who had serious complications. One patient had a pulmonary embolus and remained in the hospital for 14 days. The other patient developed a wound infection and was hospitalized on two occasions for a total of 28 days. The remainder of the complications were atelectasis and minor wound infections and did not result in prolongation of the hospitalization. There were no deaths in this group with negative findings at laparotomy. Thus, we believe that a policy of exploration of stab wounds is appropriate. The rate of 20% for negative findings at laparotomy is considered acceptable for another potentially lethal illness, appendicitis, and we believe that the potential lethality and much of the morbidity of penetrating wounds is reduced to a bare minimum by this policy of prompt exploration. Retroperitoneal and diaphragmatic injuries, for example, are frequently asymptomatic and peritoneal lavage and computerized tomography (CT) are often negative in this group as well.[25,37,40] Not only can immediate complications occur from diaphragm injuries (Fig. 4–1), but delayed complications can and do result and compromise the patient years later.[24] Although the production of adhesions that can result in the delayed complication of bowel obstruction can theoretically occur after a negative exploration, this has been most unusual in our experience; only one such patient has been encountered during the period of review for this series. In a large review of patients who had undergone negative laparotomy for trauma, the overall

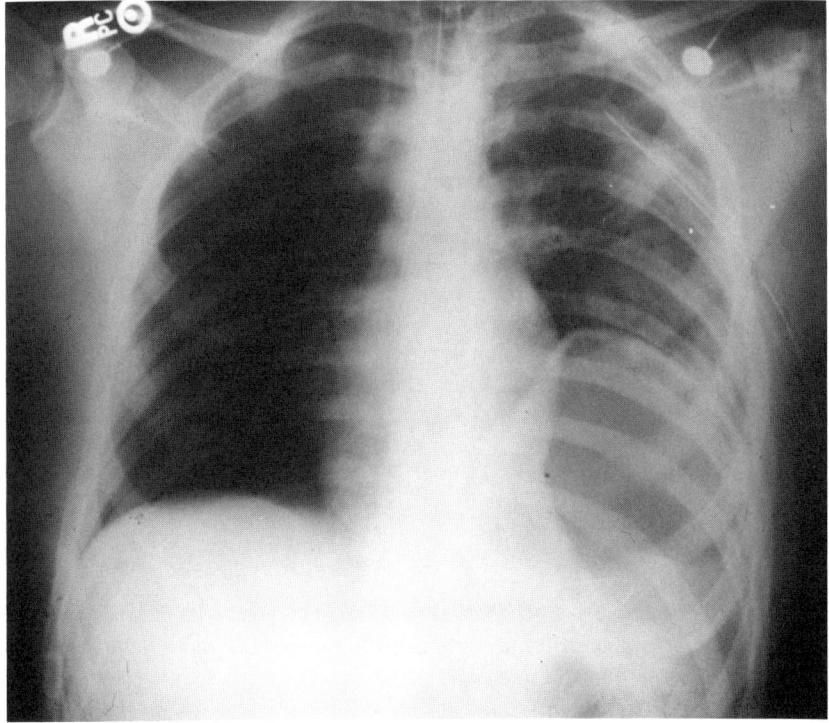

Figure 4–1. Diaphragm injury unrecognized until major gastric herniation developed.

incidence of subsequent bowel obstruction was 3% and was only 2% in patients in whom only operative inspection of the abdominal cavity was needed to rule out intraabdominal injury.[43]

Blunt Abdominal Trauma

These injuries are more subtle than penetrating trauma. The degree of injury is difficult to establish and findings even with serious injury may be minimal. In addition, patients with blunt abdominal injury are more likely than penetrating trauma patients to have altered mental status from closed head injury.

In blunt trauma, the organs most likely to be injured are solid organs such as the liver, spleen, kidney, pancreas, and mesentery (Table 4–2). Hollow viscera are less commonly injured, and the diagnosis of hollow viscus injury is not particularly difficult, especially in the conscious patient. The reason for this relates to the fact that an empty hollow viscus is relatively hard to injure. The most common hollow viscus injury is to the small bowel and is probably due either to compression of the bowel between the abdominal wall anteriorly and the vertebral column posteriorly with a resultant blow-out injury or a traction injury with disruption of the bowel mesentery and devascularization.[1] Colon is ruptured or devascularized less commonly. In the conscious patient, these injuries are almost always

Table 4-2 Blunt Trauma (Relative Incidence of Organ Injury)
Collected Series

ORGAN	PERCENTAGE
Spleen	25
Liver	15
Retroperitoneal hematoma	13
Kidney	12
Small bowel	9
Bladder	6
Mesentery	5
Large bowel	4
Pancreas	3
Urethra	2
Diaphragm	2
Vascular	2
Stomach	1
Duodenum	1

accompanied by obvious signs of peritoneal irritation. In patients with altered mental status, diagnostic peritoneal lavage is highly reliable.[10,45] Somewhat more subtle blunt bowel injuries that have increased in frequency with the use of seat belts are tears of the bowel serosa. The increased incidence of high speed motor vehicle trauma and the increased use of seat belts has increased the incidence of blunt mesenteric and bowel injuries to the point where they are now the third most commonly injured intraabdominal structures after the liver and spleen (Table 4-2).

The next most common hollow viscus to be injured is the full bladder, which when it ruptures through its weakest point at the dome leads to lower abdominal tenderness in association with gross hematuria. The bladder can also be injured directly by pelvic fractures. These injuries are generally lateral and retroperitoneal and will not lead to abdominal findings. This is of little consequence, however, as retroperitoneal bladder ruptures can usually be treated nonoperatively with bladder decompression via a urethral catheter.[8,9]

The stomach and duodenum are less commonly involved with blunt trauma.[21,38] Blunt gastric injuries require a great deal of force and generally are associated with multisystem injury and severe injuries to other intraabdominal organs. They behave similarly to small bowel injuries with respect to findings on physical exam and the reliability of peritoneal lavage. Duodenal injuries, because of the retroperitoneal location of the duodenum, are more subtle in their presentation and may be manifest only by minimal abdominal tenderness, progressive elevation of the serum amylase, or air in the retroperitoneum on an abdominal x-ray.

An injury that does not fit easily into either the blunt or hollow viscus group is blunt rupture of the diaphragm. These injuries are often but not always associated with an injury to the liver or spleen. The findings on chest x-ray can be subtle and these injuries are easily missed if there is not a high index of suspicion for them.[4]

Since a primary manifestation of solid organ injury is bleeding, the presence of unexplained blood loss is an indication for further investigation of the abdomen. Ordinarily, blood in the belly is irritating and intraperitoneal bleeding is associated with peritoneal signs. This produces a secondary ileus with overt abdominal distention. However, on occasion the blood is bland and minimal peritoneal irritation results. The reason for this is that blood in itself is not irritating. It is the clotting of blood that releases inflammatory enzymes that result in irritation. A fully anticoagulated patient will not develop peritoneal irritation. When bleeding is slow, all clotting and irritation is local so that the pain from a slow splenic or liver bleed may be ascribed to overlying rib fractures. The abdomen can accommodate most of the blood volume with a change in girth of only 4 to 5 cm. When blood in the abdominal cavity does not produce peritoneal irritation, there is little associated ileus and distention may not be particularly impressive, even though several liters of blood have been lost into the abdominal cavity.

Thus, an unexplained fall in the hematocrit, together with evidence of cardiovascular instability, means bleeding into the abdomen until proven otherwise. Unless some other source for the blood loss has been established, this is an indication for laparotomy. In patients with minimal abdominal findings who have been stable for several hours, a less aggressive approach using diagnostic peritoneal lavage or CT of the abdomen can be used.

ROLE OF "CONSERVATIVE (NONOPERATIVE) MANAGEMENT"

With the advent of peritoneal lavage and CT, the sensitivity of preoperative evaluation of blunt abdominal injuries has increased.[25] As an inevitable result, minor injuries such as small hepatic and splenic lacerations that were never diagnosed previously are now being identified. This has tended to support the concept that many significant injuries can be managed nonoperatively, particularly in the management of the resilient pediatric population where conservative treatment of splenic injuries has become policy even to the point of transfusing patients to maintain blood volume.[28,31,34,44]

Certainly there is no question that some minor injuries that are identified by lavage or CT can be managed nonoperatively. Indeed, they have often been managed nonoperatively in the past without knowledge of their presence. For this reason, in the awake responsive patient with injuries limited to the abdomen, clinical assessment should be the bottom line. In the absence of significant clinical findings and with stable hematocrit and white blood cell count values, operation is not indicated. On the other hand, increasing abdominal tenderness, a hematocrit that falls markedly without an obvious source of blood loss, and a white blood cell count that doubles are indications for exploration. The risk of laparotomy in a previously healthy trauma patient is negligible and the risk to the patient lies not only in the presumed primary pathology but also in the inability to rule out potentially lethal associated injuries such as those to the bowel or pancreas, which can and do occur in association with liver and splenic injuries. Moreover, the risk of transfusion, should it ultimately prove necessary for unchecked bleeding, exceeds that of laparotomy or postsplenectomy sepsis.[5,23] The fundamental surgical principle of obtaining hemostasis should not be abandoned.

The primary value of ancillary testing is to facilitate diagnosis in multiply injured patients or in those with altered mental status. Associated injuries, particularly when there is injury to the chest or pelvis, may render it difficult to assess the abdomen. In these circumstances, the hematocrit and white blood cell count are no longer reliable guides to the presence of intraabdominal injury and appropriately used peritoneal lavage or CT scanning provide valuable ancillary diagnostic information regarding the probable nature of injury and the need for abdominal surgery.[12,19,45]

PREOPERATIVE PREPARATION

A low threshold should be maintained for endotracheal intubation of trauma patients. Many trauma victims, because of intoxication or head injury, are unable to maintain a patent upper airway and protect themselves from aspiration. Loss of blood volume and red blood cells decreases oxygen delivery and it is important to ensure that the blood is maximally oxygenated. Head-injured patients, particularly those with mass lesions, benefit from hyperventilation. For these reasons, early intubation and positive pressure ventilation with 100% oxygen should be done in patients with abdominal injury if there is any doubt about hemodynamic stability or ability to protect the airway. This is especially true if the patient is to undergo abdominal exploration, since intubation will be necessary for the operative procedure anyway. In patients who are to undergo operation, liberal use of intubation in the emergency room should be followed. Intubation and the initiation of positive pressure ventilation is not without drawbacks, however. "Bucking" on the endotracheal tube can cause further increases in intracranial pressure in patients who already have intracranial hypertension. When blood volume is decreased, initiation of positive pressure ventilation leads to increased intrapleural pressure and further decreases an already compromised venous return. This can exacerbate hypotension. Similarly, the presence of pericardial blood and tamponade increases the pressure against which venous return must work to fill the heart. Initiation of positive pressure ventilation exacerbates the negative effects on venous return. Bleeding from injuries to the inferior vena cava or hepatic veins can also be exacerbated by positive pressure ventilation because of an increase in the back pressure in the venous system. The benefits of intubation and positive pressure ventilation outweigh the risks in patients with intracranial hypertension or those with hypovolemia. A similarly low intubation threshold should be used in unstable patients with suspected tamponade or caval/hepatic venous injuries because, once again, the benefits of intubation and positive pressure ventilation outweigh the risks. In stable patients with suspected tamponade or caval/hepatic venous injuries, the patient should be intubated if possible in the operating room after the surgeons are scrubbed and gowned and the patient has been prepped and draped in the event of a sudden hemodynamic decompensation from the initiation of positive pressure ventilation.

Preoperative antibiotics are useful adjuncts in the management of abdominal injuries.[11,15] This is particularly true for penetrating abdominal injuries where the likelihood of a bowel injury is high but it is also wise to give a preoperative dose of antibiotics to patients with blunt abdominal injury in case the bowel is found to be perforated or a bowel resection is necessary. Broad spectrum antibiotic coverage such as a second generation cephalosporin should be administered in the emergency room before operating room transfer or alternatively in the operating room. Antibiotics should be discontinued after no more than 24 hr unless major contamination was found, in which instance they should be used as therapeutic antibiotics and continued for 3 to 7 days.

Patients who require peritoneal lavage or laparotomy for blunt trauma will often have associated orthopedic injuries requiring treatment on a fracture table for optimal orthopedic exposure, manipulation, and radiography. The abdominal procedure should be done first on a regular operating table and the patient subsequently transferred to the fracture table. Although this approach means that the patient requires an additional transfer before the beginning of the orthopedic procedure, performance of an adequate laparotomy can prove extremely difficult when done on a fracture table. Options for extension of exposure into the chest are also limited.

When dealing with trauma, the possibility that any body cavity may be opened exists and that drains or chest tubes may be required at many sites. The patient should therefore be scrubbed and prepped with iodide paint from the clavicles to the groins and from table line to table line. This allows for sterile entry into the chest via either a sternotomy or a thoracotomy as well as exposure of the femoral vessels if necessary for distal control of the vasculature or arterial bypass. Draping should be done with similar considerations in mind.

CONDUCT OF THE OPERATION

For rapid access, wide exposure, and maximal flexibility, a midline abdominal incision is the incision of choice (Fig. 4–2). Only rarely will transverse or oblique incisions be appropriate for trauma. The midline incision allows for the best exposure of the entire abdomen and pelvis and can be easily and rapidly extended into the chest as either a sternotomy or thoracotomy. An upper midline approach is most appropriate for blunt trauma because this gains maximal exposure to the liver and spleen. Exposure of these organs, the spleen in particular, is facilitated by extending the upper margin of the incision as far as possible into the paraxiphoid area. If further exposure of the lower abdomen or pelvis proves to be necessary, the incision can be extended inferiorly as needed. If a peritoneal lavage has been done in the emergency room, this incision should be left open and the subcutaneous tissue prepped along with the rest of the abdomen to minimize the chance of subsequent wound infection. The upper midline incision should be extended inferiorly to include the lavage site. The fascial incision of the lavage site will therefore be subsequently included in the closure of the rest of the abdomen. This minimizes the chance of hernia formation at the lavage site.

For penetrating trauma, the incision should still be in the midline but should be located to maximize exposure to possible areas of injury. If peritoneal penetration is documented after entry into the abdomen, the incision should be large enough to allow for evisceration of the small bowel. In critically injured patients, a lengthy incision should be done at the outset to ensure maximal exposure.

In some instances, especially after blunt trauma, urgent neurosurgical or orthopedic intervention is necessary before there has been adequate time to rule out abdominal injury. In instances where the probability of abdominal injury is low either peritoneal lavage in the operating room or a "mini-laparotomy" can be used. The mini-laparotomy is a small incision in the upper midline made sufficiently long so that with the aid of sponge sticks and retractors the gastrohepatic area can be inspected for a central upper abdominal hematoma. The remainder of the procedure consists of aspirating all four quadrants of the abdomen. The absence of blood or fluid dictates closure. Although this procedure is sometimes useful, it does not allow for evisceration and inspection of the bowel. In obese patients, adequate visualization of the upper abdomen for a central hematoma can also prove difficult.

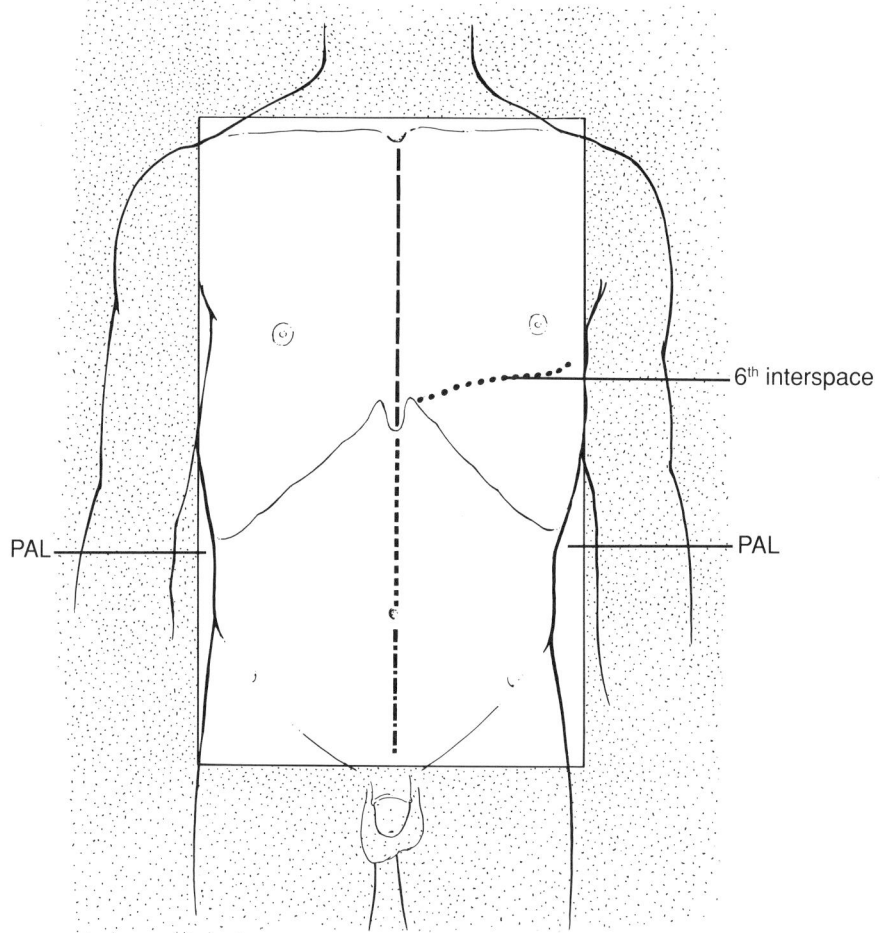

Figure 4–2. Standard trauma incision is indicated by (– –) line. It can be extended to the pubis (– · –), upward as a midline sternotomy (— —) or into the left or right chest (· · ·).

Upon entry into the abdomen, all four quadrants should be rapidly packed to control bleeding, especially if the patient is *in extremis*. During this packing, note should be taken of any obvious active bleeding and the location of any clot, which will tend to be located at sites of active bleeding, while defibrinated, nonclotting blood may be found throughout the peritoneal cavity. An abdomen filled with bright red blood is highly indicative of an arterial injury.

After packing, all four quadrants should be rapidly inspected for ongoing major hemorrhage. This can be done within a minute or two so that the major sources of hemorrhage can be identified and dealt with first. Minor injuries and sources of bleeding should not distract attention from dealing with major ongoing hemorrhage. Venous bleeding may not be obvious unless looked for since it is low pressure and is not as dramatic or as evident as arterial hemorrhage. Once all major sites of hemorrhage have been identified, they should be controlled. Almost all venous bleeding can be controlled by the judicious application of packs, which permits time for restoration of volume. This is also true of many arterial injuries and injuries of the liver. If the injury can be controlled by packing or direct pressure this should be done while intravascular volume is restored if the patient is hypovolemic. The reason for not entering the area of injury immediately and directly is that the vascular system may suddenly decompress. Massive blood loss in a previously hypovolemic patient increases the possibility of cardiac arrest.

If the injury appears to be arterial and in the upper abdomen, the possibility of injury to the visceral portion of the aorta or one of its major upper abdominal branches should be considered and proximal control should be obtained. If there is hematoma extending up to the level of the diaphragm, the left chest should be opened and the aorta encircled. If there is no hematoma at the level of the aortic hiatus, dissection can be carried down around the aorta by severing the crura of the diaphragm as they wrap around the aorta and placing an occluding clamp at this region (see Chapter 20). A safer alternative approach is to use an arterial occluder (Fig. 4–3), which when properly placed affords good temporary proximal control until dissection permits the application of a vascular clamp above the level of injury. If time permits, still a third approach to gain proximal aortic control at the diaphragm is to mobilize the left kidney, spleen, and tail of the pancreas from lateral to medial to gain lateral access to the aorta at the hiatus.

As soon as bleeding has been identified and controlled, the next priority is preventing gross contamination from hollow viscus injury. When bowel injuries are encountered as part of the routine exploration, time should not be taken to suture them initially. Instead, they should be closed temporarily with the application of a Babcock or Allis clamp if the injury is small or occluding intestinal or Kocher clamps if the disruption is major.

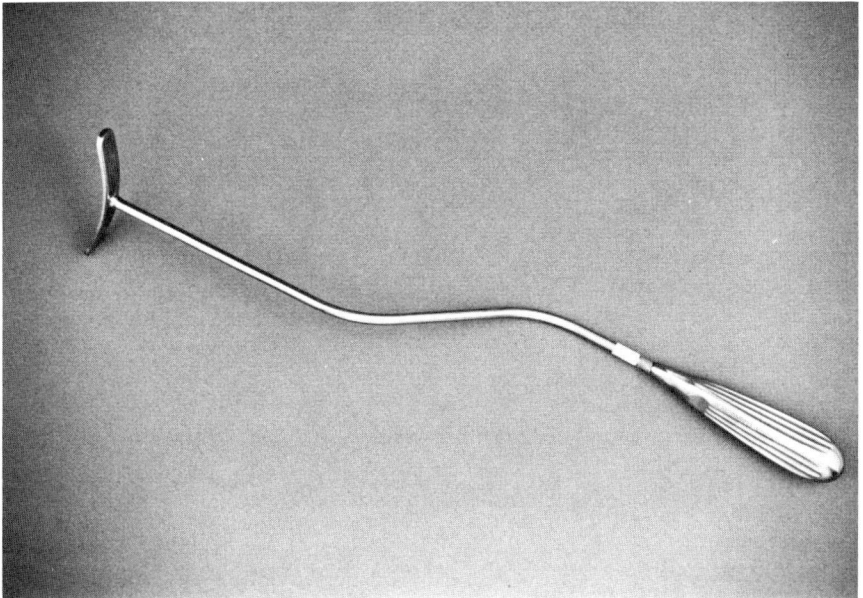

Figure 4–3. This occluder is useful to control the aorta in the upper abdomen by compression against the vertebral column.

The abdominal incision should be long enough for evisceration of the entire small bowel and visualization of all of the length of the colon. After evisceration, careful inspection of the small bowel should begin at the ligament of Treitz and be carried distally. Each bowel loop should be inspected and both sides of the mesentery inspected by fanning it out and flopping it back and forth to look at first one side and then the other. A laparotomy pad should be used to wipe away debris from the serosal surface to expose any underlying injury. This is especially important in penetrating injuries, as is exposure of the mesenteric surface of the bowel in areas of adjacent hematoma of the mesentery. After the small bowel has been inspected in its entirety, the colon should be checked from the cecum to the sigmoid colon. The transverse colon and omentum should be retracted upward for better exposure of both the base of the mesocolon and the transverse colon itself. When there is the suspicion of injury to the retroperitoneal portions of the colon, these should be mobilized by severing the lateral attachments of the colon and bringing the bowel medially and upward into the wound.

After major bleeding and gross contamination have been taken care of, the abdomen can be examined in greater detail. The specific method by which this is done is not as important as making sure that the inspection is systematic and thorough.[35] Our method is described below.

The left upper quadrant is examined first. The presence of clot strongly suggests injury to the spleen or left lobe of the liver. Careful inspection should be done by exerting gentle traction on the spleen while inspecting first the hilar area, then the outer convex surface. If an actively bleeding injury is discovered and either splenectomy or splenorrhaphy is contemplated, the spleen should be mobilized into the wound by dividing any lateral attachments sharply and any attachments to the splenic flexure of the colon between clamps. Mobilization of the spleen is most complete when the plane underneath the tail of the pancreas is developed so that it is mobilized along with the splenic pedicle. While looking at the spleen, the left hemidiaphragm should also be inspected and palpated. If no clot or overt injury to the spleen is seen, the left lobe of the liver should be bimanually palpated and the left kidney visualized. Perinephric hematomas do not require exploration unless they are tense, pulsatile, or expanding.[19,27] If a perinephric hematoma is to be entered, control of the renal artery and vein should first be obtained if possible (see chapter 20). The anterior surface of the stomach should also be inspected. This is facilitated by placing traction on the greater curvature with Babcock clamps placed far enough apart so that the surface is spread out as it is pulled down. This maneuver is easier when the stomach is empty and the anesthesiologist should be encouraged to place a nasogastric tube if one is not already down and to apply suction to it. The nasogastric aspirate can also be checked for gross blood, an important clue to the presence of gastric injury.

Attention is then directed to the right upper quadrant. The right lobe of the liver should be visualized and bimanually palpated. If injury is suspected, visualization is enhanced by dividing the triangular ligaments and mobilizing the right lobe medially. If this is done, attention should be paid to possible effects on blood pressure because mobilization of the right lobe places its weight directly on top of the inferior vena cava, which can significantly compromise venous return. Inspection of the right upper quadrant should also include a look at the pylorus and the duodenal sweep. Periduodenal blood or bile staining should prompt mobilization of the duodenum with a Kocher maneuver. The right kidney and gall bladder should also be examined at this point.

The lower quadrants are then inspected, first on the right and then on the left. Injuries to the ascending or descending colon and retroperitoneal and pelvic hematomas should be looked for. Hematomas in the pelvis generally result from pelvic fractures and usually should be left intact unless arterial injury is suspected (see Chapter 20). Penetrating injuries that result in retroperitoneal or pelvic hematomas should generally be explored. Most of the time this should be done immediately except in stable patients in whom there is a large hematoma and uncertainty about the location and nature of underlying injury. In these instances, associated intraabdominal injuries should be managed, the abdomen closed, and angiography obtained to define better the pathologic anatomy and plan the operative approach. Penetrating injuries that pass in the vicinity of the ureter dictate its exploration by mobilizing the right or left colon and entering the retroperitoneum, as described in Chapter 20. The dome of the bladder should also be inspected by placing a large retractor at the lower margin of the abdominal wound. The balloon of the urethral catheter should also be palpated and the bladder checked to be sure that it is adequately drained.

If the bowel has not already been systematically run from the ligament of Treitz to the sigmoid colon, this should be done at this point.

Finally, the lesser sac is explored if there is any suspicion of an injury to the pancreas or posterior wall of the stomach. If there is not too much intraperitoneal fat, the pancreas can be quickly checked through the gastrocolic ligament with the stomach placed on downward traction or through the gastrocolic ligament with the transverse colon placed on traction. If the lesser sac is to be explored, this is done by severing the attachment of the omentum to the transverse colon or by dividing the gastrocolic ligament. If the gastrocolic ligament is divided, this should be done to the left of the midline because this area is less vascular. In many patients, the gastrocolic ligament is avascular enough that it can be divided bluntly. In other patients, the ligament must be divided between clamps. Once the lesser sac is entered, the posterior wall of the stomach is inspected by lifting it up and putting the greater curvature on upward traction. The pancreas can also be inspected. Hematomas around the body or tail of the pancreas require further mobilization of the pancreas, further clearing of the anterior surface of the organ, and careful palpation. The head of the pancreas can be bimanually palpated by performing an extensive Kocher maneuver, placing one hand behind the head of the pancreas through the plane developed with the Kocher maneuver and the other hand through the hole made for entry into the lesser sac. Careful palpation of the pancreas is important because a small hematoma can fill out the contour of even a completely disrupted gland. If there is any loss of integrity, the pancreas should be completely mobilized by severing the lateral attachments and mobilizing the spleen and the tail of the pancreas as a unit from lateral to medial. This is facilitated by completely dividing the attachment of the omentum to the splenic flexure so this can be swung upward.

Visualization of the rectum below the peritoneal reflection can be difficult and extensive dissection can result in long-term sexual dysfunction in male patients. Sigmoidoscopy either preoperatively or in the operating room is a helpful adjunct to diagnosis. Proximal diversion with rectal washout alone should be the general rule if an injury below the peritoneal reflection is discovered.[7,36] Proximal diversion may also be necessary on occasion to prevent fecal soilage of large open perineal wounds, especially when they are associated with open fractures of the pelvis.[26,33]

After completion of the abdominal exploration, the abdominal incision is closed. We use a heavy absorbable suture for the fascia placed in a running fashion. Retention sutures are added if abdominal wall tension is increased or if severe ileus or bleeding is anticipated.

On rare occasion, because of massively distended bowel or large retroperitoneal hematomas, closure of the abdominal wall is impossible. In these instances, mesh graft can be used as a temporary closure.

PRIORITIES FOR ASSOCIATED INJURIES

In many patients, particularly those with blunt trauma, exploration of the abdomen is only the beginning of extensive surgery for associated maxillofacial, neurosurgical, soft tissue, or orthopedic injuries. Many of these procedures are lengthy and result in significant blood loss. At the completion of the abdominal exploration, priorities should be set with other operating consultants and anesthesiology about the order in which extraabdominal injuries should be fixed. This is important in the event that the patient's condition subsequently deteriorates to the point where further operative intervention must be abandoned. In general, neurosurgical procedures for the treatment of intracranial mass lesions or the monitoring of intracranial pressure take first priority, followed by stabilization of pelvic fractures and long-bone fractures of the lower extremities. Repair of upper extremity fractures, ankle fractures, facial fractures, and soft tissue injuries is of lower priority. The trauma surgeon's responsibility does not end with closure of the abdomen. In addition to coordinating the decision-making process about priorities for further operative procedures, he should make frequent subsequent visits to the operating room in critically ill patients to assess their cardiac, pulmonary, renal, and coagulation status. Sometimes it is necessary to cut short or abandon the treatment of associated injuries because of general instability of the patient. The risks of untreated injuries must be weighed against the risks of further blood loss, hypothermia, and anesthesia in such situations. On rare occasion, a patient will be so unstable at the conclusion of abdominal exploration that the trauma surgeon should insist on no further immediate surgery.

REFERENCES

1. Asbun HJ, Irani H, Roe EJ, et al. Intraabdominal seatbelt injury. *J Trauma*. 1990; 30:89.
2. Bailey H. *Surgery in Modern Warfare*. 3rd ed. Baltimore, Md: Williams & Wilkins; 1944:II.
3. Barnes JK. *The Medical and Surgical History of the War of the Rebellion*. Washington, DC: Government Printing Office; 1870:I–IV.
4. Beal SL, McKennan M. Blunt diaphragm rupture: a morbid injury. *Arch Surg*. 1988; 123:828–832.
5. Beal SL, Spisso JM. The risk of splenorrhaphy. *Arch Surg*. 1988; 123:1158.
6. Bull JC, Mathewson CF. Exploratory laparotomy in patients with penetrating wounds of the abdomen. *Am J Surg*. 1968; 116:223.
7. Burch JM, Feliciano DV, Mattox KL. Colostomy and drainage for civilian rectal injuries: is that all? *Ann Surg*. 1989; 209:600–610.
8. Cass AS, Johnson CF, Khan AU. Nonoperative management of bladder rupture from external trauma. *Urology*. 1983; 22:27–29.
9. Corriere JN Jr, Sandler CM. Management of the ruptured bladder: seven years of experience with 111 cases. *J Trauma*. 1986; 26:830–833.
10. Dauterive AH, Flancbaum L, Cox EF. Blunt intestinal trauma: A modern-day review. *Ann Surg*. 1985; 201:198–203.
11. Demetriades D. Penetrating injuries of the abdomen. *Surg Ann*. 1989; 21:201.
12. Fabian TC, Mangiante EC, White TJ. A prospective study of 91 patients undergoing both computed tomography and peritoneal lavage following blunt abdominal trauma. *J Trauma*. 1986; 26:602–608.
13. Feliciano DV, Burch JM, Spjut-Patrinely V, et al. Abdominal gunshot wounds: an urban trauma center's experience with 300 consecutive patients. *Ann Surg*. 1988; 208:362–370.

14. Forde KA, Ganepola GAP. Is mandatory exploration for penetrating abdominal trauma extinct? The morbidity and morality of negative exploration in a large municipal hospital. *J Trauma.* 1974; 14:764–766.
15. Fullen WD, Hunt J, Altemeier WA. Prophylactic antibiotics in penetrating wounds of the abdomen. *J Trauma.* 1972; 12:282.
16. Garrison FW. *History of Medicine.* Philadelphia: WB Saunders; 1929.
17. Grant HH. The practical management of bullet wounds of the abdominal viscera. *Trans South Surg Gynecol Assoc.* 1899; 12:37–52.
18. Heaton LD, et al. Military surgical practices in the U.S. Army in Vietnam. *Curr Probl Surg.* 1966.
19. Holcroft JW, Trunkey DD, Minagj, H, et al. Renal trauma and retroperitoneal hematomas: Indications for exploration. *J Trauma.* 1975; 15:1045–1052.
20. Holcroft JW, Blaisdell FW. Trauma to the torso. In: Wilmore DW, Brennan MF, Harken AH, Holcroft JW, Meakins JL, eds. *American College of Surgeons Care of the Surgical Patient.* New York: Scientific American; 1989:1–56.
21. Levison MA, Peterson SR, Sheldon GF, et al. Duodenal trauma: experience of a trauma center. *J Trauma.* 1984; 24:475.
22. Loria FL. *Historical Aspects of Abdominal Injuries.* Springfield, Ill: Charles C Thomas; 1968.
23. Luna GK, Dellinger EP. Nonoperative observation therapy for splenic injuries: a safe therapeutic option? *Am J Surg.* 1987; 153:462–468.
24. Madden MR, Paull DE, Finkelstein JL, et al. Occult diaphragmatic injury from stab wounds to the lower chest and abdomen. *J Trauma.* 1989; 29:292–298.
25. Matsubara TK, Fong HMT, Burns CM. Computed tomography of the abdomen (CTA) in management of blunt abdominal trauma. *J Trauma.* 1990; 30:410.
26. Maull KI, Sachatello CR, Ernst CB. The deep perineal laceration—An injury frequently associated with open pelvic fractures: a need for aggressive surgical management. *J Trauma.* 1977; 17:685–696.
27. McAninch JW, Carroll PR. Renal exploration after trauma: indications and reconstructive techniques. *Urol Clin North Am.* 1989; 16:203–212.
28. Mucha P, Daly R, Farnell M. Selective management of blunt splenic trauma. *J Trauma.* 1986; 26:970.
29. Nance FC. Abdominal trauma at the Southern Surgical Association, 1888–1987. *Ann Surg.* 1988; 207: 742–753.
30. Nance FC, Wenner WH, Johnson LW, et al. Surgical judgement in the management of penetrating wounds of the abdomen: experience with 2212 patients. *Trans South Surg Assoc.* 1973; 85:117–124.
31. Oakes DD, Charters AC. Changing concepts in the management of splenic trauma. *Surg Gynecol Obstet.* 1981; 153:181.
32. Petersen SR, Sheldon GF. Morbidity of a negative finding at laparotomy in abdominal trauma. *Surg Gynecol Obstet.* 1979; 148:23–26.
33. Richardson JD, Harty J, Amin M, et al. Open pelvic fractures. *J Trauma.* 1982; 22:533–538.
34. Robin AP, Andrews JR, Lange DA, et al. Selective management of anterior abdominal stab wounds. *J Trauma.* 1989; 29:1684.
35. Scalea TM, Philips TF, Goldstein AS, et al. Injuries missed at operation: nemesis of the trauma surgeon. *J Trauma.* 1988; 28:962.
36. Shannon FL, Moore EE, Moore FA, et al. Value of distal colon washout in civilian rectal trauma: reducing gut bacterial translocation. *J Trauma.* 1988; 28:989–994.
37. Sherck JP, Oakes DD. Intestinal injury missed by computed tomography. *J Trauma.* 1990; 39:1.
38. Siemens RA, Fulton RL. Gastric rupture as a result of blunt trauma. *Am Surg.* 1977; 43:229.
39. Sims JM. Careful aseptic invasion of the abdominal cavity. *Br Med J.* 1881; ii:925.
40. Sokya JM, Martin M, Sloan EP, et al. Diagnostic peritoneal lavage. *J Trauma.* 1990; 30:874.
41. Stein A, Lisoos I. Selective management of penetrating wounds of the abdomen. *J Trauma.* 1968; 8:1014.
42. Surgery in World War II, General Surgery, Office of the Surgeon General, Department of the Army, Washington, DC, 1955.
43. Weigelt JA, Kingman RG. Complications of negative laparotomy for trauma. *Am J Surg.* 1988; 156: 544–547.
44. Wesson DE, Filler RM, Hin SH, et al. Ruptured spleen: when to operate? *J Pediatr Surg.* 1981; 16:324–326.
45. Wisner DH, Chun Y, Blaisdell FW. Blunt intestinal injury: keys to diagnosis and management. *Arch Surg.* 1990; 125:1319–1323.

5
Chest and Abdominal Wall Injuries

F. WILLIAM BLAISDELL, M.D.

> HISTORY: The first recorded survival of a major abdominal wall injury appears in Xenophon's history of the Anabasis. The Greek generals went to the Persian camp to assure Tissaphernes that the Greeks were not plotting to kill him. What followed was one of history's most daring acts of treachery. The Persians turned on the Greek generals and killed all but Nicarcus, the Arcadian, who escaped and warned the other Greeks. He "came there with a wound in his stomach and holding his intestine. He told them everything which happened." Nicarcus somehow survived this wound, possibly with the aid of one of the eight doctors assigned to the Greek soldiers, who may have bandaged and attended the injury.
>
> However, laparotomy for trauma lagged well behind that for elective conditions. Baudens is given credit for introducing laparotomy for abdominal trauma in 1836.[1] Despite that, it was not used during the American Civil War except when a penetrating wound required treatment of eviscerated bowel. Although used intermittently from the late 1880s,[2] it was still considered controversial in World War I and it was not until World War II that laparotomy became established as definitive treatment for penetrating abdominal wounds.

Injuries that are limited to the abdominal wall are often taken lightly but the significance of what initially appears to be a trivial injury may be great. This is because underlying injuries may be masked or conversely, underlying injuries may be simulated and lead to abdominal exploration. Moreover, when there is a considerable degree of soft tissue injury, secondary complications involving the abdominal wound may on occasion compromise survival.

MECHANISM AND SIGNIFICANCE OF INJURY

The incidence of abdominal wall injury independent of other injuries is not well documented. In our experience, approximately 50% of stab wounds of the abdomen are not associated with significant intraabdominal injury.[3] Therefore, it would be our estimate that there are approximately twice as many abdominal wall injuries as there are viscus injuries reported in association with stab wounds. On the other hand, we have found that 92% of gunshot wounds are associated with significant intraperitoneal injury and therefore in only a minor number of gunshot wounds are the injuries limited to the abdominal wall. However, certain gunshot wounds or shotgun blasts producing tangential lesions limited to the chest wall or abdominal wall can still be devastating.[4]

Blunt trauma may produce contusion of the abdominal wall in the absence of significant abdominal injury but the abdominal wall is so resilient that most abdominal wall injuries of any significance are associated with intraperitoneal injury. One exception is perhaps related to the rectus muscle where the largest vessels of the abdominal wall, the superior and the inferior epigastric arteries, meet. Severe contusions of this muscle may result in significant hemorrhage or result in the development of a rectus muscle hematoma, which produces disability or may simulate intraabdominal injury.[5,6] Another injury that can be associated with a high complication rate is avulsion injury (Fig. 5–1). In this instance, for example, the wheels of the car passing over the back produced a shearing force that separated skin and underlying subcutaneous tissue from the fascia.[8] In most instances of avulsion injury, a large laceration is produced particularly when the injury is central on the anterior abdominal wall as the umbilicus provides a point of fixation from which skin and subcutaneous tissue are torn. When the flank or back is involved and particularly when

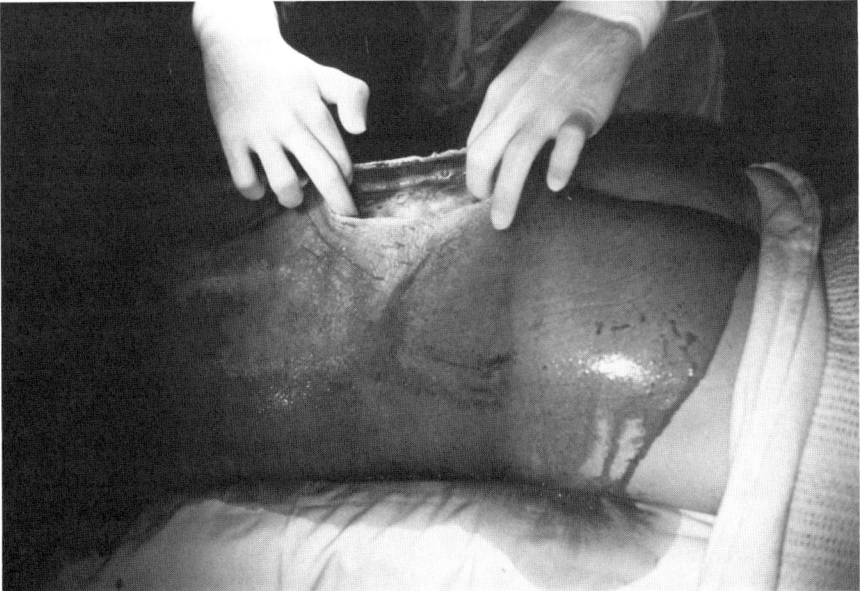

Figure 5–1. Avulsion injury of the back. The undermining extends well around the flank.

there is obesity, extensive shearing may occur without skin disruption. All of these injuries impair skin viability and subcutaneous bleeding can be sufficient to result in shock.

Another injury being seen with increasing frequency is abdominal wall muscle and fascial disruption secondary to seat belt trauma.[9-11] These injuries are often associated with intraabdominal injury and are usually associated with the "seatbelt sign." This consists of a mark on the abdominal wall that may vary from a minor abrasion to overt bruising with ecchymosis and hematoma. This can consist of muscle contusion all the way to complete separation of all underlying muscles and fascia.

Injuries to the chest wall involving the lower six ribs should also be considered to be related to abdominal injury because the mass of underlying lung is minimal and major abdominal structures, including liver, spleen, and both kidneys, lie subadjacent. In a recent review of ours, which consisted of 287 patients with fractures of the lower six ribs without any initial evidence of abdominal injury, 13, or 7%, subsequently proved to have significant intraabdominal pathology. In our experience, one in five, or 20%, of all fractures of the ninth and tenth ribs on the left side are associated with splenic rupture and it is probable that a corresponding incidence of liver damage occurs in association with right lower rib fractures. Many minor liver injuries are probably not recognized clinically and have no significance, whereas for all practical purposes, there is never a minor splenic injury. The incidence of major splenic injury associated with left rib fractures appears to correspond to or be actually higher in incidence than corresponding right rib fractures associated with injuries to the liver. The greater mass of the liver, however, more than compensates for its decreased vulnerability to injury so that the incidence of serious injury is similar.

ANATOMY

The anatomy of the lower six ribs and overlying musculature is not particularly complex and does not require definition in this text except to indicate that posteriorly the right kidney overlies the 10th, 11th, and 12th ribs. The spleen centers on the posterior axillary line with the normal spleen under the 9th and 10th ribs. The liver can be found under ribs 8 through 11. The exact relationship for both liver and spleen varies with the respiratory cycle.

The abdominal wall, over approximately 40% of its surface, consists of three muscle groups: transversus abdominis, internal oblique, and external oblique (Fig. 5–2). The muscular aponeurosis of these muscles surrounds the anterior longitudinally placed rectus muscle, the external oblique always passing in front, the internal oblique dividing and passing both back and front in the upper two-thirds of the abdomen and completely in front of the rectus muscle in the lower one-third of the abdomen. The lower edge of this change in relationship is the semicircular line on the posterior sheath of the muscle. The transversus abdominis and its inserting fascia passes posterior to the rectus muscle throughout its extent. The direction of the external oblique musculature parallels the inguinal ligament, and the internal oblique in the upper two-thirds of the abdomen passes obliquely in the opposite direction, paralleling the costal margin down to the level of the iliac crest. Just below this, the internal oblique passes transversely and, below the iliac crest, passes obliquely downward as its fibers insert with those of the transversus abdominis on the pubic tubercle. The transversus abdominis, as its name indicates, takes origin from the lumbosacral fascia with the other two muscles and passes transversely across the abdomen over most of its extent, although below the anterior superior spine of the ilium its fibers curve

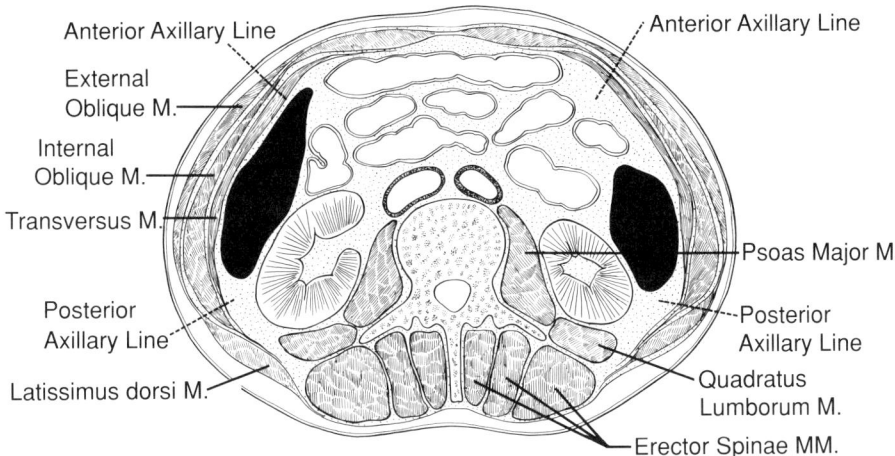

Figure 5–2. Abdominal wall muscular layers at the level of the umbilicus.

downward to insert on the pubic tubercle with those of the internal oblique as the conjoined tendon. An areolar plane separates these three muscles and the preperitoneal fat, and in the lower abdomen, the transversalis fascia separates the transversus abdominis from the underlying peritoneum.

The rectus muscle passes downward from its origin on the costal cartilages of the lower anterior ribs and sternum and inserts on the symphysis pubis and the pubic tubercle. It comprises multiple segments corresponding to the vertebrae. These segments in the upper abdomen are marked by fibrous bands, "inscriptions," that adhere to the anterior fascia but are free posteriorly so there is an areolar plane deep to the muscle and anterior to the deep fascia through which blood can dissect.

The rectus muscles are in close proximity in the lower abdomen; the separation between the right and left rectus muscles is often difficult for the surgeon to find below the umbilicus. Above the umbilicus, the rectus muscles progressively diverge from one another and at the level of xiphoid are normally separated by a distance of approximately 1 cm by a fascial line, the linea alba. The linea alba comprises anterior and posterior fascial layers that encircle the rectus muscle and join in the midline as an avascular fascial layer. The umbilicus constitutes a full thickness scar involving the peritoneum, fascia, and overlying skin. This contains the remnant of the obliterated umbilical vein, which passes upward under the linea alba in a fold of peritoneum as the ligamentum teres. Along the lateral margin of the rectus muscle is the semilunar line, an avascular area comprising the interweaving fascia of the more lateral flat muscles as they converge to surround the rectus muscle.

Posterior to the posterior axillary line, the lumbodorsal fascia, the fascia of the insertion of the anterior flat muscles of the abdomen covers the quadratus lumborum muscle, which runs between the 12th rib above and the iliac crest below. The latissimus dorsi muscles take origin from the iliac crest and the sacral fascia and pass obliquely upward along the back, the anterior edge forming the posterior axillary line. The thick extensor muscles of the back fill in the gutter between the spinous process of the vertebrae and the angles of the ribs.

The only major vessels of the abdominal wall, the superior and inferior epigastric arteries, run through the posterior aspect of the rectus muscle. The superior epigastric artery is a continuation of the internal mammary artery above, which becomes the former as the vessel passes through the mammary foramen of the diaphragm. It enters the center of the body of the rectus muscle and passes downward to meet the inferior epigastric artery coming up from below. The inferior epigastric artery takes origin from the external iliac artery at the inguinal ligament and curves upward in a plane between the peritoneum and transversalis fascia in the preperitoneal fat on an oblique course toward the umbilicus, joining the rectus muscle to anastomose with the superior epigastric artery. Additional blood supply to the abdominal wall is provided by the lower intercostal, lumbar, and iliac circumflex arteries.

The innervation of the abdominal wall muscles is by the segmental intercostal nerves 8 through 12 (Fig. 5–3). The 10th intercostal nerve passes through the corresponding thoracic vertebral foramen and encircles the abdomen in nearly a transverse direction supplying the musculature opposite the umbilicus and the sensory nerves to the overlying skin. The 9th nerve lies just above and parallels the 10th nerve in its course and, anterior to the anterior axillary line, curves obliquely upward to reach the rectus muscle. The 8th thoracic nerve innervates the abdomen below the costal margin and therefore, anterior to the anterior axillary line, passes obliquely upward paralleling the costal margin to reach the rectus

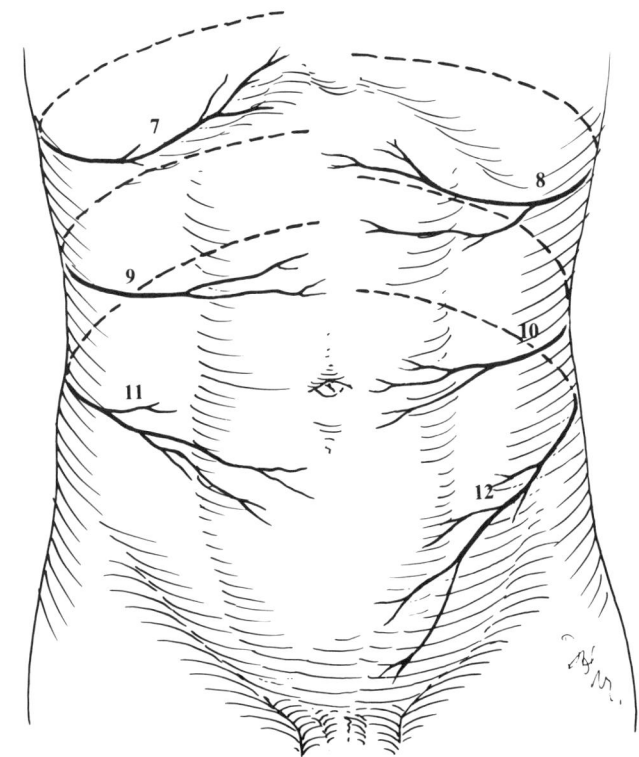

Figure 5–3. Anatomy of the nerves of the abdominal wall.

muscle. The course of T-11 is obliquely downward to innervate the lower abdomen and rectus muscle. T-12 innervates the suprainguinal and suprapubic regions of the lower abdomen before ending in the rectus muscle. When transverse incisions are made in the abdominal wall, the course of these nerves should be recognized and optimal location of incisions should be parallel to the direction of the abdominal wall nerves.

The parietal peritoneum underlies the muscles and fascia of the abdominal wall, separated from them by a variable degree of preperitoneal fat. The peritoneum underlying the abdominal wall is richly innervated by somatic nerves, whereas that lining the pelvis and that surrounding the viscera has little or no innervation. That covering the peripheral portion of the diaphragm is innervated by the local intercostal nerves, whereas the peritoneum overlying the central tendon of the diaphragm is innervated from C5. Pain in the instance of central tendon irritation is referred to the shoulder (Kehr's sign).

A midline longitudinal abdominal wall incision that permits entry and exposure of all corners of the abdomen is the standard incision used for exploratory laparotomy in trauma cases. This has the advantage of avoiding all critical anatomy, both blood vessels and nerves. The abdominal cavity can generally be likened to a barrel and the incision of the linea alba corresponds to the removal of a stave of a barrel permitting access to all segments of the interior. A transverse incision, unless very generous, limits exposure to upper or lower portions of the abdomen depending on its location. A midline incision is rapid and quick to make; a transverse incision requires longer. However, transverse incisions have a major advantage over longitudinal incisions as the stresses on the abdominal wall are such that they tend to close transverse incisions and disrupt longitudinal incisions (Fig. 5–4). The rectus abdominal muscle is the one longitudinal muscle in the abdominal wall, but its effective force is negligible compared to the lateral flat muscles. The vector of forces of these muscles that pass obliquely upward, obliquely downward, and transverse is in a transverse direction. Therefore, a transverse wound that is left open will tend to close as abdominal muscles tense, whereas a longitudinal wound will tend to gape. This is a consideration primarily when incisions are planned to drain or explore infected or heavily contaminated areas. Under these circumstances, when there is a possibility of secondary wound disruption, a transverse rather than a longitudinal incision may be optimal.

ASSESSMENT

The assessment of injuries to the lower six ribs is relatively easy. An excellent screening maneuver is to ask the patient to take a deep breath and cough. The ability to do both of these without discomfort indicates that there has been no compromise in the integrity of the lower six ribs, since fractures of the ribs are almost inevitably associated with pleural injury and severe pain with ventilation. In an uncooperative patient, compression of the lower rib cage can be used. If acute discomfort is elicited, rib fracture is likely, whereas minimal discomfort usually rules out the possibility of significant chest wall injury. If chest wall injury is documented by the above maneuvers, then the individual ribs can be palpated and the extent of the injuries noted. X-ray is frequently misleading and underdiagnoses the severity of chest wall injury, since many rib fractures cannot be seen and separation of costal cartilages cannot be diagnosed on any film.

Trauma to the abdominal wall is often evident on inspection. There may be abrasions,

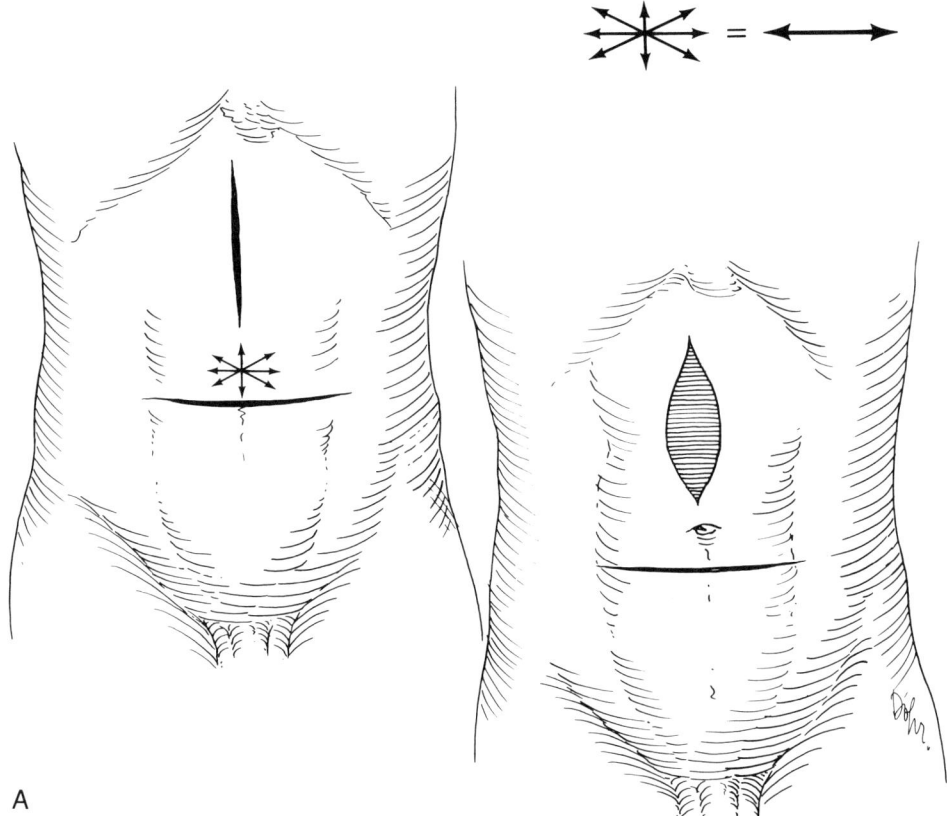

Figure 5–4. **A:** Vectors of forces acting on wounds of the abdominal wall. **B:** The effective force of these vectors is in a transverse direction tending to result in gaping at longitudinal wounds while closing transverse wounds.

ecchymosis, or splinting as the patient breathes. In the normally nourished patient, a rectus hematoma is often evident as a mass that usually increases in prominence as the patient tenses his abdominal wall. Lacerations of the thorax or abdominal wall are also evident on inspection. Palpation of the abdomen after blunt injury is generally associated with tenderness and the patient is unable to splint or tighten the muscles without aggravating the discomfort.

Injuries sufficient to produce abdominal wall damage are associated with difficulty in recognizing underlying pathology within the abdomen. Signs of peritoneal irritation should always be interpreted as irritation coming from within the abdominal cavity since, statistically, it is the most likely probability. The probing of penetrating wounds is of little value unless the probing results in the dropping of the instrument into the abdominal cavity, since the abdominal wall muscles change with the position of the patient (Fig. 5–5). Therefore, the probing object may not reveal the true depth of the injury because deeper muscle layers of the abdominal wall may change an inch or more in relation to the injury to the outermost muscle layer. Therefore, once a penetrating wound has passed through fascia, penetration of the full thickness of the abdominal wall must be assumed.

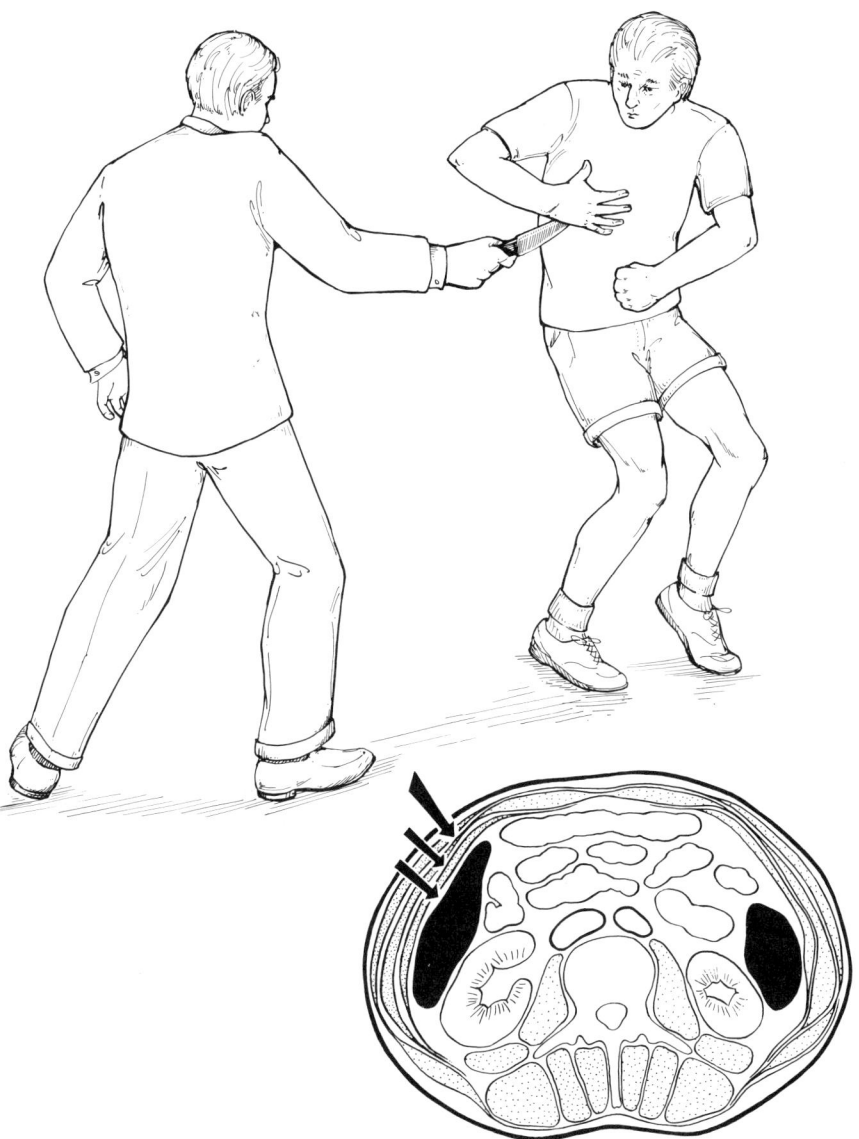

Figure 5-5. The type of change that can occur in the relationship of the abdominal walls muscles after a penetrating injury.

Occasionally, contusion of the lateral portion of the abdominal wall may be associated with relatively large hematomas. However, this is unusual because of the lack of large blood vessels in most of the abdominal wall. In the central abdomen, as indicated previously, rectus muscle injury that involves the epigastric vessels can be a significant clinical problem. Because of the presence of inscriptions and a fascial envelope that prevents the hematoma's spreading longitudinally and laterally, a rectus hematoma may appear as a specific mass. In patients with thick subcutaneous layers, this may be difficult to differentiate from an abdominal wall tumor. A mass from rectus abdominis hematoma occurs below the umbilicus in more than 80% of cases. To distinguish this mass from an intraabdominal mass, the patient should be instructed to raise his head against resistance. The mass should disappear if it is intraabdominal and remain the same or become more prominent if it is in the abdominal wall (Bouchacourt's sign). If tenderness and peritoneal irritation exist, abdominal exploration may well be indicated to rule out intraperitoneal injury, as this is the only way to differentiate between abdominal wall injury and intraperitoneal injury, particularly when peritoneal irritation exists. Ultrasound has also been established to be of diagnostic help in this condition.[12]

Avulsion injuries inevitably are associated with irregular lacerations and subcutaneous tissue separation that usually extend down to fascia. Usually there is considerable ecchymosis. Exploration of the laceration will reveal extensive undermining of the skin and subcutaneous tissue.

The seat belt sign, which may be associated with abdominal wall disruption, has already been referred to.[13,14] Careful palpation may verify a muscular defect and large hematomas also suggest a high probability of underlying injury.

INDICATIONS FOR OPERATION

Operation is not necessarily required for blunt injuries of the abdominal wall unless there is a major devitalizing injury or there is an open wound with major contamination. In addition, surgery may be required to rule out intraabdominal injury, to drain large hematomas, or to repair gross disruption. Avulsion injuries are usually followed by skin necrosis and infection of the elevated flap. If trauma to the subcutaneous tissue is extensive, removal of devitalized fat from the skin flap is often indicated with the skin reapplied to the abdominal wall as a full thickness graft.

A stab wound in the anterior abdominal wall that is 2 cm or more in transverse diameter, if anterior to the anterior axillary line, should have the fascial and peritoneal defect closed, if only to prevent subsequent evisceration or hernia. Shotgun and high velocity tangential injuries of the abdominal wall require debridement of all dead and devitalized tissue.[4] Penetrating injuries always carry the possibility of hollow viscus injury and should be treated with preoperative antibiotics.

DEFINITIVE TREATMENT

Multiple rib fractures do not, as a rule, require operative treatment; however, if a flail segment is present that results in compromised ventilation, the early institution of endotracheal intubation and mechanical ventilation is appropriate (Table 5–1). Pain relief can then be provided by oral or injectable narcotics since the adequacy of ventilation can be ensured. Alternatively, in lesser injuries, injection of isolated rib fractures with a long-acting local anesthetic may provide considerable symptomatic relief and permit the patient to cough, deep breathe, and clear secretions. When multiple fractures are present, epidural narcotic administration is appropriate. This has constituted a major advance in pain control

Table 5–1 Indications for Continuous Mechanical Ventilation

Ventilatory (mechanical failure)
    Respirations $\geq 35-40$/min
    Inadequate alveolar ventilation with $Pa_{CO_2} \geq 48$ mm Hg
    Vital capacity $\leq 10-15$ ml/kg body weight
    Maximal inspiratory force ≤ -25 cm H_2O
Pulmonary (parenchymal) failure
    Alveolar-arterial oxygen gradient $(A - aDO_2) \geq 300$ mm Hg
    Right to left shunt fraction $(Q_s/Q_t) \geq 15-20\%$
    Wasted ventilation $(V_d/V_t) \geq 0.6$
    Compliance less than 30 ml/cm H_2O

and in older patients with isolated fractures can be life-saving.[15] Patients can ventilate normally without discomfort and atelectasis, hypoxemia, and pneumonitis are thereby prevented.[15] Operative treatment with internal fixation of rib fractures may be indicated in isolated instances when there are severe compound injuries, major flail segments, or underlying intrathoracic injury that requires thoracotomy.

Penetrating abdominal wall injuries such as stab wounds of 1 cm or larger are best treated by laparotomy with closure of peritoneum and fascia from inside the abdomen, after verifying the absence of intraperitoneal injury. Even though the external fascial defect is closed, it is possible for a knuckle of bowel to herniate into the deeper layer of the abdominal wall.

Shotgun injuries and other high velocity injuries that produce devitalization of the abdominal wall should be explored and all overtly necrotic tissue debrided.[4] If this involves full thickness of the abdominal wall, some type of plastic procedure or prosthesis may be appropriate to prevent evisceration of abdominal contents. It may be possible to mobilize skin flaps to close a fascial defect. If the defect is large, Marlex mesh can be sutured circumferentially to viable fascia and later covered with split thick skin grafts. In desperate circumstances, particularly when there are associated injuries, the abdominal wound can be packed open and evisceration prevented with an abdominal binder.

Abdominal wall hematomas rarely require operation, although a large rectus hematoma may be treated operatively with resultant less morbidity overall than conservative management.[6] This permits ligation of the injured epigastric artery and evacuation of the hematoma. If exploratory laparotomy is indicated, the standard midline incision can be used and the rectus sheath opened, or the hematoma decompressed using the paramedian incision, which provides direct access to the injured muscle.

Avulsion-type injuries should be explored and the degree of undermining determined. If the flaps raised exceed a hand's breadth, or 12 to 15 cm,[2] the flap is best elevated, defatted, and all underlying devitalized tissue removed.[8] The skin can then be put back as a full thickness graft. If this does not take, the wound should be allowed to develop vascularity and then covered with split thick skin grafts.

Abdominal wall disruption such as that associated with seatbelt injury can be treated with direct fascial repair, repair reinforced with Marlex mesh, or by Marlex mesh replacement. If there is major enteric contamination associated with muscle damage, the wound should be debrided, packed open, and closed electively at a later date.

COMPLICATIONS

The thoracic complications associated with rib fractures can be pneumothorax, hemothorax, or respiratory complications. These can be manifest acutely as a tension pneumothorax, which is a life-threatening problem. If not present initially, pneumothorax can complicate the patient's course at any time, particularly when mechanical ventilation is instituted for anesthesia or for postoperative management. This should be considered as a possibility whenever there is sudden unexplained deterioration of the patient. For this reason, chest tubes are used liberally when chest wall injury is present.

Hemothorax, which results in significant obliteration of the sulcus in the upright chest x-ray or partial opacification of the chest in the supine position, should be treated also by the placement of a chest tube for evacuation and monitoring of intrapleural bleeding.

Atelectasis and/or pneumonia should be prevented or treated by encouraging the patient to deep breathe and cough. Should major pulmonary collapse occur, this should be treated with tracheobronchial aspiration or bronchoscopy as necessary to remove mucous plugs. The ability of the patient to deep breathe and cough may be facilitated by appropriate application of intercostal nerve block and/or titration with small doses of narcotic.

The complications of abdominal wall injuries may also be pulmonary since the patient may have difficulty deep breathing or coughing as well. Abdominal wall defects with herniation may occur after penetrating injuries if the fascial defect is not repaired. Blunt injuries with musculofascial disruption are also associated with immediate or delayed defects. Septic complications are relatively rare in clean injuries in which abdominal contamination has not occurred but are always a possibility when there has been contamination from within or from without. These can vary from benign abscesses to lethal necrotizing synergistic infections or clostridial infections.

REFERENCES

1. Loria FL. *Historical Aspects of Abdominal Injuries*. Springfield, Ill: Charles C Thomas; 1968.
2. Coley WB. The treatment of penetrating wounds of the abdomen. *Am J Med Sci*. 1891; 101:243–247.
3. Peterson FR, Sheldon CF. Morbidity of negative findings at laparotomy in abdominal trauma. *Surg Gynecol Obstet*. 1979; 148:23.
4. Sherman RT, Parrish RA. Management of shotgun injuries. *J Trauma*. 1963; 3:36.
5. Cullen TS, Bordel M. Lesions of the rectus abdominis muscle simulating acute abdominal conditions. *Bull Johns Hopkins Hops*. 1937; 61:295.
6. Zainea GG. Rectus sheath hematomas: their pathogenesis, diagnosis and management. *Am Surg*. 1988; 54:630.
7. Gocke JE, MacCarty RL, Foulk WT. Rectus sheath hematomas: diagnosis by computed tomography scanning. *Mayo Clin Proc*. 1981; 56:757.
8. Kalisman M, et al. Treatment of extensive avulsions of the skin and subcutaneous tissues. *J Dermatol Surg Oncol*. 1978; 4:322.
9. Payne DD, Resnicoff SA, States JD. Seatbelt abdominal wall muscular avulsion. *J Trauma*. 1973; 13:262.
10. Johnstone BR, Waxman BP. Transverse disruption of the abdominal wall—a tell tale sign of seatbelt related hollow viscus injury. *Aust NZ J Surg*. 1987; 57:455.
11. Wagner AC. Disruption of abdominal wall musculature: unusual feature of seat belt syndrome. *AJR*. 1979; 133:753.
12. Wyatt CM, Spitz HB. Ultrasound in the diagnosis of rectus sheath hematoma. *JAMA*. 1979; 241:1499.
13. Ashbun HJ, Irani H, Roe EJ, Bloch JH. Intraabdominal seatbelt injury. *J Trauma*. 1990; 30:189.
14. Dardik H, Warren A, Dardik F. Diaphragmatic, visceral and somatic injuries following rear lap seatbelt trauma. *NY State J Med*. Vol 73. 1973; 557–580.
15. MacKersie RC, Shackford SR, Hoyt DB, Karagianis TG. Continuous fentanyl analgesia: ventilatory function improvement with routine use in the treatment of blunt trauma. *J Trauma*. 1987; 27:1207–1213.

6
Diaphragm Rupture

SANDRA L. BEAL, M.D.

HISTORY: Posttraumatic herniation of the stomach through the diaphragm was first described by Sennertus in 1541, from the autopsy findings of a man who had sustained a stab wound to the chest 7 months previously.[1] The devastating outcome of gangrenous colon, strangulated through a defect in the diaphragm, was first reported by Paré in 1579 in a patient who initially survived a gunshot wound, but died 8 months later.[2] Blunt diaphragmatic rupture with post mortem findings of gastric incarceration occurring in a stone mason several months after severe blunt abdominal trauma was also reported by Paré.[2] Congenital and acquired diaphragmatic hernias were differentiated by Petit (1674–1750).[3]

Morgagni in 1769 wrote a monograph on diaphragmatic hernia, describing those varieties of hernias passing through natural diaphragmatic openings.[4] A case of posttraumatic diaphragmatic hernia established before death was first reported by Bowditch in 1853.[5]

Specific criteria for the diagnosis of posttraumatic diaphragmatic hernia were developed by Bowditch.[5] Riolfi in 1886 repaired a laceration of the diaphragm through which omentum had prolapsed. Naumann in 1888 operated on a patient who had stomach herniated into the left chest through a traumatic diaphragmatic hernia.[6] Multiple reports of diaphragm injury began to appear in the literature in the 1940s. With the increase of overall incidence and severity of trauma over the years, there has been a parallel rise in the incidence of diaphragmatic injury.[7] Blunt diaphragm rupture occurs in 7% of persons who die of blunt thoracic trauma.[8] Two to 7% of patients with major chest trauma have been found to have a diaphragmatic injury.

ANATOMY OF THE REGION

The diaphragm is formed by the fusion of five embryologic structures: the septum transversum, the pleuroperitoneal and pleuropericardial folds, the dorsal mesentery, and a mesodermal rim from the lateral body wall.[9] The diaphragm is arched, culminating superiorly in the inferior pericardial surface and central tendon, surrounded by radially arranged muscle fibers attached to the lateral chest wall (Fig. 6–1). The most posterior portion of diaphragm inserts on the periosteal surfaces of the first, second, and third lumbar

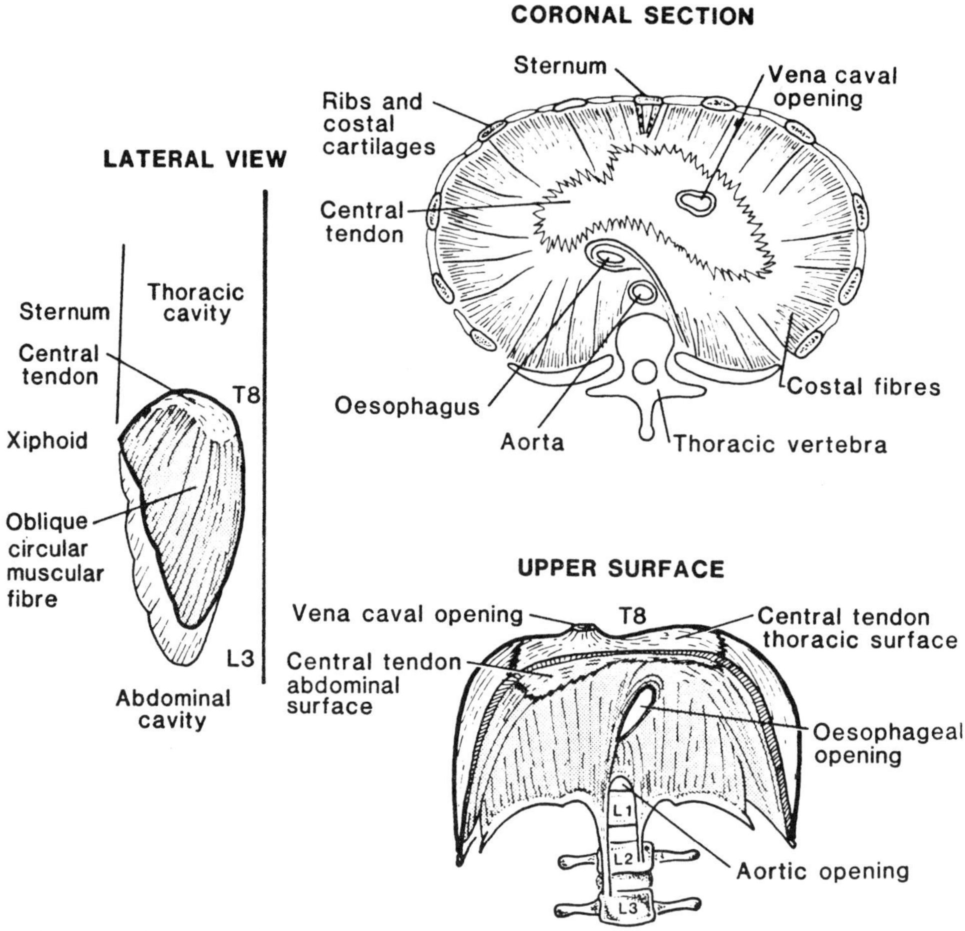

Figure 6–1. Anatomy of the diaphragm.

vertebral bodies. The most anterior portion attaches to the lowermost sternum at the junction with the xiphoid. The diaphragmatic muscle spans laterally where it inserts on the 12th rib posteriorly to the 6th rib anteriorly. The undersurface covers the liver, stomach, spleen, kidneys, and, to some extent, the pancreas and transverse colon.

There are three major orifices in the diaphragm. These are the aortic, vena caval, and esophageal apertures. The aorta, azygos vein, and thoracic duct pass through the aortic aperture. The esophagus and vagus nerves pass through the esophageal hiatus. The vena caval opening transmits only the vena cava.

The diaphragm is innervated by the phrenic nerves (Fig. 6–2). The phrenic nerve courses from the neck anterior to the medial border of the scalenus anticus muscle, through the chest along the posterolateral mediastinum on the pericardial surface. The phrenic nerve inserts into the diaphragm, at the junction of the pericardium and central tendon. At this point, on each side a crow's foot configuration splays out laterally with anterior and posterior branches that pass circumferentially through the peripheral ring of muscle.

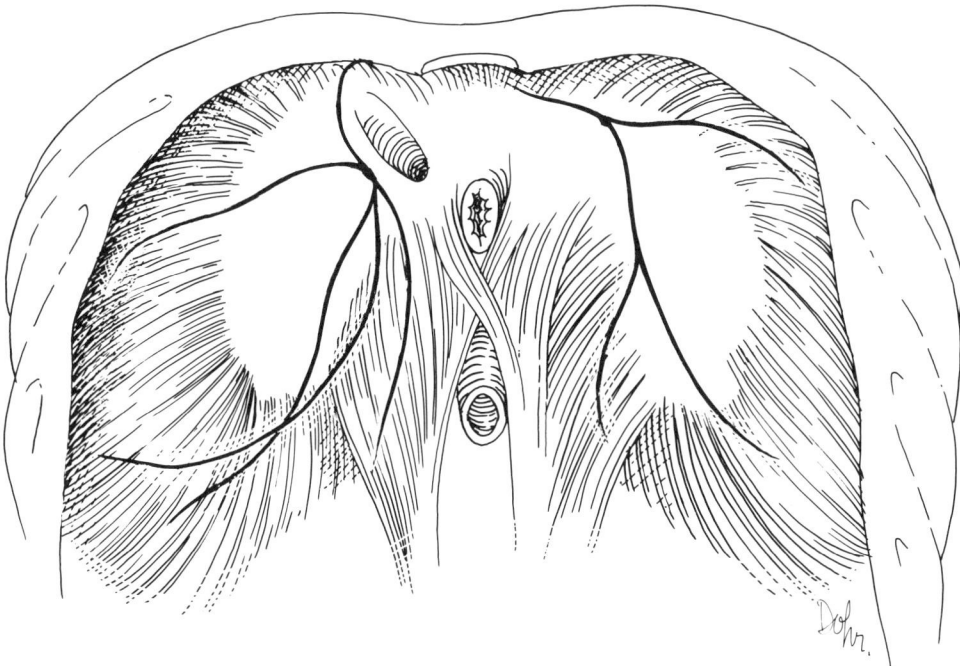

Figure 6–2. Anatomy of the diaphragm showing location of the phrenic nerves.

Arterial supply to the diaphragm arises inferiorly from direct branches off the aorta and superiorly from companion vessels traveling with the phrenic nerves. Peripheral blood supply from intercostal vessels is abundant.

Normal breathing causes a 3- to 5-cm shift, with the right leaflet rising anteriorly to the fourth intercostal space whereas the left leaflet rises to the fifth intercostal space. Posteriorly both diaphragms ascend to the eighth intercostal space.

GENERAL MECHANISM OF INJURY

Penetrating trauma is the most common cause of diaphragmatic injury. Diaphragmatic injuries account for 6% of the injuries found at laparotomy from penetrating trauma.[10] Penetrating injuries occur most commonly from stab or gunshot wounds in the vicinity of the lower chest or upper abdomen.

Blunt diaphragmatic injury requires considerable force and is almost always accompanied by associated thoracoabdominal injuries. The most common cause of blunt diaphragm rupture is violent vehicular trauma.[11] It may also result from other crushing injuries, such as a fall or from blows to the lower chest or abdomen. Among patients requiring laparotomy and/or thoracotomy, the diaphragm will be injured 5.8% to 8% of the time.[12,13]

The exact mechanism of blunt rupture of the diaphragm is not known. The fusion lines of the individual leaflets during development of the diaphragm are postulated to be weak points that may be predisposed to rupture. However, disruption has been observed at every site of the diaphragm. It has been postulated that a sudden rise in intraabdominal pressure created during the traumatic impact to the abdomen is transmitted to the diaphragm and is the main cause of rupture. Marchand demonstrated that intraperitoneal pressure fluctuates during quiet respiration from $+2$ cm H_2O to $+10$ cm H_2O while the corresponding pleural pressure varies from -5 cm H_2O to -10 cm H_2O.[14] In the supine position, the pleuroperitoneal gradient fluctuates from 7 cm H_2O to 20 cm H_2O. With maximal inspiration, the gradient may exceed 100 cm H_2O.

PATTERNS OF INJURY

The position of the diaphragmatic dome in the chest varies with inhalation and exhalation during respiration. During forced expiration, the diaphragm rises as high as the fifth interspace anteriorly and on deep inspiration falls to the lower level of the rib cage. The right half tends to be a littler higher than the left.

Penetrating wounds of the lower chest and upper abdomen are the most frequent cause of injury to the diaphragm. Wounds in remote areas of the body, however, may cause diaphragmatic injury. Penetrating injuries from gunshot wounds involve the right and left diaphragms in equal frequency.[1,4] Stab wounds injure the left hemidiaphragm more frequently, presumably because more assailants are right-handed.[15]

Herniation of abdominal viscera into the pleural space may not occur immediately after penetrating trauma unless the defect is large. In these smaller injuries (1–2 cm) the hole may be temporarily "corked" by the adjacent abdominal viscus, then gradually over weeks or months, more and more of that viscus is sucked up into the chest.

Associated injuries occur commonly with penetrating diaphragm lacerations. Symbas et al., reporting on 185 patients with penetrating diaphragmatic injuries, noted 11% had isolated diaphragmatic lacerations.[15] Forty-three percent had injury to an additional organ, 45% had sustained injury to two to four additional organs, and 2% had greater than four organs injured.

Blunt rupture results in a tear that is frequently in a radial direction involving the posterolateral diaphragm (Fig. 6–3). Blunt rupture may occur in various locations without a particular pattern. The pericardial and central portions of the hemidiaphragm are infrequently ruptured.

Abdominal viscera tend to herniate into the pleural space after blunt injury (Fig. 6–4). This is because the defect resulting from blunt trauma is usually large and the transiently elevated pleuroperitoneal pressure gradient with blunt abdominal trauma promotes herniation. The stomach is the most commonly herniated organ followed in decreasing order of frequency by the colon, spleen, small intestine, liver, kidney, and omentum.[11] One-third of patients simultaneously have herniation of three abdominal viscera.[11]

Whereas two-thirds of the injuries occur on the left, one-third to 48% of diaphragm ruptures occur on the right side as occasionally bilateral rupture occurs.[1,11,16,17] The site of diaphragm rupture correlates with the site where the blunt force had been sustained. Many right-sided diaphragm ruptures also had right-sided rib fractures, pulmonary contusion, pneumothorax, hemothorax, and liver injuries. This is similar for left-sided ruptures that had associated left-sided injuries.

Patients sustaining a ruptured diaphragm are critically injured. In Beal's series of 39

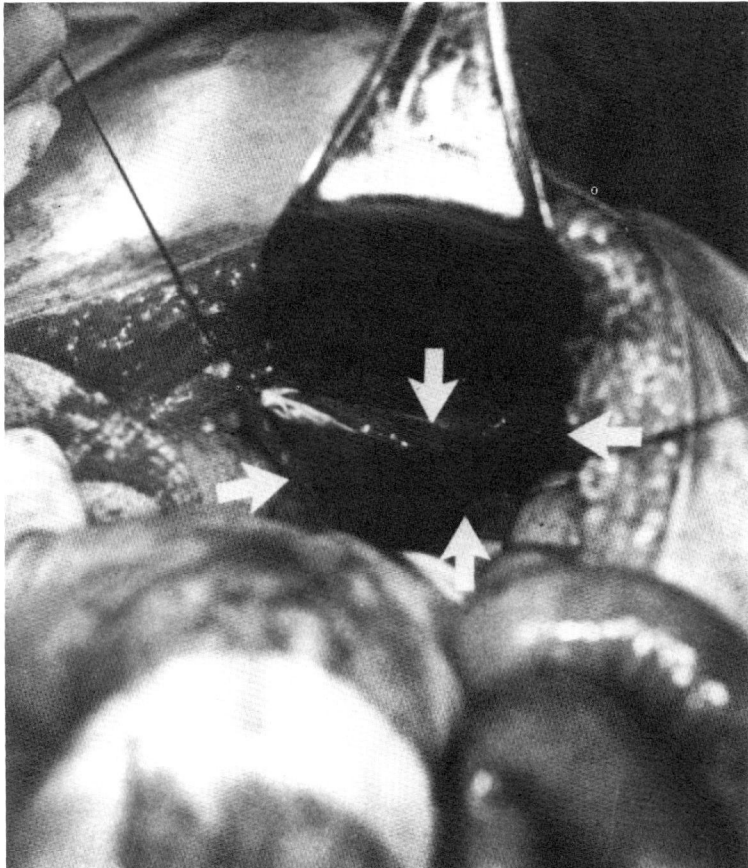

Figure 6–3. Example of typical ruptured diaphragm (*arrows* outline diaphragm rupture).

and Hood's collective review of 261 cases, all but one patient had severe associated injuries.[11,18]

ASSESSMENT OF INJURY AND PREOPERATIVE WORK-UP

The diagnosis of diaphragmatic injury remains elusive. Penetrating diaphragmatic injuries often do not produce early symptoms unless the laceration is large enough to permit immediate herniation of abdominal viscera. If there is not herniation of viscera and no other significant injuries, the diagnosis may be overlooked initially. Most patients with penetrating diaphragmatic wounds have injuries to other organs. Early symptoms and signs are related to the more readily apparent coexisting injuries. It is the trajectory of the penetrating object that should suggest the injury.

The likelihood that a penetrating wound of the diaphragm will be visualized on chest

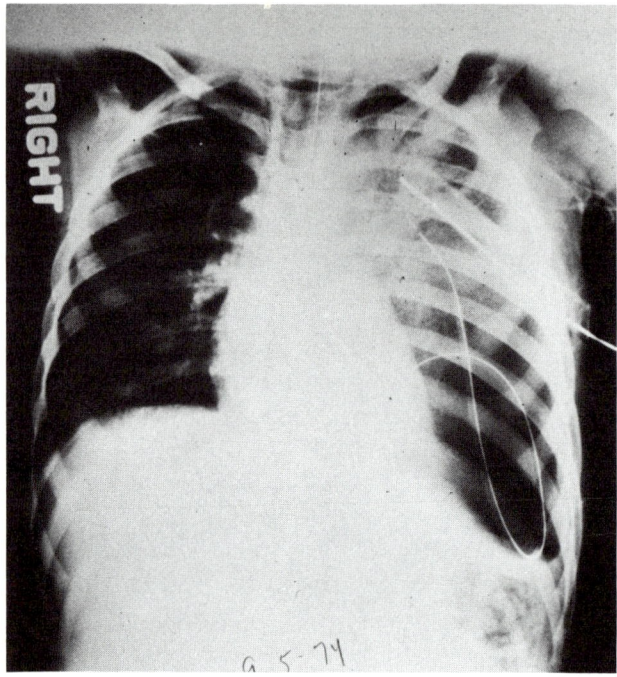

Figure 6–4. The presence of the nasogastric tube in the left pleural space documents the presence of diaphragmatic laceration.

x-ray is small. Careful scrutiny of the admission chest film still affords the best tool for prompt diagnosis but is highly imperfect. Chest roentgenograms are interpreted as normal in approximately 50% of patients with penetrating diaphragm injuries, and the radiographic findings in the remaining are usually limited to a small pneumothorax or hemothorax.[19] Diaphragmatic injury should be suspected when the chest roentgenogram shows an obscured or abnormal diaphragmatic shadow, a radiodensity or radiolucency, or one or more air/fluid levels in the lower lung field. In the acute situation, often only an anteroposterior chest film is initially obtained. Additional erect posteroanterior and lateral views with the affected side to the film may be more revealing.

Diagnosis depends on a high index of suspicion and careful scrutiny of the chest roentgenogram. Repeated evaluation hours and days after injury may be necessary to discern injury in those patients who did not originally have exploratory operation.

Falsely negative peritoneal lavage has been noted in 12% to 40% of patients with penetrating diaphragmatic injuries.[11,19,20,21] Classic diagnostic peritoneal lavage criteria do not rule out an isolated diaphragmatic injury. This is because the laceration is promptly tamponaded by an abdominal viscus and the bleeding that did occur will be sucked into the chest.

In most patients the diagnosis of diaphragmatic injury is established during an emergency laparotomy or a thoracotomy for suspected injuries to other organs. During such exploratory procedures, the diaphragm should be thoroughly inspected and palpated for an injury before the procedure is concluded.

Penetrating injuries to the diaphragm can be especially treacherous because they are frequently missed and enlarge over time. Intestinal obstruction and strangulation subsequently occur, usually in 85% of cases by 3 years.[18,22] When patients develop gastrointestinal obstruction, the herniated viscus usually expands rapidly and the diagnosis can be made from the erect posteroanterior and lateral chest x-ray films.

The diagnosis of blunt diaphragm rupture also remains elusive. In our series of 39 ruptures seen over 13 months, the diagnosis was not made preoperatively in 69% of cases and was again missed at laparotomy in two cases.[11]

Patients who sustain a ruptured diaphragm from blunt trauma are severely injured. Half of the patients in our series arrived in the emergency room in profound shock. The vast majority, 81%, manifested respiratory embarrassment, often necessitating early intubation with ventilatory support. The only consistent findings in this group of patients were the respiratory distress and decreased breath sounds. Neither is sensitive nor specific for diaphragm injury. The diaphragm rupture was obscured by other coexisting and life-threatening injuries. Of the 37 chest roentgenograms obtained on admission, one was interpreted as normal and 24, although not normal, were not pathognomonic of a diaphragm injury. This includes nine patients in whom abdominal viscera were found in the chest at the time of operation. Roentgenographic findings included indistinctness and/or elevation of a hemidiaphragm, marked lower lobar atelectasis or collapse, air/fluid levels, hemothorax, pneumothorax, pulmonary contusion, and/or multiple rib fractures (Figs. 6–5 and 6–6).

Numerous methods to diagnose diaphragm injury have been proposed. These include chest roentgenography in combination with fluoroscopy, arteriography for persistent bleeding from chest tubes, pneumoperitoneum, upper and lower gastrointestinal barium

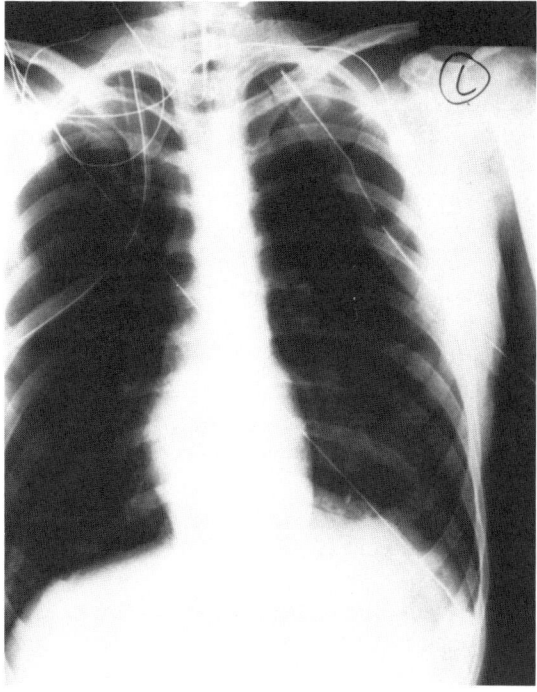

Figure 6–5. Roentgenogram showing left hemidiaphragm rupture.

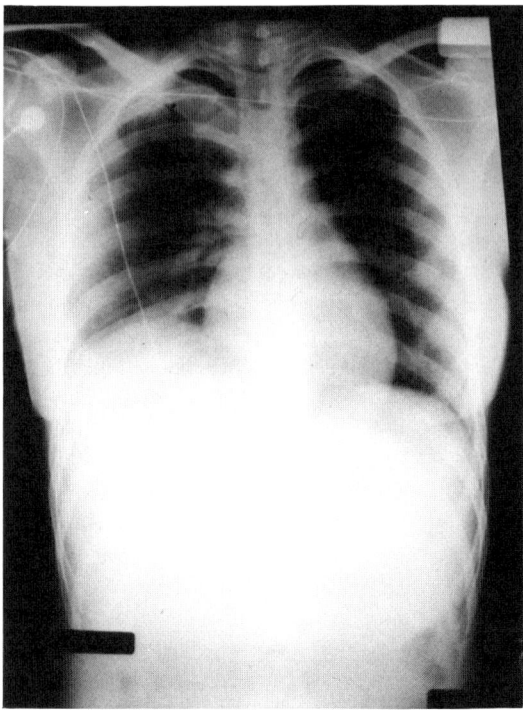

Figure 6–6. Roentgenogram showing right hemidiaphragm rupture.

studies, cholangiography, and liver–spleen scans.[11,23–28] None of these, however, have proven to be entirely reliable. These additional diagnostic modalities, although innovative, are of limited value in the early assessment of the critically injured trauma patient.

Although often not pathognomonic, chest roentgenography remains the best screening examination and is more often diagnostic in blunt trauma than penetrating trauma. Retrospective review of admission chest roentgenograms "revealed that the injured diaphragm was consistently abnormal." The hemidiaphragm often could not be visualized in its entire course. The absence of the entire hemidiaphragmatic shadow should raise suspicion for a diaphragm injury. The lack of a normal diaphragmatic shadow should lead to further evaluation, resulting in the diagnosis or exclusion of a diaphragm injury.

Peritoneal lavage is unreliable in establishing the diagnosis of blunt diaphragm rupture. It was falsely negative in 60% of our patients who underwent lavage. This injury is consistently missed with lavage.[11,24,28–30]

The most consistent way to diagnose a ruptured diaphragm acutely is at laparotomy. An exploratory laparotomy or thoracotomy for trauma should always include inspection and palpation of both hemidiaphragms.

PREOPERATIVE PREPARATION

Patients with diaphragmatic injury require resuscitation and evaluation, including airway control and ventilation as well as restoration of circulation. This includes stopping external hemorrhage and providing volume restoration. Military antishock trousers should not be applied to those patients suspected of having diaphragmatic damage. Dramatic deterioration in cardiopulmonary function, when the trousers were used, has been reported.[31,32] Hypotensive patients should be resuscitated with volume, not with the military antishock trousers, when the status of the diaphragm is unknown. A nasogastric tube should be inserted in any patient in whom there is a possibility of diaphragmatic injury.

The injuries associated with the blunt diaphragm rupture usually take priority. Massive herniation of abdominal contents into the pleural cavity or pericardial sac can cause cardiorespiratory embarrassment or luxation of the heart. When this occurs, the diaphragmatic injury requires urgent attention. Otherwise, the diaphragm injury should be repaired after the other intraabdominal organs have received appropriate operative care.

TREATMENT

The treatment for diaphragmatic injury is repair of the laceration as soon as possible, to avoid progressive respiratory embarrassment, thoracic contamination, and possible future complications from herniation of the abdominal viscera into the thoracic cavity.

We use a transabdominal approach for repair of acute diaphragm injuries, resulting from either penetrating or blunt injuries. This approach is used because of the high incidence of associated abdominal injuries and the fact that herniated organs are more easily reduced.

In those infrequent penetrating diaphragm injuries with associated hemothorax massive enough to require operative intervention, a thoracotomy is performed. In this instance, the hole in the diaphragm can be enlarged, permitting limited abdominal exploration. The diaphragm can be repaired from the thorax. Laparotomy may also be indicated to rule out or treat associated abdominal injuries.

Patients with combined gastric and diaphragm lacerations from penetrating trauma, in our experience, have a high incidence of subsequent empyema formation. This is because many patients at the time of injury have a full stomach. The penetrating weapon simultaneously lacerates the diaphragm and adjacent stomach. The negative intrathoracic pressure facilitates drainage of gastric contents into the thoracic cavity. Simple closed thoracostomy has been insufficient to drain the particulate material. In these cases with concomitant gastric and diaphragm laceration we routinely perform a limited anterior thoracotomy for copious lavage of the pleural cavity. The thorax is drained with a chest tube. The patient is started on therapeutic antibiotics.

Laparotomy is also the operative approach for blunt diaphragm rupture, including patients with a hemothorax.[11,33] In most patients who undergo emergency thoracotomy for massive hemothorax, the source of blood loss is most often found in the abdomen, usually from a ruptured spleen or liver. With initial laparotomy, a potentially treatable lesion such as a ruptured spleen or liver can be immediately dealt with, controlling the life-threatening hemorrhage and thus improving the patient's chances for survival. Should the decision be made to perform a thoracotomy first, valuable time is lost. The principle should be to look for and deal with the salvageable injuries first. Massive hemothorax from blunt great-vessel rupture or pulmonary hilar injury is exceedingly rare in a patient arriving alive and is often fatal at the scene. The rare bilateral diaphragm injury also will not be missed with this transabdominal approach.

Diaphragm tears are repaired in the following manner. The enteric organs are returned to their normal position. If reduction is difficult because of the negative intrathoracic pressure, the laceration is extended in a radial direction to avoid injury to the phrenic nerve. The diaphragm can be repaired with #1 or #0 absorbable or permanent sutures placed in a simple running fashion. Each stitch should include 1 to 2 cm of muscle on each side. If the muscle is actively bleeding, a running, locking stitch is used for hemostasis. Before completion of the repair, a Red Robinson catheter is passed into the pleural cavity for aspiration. The catheter is removed under suction at the completion of the repair. A chest tube, if not previously placed, is usually not necessary if there has been no associated abdominal viscus injury.

Because of difficulty in diagnosis, a diaphragmatic injury may not become evident until days to years after the injury. In this circumstance, the operation is done solely for diaphragmatic repair. A delayed repair within the first few days can be done via laparotomy or thoracotomy. On the right side, a thoracotomy is preferable. After about 7 to 10 days, there may be intrathoracic adhesions of the herniated abdominal organs. The preferable approach is a thoracotomy on the affected side, but simultaneous abdominal approach is often necessary. Dissection of intrathoracic adhesions can vex even an experienced surgeon. Gangrenous viscera may require resection or proximal colostomy. Usually the edges of the diaphragmatic rent can be approximated. Long-standing hernias may on a rare occasion necessitate the use of Dacron, Marlex, or other prosthetic material.[34,35]

POSTOPERATIVE MANAGEMENT

Meticulous attention to vigorous pulmonary toilet is required. Almost all patients with blunt diaphragm rupture have an associated pulmonary contusion. In addition, diaphragm dysmotility, a direct result of muscle injury and associated phrenic nerve contusion, contributes to and exacerbates the pulmonary problems encountered. Diaphragmatic action accounts for two-thirds of the tidal volume in the standing position.[36] Paralysis on one side results in a 25% to 50% decrease in pulmonary function.[37] Lobar collapse occurs frequently in the blunt diaphragm rupture patient. The collapse often does not respond to vigorous pulmonary toilet, necessitating bronchoscopy for reexpansion.

COMPLICATIONS

There is around a 40.5% mortality rate associated with blunt diaphragm rupture.[11] This is consistent with the mortality rate after blunt thoracic trauma.[38] Most deaths occur in the acute injury period. The deaths are due to associated injuries and not a result of the ruptured diaphragm. The majority, around 82%, of patients have complications, the most common being pulmonary. The high incidence of complications is related to the associated injuries.

The complications in penetrating diaphragm injury are due primarily to the associated injuries.

REFERENCES

1. Schneider CF. Traumatic diaphragmatic hernia. *Am J Surg*. 1956; 91:290.
2. Hamby WB. *The Case Reports and Autopsy Records of Ambrose Paré*. Springfield, Ill: Charles C Thomas; 1960.

3. Allison PR. In: *Gibbon's Surgery of the Chest*. 2nd ed. Philadelphia: WB Saunders; 1969.
4. Morgagni GB. *Seats and Causes of Diseases*. Zellts 54, Monograph on Hernia of the Diaphragm; 1769.
5. Bowditch HI. Diaphragmatic hernia. *Buggalo Med J*. 1853; 9:1,65.
6. Grage TB, MacLean LD, Cambell GS. Traumatic rupture of the diaphragm, a report of 26 cases. *Surgery*. 1959; 46:669.
7. Wren HB, Texada PJ, Krementz ET. Traumatic rupture of the diaphragm. *J Trauma*. 1962; 2:117.
8. Besson A, Saegesser F. *Color Atlas of Chest Trauma and Associated Injuries*. Oradell, NJ: Medical Economics Books; 1983; 1.
9. Patten BM. *Foundations of Embryology*. 2nd ed. New York: McGraw-Hill Book Co; 1964.
10. Cevese PG, Becchioni R, D'Amico DF. Postoperative chylothorax. *J Thorac Cardiovasc Surg*. 1975; 69(6):966.
11. Beal SL, McKennan M. Blunt diaphragm rupture: a morbid injury. *Arch Surg*. 1988; 123:828–832.
12. Waldschmidt ML, Laws HL. Injuries of the diaphragm. *J Trauma*. 1980; 20:587–592.
13. Drews JA, Mercer EC, Benfield JR. Acute diaphragmatic injuries. *Ann Thorac Surg*. 1973; 16:67–77.
14. Marchand P. A study of the forces productive of gastrooesophageal regurgitation and herniation through the diaphragmatic hiatus. *Thorax*. 1957; 12:189–194.
15. Symbas PN, Vlasis SE, Hatcher CR Jr. Blunt and penetrating diaphragmatic injuries with or without herniation of organs into the chest. *Ann Thorac Surg*. 1986; 42:158.
16. Mansour KA, Clements JL, Hatcher CR Jr, et al. Diaphragmatic hernia caused by trauma: experience with 35 cases. *Am Surg*. 1975; 41:97.
17. Meads CE, Carroll SE, Pitt DF. Traumatic rupture of the right hemidiaphragm. *J Trauma*. 1977; 17:797.
18. Hood RM. Traumatic diaphragmatic hernia. *Ann Thorac Surg*. 1971; 12:311–324.
19. Miller OL, Bennett EV, Root HD, et al. Management of penetrating and blunt diaphragmatic injury. *J Trauma*. 1984; 24:403.
20. Aronoff RJ, Reynolds J, Thal ER. Evaluation of diaphragmatic injuries. *Am J Surg*. 1982; 144:671.
21. Thal ER. Evaluation of peritoneal lavage and local exploration in lower chest and abdominal stab wounds. *J Trauma*. 1977; 17:642.
22. Pomerantz M, Rodgers BN, Sabiston DC Jr. Traumatic diaphragmatic hernia. *Surgery*. 1968; 64:529.
23. Ward RE, Flyn TC, Clark WP. Diaphragmatic disruption secondary to blunt abdominal trauma. *J Trauma*. 1981; 21:35–38.
24. Brooks JW. Blunt traumatic rupture of the diaphragm. *Ann Thorac Surg*. 1978; 26:199–203.
25. McElwee TB, Myers RT, Pennell TC. Diaphragmatic rupture from blunt trauma. *Am Surg*. 1984; 50:143–149.
26. Ebert PA, Gaertner RA, Zuidema GP. Traumatic diaphragmatic hernia. *Surg Gynecol Obstet*. 1967; 125:59–65.
27. Fallazadeh H, Mays ET. Disruption of the diaphragm by blunt trauma: new dimensions of diagnosis. *Am Surg*. 1975; 41:337–341.
28. Soderstrom CA, DuPriest RW, Cowley RA. Pitfalls of peritoneal lavage in blunt abdominal trauma. *Surg Gynecol Obstet*. 1980; 151:513–518.
29. Brotman S, Clayton HS, Cowley RA. False negative peritoneal lavage. *Am Surg*. 1981; 47:309–310.
30. Freeman T, Fischer RP. The inadequacy of peritoneal lavage in diagnosing acute diaphragmatic rupture. *J Trauma*. 1976; 16:538–542.
31. Dronen SC. Disorders of the chest wall and diaphragm. *Emerg Med Clin North Am*. 1983; 1(2):449–468.
32. Maull KI, Krahwinkel DJ, Rozycki GS, et al. Cardiopulmonary effects of the pneumatic anti-shock garment on swine with diaphragmatic hernia. *Surg Gynecol Obstet*. 1986; 162:17–24.
33. Shuck JM, Schiller WR. Median sternotomy: extension of laparotomy for ruptured right hemidiaphragm. *J Trauma*. 1980; 20:806–808.
34. Juttner F, Pinter H, Kampler D, et al. Triple diaphragmatic rupture with disruption of the pericardium: Pericardial reconstruction by lyophilized dura allograft. *Ann Thorac Surg*. 1984; 38:526–528.
35. Feigenberg Z, Solomon J, Long MJ. Traumatic rupture of the diaphragm: surgical reconstruction with special reference to delayed closure. *J Thorac Cardio Surg*. 1977; 74:249–252.
36. Campbell EJM, Agostini E, Davie JN. *The Respiratory Muscles: Mechanics and Neural Control*. 2nd ed. Philadelphia: WB Saunders; 1970.
37. Hill LD. Injuries of the diaphragm following blunt trauma. *Surg Clin North Am*. 1972; 52:611–624.
38. Schall MA, Fischer RP, Perry JF. The unchanged mortality of flail chest injuries. *J Trauma*. 1979; 19:492.

7
Pelvic Fractures

FELIX BATTISTELLA, M.D.

HISTORY: Fractures of the pelvis must have been known since antiquity, but in modern history their management is first dealt with in the third book by Albucasis (1013–1106).[1] Recognition of the complexity of pelvic fractures was provided by Joseph François Malgaigne in his textbook on fractures in 1847. He stated that the injury that now bears his name occurred from direct forces such as crushing of the pelvis between two carriages or from a wheel passing over this region.[2] The most satisfactory treatment for unstable pelvic fractures was that advocated by Sir Astley Cooper in 1842, who suggested the use of a pelvic sling.[3] This involved placing the patient's pelvis in a stout sling with ropes crossing from the right to be suspended on the left side of the patient and vice versa so that when sufficient weight was applied to the sling to lift the patient off the bed, the sling tended to compress and close the fracture. This method of managing pelvic fractures is still being used.[4,5]

The mortality of pelvic fractures has always been high. Holdsworth first noted in 1948 that retroperitoneal hemorrhage was a major source of mortality and morbidity.[6] The concept of the need for early operative reduction and fixation of these fractures is a modern development. In 1943 Levine reported the first case of open reduction with internal plate and screw fixation of fractures of the pelvis and acetabulum.[7] Although a good result was obtained, this method of treatment was not immediately adopted and was used only sporadically. It was not until the early 1960s when the Judet brothers published their results of open reduction internal fixation, which they had been using routinely since the mid-1950s, that this technique was widely accepted.[8]

Significant pelvic injuries rarely result from penetrating trauma; when these do occur they are inevitably the result of high velocity gunshot wounds.[9] Almost all injuries result from blunt trauma with the most frequent being crushing types of injuries associated with motor vehicle accidents.[10,11] Two-thirds of all pelvic fractures are the result of auto accidents with the incidence of pelvic fractures in fatal motor vehicle accidents being as high as 24%,[11] and approaching 50% for fatal pedestrian accidents.[12] Because of the high incidence of pelvic fractures, an anteroposterior pelvis x-ray should be used in the initial evaluation of all victims of high velocity blunt trauma.[13] The significance of pelvic fractures is more than just the fracture itself. Injury to the anterior elements is associated with a high likelihood of injury to the urethra and bladder and rarely the rectum. Disruption of the posterior bony elements or ligaments requires tremendous force so that the associated soft tissue injuries and accompanying hemorrhage are major. Associated injuries, particularly intraabdominal injuries, are likely and often can be ruled out only by operative intervention.

ANATOMY

The pelvis constitutes a bony box that protects the lower abdomen. It consists of the false pelvis comprising the iliac wings and the true pelvis, which is that portion of the lower abdominal cavity enclosed by the pubic rami anteriorly, the ischium laterally, and the sacrum posteriorly. As a result of this protection, the pelvic peritoneum requires minimal innervation compared to the parietal peritoneum of the upper abdomen. Therefore, the patient with pelvic irritation, whether due to blood or bowel contents, is unable to localize the source of irritation and may feel little, if any, discomfort.

The bony ring of the pelvis comprises the sacrum posteriorly, a large wing or ilium posterolaterally, the pubis anteriorly, and the ischium inferiorly. The ischium, ilium, and pubis merge in the acetabulum. The superior and inferior rami of the pubis pass around the obturator foramen and join at the symphysis pubis. Injuries that disrupt the bony ring, anterior to the acetabulum, are stable fractures since weight is transmitted through the acetabulum to the sacrum and vertebral column. If the acetabulum, the posterior structures, and the sacroiliac joint are intact, the patient can usually bear weight without compromise of healing and with minimal discomfort. Fractures involving the acetabulum and posterior elements, including the sacroiliac joints, often are unstable and must be treated in a non–weight-bearing fashion until bony union or integrity of ligamentous structures has developed.

Blows to the anterior abdominal wall may result in diastasis of the symphysis or fractures of the superior or inferior rami of the pubis and, as indicated previously, may be associated with injuries to the underlying bladder or urethra. The anterior components of the pelvis are relatively fragile and the mass of soft tissue overlying them is minimal; therefore, minimal force is required to produce fractures in this area. These injuries generally have a good prognosis and there is a relatively low incidence of secondary complications once bladder and urethral injuries have been ruled out.

In contrast, the posterior elements of the pelvis are strong, stable structures and violent trauma is required to produce disruption. Therefore, when posterior elements of the pelvis are injured, the associated soft tissue injury is usually considerable. Moreover, major blood vessels and the common iliac arteries and veins overlie the sacroiliac joint, and the internal iliac arteries and veins spread fanwise over the lateral pelvic wall to supply adjacent abdominal organs. These vessels may be disrupted by posterior element injuries and result in major bleeding and large pelvic hematomas. The rectum occupies the hollow of the pelvis and the perineum and levator sling close the true outlet. Injuries that tend to avulse or abduct the thigh violently may produce a tear of the rectum and/or muscles and ligaments of the pelvic outlet. The presence of a perineal laceration in association with pelvic fractures likely indicates that a serious avulsion type of compound fracture is present.

The sacroiliac ligament, the strongest ligament in the body, serves to tie the sacrum onto the anterior components of the pelvic ring. The posterior portion of the ligament resists internal rotation while the anterior complex helps resist pelvic external rotation or springing open of the pelvis.

The iliolumbar ligament enhances the stability of the pelvis and sacrum because its attachment to the lumbar spine prevents cephalad–caudad shift on the hemipelvis. The sacrotuberous ligaments also prevent this instability from vertical shear along with the iliolumbar ligament. The sacrospinous ligaments are arranged at a 90° orientation to the sacrotuberous ligaments and prevent external rotation and springing open of the pelvis along the weaker anterior sacroiliac complex.

The pelvis is usually fractured by direct compression by a force directed in an anteroposterior direction or as a result of a lateral impact. Fractures associated with the former mechanism give rise to injuries of the anterior components of the pelvis with a disruption of the posterior elements such that the pelvis opens by hinging on the posterior elements, resulting in an "open book" fracture of the pelvis. Lateral compression of the pelvis usually leads to fractures of the sacrum associated with concomitant disruption of the anterior elements.

Exceptions to the compression mechanism result from a shearing force to the thigh in which the leg is literally torn from the body; the extreme injury being traumatic hemipelvectomy. These are compound fractures of the pelvis in which there is a perineal tear in association with an unstable fracture, and result from an abduction of the leg most commonly associated with motorcycle accidents. Mortality for these injuries is extremely high because of the problems of hemorrhage, soft tissue injury, and multiple organ damage.[14]

Since the pelvis is a ring structure, in order to have a break in one area it is necessary to have secondary failure elsewhere. A second lesion may not be evident on x-ray because it may be through the ligamentous regions such as the pubic symphysis or the sacroiliac ligament.

Finally, acetabular fractures result from impaction of the femoral head into the acetabulum. Although this group of fractures can be quite complex, they will not be dealt with in this chapter because when isolated they represent a different entity as they are usually not associated with extensive hemorrhage or tissue damage.

FRACTURE TYPES

It is helpful to classify pelvic fractures because this facilitates prognosis, as the pattern of bony injury can predict the severity of injury and extent of soft tissue disruption. Many classification systems of pelvic fractures have been described over the years.[10,15–20] The common thread of these classifications is that unstable pelvic fractures are more likely to have associated pelvic arterial injuries leading to increased blood loss as well as an increased incidence of associated injuries, especially intraabdominal. Patients with "unstable" fractures, defined by Cryer et al. as a diastasis of the pubic symphysis greater than 5 mm or a fracture displacement greater than 5 mm based on an anteroposterior x-ray, had associated intraabdominal injuries and arterial injuries in 45% and 11%, respectively.[15] The classification described by Trunkey et al. is summarized in Table 7–1.[10] Class I injuries are comminuted unstable fractures in which there has been injury to three or more structures of the pelvic ring (Fig. 7–1). Class II injuries are unstable fractures that are often referred to as diametric fractures, as originally described by Malgaigne in 1847. A diametric fracture is

Table 7–1 Classification of Pelvic Fractures

I. Comminuted (crush) injuries
   Three or more major components involved (rami, ilium, acetabulum, sacrum)
   Often unstable
   Usually are combinations II—A, B, C, D
II. Unstable
   A. Diametric fractures with cranial displacement of hemipelvis (Malgaigne, 1847)
   B. Diametric fractures, undisplaced
   C. Open-book (sprung) pelvis
   D. Acetabular fractures
III. Stable
   A. Isolated fractures
   B. Fractures of the pubic rami

any fracture in which the fracture lines extend through the pubic rami or pubic symphysis anteriorly and through either the sacroiliac joint or ilium posteriorly such that there is potential or actual cranial displacement of the hemipelvis (Fig. 7–2). Class II-a is the diametric fracture with displacement. Class II-b is a diametric fracture without displacement. Class II-c is the open-book or sprung pelvis, in which because of anterior disruption, the pelvis is open like a book, hinging on intact posterior structures but with some disruption of these. The classic injury is separation of the pubic symphysis accompanied by separation of the sacroiliac joint, but the open-book injury can also occur with fractures of the pubic rami. When pelvic fractures are associated with perineal or other overlying lacerations, a compound fracture of the pelvis is present. This is most commonly associated with Class II-c injuries. Because of the instability of Class II fractures, persistent hemorrhage is often a problem. To reduce or control hemorrhage, these fractures usually require immobilization by sling, external or internal fixation, or other techniques necessary to hold it stable. Class II-d fractures are fractures of the acetabulum that can be either

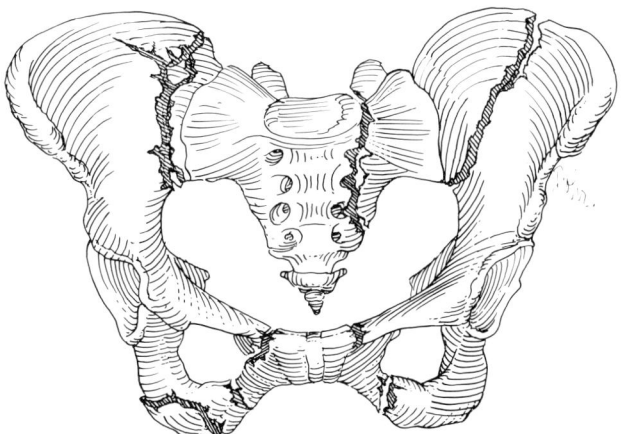

Figure 7–1. Class I injuries—comminuted, unstable fractures.

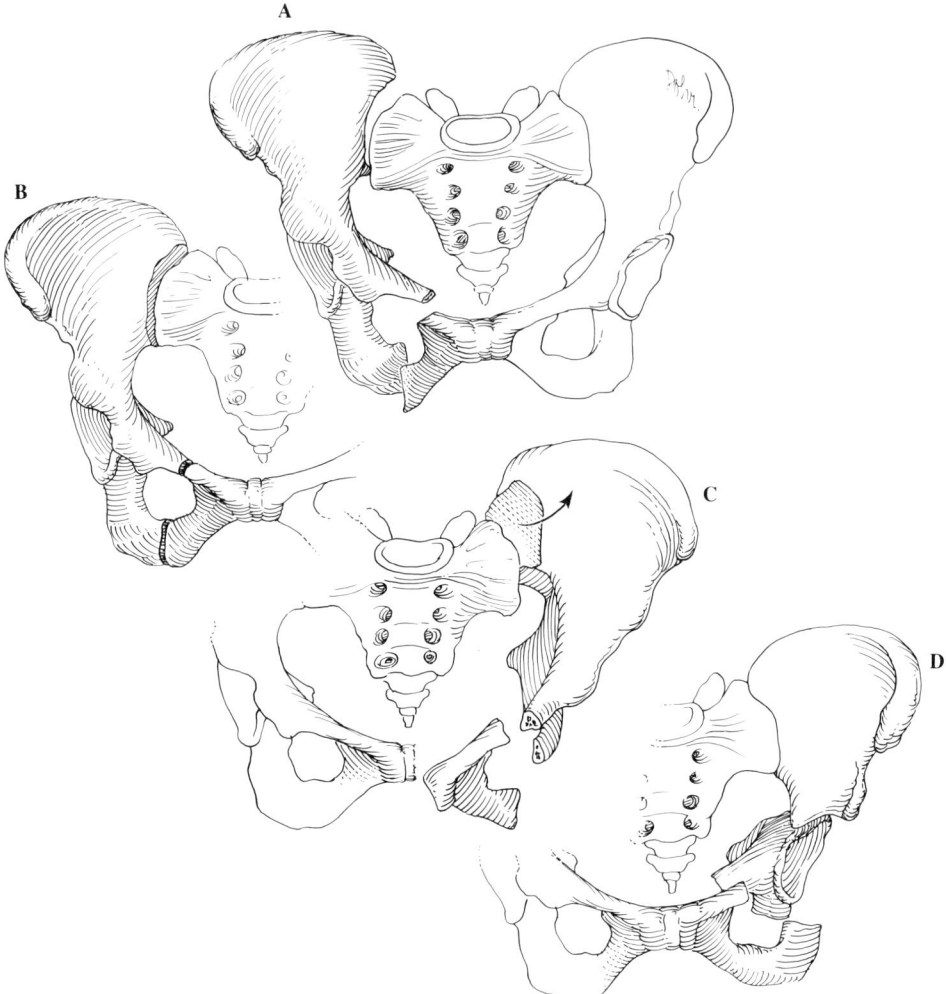

Figure 7–2. Class II diametric fractures—extend through the pubic rami or pubic symphysis. **A:** Displacement; **B:** undisplaced; **C:** open-hook; **D:** acetabular.

displaced or undisplaced. The displaced fractures are accompanied by a simple central dislocation of the femoral head. Posterior dislocation of the femoral head with fracture of the acetabulum may also be present. These fractures usually require longitudinal and horizontal traction to reduce the fracture and maintain adequate position of the acetabular fragments.

Class III fractures are stable fractures that can be divided into two types: the isolated fractures (Type A) and fractures of the pubic rami (Type B) (Fig. 7–3). An example of an isolated fracture is an avulsion fracture of the iliac wing. With the exception of comminuted fractures of the iliac wing, these usually present no problem from the standpoint of either hemorrhage or the need for immobilization. Mortality for Class I and II fractures is 14% to 26%, whereas Class III injuries carry a mortality of 2.2% to 7.2%.[10,21–23]

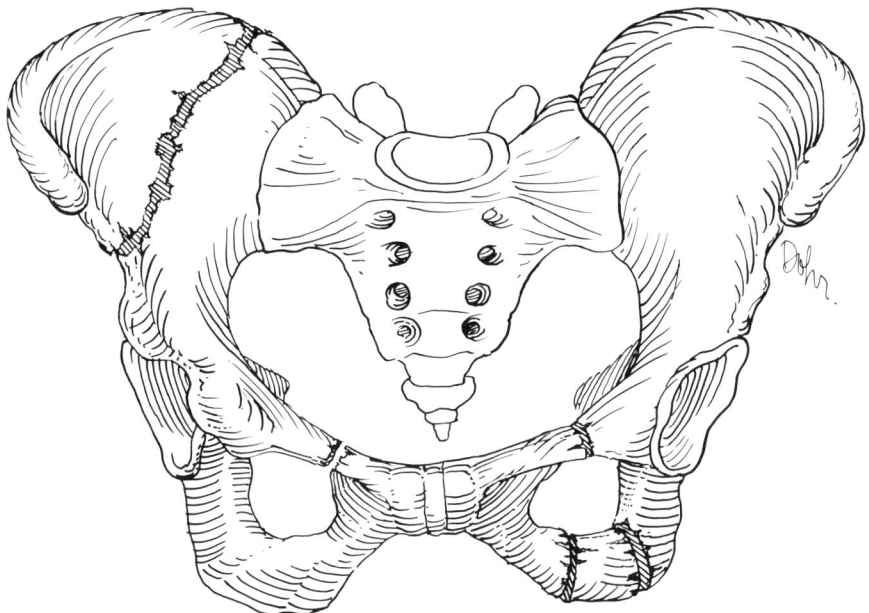

Figure 7–3. Class III fractures—two types of stable fractures.

ASSESSMENT

The patient who may have pelvic injury should be questioned regarding the presence and the location of pain. Pain or discomfort in the sacral area, in the hips on movement of the legs, or lower abdominal discomfort may be a manifestation of sacral, hip, or anterior pelvic injury, respectively.

The examination should be directed at assessing: (1) the integrity of the bony pelvis, (2) presence of vascular injuries, (3) assessment of neurologic systems, and (4) assessment of the skin. The initial maneuver should be to stress the pelvis gently to assess its stability. This can be done by leaning gently with increasing force on the iliac wings. It is not necessary to demonstrate gross movement—the elicitation of pain by posterior or lateral iliac wing compression is evidence of fracture. Next, gentle compression over the symphysis pubis will establish likelihood of anterior pelvic injuries if pain or tenderness is present. The examining hand can then be passed posteriorly under the patient to check for tenderness of the sacral and perisacral regions. Tenderness in this location is presumptive evidence of a posterior disruption. Next, the hip joint should be assessed by grasping the leg and thigh and gently flexing and abducting the thigh. Acetabular injury or hip fracture is likely if there is hip pain with this maneuver. If there is suspicion of injury, appropriate x-rays should be taken to assess the nature of the injury. On occasion, stress films may be required to document posterior instability.

When there is presumptive evidence of pelvic injury, the pelvic organs should be assessed. Gentle rectal examination should be carried out to assess the presence of blood or to verify gross bony deformity. Associated urologic injuries occur in 10% of pelvic fractures.[4] Examination might reveal blood at the urethral meatus indicating an underlying urethral tear. Rectal exam can reveal a high-riding prostate gland or soft, mushy feel anteriorly, consistent with a hematoma and indicating urethral injury as well. The presence of gross hematuria suggests the probability of a bladder injury.

A crucial part of the examination is the neurovascular assessment. The incidence of concomitant injury to pelvic and or lower extremity nerves is high, and at least 5% of patients with pelvic fractures are left with permanent neurologic sequelae.[24]

Nerve injury is especially common when there are fractures of the sacral ala traversing the sacral foramina or the sciatic notch. The presence of a sciatic palsy dictates the need for early reduction and fixation to decompress the sciatic nerve when there is fracture displacement. The sciatic nerve will often be found tented over a displaced fracture fragment or even caught between fracture fragments at a disrupted sciatic notch. A patulous rectal sphincter suggests injury to the lower sacral nerve roots.

Finally, it is important to assess the status of the skin as this is often forgotten or ignored. The patient should be log-rolled to inspect both the spine and the sacral region to look for areas of abrasion, laceration, or contusion. The sacral area overlying a pelvic fracture is often contused and hemorrhagic. The soft tissues are often sheared from the bone by the force of injury; as a result, there is danger of skin breakdown and sloughing.

Most importantly, the cardiovascular status should be assessed and serial hematocrits followed. Pelvic fractures, depending on their nature, can be associated with extensive blood loss and even exsanguination. Retroperitoneal hematomas are common particularly after posterior element fractures. These result from lacerations of major branches of the internal iliac artery or vein and, more rarely, lacerations of the iliac artery or vein itself. If the patient is unstable, laparotomy should be carried out to assess the status of intraperitoneal bleeding and to verify the magnitude of the retroperitoneal hematoma. In the stable patient diagnostic peritoneal lavage should be performed followed by urgent laparotomy if grossly positive. Stable patients with microscopically positive lavages should also undergo exploration as 50% may have associated intraabdominal injuries[25]; however, time may permit obtaining a cystogram and possibly a computer tomographic (CT) scan of the head if indicated before laparotomy (Fig. 7–4). False positive results obtained with peritoneal lavage can be reduced by performing the lavage supraumbilically, which reduces the likelihood of entering the retroperitoneal hematoma.

Immediate stabilization of pelvic fractures will, more than any other factor, control ongoing hemorrhage and, therefore, in major pelvic fractures, prompt orthopedic consultation should be obtained.

IMAGING

An anteroposterior pelvic film is part of routine assessment of any victim of blunt trauma when multiple injuries are present. This, in conjunction with the physical examination, is extremely accurate in establishing the presence or absence of a pelvic fracture. Anterior element fractures are relatively benign injuries but a posterior element fracture carries serious risk of morbidity and mortality and benefits from early, if not immediate, diagnosis and stabilization.

If a fracture is identified or strongly suspected, a Judet view taken at 45° of obliquity bilaterally is often helpful. It is particularly useful in diagnosing acetabular fractures but also can further delineate the pattern of a pelvic fracture. The iliac oblique view is

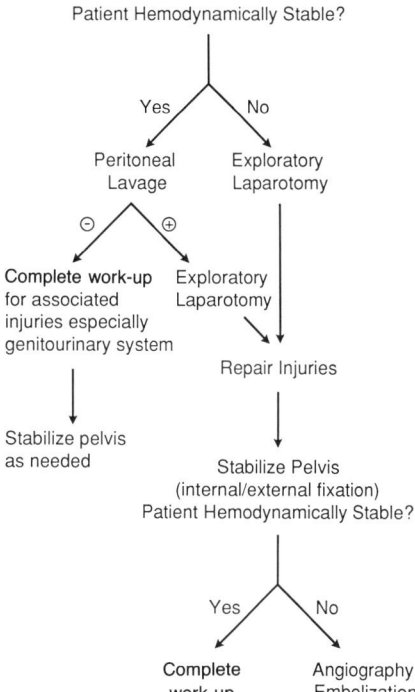

Figure 7–4. Management of pelvic trauma.

optimal for showing the posterior column and the obturator oblique shows the anterior column of the pelvis. These are often helpful supplemental films. When a sacroiliac complex injury is suspected, sacroiliac films can be helpful to compare widening of the site of presumed injury with the contralateral joint. The CT scan is helpful and will confirm the amount of sacroiliac joint widening and can be used as the definitive test in cases of questionable widening on plain films. Other important films for evaluating the stability of the sacroiliac joints are the pelvic inlet and outlet views. Since the sacrum is positioned obliquely in the body, fractures of sacroiliac area can be significantly displaced but the displacement may not be demonstrated on the anteroposterior view.

Significant pelvic instability is present when there is sacroiliac joint widening of greater than 1 cm, a pubic diastasis separation of greater than 2.5 cm, a sacral or iliac fracture showing a displacement greater than 0.5 cm, or a vertical shear fracture with cephalad or caudad migration greater than 0.5 cm.

If there is a question of instability based on examination of the plain films, and in particular, if attempts at weight-bearing are associated with extreme pain, stress films may be appropriate. Occasionally push-pull stress films carried out under anesthesia may be necessary. The pelvic outlet view is obtained with the assistant maximally pushing the foot on the injured side with actively directed force while pulling on the foot on the uninjured side to provide counter-resistance. The second film is obtained after reversing the maneuver. Open-book pelvic fractures can be evaluated and emphasized by frogging the leg into a figure-4 position and applying additional vertical direction force on the bent knee to rotate the hip externally. An anteroposterior film will document the amount of opening produced. The corresponding reduction film can be taken by an anteroposterior film with the patient in the later decubitus position. The force of gravity then acts to reduce the fracture. When the two films are compared, changes document the lesion.

Indications that a urethral injury may be present, such as blood at the meatus or a high-riding or mushy prostate mandate evaluation with a retrograde urethrogram before insertion of an indwelling bladder catheter to prevent further disruption of a partially transected urethra.

If a bladder injury is suspected, a cystogram with anteroposterior, lateral, and postvoid views should be obtained. Intraperitoneal bladder ruptures require repair via a laparotomy, whereas retroperitoneal ruptures can be managed nonoperatively with decompression of the bladder and a follow-up cystogram in 10 to 14 days.

PREOPERATIVE PREPARATION AND INDICATION FOR OPERATION

Pelvic fractures in themselves do not necessarily require operation. A stable fracture with no involvement of the urethra, bladder, or rectum can be safely observed. A problem arises when the patient's hematocrit falls or he/she becomes unstable from a cardiovascular standpoint. This is far more common with unstable pelvic fractures but can result from any form of pelvic fracture. Under these circumstances it may be appropriate to conduct an exploratory laparotomy and to verify that the hemorrhage is confined to the pelvic retroperitoneum. Peritoneal lavage or CT scan may be helpful but in the face of continued hemorrhage a last-analysis judgment is required since both of these tests can be negative when there is ongoing bleeding that is benefitted by operative control. Moreover, there can be disruption of major iliac arteries or veins with catastrophic retroperitoneal bleeding or bleeding into the pelvic cavity that requires surgical treatment.

When the patient's injuries are confined to the pelvis, it is appropriate to observe the patient, monitor hematocrits, and make decisions based on the magnitude of blood loss and the nature of the pelvic injury. Ongoing blood loss in a stable fracture dictates laparotomy to rule out associated injury since stable fractures are not necessarily associated with major bleeding in themselves.

Although continued bleeding is rare after pelvic stabilization, should this occur arteriography should be carried out and embolization used to treat small vessel arterial bleeding. Although larger vessels can be involved, arterial injuries after blunt pelvic trauma usually involve the superior gluteal arteries.[26] The latter can be treated with embolization at the time of arteriography, whereas large vessel injury should be treated by proximal arterial control and repair. Preoperative preparation of patients with unstable pelvic fractures should include early transfusions, with the use of universal donor blood in the emergency and operating rooms before the availability of type-specific or fully cross-matched blood in patients who are hemodynamically unstable.

TREATMENT

The specific management of the various fractures of the pelvis are described in a companion volume on extremity trauma. Various maneuvers used are anterior plating for separation of the symphysis pubis, screws and plates for posterior sacral stabilization, and external fixation for certain unstable posterior element fractures and comminuted fractures. Occasionally, traction is the only initial treatment possible for some complex acetabular fractures. Stable fractures should be treated with early mobilization and ambulation as tolerated. This will minimize morbidity associated with immobilization.

Unstable pelvic fractures in patients who are hemodynamically stable should be externally/internally fixed within the first 12 to 24 hr because the risk of developing multiorgan system failure can be reduced by early reduction and rigid fixation of fractures.[27,28] Use of external pelvic fixators should be limited to fixation of pelvic ring fractures with intact posterior sacral ligaments. The external fixators are applied to the iliac wings and rely on the sacral ligaments to keep the posterior elements of the pelvis from rotating externally. In patients with disruption of the posterior ligaments, application of the external fixators can lead to increased bleeding due to distraction of the posterior pelvic fragments. These patients should undergo early internal fixation, which can be accomplished via a retroperitoneal approach.[29] Most of the bleeding encountered with this approach is venous and originates from the fracture site; thus, reduction and fixation of the bony injuries lead to control of the hemorrhage. With intraoperative use of a cell saver, early skeletal stabilization may lead to a reduction in the total blood loss and the need for transfusions.[30]

Stabilization of posterior element fractures is the best way to control pelvic bleeding. Thus, if the patient manifests ongoing blood loss, the best treatment is immediate orthopedic stabilization. Before stabilization it may be appropriate to carry out a laparotomy to rule out intraperitoneal bleeding or injury. This can be done under the same anesthetic used for the orthopedic reduction. If there is a large arterial hematoma, the pelvis can be packed and the patient taken to x-ray for arteriography and embolic treatment, or proximal aortic control can be obtained and the vessels then exposed to establish the nature of the injury for direct treatment. Large venous hematomas are best left intact since opening of a venous hematoma may result in uncontrollable bleeding from the proximal pelvic veins. If there is an open pelvic laceration with major venous bleeding, the options available are similar and include packing the pelvis to control the bleeding with removal of the packs 24 hr later or exposure and repair of the venous injury. The latter requires exposure of the external iliac vein at the inguinal ligament, control of the proximal common iliac vein at the cava, and then opening the hematoma to gain control of the internal iliac veins. Such an approach is best undertaken in conjunction with orthopedic surgeons who are prepared to reduce and stabilize the pelvis internally.

The role of the MAST garment should be limited to the prehospital setting where it serves as a splint. Long-term use of the trousers has been associated with numerous complications and they are not as effective at stabilizing the pelvis when compared to external/internal fixation.

Specific fractures that require management by the general surgeon consist of those that are associated with perineal lacerations. These may involve minimal bony injury or near-complete traumatic hemipelvectomies. These types of injury can be challenging even to the most experienced traumatologist. The mortality for open pelvic fractures remains high, with recent series reporting a decrease in mortality from 50% to 30% with the use of early fixation.

Perineal laceration, which occurs in association with pelvic fractures, is an indication for colostomy to avoid and control perineal contamination. Any rectal perforations or vaginal lacerations associated with stable fractures may also benefit from proximal fecal diversion. Using a midline laparotomy, a sigmoid colostomy can be carried out after division of the sigmoid loop at its apex. The proximal bowel should be brought out in the mid–left lower quadrant. The distal end can be brought out of the lower end of the midline wound as a mucous fistula. This permits the insertion of a catheter and gentle irrigation and cleansing of the distal rectal segment. It is essential when this irrigation is carried out that it be done gently using low pressures. The anal sphincter is dilated so that, should any perforation of the rectum be present, contamination is not forced out into the perirectal tissues. Once irrigations are clear, 500 mg of neomycin or kanamycin and 500 mg of erythromycin base are instilled into the rectal segment. The patient should be placed on perioperative systemic antibiotics. The perineal laceration should be irrigated vigorously with saline solution to remove any additional contamination.

Definitive management of the colostomy requires that it either be matured immediately or the bowel simply brought out, the colostomy clamp left in place, and Vaseline gauze placed about the colostomy with the stoma being matured 2 to 4 days later. If the patient has major associated injuries and particularly requires large volumes of fluid and blood, progressive abdominal swelling may result in disruption of the colostomy and therefore initial maturation is often not indicated. After creation of the colostomy, fixation of the bowel to the peritoneum and fascia may be helpful in preventing tension on the ostomy should abdominal distension develop.

TRAUMATIC HEMIPELVECTOMY

Early completion of a traumatic hemipelvectomy may lead to improved survival in patients with such devastating injuries. Thanks to rapid transport and resuscitation en route, an occasional patient who has suffered an avulsion of the hemipelvis may present to the emergency department alive. In many instances the magnitude of the pelvic separation may not be obvious as apparent integrity may be provided by skin alone. Ultimately, because of bleeding problems or subsequent complications, investigation of the fracture site may reveal essentially complete hemipelvic separation.

There are three indications for completion of a hemipelvectomy. These consist of (1) uncontrollable hemorrhage, (2) loss of limb circulation and/or neurologic function, and (3) development of uncontrollable pelvic sepsis.[14]

Occasionally despite attempts at stabilization, hemorrhage may be uncontrollable. When near amputation is present, bleeding may often be controlled only by exposure of the entire area of the injury requiring removal of the leg and hemipelvis. The second indication exists when the patient has had prolonged limb ischemia and/or no neurologic function. Attempts at revascularizing limbs in which there has been sciatic nerve disruption will not result in a functional limb and, moreover, reperfusion when the limb has been ischemic for more than 4 to 6 hr may either result in DIC or overwhelming septic complications.

Finally, septic complications such as necrotizing infections or Clostridial infections may supervene, requiring completion of the amputation. Usually the injury has resulted in avulsion of the internal iliac vessels such that the gluteal flap is nonviable. As a result, no immediate coverage may be readily available. In this instance, the wound can be packed and a pressure dressing applied. If there is a viable gluteal flap, this can be used to close the wound (Fig. 7–5); however, even these flaps will often necrose and slough. As local muscle flaps are usually unavailable, coverage of these large hemipelvectomy defects is

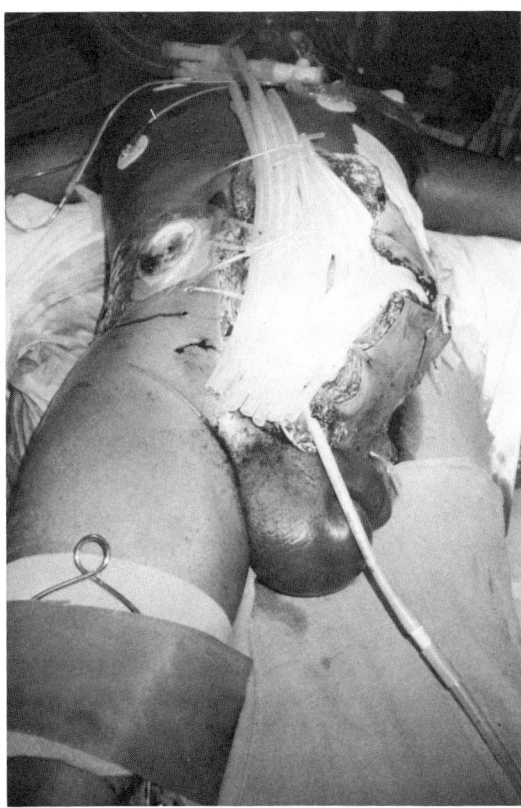

Figure 7–5. Traumatic hemipelvectomy. The abdominal wound has been left open. The bowel has been contained by silastic tubing placed under silastic retention sutures. A gluteal flap has been used to partially close the wound.[14]

often difficult, necessitating various types of rotational or free myocutaneous flaps. Rarely skin grafting alone may be appropriate (Fig. 7–6).

Colostomy and cystostomy are usually necessary with the traumatic hemipelvectomy because these organs are usually injured in parallel and gross incontinence is common. Moreover, the risk of contamination of the wound itself dictates the need for diversion of the fecal stream.

POSTOPERATIVE MANAGEMENT

Management of the patient postoperatively will be dictated by the severity of the pelvic injury and by the presence or absence of associated injuries. In closed injuries where there has been no contamination, a 24-hr antibiotic coverage started preoperatively and continued postoperatively is all that is indicated. For open fractures, broad spectrum coverage should be continued for at least 3 to 4 days. With major injuries such as hemipelvectomy, mechanical ventilation should be continued and the patient monitored for 24 hr anticipating possible development of the respiratory distress syndrome. If the patient is able to ventilate and oxygenate spontaneously, extubation can be carried out the following day.

The patient should be monitored in all instances for bleeding complications with

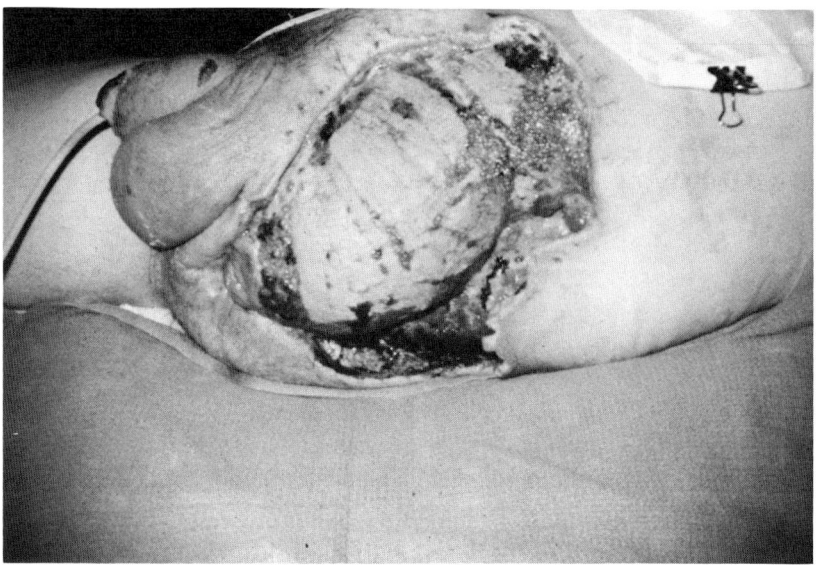

Figure 7–6. Late maturation of a hemipelvectomy wound in which a split thickness skin graft has been used to close the wound partially. A latissimus flap was subsequently used for definitive closure.[14]

hematocrits being followed every 4 hr, and transfusion should be used as necessary to maintain the hematocrit between 25 and 30. Urine output should be monitored to assure adequate cardiac output and perfusion.

COMPLICATIONS

Pelvic fractures are complicated by respiratory failure, infection, and thromboembolic problems. If the patient is extubated early because the nature of the injuries appears minimal, respiratory function should be monitored closely. As long as respirations are slow, full, and even, at a rate under 25, it can be assumed the patient is doing well. Respiratory rates above 25 and certainly those above 30 require attention to clearing of secretions, positional changes to prevent atelectasis, and repeated blood gas sampling. Serious consideration should be given to endotracheal intubation and mechanical ventilatory support if respiratory rates remain above 30 to 35, even in the presence of reasonably good gases. If the arterial oxygen tension deteriorates, this constitutes an obvious indication for intubation and continued mechanical ventilation.

Infection can complicate any case of major injury. Since posterior pelvic fractures are inevitably associated with extensive soft tissue injury and since septic complications correlate well with the magnitude of soft tissue injury, these patients should be monitored carefully in the postoperative period. Decreased urine output, increased fluid requirements, and other systemic manifestations of sepsis require investigation of any wounds that are present. When infection is documented, open drainage and specific antibiotic therapy are indicated. Specific antibiotics can be selected based on the appearance of the organisms on Gram stain, and modified subsequently based on sensitivity studies. If the patient has open fractures or has had bladder, urethral, or rectal injury and is at high risk for infection, the wound should be monitored and repeatedly cultured.

Patients with posterior element pelvic fractures are at high risk for thromboembolic complications, with the incidence of deep venous thrombosis (DVT) being at least 15% in patients with severe pelvic fractures, as documented by serial duplex ultrasound screening.[31] The extensive soft tissue injury leads to the release of procoagulants and tissue breakdown products into the vascular system. In addition, the iliac veins are often stretched as part of the injury and any intimal lesions present may be the source of lethal embolism. Unless specifically contraindicated by associated fractures, intermittent pneumatic compression stockings should be used on both legs as part of routine postoperative care, particularly if the patient is in a critical care setting. Low dose heparin therapy can be instituted 24 to 48 hr after the injury and is best used by administering an initial intravenous (IV) bolus followed by continuous IV infusion sufficient to produce a slight elevation in the partial thromboplastin time. Should the patient develop clinical evidence suggesting pulmonary embolism, this can be confirmed by angiography or, if no contraindication exists, simply treated by anticoagulation. Thrombophlebitis should be treated with moderate dose heparin, i.e., heparin sufficient to elevate the partial thromboplastin time to approximately two times normal, whereas major pulmonary embolism should be treated initially with high dose heparin while the patient is unstable. This consists of a 20,000-unit bolus and 4000 to 5000 units an hour for at least the first 24 to 48 hr. At this point, if the patient's condition has improved, he/she can be titrated down to more conventional moderate dose heparin. When moderate to high dose heparin is used, the partial thromboplastin time should be monitored to ensure heparin effect. The hematocrit should be monitored every 4 hr and the platelet count at least once a day, the latter because the patient may on rare occasion develop an immunologic response to heparin and develop the white clot syndrome or diffuse intravascular platelet thrombosis. This is recognized by a fall in platelet count to below 50,000. At this point alternate forms of treatment should be considered such as warfarin, dextran, or caval interruption. Prophylactic use of the Greenfield filter should be considered in these high risk patients in whom anticoagulation is contraindicated.[32]

Reported complications after pelvic fractures include entrapment of bowel within the fracture fragments. If unrecognized and untreated early, this can lead to fatal complications.[33] Lumbosacral plexus injuries after pelvic fractures are found in approximately 1% of pelvic fractures.[34] Impotence after pelvic fractures associated with urethral injuries is reported in 32% to 42% of patients.[35] Some pelvic fractures are associated with injuries to the vagina resulting in an open fracture and/or injuries to the female reproductive organs.[36] Chronic pain occurs in approximately 50% of pelvic fractures and it has been shown that good quality sacroiliac joint reduction decreases the incidence.[4,37,38] Neurologic injury manifested by paresthesias and weakness occurs in 32% to 46% of severe pelvic fractures, especially those associated with sacral ala fractures. Impaired gait after severe pelvic fracture is found in approximately 31% to 41%.

RESULTS

Gunshot wounds to the pelvis present a complex challenge because of the likelihood of concomitant vascular and intestinal injuries; even though the mass of tissue injured may be less and the associated injuries (i.e., head and thoracic injury) fewer than in pelvic fractures due to blunt trauma, mortality for these injuries remains comparable to that for blunt injuries, with a recent series reporting an overall mortality of 12.2%.[39]

Currently the overall mortality rate for pelvic fractures after blunt trauma ranges between 7.6% and 15.5%.[4,16,20,25,40,41] Although pelvic fractures are a marker of injury severity, final outcome is determined by associated injuries as 80% to 90% of patients with severe pelvic fractures have concomitant injuries, with as many as 50% having intraabdominal injuries.[25,41] In a series reported by Burgess et al., closed head injury was present in 66.1%, hemopneumothorax in 16.1%, bladder injury in 6.1%, pulmonary injuries in 9.3%, spleen injuries in 9.3%, retroperitoneal hematoma in 8.6%, bowel injury in 6.8%, liver in 5.6%, renal in 5.6%, diaphragm in 4.3%, urethra in 3.7%, and other in 6.8%.[20]

Recent series of open pelvic fractures by Birolini et al.[42] and Hanson et al.[43] revealed mortality rates of 31.5% and 30%, respectively, when immediate fixation was carried out, compared to previous rates of approximately 50%.[14] This as well as other evidence demonstrates an improved outcome with early reduction and stabilization of pelvic fractures.[30]

Not only is mortality improved, but long-term disability can also be reduced significantly with early (within 24 hr) anatomical reduction and fixation of unstable pelvic fractures. The incidence of chronic pain and of gait impairment after early fixation are reduced from approximately 50% and 36% to 5% and 10%, respectively.[4,44,45]

Best results are achieved with a cooperative effort between the general surgeon and the orthopod to (1) rule out and correct associated injuries, (2) stabilize the pelvis early including internal fixation if needed, and (3) effect aggressive postoperative management with early mobilization.

REFERENCES

1. Garrison FH. *History of Medicine*. 4th ed. Philadelphia: WB Saunders; 1929.
2. Peltier LF. Joseph François Malgaigne and Malgaigne's fracture. *Clin Orthop*. 1980; 151:4.
3. Cooper A. *A Treatise on Dislocations and Fractures of the Joints*. London: Churchill Publishers; 1842.
4. Monahan PRW, Taylor RG. Dislocation and fracture-dislocation of the pelvis. *Injury*. 1975; 6:325.
5. Holm CL. Treatment of pelvic fractures and dislocations. *Clin Orthop*. 1973; 97:97.
6. Holdsworth FW. Dislocation and fracture dislocation of the pelvis. *J Bone Joint Surg*. 1948; 30-B:461.
7. Levine MA. A treatment of central fractures of acetabulum. *J Bone Joint Surg*. 1943; 25:902.
8. Judet R, Judet J, LeTournel E. Fractures of the acetabulum. Classification and surgical approaches for open reduction. *J Bone Joint Surg*. 1964; 46-A:1615.
9. Lucas GL. Missile wounds of the bony pelvis. *J Trauma*. 1970; 10:624.
10. Trunkey DD, Chapman MW, Lim RC Jr, Dunphy JE. Management of pelvic fractures in blunt trauma injury. *J Trauma*. 1974; 14:912.
11. Sevitt S. Fatal road accidents. Injuries, complications, and causes of death in 250 subjects. *Br J Surg*. 1968; 55:481.
12. Braunstein PW, Skudder PA, McCarroll JR, et al. Concealed hemorrhage due to pelvic fractures. *J Trauma*. 1964; 4:832.
13. Shaftan GW. The initial evaluation of the multiple trauma patient. *World J Surg*. 1983; 7:19.
14. Beal SL, Blaisdell FW. Traumatic hemipelvectomy: a catastrophic injury. *J Trauma*. 1989; 29:1346.
15. Cryer HM, Miller FB, Evers BM, et al. Pelvic fracture classification: correlation with hemorrhage. *J Trauma*. 1988; 28:973.
16. Dalal SA, Burgess AR, Siegel JH, et al. Pelvic fracture in multiple trauma: classification by mechanism is key to pattern of organ injury, resuscitative requirements, and outcome. *J Trauma.*. 1989; 29:981.
17. Tile M. *Fractures of the Pelvis and Acetabulum*. Baltimore: Williams & Wilkins; 1984.
18. Looser KG, Crombie HD Jr. Pelvic fractures: an anatomic guide to severity of injury. *Am J Surg*. 1976; 132:638.

19. Pennal GF, Tile M, Waddell JP, Garside H. Pelvic disruption: assessment and classification. *Clin Orthop*. 1980; 151:12.
20. Burgess AR, Eastridge BJ, Young JWR, et al. Pelvic ring disruptions: effective classification system and treatment protocols. *J Trauma*. 1990; 30:848.
21. Conolly WB, Hedberg EA. Observations on fractures of the pelvis. *J Trauma*. 1969; 9:104.
22. Rothenberger DA, Fischer RP, Strate RG, et al. The mortality associated with pelvic fractures. *Surgery*. 1978; 84:356.
23. Flint LM Jr, Brown A, Richardson JD, Polk HC. Definitive control of bleeding from severe pelvic fractures. *Am Surg*. 1979; 189:709.
24. Dickinson D, Lifeso R, McBroom R, Tile M. Disruptions of the pelvic ring. *J Bone Joint Surg*. 1982; 64-B:635.
25. Flint L, Babikian G, Anders M, et al. Definitive control of mortality from severe pelvic fracture. *Ann Surg*. 1990; 211:703.
26. Smith K, Ben-Menachem Y, Duke JH, Hill GC. The superior gluteal: an artery at risk in blunt pelvic trauma. *J Trauma*. 1976; 16:273.
27. Seibel R, LaDuca J, Hassett J, et al. Blunt multiple trauma (ISS 36), femur traction, and the pulmonary failure-septic state. *Ann Surg*. 1985; 202:283.
28. Riska EB, von Bonsdorff H, Hakkinen S, et al. Prevention of fat embolism by early internal fixation of fractures in patients with multiple injuries. *Injury*. 1976; 8:110.
29. Simpson LA, Waddell JP, Leighton RK, et al. Anterior approach and stabilization of the disrupted sacroiliac joint. *J Trauma*. 1987; 27:1332.
30. Latenser BA, Gentilello LM, Tarver AA, et al. Improved outcome with early fixation of skeletally unstable pelvic fractures. *J Trauma*. 1991; 31:28.
31. White RH, Goulet JA, Bray TJ, et al. Deep-vein thrombosis after fracture of the pelvis: assessment with serial duplex-ultrasound screening. *J Bone Joint Surg*. 1990; 72-A:495.
32. Golueke PJ, Garrett WV, Thompson JE, et al. Interruption of the vena cava by means of the Greenfield filter: expanding the indications. *Surgery*. 1988; 103:111.
33. Ashai F, Ortho MS, Mam MK, et al. Ileal entrapment as a complication of fractured pelvis. *J Trauma*. 1988; 28:551.
34. Patterson FP, Morton KS. Neurologic complications of fractures and dislocations of the pelvis. *Surg Gynecol Obstet*. 1961; 112:702.
35. Ellison M, Timberlake GA, Kerstein MD. Impotence following pelvic fracture. *J Trauma*. 1988; 28:695.
36. Doman AN, Hoekstra DV. Pelvic fracture associated with severe intra-abdominal gynecologic injury. *J Trauma*. 1988; 28:118.
37. Henderson RC. The long term results of nonoperatively treated major pelvic disruptions. *J Orthop Trauma*. 1989; 3:41.
38. Kellem JF. The role of external fixation in pelvic disruptions. *Clin Orthop*. 1989; 241:66.
39. Duncan AO, Phillips TF, Scalea TM, et al. Management of transpelvic gunshot wounds. *J Trauma*. 1989; 29:1335.
40. Evers BM, Cryer HM, Miller FB. Pelvic fracture hemorrhage. *Arch Surg*. 1989; 124:422.
41. Poole GV, Ward EF, Muakkassa FF, et al. Pelvic fracture from major blunt trauma. *Ann Surg*. 1991; 213:532.
42. Birolini D, Steinman E, Utiyama EM, Arooyo AA. Open pelviperineal trauma. *J Trauma*. 1990; 30:492.
43. Hanson PB, Milne JC, Chapman MW. Open fractures of the pelvis. *J Bone Joint Surg*. 1991; 73-B:325.
44. Raf L. Double vertical fractures of the pelvis. *Acta Chir Scand*. 1966; 131:298.
45. Slatis P, Karaharju EO. External fixation of unstable pelvic fractures: experiences in 22 patients treated with a trapezoid compression frame. *Clin Orthop*. 1980; 151:73.

8
Esophageal, Gastric, and Omental Injuries

RICHARD A. CRASS, M.D.
RICHARD J. MULLINS, M.D.

HISTORY: *Although Celsus, in the first century, advocated excising devitalized omentum that herniated through a stab wound, reports of surgical management of penetrating wounds of the upper abdomen were rare before the 18th century.[5] In the late 16th century Schenk treated a spear wound to the abdomen accidentally inflicted during a Bohemian hunt that resulted in a gastric fistula with survival of the victim.[13] Two centuries later, a shotgun wound sustained by Alexis St. Martin produced a similar outcome and was to provide Beaumont with a means of making his pioneering observations on gastric physiology. Nolleson in 1767 reported that a Palatine soldier named Rumpf had received a piercing stomach wound by a saber. The gastric wound was sutured and the patient survived.[11] In most of the cases of penetrating abdominal trauma reported in the 19th century, the surgeon limited repairs to the injured bowel that had eviscerated through the victim's wound. A surgically performed laparotomy to gain access to the peritoneal cavity and to repair injured stomach was not reported in the encyclopedic review of surgery performed during the Civil War.[14] During the First World War, the frequently fatal outcome of exploratory laparotomy still convinced surgeons that nonoperative management of penetrating abdominal injuries was appropriate, despite the generally recognized high mortality rate if a perforated viscus was left untreated. Routine prompt abdominal exploration, improved operative technique, and superior postoperative care reduced the mortality rate from isolated gastric injuries from 29% during World War I to essentially zero during World War II.[10]*

The sheltered location of the intraabdominal esophagus and pliability of the stomach and omentum make penetrating injury to these organs more common than blunt injury. However, a distended stomach can rupture after a sharp blow to the epigastrium, and gastric rupture has been reported as a complication of cardiopulmonary resuscitation in which the stomach was inflated and chest compressions were overvigorous and incorrectly applied.[3-5,9,18,20] In most large series of penetrating abdominal trauma, the prevalence of gastric injury is 20% whereas the prevalence of injury from blunt trauma is less than 1%.[2,9]

Gastric necrosis with perforation can result from corrosive ingestion, particularly when a bolus of caustic fluid is gulped in a suicidal gesture.[17] Laparotomy should be undertaken without delay in any patient who develops peritonitis after ingestion of a corrosive.[1,6]

The prognosis for isolated gastric perforations is good because of a combination of plentiful blood supply, relative sterility of the empty organ, and early diagnosis due to the rapid onset of peritoneal signs from leak of acid contents. The results of treatment, of course, can be disastrous when a gastric perforation is overlooked and operative treatment is delayed for 24 hr or more.

Injuries to the intraabdominal esophagus are rare and usually result from penetrating trauma.[10,21] However, blows to the abdomen in the presence of a full stomach can result in rupture of the esophagus akin to emetogenic injury (Boerhaave syndrome).[19]

The most serious consequence of omental injury is bleeding. The omentum is most commonly injured by penetrating trauma, but bleeding from it can occur when the omentum is fixed by adhesions and avulsion occurs during a sudden deceleration.

ANATOMY

The abdominal esophagus emerges from the esophageal hiatus, where it is supported by the phrenoesophageal ligament, to course for 2 to 4 cm within the abdominal cavity before joining the stomach. Only the anterior surface of the esophagus is covered by the peritoneum, making it a retroperitoneal structure. The posterior surface overlies the aorta. Accompanying the esophagus through the hiatus are the vagal trunks. The left vagus nerve lies on the left anterior surface of the esophagus as it passes through the esophageal hiatus. The right vagus lies on the posterior right side of the esophagus.

The empty stomach occupies the left upper quadrant of the abdomen, where much of it is sheltered by the lower rib cage. Topographically, the stomach is divided into the cardia, adjacent to the esophageal junction, the fundus, that portion craniad to the esophagastric junction, and the body and the pyloric antrum, extending from the angular incisure to the pylorus. The stomach is suspended from the gastrohepatic ligament on the right and from the crural attachments and esophagus from above. The stomach attaches by a wide segment of the omentum, the gastrocolic ligament, to the transverse colon below. The splenic ligament, including the short gastric vessels, attaches the greater curvature to the spleen on the left. Aside from these attachments on the greater and lesser curvatures, the stomach is totally invested in peritoneum with the anterior surface facing the general peritoneal cavity and the posterior surface forming a large surface area of the lesser sac. The generous blood supply of the stomach includes the left and right gastric arteries to the lesser curve and the left and right gastroepiploic arteries and the short gastric branches to the greater curvature (Fig. 8–1). The left gastric artery is a branch of the celiac axis, the right gastric artery arises from the common hepatic artery, the right gastroepiploic from the gastroduodenal artery, and the left gastroepiploic and short gastric arteries from the splenic artery. The venous drainage is through the coronary vein to the portal vein for the lesser curvature and right and left gastroepiploic and short gastric veins for the greater curvature, the last two emptying into the splenic vein (Fig. 8–1).

The omentum is a double layer of peritoneum and adipose tissue that originates from the greater curvature of the stomach. The blood supply consists of arcades extending outward from the gastroepiploic vessels along the greater curvature of the stomach. Two

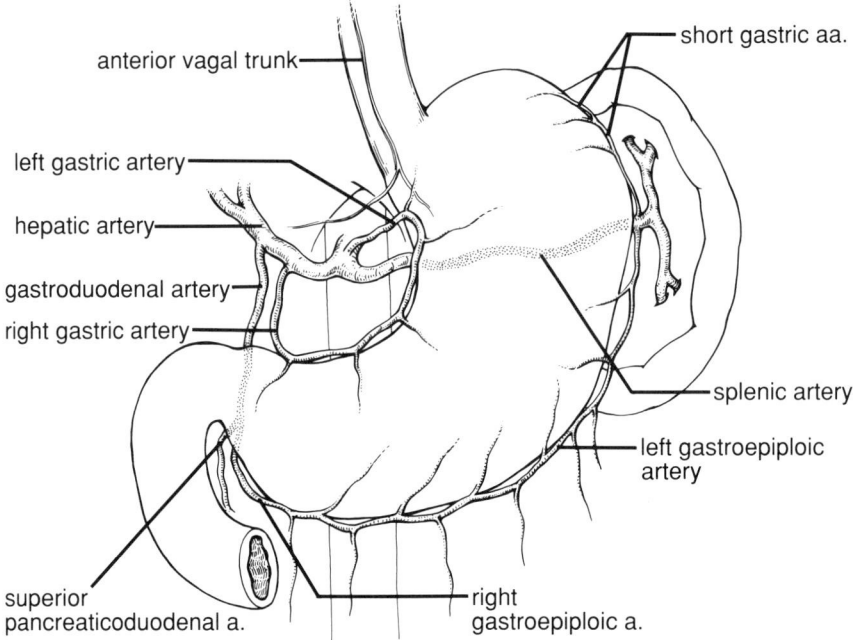

Figure 8–1. Gastric blood supply. The left and right gastric arteries supply the lesser curvature; the right and left gastroepiploic and the short gastric arteries, the latter from the splenic hilum, supply the greater curvature.

major vascular trunks arise from the right gastroduodenal and splenic arteries and arch across the inferior edge of the omentum. Understanding of the vascular anatomy of the omentum enables the surgeon to prepare large pedicled flaps that can be mobilized to cover bleeding liver wounds and other injuries.[16] The omentum drapes from the greater curvature of the stomach as an apron over the transverse colon, to which it has nearly avascular attachments. To the left side of the epigastric abdomen, the omentum bridges over the space anterior to the pancreas delimiting the lesser sac. On the right side the sheet of omentum is fused as the anterior layer with the mesocolon. As the posterior layer, which includes the middle colic vessels, the mesocolon can be separated by careful blunt dissection from the omentum.

ASSESSMENT

Most patients with gastric perforation will develop peritoneal signs rapidly from the leaking gastric acid. However, in patients with head injury or spinal cord lesions, the findings of peritoneal irritation may be absent or negligible and the physical examination unreliable. Perforation of the intraabdominal esophagus at or near the hiatus may cause minimal peritonitis as the leakage is often retroperitoneal. Esophageal contamination may dissect upward in the periesophageal alveolar plane and produce mediastinitis, which can be an elusive diagnostic challenge. A plain abdominal film in trauma patients with a perforated stomach or esophagus usually does not demonstrate free air. A computed tomographic (CT) scan is more sensitive in demonstrating small amounts of extraluminal air. An essential step in obtaining a CT scan is administration of an endoluminal contrast agent 30 min before the scan. Patients able to swallow may drink the contrast, although most patients will be given it down a gastric tube. In addition, the presence of gross blood in the aspirate of the nasogastric tube should raise the surgeon's suspicion of a gastric perforation.

Penetrating injuries to the lower chest and upper abdomen, as well as flank and back, can injure the stomach and intraabdominal esophagus. Esophageal injury is a possibility in patients with transmediastinal penetrating chest injuries, and part of the work-up of these patients should include esophagoscopy with a fiberoptic scope or a water-soluble contrast swallow. A carefully performed esophagoscopy with a flexible fiberoptic instrument should be performed immediately on patients who have ingested corrosives. If the procedure is delayed by more than 6 to 8 hr from the time of injury, organ integrity may be lost. The endoscopist should not pass the scope beyond necrotic mucosa because of the risk of perforation.[17]

There is nothing specific to implicate an omental injury except for evisceration. Occasionally, substantial intraperitoneal bleeding occurs after injury to a major omental vessel that results in hypotension or peritoneal irritation. Diagnostic peritoneal lavage has been established as a highly specific and sensitive test for significant intraabdominal bleeding.

PREOPERATIVE CARE

Before exploration of the abdomen for traumatic injuries, antibiotics should be given. A first generation cephalosporin is preferred by many surgeons if the patient is not allergic to the drug. A critical step in the preparation of any patient for emergency surgery is resuscitation, including infusion of sufficient volumes of fluid and, when appropriate, blood to restore intravascular blood volume before induction of anesthesia. If the probability of gastric perforation is recognized preoperatively, a large-bore gastric tube should be inserted to initiate gastric decompression. Moreover, the presence of blood will also provide diagnostic information and will encourage thorough gastric and esophageal exploration.

INITIAL OPERATIVE EXPOSURE AND TREATMENT

The trauma patient should be prepped and draped from the neck to the knees and from one posterior axillary line to the other. An upper midline incision provides access to the epigastrium; however, an extension up to the side of the xiphoid and continuation of the incision below the umbilicus is often required. The stomach should be decompressed, but in trauma victims with a stomach filled with solid food, this often is only accomplished by the patient either vomiting preoperatively or the anesthesiologist passing a large Ewald transoral tube into the stomach. To visualize the stomach's entire anterior surface it must be flattened out with the surgeon's hand while an assistant retracts on the greater curvature with Allis or Babcock clamps or applies traction on the omentum. The esophagus, cardia, and fundus can be difficult to examine completely, and often in these areas flattening of gastric folds with sponge sticks is required. Inspection before dissection is important because any serosal blood staining or retroperitoneal air bubbles alert the surgeon that detailed inspection of that area is required. Complete inspection of suspicious hematomas in the greater or lesser curvatures often requires ligation and division of vessels and excision of adherent omental fat to expose a small concealed perforation.

Examination of the posterior surface of the stomach requires entrance into the lesser sac. This can be done by incising the gastrocolic omentum below the gastroepiploic arcade (Fig. 8–2) or by detaching the avascular attachments of the omentum to the transverse colon. The gastroepiploic arcade should be preserved to minimize the risk of devascularization of the stomach. Filmy adhesion between the posterior stomach and the pancreas should be taken down sharply to expose the entire posterior gastric surface. To examine the back surface of the stomach often requires the use of narrow retractors or sponge sticks to flatten folds and creases. If injury is suspected in the cardia or fundus, the upper portion of the greater curvature should be mobilized. This can be accomplished by sequentially dividing the short gastric vessels to the spleen and mobilizing the fundus medially and anteriorly. Alternatively, the spleen and tail of the pancreas can be mobilized anteriorly into the midline incision delivering with them the greater curvature of the stomach for direct inspection. Splenic injury is a risk with this procedure, but is usually avoided by carefully dividing the splenocolic attachments before mobilization. During a laparotomy large perforations of the intraabdominal esophagus or stomach are easily identified. However, small perforations, for example from low velocity bullets, may be occult and only identified if the stomach is inflated with a liter or more of air while the surgeon looks for bubbles leaking from a perforation into the saline-filled peritoneal cavity.

The lower esophagus must be exposed and mobilized when there is evidence of hemorrhage or staining in the esophagocardiac area. Both the anterior and posterior surfaces must be examined. When there is uncertainty regarding esophageal injury, complete mobilization of the intraabdominal esophagus similar to what is done during a truncal vagotomy is required. The left lobe of the liver is retracted out of the way after

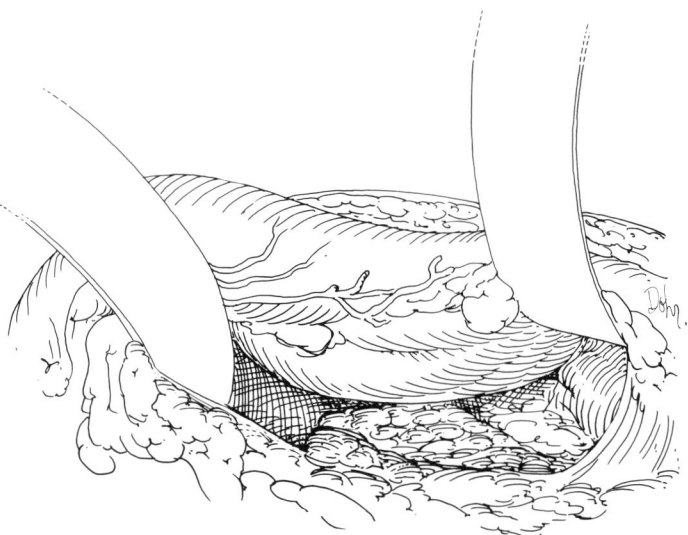

Figure 8–2. Exposure of the posterior wall of the stomach through the lesser sac.

its triangular ligament is divided. The peritoneum, anterolateral to the esophagus, is opened sharply. Above the fundus the esophagus is encircled by blunt dissection with the index finger and then a second finger, which are used to grasp a Penrose drain and pull it around the esophagus. With downward and anterior traction the entire esophagus can be inspected. Exposure of a small puncture can be facilitated by having the anesthesiologist pass a large-bore tube, such as 36 to 40 F Maloney dilators or an Ewald tube, while the surgeon is observing the esophagus. The esophagus then can be rotated about the tube with the perforation easier to recognize and repair in the distended esophagus.

DEFINITIVE OPERATIVE TREATMENT

Esophageal injuries are best closed over a large-bore oral gastric tube or Maloney dilator to assure that the lumen is not compromised by the closure. One layer of interrupted nonabsorbable or synthetic collagen 3-0 or 4-0 through-and-through suture is sufficient. A second layer does not add to the strength of the closure, owing to the absence of serosa, and may narrow the lumen. The closure can be secured by a patch of gastric fundus or omentum or alternatively encircling the esophageal repair with a gastric wrap in a fashion similar to a Nissen fundoplication. If a portion of esophageal wall is lost because of injury or debridement, the closure of the defect can be secured without narrowing the esophageal lumen with the fundus of the stomach, which is mobilized and wrapped around the defect as a Thal patch. As an alternative, tenuous closures can be enveloped with a vascularized pedicle of omentum.

In most cases of these distal esophageal wounds, a gastrostomy tube would be inserted to permit gastric decompression so that an esophageal foreign body can be avoided. Early institution of enteral feedings can be achieved if the surgeon places a feeding jejunostomy.

Devitalized tissue in the edges of a gastric wound must be excised before closure. A two-layer closure of stomach wounds is optimal, with the inner layer being run with absorbable 3-0 suture, which achieves hemostasis. If the mucosa cannot be visualized because of a small serosal wound, one should not hesitate to extend the length of the wound to assure an accurate hemostatic closure. The outer layer should be interrupted 3-0 or 4-0 Lembert nonabsorbable sutures. The presence of one gastric wound demands a thorough search for a second. The occasional complex wound involving antrum, duodenum, and pancreas presents a formidable challenge. Management of this type of wound is discussed in Chapter 9. If the stomach is necrotic after ingestion of corrosive material, total gastrectomy without reconstruction is prudent. A duodenostomy and feeding jejunostomy will decompress the bowel and permit enteral alimentation during recovery and up to the time of elective reconstruction. A transnasal sump tube can be left above the esophageal closure for proximal decompression. Alternatively, the distal esophagus can be drained to the flank, using a right-angled chest tube inserted into the esophagus from below, or a cervical esophagostomy can be carried out.

The surgeon usually has no problem identifying bleeding omental vessels. Vessels in the omentum draped beneath the greater curvature of the antrum are in close proximity to the middle colic vessels, and mass ligatures in that area should be avoided. Omental tears are openings that are best eliminated by either closure or dividing the omentum from the hole to its edge to prevent intestinal hernias and obstruction.

When bleeding in the omentum has been controlled by ligature, residual devitalized omentum should be excised. Before closure of the abdomen at the end of an exploratory laparotomy at which peritoneal contamination was significant, lavage with 2 to 4 liters of balanced salt solution, with or without topical antibiotics, is performed. Fascial closure depends on the judgment of the surgeon. We use interrupted nonabsorbable sutures in patients with serious visceral injuries, although data support closing the abdomen with a running absorbable #1 suture. Skin is routinely closed with staples unless contamination has been heavy and prolonged. Closed suction drains are rarely placed near repairs and only when esophageal or gastric closures are tenuous.

POSTOPERATIVE MANAGEMENT

The gastric tube is used to decompress the stomach for 3 to 4 days after repair of gastric injuries. If the patient has multiple injuries, antacids or H2 blockers are used to prevent stress ulceration. These are continued until the patient is eating. Diet is begun when the patient passes flatus and is hungry. After esophageal repairs, a contrast study is obtained 1 week postoperatively to assure there is no leak or obstruction before instituting oral intake. Solid food should be initiated cautiously.

Antibiotics are not continued for more than 24 hr unless there is a colonic perforation, in which case the antibiotics are continued for 5 days. When the skin wound is packed open, saline-soaked dressings are continued for 4 days, and if the wound does not appear infected, a delayed primary closure is performed with tapes.

COMPLICATIONS AND RESULTS

Simple gastric injuries in the absence of other serious injuries do well and complications are minimal. Esophageal injuries carry a greater risk of complications related to leak or obstruction. When recognized early and treated appropriately the prognosis is excellent and most life-threatening complications of esophageal and gastric injury result either from treatment delays, associated injuries, or failure to recognize and treat complications when they do develop. Suture line bleeding is extremely unusual if proper closure of gastric wounds is accomplished. When bleeding occurs and persists, reexploration for control may be required. Preoperative or intraoperative endoscopy is useful to exclude hemorrhage from other locations such as stress gastritis, duodenal ulcers, or hemobilia.

The major risk after repair of esophageal or gastric injuries is failure of the closure with leakage of enteric contents. Generalized peritonitis can result, but a more common presentation is an intraabdominal abscess which, when drained, can lead to a gastric or esophageal fistula. CT with endoluminal water-soluble contrast is the diagnostic procedure of choice in patients who develop fever leukocytosis, sympathetic pleural effusions, and epigastric tenderness. When intraabdominal collections are identified, antibiotics and drainage are indicated. In selected cases this can be performed percutaneously. Although a direct extraperitoneal posterior approach is preferred if the collection is in the right subphrenic or subhepatic space, left subphrenic or lesser sac abscesses usually require exposure through the midline laparotomy and careful dissection to avoid injury to the spleen, pancreas, or splenic flexure of the colon. After the abscess has been identified, posterior-dependent drainage can be accomplished through the bed of the 12th rib or a generous lateral subcostal incision. Silastic drains are preferred because these soft drains seldom erode bowel or blood vessels.

When a gastric or esophageal repair disrupts, closure of the leak is seldom possible. Attempts to suture the friable tissue will usually lead to further breakdown. Thus, the surgeon's goal should be to obtain unobstructed drainage. The fistula will usually close spontaneously with adequate drainage, gastric suction, and nutrition if there is no distal obstruction. Although intravenous nutrition can be used, if the surgeon can place a proximal small bowel feeding tube, management of these often septic fistula patients is usually simplified.

REFERENCES

1. Allen RE, et al. Corrosive injuries of the stomach. *Arch Surg.* 1970; 100:409.
2. Anderson CR, Ballinger WF. Abdominal injuries. In: Zuidema GF, Rutherford RB, Ballinger WF, eds. *The Management of Trauma.* Philadelphia: WB Saunders; 1979:431.
3. Asch MJ, Coran AG, Johnston PW. Gastric perforation secondary to blunt trauma in children. *J Trauma.* 1975; 15:187.
4. Brunsting LA, Morton JH. Gastric rupture from blunt abdominal trauma. *J Trauma.* 1987; 27(8):887–891.
5. Bussey HJ, McGehee RN, Tyson KRT. Isolated gastric rupture due to blunt trauma. *J Trauma.* 1975; 15:190.
6. Celsus. *De Medicina* (Spencer WC, Trans.). Harvard University Press; 1938; VII:16.
7. Citron RP, et al. Chemical trauma of the esophagus and stomach. *Surg Clin North Am.* 1958; 48:1303.
8. DiVincenti FC, et al. Blunt abdominal trauma. *J Trauma.* 1968; 8:1004.
9. Garfinkle ES, Matolo NM. Gastric necrosis from blunt abdominal trauma. *J Trauma.* 1975; 16:406.
10. Glatterer MS, Toon RS, Ellestad C, et al. Management of blunt and penetrating external esophageal trauma. *J Trauma.* 1985; 25(8):784–792.
11. Griswold RA, Collier HS. Blunt abdominal trauma. Int. *Abstr Surg.* 1961; 112:309.
12. Howard JM, et al. Studies of adrenal function in combat and wounded soldiers: a study of the Korean Theatre. *Ann Surg.* 1955; 141:314.
13. Nolleson Le Fils. Surg une plaie d'gastromac guerie la suture de pelletier. *J Med Chir Pharm.* 1767; 27:595.
14. Otis GA. *The Medical and Surgical History of the War of the Rebellion, Part II, Vol. II, Surgical History.* Washington, DC: U.S. Government Printing Office; 1877.
15. Schenk J. *Observationum medicarum, rosarorum, novarum, admirabilium, et monstrosatum.* Frankfurt; 1609:38.
16. Stone HH, Lamb JM. Use of pedicled omentum as an autogenous pack for control of hemorrhage in major injuries of the liver. *Surg Gynecol Obstet.* 1975; 141:92.
17. Sugawa C, Mullins RJ, Lucas CE, Leibold WC. The value of early endoscopy following caustic ingestion. *Surg Gynecol Obstet.* 1981; 153:553–556.
18. Vassy LE, et al. Traumatic gastric perforation in children from blunt trauma. *J Trauma.* 1975; 16:184.
19. Worman LW, et al. Rupture of the esophagus from external blunt trauma. *Arch Surg.* 1962; 85:333.
20. Yajko RD, Seydel F, Trimble C. Rupture of the stomach from blunt abdominal trauma. *J Trauma.* 1975; 16:177.
21. Yap RG, Yap AG, Obeid FN, Horan DP. Traumatic esophageal injuries: 12-year experience at Henry Ford Hospital. *J Trauma.* 1984; 24(7):623–625.

9
Trauma to the Pancreas and Duodenum

CHARLES FREY, M.D.
TATSUO ARAIDA, M.D.

HISTORY: An intoxicated woman struck in the chest and abdomen by a stagecoach wheel and brought to St. Thomas' Hospital was reported by Travers in the 1827 Lancet.[117] *She was the first recorded victim of blunt injury to the pancreas. At autopsy, hours after the injury, a transverse tear of the pancreas as well as a hepatic laceration were found. The cause of death was intraabdominal hemorrhage from an associated hepatic injury.*

The first recorded description of a penetrating injury and surgical resection of a portion of the pancreas is credited by Otis (who edited the Medical and Surgical History of the War of the Rebellion *[Civil War] in 1876) to Kleberg of Odessa.[88] Kleberg described in 1868 a 60-year-old soldier who fell among thieves and was stabbed in the abdomen. The protruding exteriorized pancreas was later ligated and excised. The patient had an uncomplicated course after discharge.*

Similarly, the only survivor among five patients reported with pancreatic injury during the Civil War had a portion of pancreas excised and ligated. The other four patients reported by Otis had survived long periods of delay (the shortest of which was 1.5 days) between the time of injury and definitive hospitalization, only to die from late complications of injury, peritonitis, and hemorrhage, which in three of the four cases resulted from associated injuries to liver, stomach, or splenic vessels.[88]

While the significance of an intact pancreatic duct was not fully appreciated by Otis, he described two patients who had at autopsy a ball (bullet) lodged in the pancreas, the main duct of which, in both cases, was intact but showed no evidence of pancreatic inflammation or necrosis, and who, in fact, died of associated injuries. Case 506, "The pancreas was perforated at about its middle but except in the immediate track of the ball, gave evidence of no departure from its healthy standard"; and Case 418, "The pancreas was rather large, seven inches long; weight five ounces except the presence of the foreign body . . . On examining the specimen microscopically, no deviation from the normal structure is found in sections made from tissue taken from the left end or tail of the viscera and from the middle part or body.

The coat of the great arteries with which the ball was in apposition were uninjured."[88] Otis then went on to quote several surgical treatises and textbooks of surgery that outline the problems and importance of diagnosing pancreatic injury, the consequences of not doing so, and what constitutes a significant pancreatic injury.[88] These concepts have been reaffirmed and generally recognized only recently as valid more than 150 to 200 years after the original publication. Bell (A System of Surgery, volume V, published in 1787) said, "As the pancreas lies deeply covered with the other viscera, wounds of it can seldom be discovered: but as a division of the duct of this gland will prevent the secretion which it affords from being carried to the bowels, this may, by interrupting or impeding digestion, do much injury to the constitution; and as the liquor will be effused into the cavity of the abdomen, it may thus be productive of collections, the removal of which may ultimately require the assistance of surgery."

Gooch (Chiurgical Works, volume I, 1792, p. 99), declares that "wounds of the pancreas are to be concluded mortal if its duct or blood vessels are injured, whence the succus pancreaticus or blood may be discharged into the cavity of the abdomen and there putrefying, cause inevitable death."

Little progress was made in both the recognition and management of pancreatic injuries during World War I. Only five cases with one survivor were described by the British, a record similar to that observed in the Civil War.

Poole's World War II report on the Second Auxiliary Surgical Group in 1944 and 1945 recorded 62 pancreatic injuries associated with a 56% mortality.[94] The importance of associated injuries as factors contributing to mortality received appropriate emphasis, as only 1 of the 62 patients was noted to have an isolated pancreatic injury. Thirteen of the 35 deaths were associated with major vascular injury and a correlation was noted between the number of viscera injured and mortality. The mortality rose progressively from 33% with one associated injury, to 50% with two viscera, to 60% with three viscera, to 100% with four viscera injured in addition to the pancreas.

During the Korean conflict, the mortality of nine pancreatic injuries was reduced to 22%, according to Sako, reporting the experiences of the surgical research team in Korea of the Army Medical Service Graduate School, United States Army.[98] There was no evidence of any enhanced awareness of the appropriate operative management of the surgical injuries included in the report. The decreasing mortality of pancreatic injury, as well as of other injury, was attributed accurately to improvements in supportive care, including resuscitation, fluid replacement, antibiotics, and improved management of associated injuries.

A major step in improved diagnosis of pancreatic injury after blunt trauma to the pancreas was the observation by Elman in 1929 that the serum amylase became elevated in some pancreatic injuries if the duct was injured or obstructed.[25] This observation was later confirmed by McCorkle and Goldman in 1942 and reaffirmed the following year in a report by Naffziger and McCorkle.[71,82]

Walton in 1923 recommended pancreatic resection of the portion of the pancreas distal to the fracture and oversewing the proximal end of the pancreas as the safest form of management of injuries to the body and tail of the pancreas in which the pancreatic duct was severed.[126] The report by

Kerry and Glas in the Archives of Surgery *in 1962 emphasized the significance of injury to the major ductal system of the pancreas through clinical and laboratory investigations and has become a landmark in establishing appropriate operative management of patients with complex pancreatic injuries and associated injuries to duodenum and common bile ducts.*[57]

The pancreas and duodenum, both retroperitoneal organs in intimate proximity to one another, present unique problems in diagnosis and treatment. These organs, because of their relatively protected location, are infrequently injured, and constitute no more than 3% to 12% of all abdominal injuries.[19,24,98,130] However, if the possibility of trauma to these structures is not considered and appropriate studies are not obtained either preoperatively or at operation, significant injuries associated with high morbidity and mortality may be missed during routine laparotomy.[4,23,67]

While the major pancreatic duct and duodenum and common duct may be injured separately, not infrequently the major pancreatic duct and duodenum are both injured (20%) or some other combination of injury, including all three structures, may occur.[51] These combined injuries, even when recognized promptly, or indeed any injury to either pancreas or duodenum missed on initial evaluation or at celiotomy, present complex challenges to the trauma surgeon's judgment and technical ability, and to intensive care support facilities. The incidence of secondary life-threatening complications with pancreatic and duodenal injury is far higher than with other comparable abdominal injuries. Delays in diagnosis are common and this increases the complexity of the treatment and greatly increases the chance of serious secondary complications.[3,18,21,67]

Mortality associated with pancreatic or duodenal trauma based on recent reports is in the range of 7% to 21%,[50,63,86,104,110,132,Moore] somewhat of an improvement over the 16% to 20%[21,51,108,114] we reported in this chapter in 1982. More than half these deaths in pancreatic trauma and 80% or more in duodenal trauma continue to be the result of massive hemorrhage and shock due to associated injuries to major vascular structures; death occurs intraoperatively or within 48 hr of injury. Duodenal and pancreatic injury have almost nothing to do with the fatal outcome in these early deaths.[21,50,51,55,63,85,104,107,108,114,135] Sepsis, the second most common cause of death after hemorrhage, is most often seen in patients with hemorrhagic shock in the preoperative and operative period and in those with colon injury or those in whom the gastrointestinal tract has been opened.[44,50,51,85,104,107,115,131,135]

PANCREATIC INJURIES

A major problem related to pancreatic injuries is the high incidence of associated injuries (Table 9–1). Mortality relates to the nature of the pancreatic injury, the number and type of associated injuries, and the wounding agent (Table 9–2). The immediate cause of death is uncontrollable hemorrhage from the pancreas and associated injury in 72.1% of the patients, as a result of the secondary complications of sepsis and abscess formation in 15.6%, organ failure in 8.3%, and miscellaneous causes such as central nervous system injury and secondary hemorrhage in the remaining 4% (Table 9–3).

Table 9–1 Pancreatic-associated Injuries

AUTHOR		NO. OF PATIENTS	MAJOR VASCULAR	LIVER	STOMACH	SPLEEN	DUODENUM	CBD/GB	KIDNEY	COLON/SB
Glancy[34]*	P	544	164	259	178	159	79	34	129	192
	B	272								
Bass[8]	B	26	—	2	—	2	1	—	1	—
Mckone[72]	P	1	1	2	—	—	5	—	1	1
	B	4								
Lauststen[61]	B	2	1	—	—	—	1	—	—	—
Whalen[128]†	P	100	16	48	44	15	69	8	14	19
	B	26								
Feliciano[26]	P	104	33	60	43	—	129	—	35	82
	B	25								
Keeling[56]	B	9	—	1	—	1	—	—	—	—
Nowak[86]	P	39	10	20	26	12	13	3	7	25
	B	3								
Wynn[134]†	P	49	3	17	12	15	6	—	10	17
Jones[50]	P	362	190	—	—	—	91	—	—	101
	B	138								
Sims[104]	P	37	—	23	—	10	14	—	—	17
	B	7								
Moore[79]†	P	19	11	17	—	—	—	7	—	12
	B	15								
Sorensen[109]	P	41	10	17	19	—	6	3	6	19
Oreskovich[87]	P	7	4	7	3	2	—	1	1	4
	B	3								
Nilsson[85]	P	2	1	3	3	7	—	—	1	—
	B	27								
Leppaniemi[63]	P	32	13	18	—	—	—	—	—	—
	B	11								
Wisner[131]‡	P	44					19			
	B	47								
Ivantury[48]	P	107	47	37	42	19	13	—	15	20
Totals		2103	(25 deaths) 504	(13 deaths) 531	(8 deaths) 370	(6 deaths) 242	(8 deaths) 446	56	(7 deaths) 220	(8 deaths) 509

*These figures exclude patients reported in the other series listed below.
†These reports also include combined pancreaticoduodenal injuries.
CBD/GB, common bile duct/gall bladder; Colon/SB, colon/small bowel.
‡Accepted for publication.

Table 9-2 Pancreatic Injury Wounding Agent and Mortality

AUTHOR	PENETRATING (% DIED)	STAB (% DIED)	GUNSHOT (% DIED)	SHOTGUN (% DIED)	BLUNT (% DIED)
Glancy[34]*	548 (19.0)	74 (5.4)	291 (7.9)	56 (39.3)	271 (26.6)
Bass[8]	—	—	—	—	26 (?)
Mckone[72]	1 (0)	—	—	—	4 (0)
Lauststen[61]	2	—	—	—	2 (0)
Whalen[128]†	100 (?)	—	—	—	26 (?)
Feliciano[26]†	104 (?)	15 (?)	82 (?)	7 (?)	25 (?)
Keeling[56]	—	—	—	—	9 (11.1)
Nowak[86]	39 (20.5)	2 (0)	34 (23.5)	3 (0)	3 (66.7)
Wynn[134]†	35 (?)	14 (?)	20 (?)	1 (?)	49 (?)
Jones[50]	362 (22)	76 (5)	252 (22)	34 (56)	138 (19)
Sims[104]	37 (10.8)	7 (?)	30 (?)	—	7 (28.6)
Moore[79]†	19 (10.5)	1 (0)	16 (6.3)	2 (50)	15 (13.3)
Sorensen[109]	41 (14.5)	13 (?)	25 (9?)	3 (66.7)	—
Oreskovich[87]	10 (0)	0	7 (0)	3 (0)	—
Nilsson[85]	2 (?)	—	—	—	27 (?)
Leppaniemi[63]	32 (7)	—	—	—	11 (45)
Wisner[131]‡	44	21	19	4	47
Ivantury[48]	107 (32)	32 (21)	69 (34.6)	—	—
Totals—1990	1483	255	845	113	660

*These figures exclude patients reported in the other series listed below.
†These reports include combined pancreaticoduodenal injuries.
‡Accepted for publication.
(?)Mortality rates or number of deaths not included in another report by etiology.

Table 9-3 Pancreatic Injury Cause of Death

AUTHOR	HEMORRHAGE-ASSOCIATED INJURIES	PANCREATIC INJURY: ABSCESS AND SEPSIS	ORGAN FAILURE	MISCELLANEOUS
Graham[37]	47	8	11	6
Whalen[128]*	11	4	—	—
Feliciano[26]*	22	9	7	—
Keeling[56]	1	—	—	—
Nowak[86]	5	3	—	2
Wynn[134]	2	—	1	—
Jones[50]	68	11	—	—
Sims[104]	3	2	1	—
Moore[79]*	2	1	—	—
Sorenson[109]	4	—	—	—
Leppaniemi[63]	7	1	—	—
Smego[107]	12	2	4	3
Wisner[131]	6	—	1	1
Ivantury[48]	27	6	0	0
Total	217 (72.1%)	47 (15.6%)	25 (8.3%)	12 (4%)

*These reports also include combined pancreaticoduodenal injuries.

DUODENAL INJURIES

Although blunt trauma to the abdomen resulting in duodenal perforation was associated with a mortality of more than 86% in the period preceding World War I, the mortality had been reduced to 50% by the time of World War II, which closely paralleled the experience with penetrating injuries of the duodenum reported in military casualties, 56%.[76,93,101] By the time of the Korean conflict, the mortality of duodenal injuries from blunt trauma had been reduced to 20%, although the mortality of penetrating injuries remained at 43% despite advances in resuscitation, fluid replacement, and antibiotic therapy.[19,98]

In 1964, Cocke and Meyer identified the retroperineal rupture of the duodenum as a special problem that if not suspected and operated on, or if not recognized at operation (as occurred in 15% of patients) was, as a result of the delay, associated with extensive retroperitoneal inflammation and an operative mortality of 71%.[18]

As is true of the pancreas, the location of the duodenum in a relatively protected position results in a high incidence of associated injuries (Table 9–4). The wounding agent plays a major role in subsequent mortality; knives are considered negligible whereas shotgun wounds are highly lethal (Table 9–5). The cause of death is similar to that after pancreatic injury consisting of hemorrhage in 47.1%, duodenal fistula in 25%, sepsis in 15.5%, organ failure in 10%, and other causes in the remaining 6.4% (Table 9–6). There has been a marked decrease in the number of deaths reported from duodenal fistula since our 1982 report, down from 38.5% to 25%, whereas the incidence of early deaths from massive hemorrhage and late deaths from sepsis has increased slightly.

COMBINED PANCREATIC AND DUODENAL INJURIES

The basis of our understanding of these complex injuries involving duodenum, pancreas, and common bile duct was derived in large part from the 1962 report of Kerry and Glas.[57] These authors defined which lesions of the pancreas or duodenum resulting from blunt or penetrating trauma required resection of the duodenum or pancreas in order to ensure survival.

ANATOMY

The junction between the stomach and duodenum is marked by the pyloric vein, which courses inferiorly upward from the pancreas, transversely across the duodenum at the distal end of the pyloric muscle. The first portion of the duodenum is that portion between the pyloric muscle and the common duct superiorly and the gastroduodenal artery inferiorly. The second portion of the duodenum extends from the common duct and gastroduodenal artery to the ampulla of Vater. The third portion of the duodenum extends from the ampulla of Vater to the mesenteric vessels and the fourth portion of the duodenum extends from the mesenteric vessels to the point at which the duodenum emerges from the retroperitoneum at the ligament of Treitz. The duodenum shares a common blood supply with the pancreas, so that although it is possible to remove the duodenum from the pancreas, it was not thought possible to remove all the head of the pancreas without irreversibly devascularizing and necrotizing the duodenum. This is why 5% of the pancreas along the rim of the inner aspect

Table 9–4 Duodenum-associated Injuries

AUTHOR		NO. OF PATIENTS (%)	MAJOR VASCULAR (%)	LUNG (%)	LIVER (%)	STOMACH (%)	SPLEEN (%)	PANCREAS (%)	CBD (%)	KIDNEY (%)	COLON (%)	SMALL BOWEL (%)
Stone[113]	P	299 (74%)	Artery (31%) Vein (33%)	21	63	33	—	34	25	21	34	50
Snyder[108]	B	27 (26%)	43	—	63	—	33	26	—	26	—	—
	P	190 (78%)		—	43	26	—	28	16	23	32	26
Flint[28]	B	54 (22%)	17	—	41	32	—	27	15	16	39	33
	P	56 (75%)										
	B	19 (25%)										
Shorr[103]	P	94 (90%)	30	—	31.4	14.2	—	24.8	7.6	19	24.8	16.2
	B	11 (10%)										
Pororny[95]	P	3 (30%)	20	—	20	20	—	60	10	10	20	20
	B	7 (70%)										
Wynn[134]		38	7.9	—	23.7	—	5.3	15.8	—	10.5	42.1	Combined with colon 8 small bowel 28
Martin[70]	P	109 (85%)	59.4	—	38	20	9	43	20.3	21.9	46.1	
	B	19 (15%)										
Ivantury[47]	P	82	9.8	—	34.1	20.7	—	12.2	6.1	20.7	17.1	23.2
Kashuk[55]	P	25 (74%)	58.2	—	35.3	32.3	5.9	52.9	8.8	8.8	38.2	20.6
	B	9 (26%)										
Stigall[112]	B	1	100	—	—	—	—	—	—	—	—	100
Reyna[96]	B	1					No associated injury					
Grindlinger[39]	P	1	—	1								

CBD, common bile duct; B, blunt; P, penetrating trauma.

Table 9-5 Duodenum: Wounding Agents and Mortal Injury

AUTHOR	PENETRATING (% DIED)	STAB (% DIED)	GUNSHOT (% DIED)	SHOTGUN (% DIED)	BLUNT (% DIED)
Stone[113]	—	31 (0)	239 (11)	24 (46)	27
Snyder[108]	—	23 (0)	143 (10)	14 (29)	44
Flint[28]	55 (20)	4	51	—	19 (11)
Shorr[103]	94 (4.3)	42 (0)	52 (7.7)	—	11 (0)
Pororny[95]	3 (0)	—	3 (0)	—	6 (0)
Ivantury[47]	60 (5)	19 (0)	41 (7.3)	—	—
Kashuk[55]	16 (6.3)	—	—	—	9 (0)
Stigall[112]	—	—	—	—	1 (0)
Reyna[96]	—	—	—	—	1 (0)
Grindlinger[39]	1 (0)	—	—	—	—
Totals	229	119	529	38	118

of the duodenal "C" is preserved during a 95% resection of the pancreas for chronic pancreatitis as penetrating within its substance are the anterior and posterior branches of the inferior and superior pancreaticoduodenal arcade. Lambert et al., however, have reported on 14 patients with chronic pancreatitis in whom total pancreatectomy was possible while preserving the duodenum. The duodenum was said to be cyanotic in some patients but contractility of the duodenum was evident and assured viability of that structure.[60]

The first portion, the distal third portion, and all of the fourth portion of the duodenum lie over the vertebrae and are particularly vulnerable to injury by abdominal trauma that compresses them against the vertebral column. The mesocolon lies over and prevents direct inspection of the third and fourth portions of the duodenum, and the omentum and transverse colon overlie much of the second and, occasionally, the first portion of the duodenum. The duodenum is essentially entirely retroperitoneal, although the anterior half of the circumference of the first and second parts of duodenum can be visualized through

Table 9-6 Duodenum Deaths

AUTHOR	HEMORRHAGE	DUODENAL DEHISCENCE OR FISTULA	INTRA-ABDOMINAL SEPSIS	ORGAN FAILURE (LIVER, LUNG, KIDNEY)	MISCELLA-NEOUS
Stone[113]	19	5	3	2	4
Snyder[108]	19	27	—	—	—
Flint[28]	5	5	5	2	—
Whalen[128]	—	1	—	—	5
Shorr[103]	—	—	2	2	—
Pororny[95]	—	—	—	—	1
Wynn[134]	4	1	4	—	1
Martin[70]	11	1	12	4	—
Ivantury[47]	14	3	—	—	—
Kashuk[55]	9	—	1	—	—
Totals	81 (47.1%)	43 (25%)	27 (15.7%)	10 (5.8%)	11 (6.4%)

the thin overlying translucent peritoneum in most patients. The third part of the duodenum can be visualized by mobilizing the cecum and distal ileum, as described by Braach.

The pancreas is divided anatomically into a head, body, and tail. The junction between the head and the body, the neck, can be identified by the groove through which the superior mesenteric artery and vein run on their way to the small bowel mesentery. The neck of the gland portion of the proximal body directly overlies the vertebral column and mesenteric vessels. The uncinate process is the posterior part of the head of the pancreas and is derived from the ventral pancreas, bulging to the patient's left posteriorly under the mesenteric vessels superficial to the aorta.[38] The body of the pancreas extends laterally, dorsally, and superiorly from the neck and blends into a distal, more narrow portion of the pancreas or tail, which constitutes approximately the lateral one-third of the length of the gland.

The distal portion of the body and the tail of the gland overlie the left adrenal and superior pole of the kidney. The tail of the pancreas, containing the highest concentration of islets in the gland, overlies the superior pole of the kidney and ends at the hilum of the spleen.[133]

The pancreatic duct, which represents the fusion of the duct of Santorini supplying the body and tail with the duct of Wirsung, which supplies the head, runs longitudinally through the gland, entering the duodenum at the ampulla of Vater. Numerous lobular ducts come off at right angles to the main duct. Both the pancreatic duct and common duct enter the duodenum through a common channel in 85% of patients at the ampulla of Vater. In another 5% of patients the two ducts enter the duodenum on the same papilla but through separate channels.[73] In 10% of patients, the bile duct and pancreatic duct enter the duodenum separately.[75] This is because the major pancreatic duct may be derived from the dorsal pancreas and enters the duodenum separately in a more proximal location closer to the pylorus.[43] In this 10% of cases, an accessory pancreatic duct, derived from the dorsal pancreas (the duct of Santorini), drains a major portion of the gland.[43,75] The duct enters the second portion of the duodenum, where it is vulnerable to injury. Injury to either of the pancreatic ducts anywhere in their course through the pancreas sets the stage for pancreatic ductal obstruction with all its attendant complications such as pancreatitis, pancreatic fistula, pancreatic pseudocyst, and pancreatic abscess.

Experience with endoscopic retrograde cholangiopancreatography has confirmed the important observation first made by Cross that there are small accessory pancreatic ducts that enter the duodenum independent of the main duct in most patients.[22] These can become dilated and form small psuedocysts that are not decompressed by filleting open the main pancreatic duct, as is done in the Puestow ductal decompression operation.

The pancreas and duodenum are abundantly supplied with blood vessels (Fig. 9–1). The largest vessel in intimate relationship with the pancreas is the splenic artery, one of the main branches of the celiac axis that joins the superior aspect of the gland near, but lateral to, the junction of the head and body and runs in the branches at right angles to the long axis of the pancreas along the way in 75% of patients. It then leaves the pancreas to enter the spleen. In 25% of patients the splenic artery gives off virtually no branches to the pancreas, except a large branch, the dorsal pancreatic, which joins the transverse pancreatic artery that supplies the pancreas.[105] Short gastric branches are given off by splenic artery to the greater curvature of the stomach as the splenic artery leaves the tail of the pancreas. Most proximal to these is the left gastroepiploic artery, which supplies the greater curvature of the stomach and the omentum, and in 75% of patients a major branch, the dorsal pancreatic, joins the transverse pancreatic artery, which runs parallel and inferior

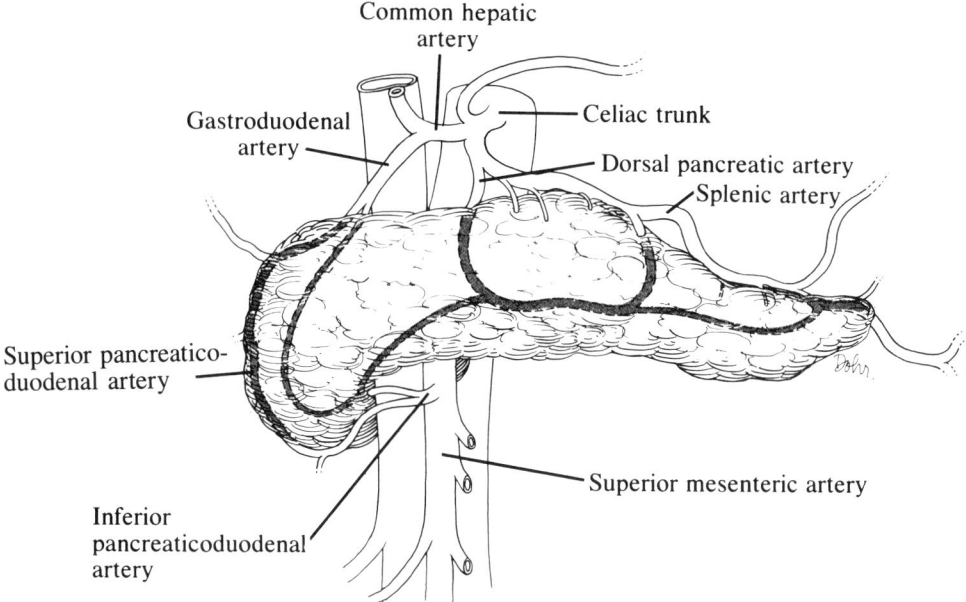

Figure 9-1. Blood supply of the pancreas.

to the splenic to the tail of the gland. The splenic artery, but not the splenic vein, may be ligated without compromising the viability of the spleen or distal pancreas.[105]

The first branch of the hepatic artery is the gastroduodenal artery. This courses from its hepatic artery origin at the superior surface of the duodenum under the second portion of the duodenum to enter the pancreas just below and opposite the common duct above the duodenum. Superior to the pancreas, this artery divides into the superior pancreaticoduodenal artery and the right gastroepiploic artery. This latter vessel leaves the pancreas adjacent to the duodenum and supplies the greater curvature of the stomach and the omentum. The pancreaticoduodenal artery curves through the head of the pancreas near the duodenum, giving off multiple branches to the pancreatic head, many of these anastomosing with inferior pancreaticoduodenal artery. The latter, a branch of the superior mesenteric artery, arises off the superior mesenteric just as it emerges from the inferior surface of the pancreas. In 5% of patients, an anomalous common hepatic artery or, in 25% of patients, an anomalous right hepatic artery arises from the superior mesenteric artery. It is crucial for the surgeon to be aware that the anomalous common or right hepatic artery may pass through the head portion of the uncinate process of the gland and be injured during resection of the uncinate process when the short, direct branches to the uncinate from the superior mesenteric artery and vein are being divided or ligated.[74,121]

The major vein draining the pancreas is the splenic vein, which runs longitudinally in a groove up the mid- to upper portion of the posterior surface of the gland from the spleen to its junction with the portal vein posterior to the pancreatic neck. The portal vein is constituted by the joining of the splenic and superior mesenteric vein. The latter vessel courses under the pancreas, following the same pathway in the opposite direction as the superior mesenteric artery. It joins the splenic vein near the superior border of the gland.

The first portion of the portal vein and distal portion of the superior mesenteric vein receive veins draining the uncinate portion of the head of the pancreas. The superior mesenteric and portal veins pass under, and are in intimate contact with, the posterior surface of the neck of the gland. The portal vein emerges from the superior surface of the duodenum most often just posterior to and between the common bile duct on the right and the hepatic artery on the left. The inferior mesenteric vein joins the superior mesenteric or splenic vein as does the coronary vein, which may, in some cases, enter the portal vein. The pancreas is entirely covered by the retroperitoneum of the lesser sac and, anterior to this, another layer consisting of the stomach and gastrohepatic ligament. Much of the body may be visible through the gastrohepatic ligament superiorly and through the base of the mesocolon inferiorly in the vicinity of the ligament of Treitz.

The common bile duct enters the posterior substance of the head of the pancreas in 83% of patients after it passes under the duodenum.[38,106] After piercing the capsule of the gland posteriorly, it courses down within the pancreatic substance a centimeter or two from the curve of the duodenum, entering the duodenal lumen at the junction between the second and third portion of the duodenum approximately 20 to 25 cm from the pylorus.[105]

ASSESSMENT OF PANCREATIC OR DUODENAL INJURY

The pancreas and duodenum are injured either by blunt or penetrating trauma. The likelihood of penetrating injury occurs whenever a missile or penetrating object passes in the vicinity of the pancreas or duodenum. Since penetrating injury is usually obvious and is usually associated with clinical findings that demand exploration, the primary problem in diagnosis is the recognition of blunt injury to the pancreas or duodenum. This is particularly true when the injury is confined to either of these two organs, both of which lie in a relatively protected position and are usually injured only by a direct blow that compresses them against the vertebral column.

Classically, with injuries to the retroperitoneal pancreas or duodenum, abdominal discomfort may be out of proportion to the abdominal findings and the patient usually has abdominal tenderness and an absence of bowel sounds. The protected position of the pancreas and duodenum does not result in peritoneal irritation as severe as more common intraabdominal injuries, as the extravasated blood, enteric contents, or enzymes are initially contained retroperitoneally. Unless the surgeon has a high index of suspicion, these injuries may not be recognized immediately. It is important for the surgeon to understand the mechanism of blunt injury to pancreas and duodenum and, therefore, to know why the presenting signs and symptoms may not reflect the seriousness of the injury.

The typical blunt trauma resulting in injury is a blow to the abdomen. Most commonly, in our experience, this has been due to impalement of a driver of a motor vehicle on the wheel of the car.[23,51,85,108,132] History of a severe blow to the upper abdomen should lead to the suspicion that pancreatic or duodenal injury may exist. In children, bicycle handlebar injuries or any fall against an object are the most common cause of pancreatic and duodenal injuries other than being a passenger in an automobile.[8,23,51,69,93,95,105] Tenderness in the anatomic location of either of these two organs should suggest the possibility of pancreatic or duodenal injury.

In blunt trauma, the duodenum or head, body, or tail of the pancreas are injured, depending on which direction the impinging force is directed at the vertebral column. If the force is sufficient, fracture of the pancreas or duodenum may result, between the steering wheel compressing the abdominal wall and the unyielding spinal column. The spinal column is like the hub of a wheel around which the pancreas is wrapped. If the patient has his left side between the steering wheel and his vertebral column, the tail of the pancreas will be injured; if his right side is forward, then the head of the pancreas and duodenum are at risk; if he is struck in the midepigastric region, the neck of the pancreas may be divided over the mesenteric vessels. The major pancreatic duct is a more rigid, brittle structure than are the vasculature, the capsule, and pancreatic parenchyma. Often the duct is fractured in the absence of appreciable hemorrhage or capsular disruption, a fact that must be appreciated if significant injury to the pancreas is not to be overlooked at operation (Fig. 9–2A). If the major duct is fractured, the injury is significant owing to the leakage of enzymes. A ductal obstruction will result, causing possible pancreatic fistula, pseudocysts, and pancreatitis. If the major duct is intact, pancreatic injury is not significant. Extravasation of pancreatic secretion from the tributary ducts or obstruction of the tributary ducts causes self-limited fistula or pancreatitis.

The duodenum may be ruptured if compression of the abdominal wall by the impinging force traps the distal end of the duodenum against the vertebral column at the time the pylorus is shut, creating a closed loop while the duodenum is full of fluid.[18,23] This type of closed loop injury leads to extravasation of digestive enzymes in the retroperitoneum and is most often associated with severe symptoms and so is usually suspected and diagnosed. However, in instances when the duodenum is crushed against the vertebral column, the nonviable crushed wall may remain intact for a period of hours or even days until it is digested by a combination of gastric juice and pancreatic enzymes. In such instances, while the necrotic wall is still intact, initial abdominal findings may be minimal.

A less common problem is intramural hematoma of the duodenal lumen. The vomiting of bile or gastric juice after epigastric trauma should lead to the suspicion of the possibility of duodenal obstruction.[49] This is particularly likely if there is little associated abdominal distention. If there is a question of intramural duodenal hematoma, a gastrointestinal series, with soluble radiopaque material demonstrating the characteristic inverted fir-tree sign due to swelling of the plicae of the duodenal mucosa will lead to the diagnosis.[49]

Pancreas injury resulting from blunt trauma should be suspected by the presence of tenderness over the anatomical distribution of the pancreas. Pancreatic injury is often associated with accompanying ileus and very frequently the serum pancreatic enzymes (amylase and lipase) are elevated. This does not provide any clues as to the magnitude of pancreatic injury and is not specific for the pancreas, since any upper gastrointestinal enteric perforation may release pancreatic enzymes in the free peritoneal cavity and their absorption by the abdominal lymphatics will result in elevation of the serum enzymes. Mild trauma that is of no clinical significance may, on occasion, be associated with amylase elevations.[80]

Patients with isolated duodenal or pancreatic compression injuries are often hemodynamically stable and sometimes may initially have no abnormal abdominal findings.[4,108] Diagnostic peritoneal lavage may well be normal (returns of which should also be checked for elevated amylase level) because of the retroperitoneal position of the pancreas and posterior aspect of the duodenum or because of an initially intact, but necrotic, duodenal wall. In such patients, where there is no immediate indication for operation, the serum amylase or urine amylase is a useful test with which to follow the patient.[3,4,130] If the serum or urine amylase is noted to increase progressively, on the basis of serial determinations every 3 to 4 hr, or remain elevated, then surgery is indicated and the duodenum and

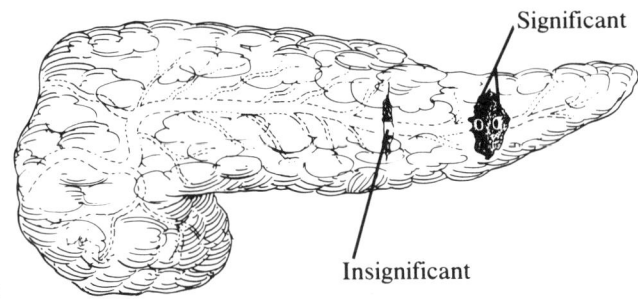

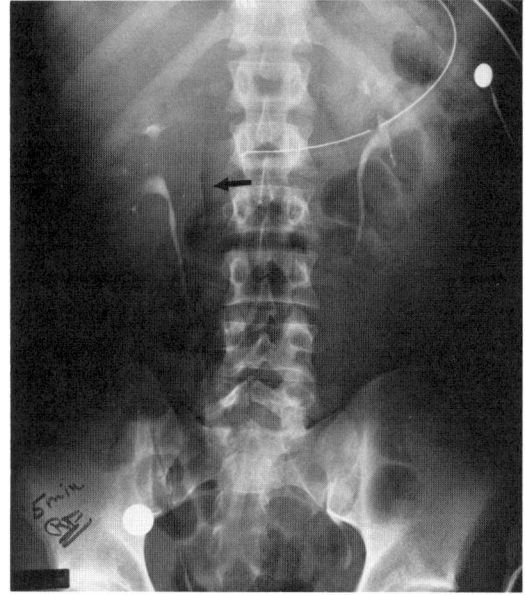

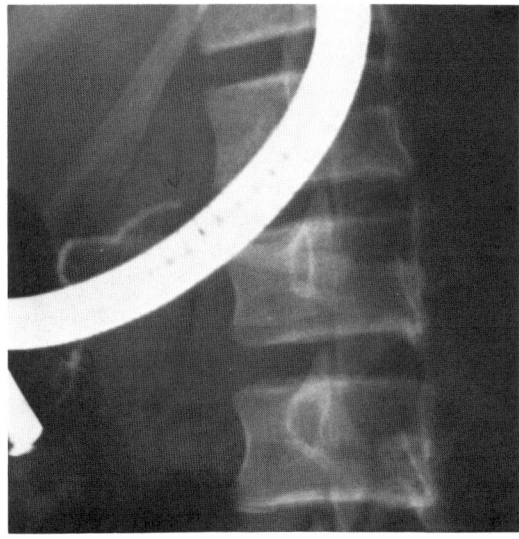

Figure 9–2. A: Demonstration of significant (disruption of pancreatic duct) versus proximal insignificant injury (in which duct is intact). **B,C:** ERCPs showing extravasation of contrast and duct cutoff. Either finding is evidence of severe injury.

pancreas should be examined at operation. If an initially elevated serum amylase declines and there is no other indication for operation, none should be undertaken. A single amylase determination should not be used as a basis for deciding whether a patient does or does not need an operation.[80] In many patients with total disruption of the pancreatic ductal system, the serum amylase will not become elevated until 24 to 48 hr after injury.[4] White has noted serum amylase levels tend to rise more with ductal injuries of the head and body than with injuries of the tail.[130] This is understandable. The serum amylase is a measure of ductal obstruction. The more proximal the fracture of the duct to the duodenum, the more gland there is secreting behind the obstruction or ductal disruption. The amylase behind an obstructed duct diffuses into the interstices of the gland and may be picked up and returned to venous stream by the pancreatic venous capillaries and lymphatics, or if the duct draining the distal pancreatic segment is pouring its contents in the abdominal cavity, the amylase will be picked up by the abdominal lymphatics and returned to the blood venous circulation, raising serum levels of amylase. Knowing these facts, it should be no surprise why the amylase may remain normal if the tail of the gland is shot away. First, there is no proximal obstruction, so that pancreatic juice in the uninjured body and head continue to flow into the duodenum, not retrograde into the area of injury. Second, with the tail shot away, there are no viable acinar cells left to produce a pancreatic secretion containing amylase, even if the duct of the distal segment was fractured and obstructed.

In patients who are hemodynamically stable and in whom there is no other indication of injury or need for celiotomy, other than a progressive increase in amylase, endoscopic retrograde cholangiopancreatography (ERCP), if available, ought to be employed to ascertain whether the suspected pancreatic ductal rupture has occurred and to ascertain its location, that is, the head, body, or tail.[35,118] Increased experience has demonstrated the value of this procedure in defining a significant ductal injury either in the form of extravasation or duct occlusions (Figs. 9–2B,C).

There are no specific diagnostic tests for pancreatic injury. CT scanners and peritoneal lavage are being used with increasing frequency to evaluate abdominal trauma and retroperitoneal edema in the vicinity of the pancreas and may lead to suspicion of pancreatic injury. However, we do not believe that injury can necessarily be ruled out should the scan or peritoneal lavage be interpreted as normal, particularly with early assessment of the injured patient.

In the final analysis, the diagnosis of pancreatic or duodenal injuries rests with a high index of suspicion leading to laparotomy. Whether the injury is due to blunt or penetrating trauma, there is no substitute for exploration of the abdomen.

PREOPERATIVE PREPARATION

As with any patient about to undergo laparotomy, good reliable access to the vascular system should be obtained for fluid and blood infusion, preferably by at least one good cutdown in an upper extremity.

A nasogastric tube should be placed preoperatively if pancreatic or duodenal injury is suspected, to decompress the stomach to prevent a leakage of gastric juice from the ruptured duodenum. In blunt trauma, preoperative antibiotics are not indicated. In penetrating trauma, broad spectrum antibiotics are usually administered before surgery in anticipation of a possible hollow viscus injury and intraperitoneal or retroperitoneal contamination. Blood should have been sent for typing and crossmatch. Routine complete blood count, white count, and urinalysis are necessary and helpful in the evaluation of associated injuries. Routine chest x-ray should be obtained in all instances of penetrating trauma and is often helpful in blunt trauma. Intravenous pyelograms should be obtained if penctrating trauma passes anywhere near the vicinity of a kidney or kidney hilum, as is usually the case when pancreatic injuries are suspected or are present. Hematuria suggests renal damage and is an indication for preoperative intravenous pyelograms, if for no other reason than to verify the presence of two functional kidneys. The patient, as is true in all trauma cases, should be prepped from clavicles to pubis and from bedline to bedline to permit posterior drainage should this be necessary.

OPERATIVE EXPLORATION AND EVALUATION OF THE PANCREAS AND DUODENUM

The routine laparotomy incision for most trauma is a midline abdominal incision. When there is tenderness in the upper abdomen, and the most likely source is in this region, the initial incision should be generous and carry at least from the xiphoid to the umbilicus. It should then be extended well below the umbilicus once the presence of injury or reasonable probability of injury has been verified.

The patient should be eviscerated promptly to permit a thorough abdominal exploration with inspection of the retroperitoneum. All blood and clots should be rapidly evacuated from the peritoneal cavity. Any injury other than catastrophic bleeding should be temporarily isolated with packs to avoid missing more major sources of hemorrhage. After verification that no injury to intraabdominal structures exists or after assessment and treatment of the injuries that do, particularly injuries to major vascular structures [which are the principal cause of mortality (Tables 9–1 and 9–2)], attention should be directed toward the retroperitoneum and the duodenum and pancreas. Since injuries of these structures rarely produce catastrophic hemorrhage in themselves, they do not have high priority in the initial exploration.[102,112] The sites of injury in duodenum and pancreas from collected reviews of pancreatic and duodenal injuries are shown in Figure 9–3.

The initial exploration of the free peritoneal cavity with the bowel eviscerated permits inspection of the inferior aspect of the base of the mesocolon from the ligament of Treitz outward to the left. Injury to the pancreatic ductal system is suspected whenever a retroperitoneal hemorrhage can be seen through the base of the mesocolon or gastrohepatic mesentery. Sometimes it is possible to visualize a ductal injury in penetrating trauma or appreciate that the duct must be fractured if the pancreas itself is more than half transected. A severely macerated gland or one that has a central perforation should be assumed to have a ductal injury until this is ruled out by pancreatogram or operative exploration.[35] In most patients, the pancreatic substance can be inspected along its inferior surface and injury to the body and tail relatively well ruled out. Attention can next be directed toward the gastrohepatic ligament because in thin patients the upper portion of the body and tail can often be visualized through the gastrohepatic ligament; once again, hemorrhage seen through the gastrohepatic ligament suggests the possibility of pancreatic injury.

Next, attention should be directed toward the duodenum, mobilizing the colon downward and, if necessary, sweeping the mesocolon down with sponges. The hepatic flexure of the colon should be mobilized when there is any reason to suspect injury to the duodenum or the head of the pancreas. By severing the lateral attachments of the hepatic

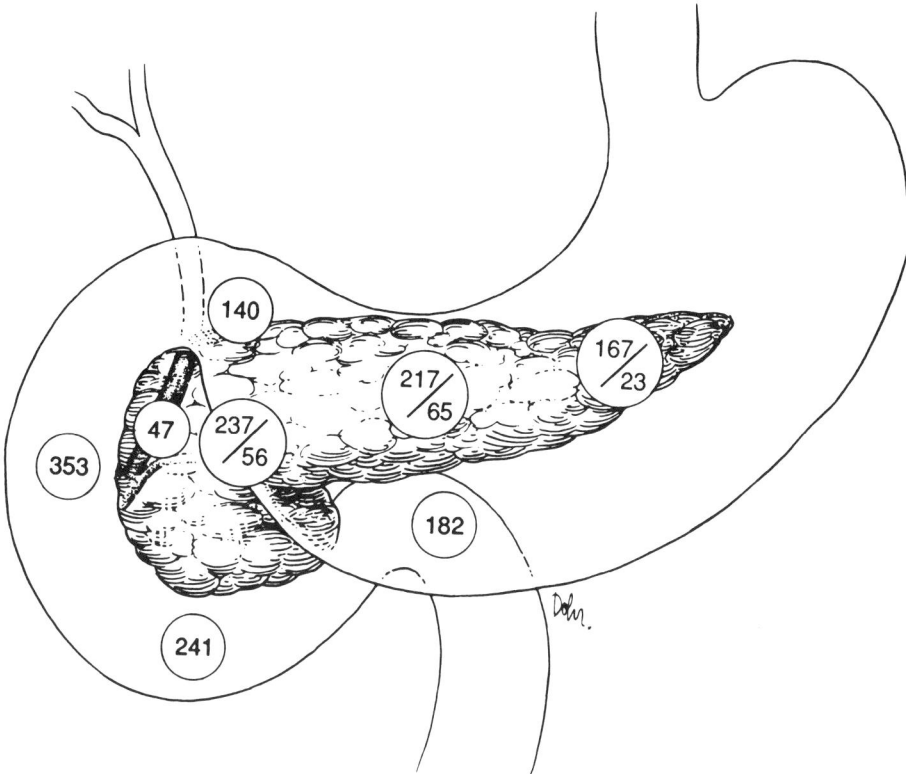

Figure 9–3. Incidence of injury to various parts of the pancreas and duodenum.

flexure of the colon, the entire mesocolon can be mobilized downward to permit inspection of the anterior or lateral surface of the first, second, and third portions of the duodenum (Kocher maneuver). These attachments should be cut from the foramen of Winslow around to the fourth portion of the duodenum. This permits the entire duodenum to be mobilized upward and the posterior surface inspected and palpated. It also permits evaluation of the head of the pancreas. If there should be even a small hematoma in the head of the pancreas, bimanual palpation should be carried out to determine whether there is loss of substance or pulpifation of the head. This finding is associated with the possibility of injury to major pancreatic ducts. The fourth portion of the duodenum can be inspected from the area of the ligament of Treitz. The absence of hemorrhage around the ligament of Treitz makes injury to the fourth portion of the duodenum unlikely. Should there be a suggestion of injury, the entire right colon and small bowel mesentery can be mobilized and swung up and medially to permit exposure of the entire sweep of the duodenum.[14] When there is any reason to suspect the possibility of injury to the body and tail of the pancreas or when there is evidence of trauma to the head of the pancreas, the lesser sac should be opened and the entire pancreas exposed. This is best done by ligating two to three arcades outside the gastric epiploic vessels in a relatively avascular area of the gastroeploic omentum and coming down on the pancreas through the lesser sac. Once the lesser sac is entered in the right plane, the entire body and tail of the pancreas are open to view.

If there should be evidence of hemorrhage in the retroperitoneum, the entire transverse colon should be separated from the omentum to permit direct inspection of the entire anterior surface of the pancreas. Ecchymosis in the area of the neck, body, or tail of the pancreas requires an exploration. Bimanual palpation is another method for evaluating a pancreatic injury. This can best be done by sweeping the mesocolon downward, separating it from the inferior surface of the pancreas or by opening the mesocolon at its junction with the retroperitoneum inferiorly. The latter maneuver, unless carefully done, risks injuring the colonic arcade that provides collateral blood flow from the middle colic artery to the left colic artery. Once the colon and the mesentery have been separated from the body and tail of the pancreas, the body and tail of the pancreas can be rotated superiorly along its length without having to mobilize the spleen. The posterior aspect of the gland can be visualized and bimanual palpation of the body of the tail of the pancreas performed. A loss of integrity of pancreatic substance provides indirect evidence of ductal injury. An alternative exploration for those experienced with pancreatic injury is accomplished by duodenotomy and retrograde pancreatogram through the ampulla of Vater using a Fogarty irrigating catheter. The pancreatic duct can also be intubated by incising the tail of the pancreas and using the Fogarty irrigating catheter to perform a pancreatogram. The importance of assessing ductal integrity and planning an appropriate operation as espoused by Kerry, Glas, and Bach in the 1960s and 1970s was more recently demonstrated by Berni who, by the use of intraoperative pancreaticography, sharply reduced the morbidity of pancreas-related complications. The liberal use of intraoperative pancreaticography has also been supported by Ivantury, who noted few complications resulting from duodenotomy and no instances of duodenal fistulization.[12,48] However, a less invasive and superior technique (if the patient is stable) is either preoperative or intraoperative ERCP to assess the integrity of the major pancreatic duct.[42]

EVALUATION OF THE PANCREATIC AND DUODENAL INJURY

Absence of any hemorrhage over the pancreas and duodenum makes injury unlikely. The only exception is the possibility of injury to the posterior aspect of the duodenum, although this is entirely unlikely if palpation of the duodenum does not reveal induration, crepitus, or bile staining nor, on inspection, the slightest trace of ecchymosis. Small, ecchymotic lesions, however, demand definitive evaluation, since injuries to the pancreas and duodenum are easily underestimated.[4,17]

Duodenal intramural hematomas and duodenal lacerations are relatively easily recognized: the former, by the presence of severe ecchymosis and induration of the duodenal contents on mobilization of the duodenum.[49,114] The consequences of the injury may be difficult to evaluate in the duodenum if the time between injury and operation is short. If 4 or 5 hr have passed and there has been no evidence of duodenal obstruction, intramural hematomas of the duodenum can be left intact.[49] If, preoperatively, there has been evidence of obstruction, manifest by biliary drainage from the nasogastric tube or by x-ray studies, the serosa should be opened through the main area of the induration and the submucosal hematoma evacuated.[49]

The pancreas is the most difficult of all abdominal organs to evaluate. In the dog the pancreas can be pounded with a hammer, squeezed and macerated, its substance and capsule lacerated, yet serious injury does not result as long as the main pancreatic duct remains intact, as Kerry and Glas demonstrated.[57] The same situation seems to apply to humans. Conversely, a seemingly relatively minor injury may result in disruption or obstruction of a brittle main pancreatic duct, resulting in a leakage of pancreatic juice causing acute pancreatitis and if untreated, pancreatic pseudocysts, fistulas, ascites, abscesses, sepsis, and chronic pancreatitis.[4,7,29,32,40,44,51,54,111,112,130]

For all practical purposes, if the major pancreatic ductal system is intact, the pancreatic injury, be it capsular tear, hematoma, or laceration of its substance, is not significant. Any leakage of pancreatic fluid from a tributary duct will resolve spontaneously, usually in less than 4 to 6 weeks, if drainage is instituted. Hematomas of the pancreas and capsular injuries of the pancreas, if encountered at operation, ought to be drained even if the pancreatic ductal system is disrupted. It is essential that the injury be recognized and treated appropriately to prevent mortality and serious morbidity.

CLASSIFICATION OF PANCREATIC AND DUODENAL INJURY

For purposes of comparing the experience of one institution with another, identifying and comparing injuries of similar severity, and as a guide to therapy, injuries have been classified into four categories. Category I injuries we manage by drainage alone. Category II injuries are best managed by distal pancreatectomy with preservation of the spleen. Category III injuries are complex problems and management individualized. Whenever possible, depending on the condition of the patient, a Roux-en-Y end-to-side pancreaticojejunostomy should be performed. Category IV injuries are best managed by pancreaticoduodenectomy.[66]

> Category I: Hematoma, contusion, or capsular tear
> Category II: Injury associated with fracture or disruption of the major duct in the body or tail of the pancreas
> Category III: Disruption of the major pancreatic duct in the head of the pancreas
> Category IV: Disruption of the major pancreatic duct in the head of the pancreas, associated with injury to the duodenum and/or common bile duct

The Abdominal Trauma Index (ATI) described by Moore et al.[77] is an attempt to quantitate the severity of injury of individual abdominal organs. The pancreas, on a scale of 1 to 5, was assigned a risk of 5, meaning it was an organ at high risk of complications if injured.

The injury to the pancreas was also graded for severity from 1 to 5. Grades I and II involved injuries in which the major duct's integrity was maintained. Grade III consisted of an injury involving the major duct in body and tail of the pancreas. Grade IV consisted of injury to the major duct in the head of the pancreas, and grade V consisted of combined injury of the major pancreatic duct and common bile duct or duodenum or both.

The injury could then be quantitated by multiplying 5 (the number assigned to the pancreas) times the severity of injury to the organ, so scores for pancreatic injury could range from $5 \times 1 = 5$ to $5 \times 5 = 25$. Duodenal injuries have also been classified into four categories:

Category I: Hematoma or contusions
Category II: Full thickness penetration
Category III: Major duodenal injury with more than 75% defect circumferentially
Category IV: Major duodenal injury and injury to the common bile duct and/or major pancreatic duct

RATIONALE FOR CHOICE OF OPERATION

We feel the rationale for the choice of operation in duodenal and pancreatic trauma, which may occur either independently or together or in association with common duct injury, should be reconstitution of enteric and ductal integrity based on the anatomy of injury and preservation of function. However, our first priority should be to save a life and, in a hemodynamically unstable patient with severe associated injuries to major vascular structures, definitive therapy of the pancreatic or duodenal injury may have to be delayed to shorten operating time.

Some useful concepts in the management of pancreatic trauma that can be applied to the individual patient are discussed below.

1. At operation, the diagnosis and management of pancreatic and duodenal injuries should be deferred in the patient with multiple injuries until hemorrhage from associated injuries, such as to major vessels or liver and spleen, is controlled. This recommendation is based on the knowledge that the single most frequent cause of death in pancreatic and duodenal injury is hemorrhage and shock from associated injuries (see Tables 9–3 and 9–6). Most of the deaths from these injuries occur with 48 hr of injury.[1,7,16,17,21,24,26,32,36,41,45,47,50,51,55,59,65,70,83,85,103,104,107,109,110,112,114,116,128,135,137]

2. Definitive management of pancreatic injuries in the absence of injury to the common duct or duodenum requires recognition of pancreatic ductal injury and, generally, either resection of the distal segment if less than 50% to 60% of the gland, or drainage of the distal segment if it exceeds 60% to 70% of the gland by means of a Roux-en-Y limb of jejunum. The pancreaticojejunostomy should be an end-to-side duct to a jejunal mucosa anastomosis.[14] Although most patients do not become diabetic unless 80% of the gland is resected, an occasional patient may do so with what is judged to be less than an 80% resection.[32] Aside from the fact that we have no way of knowing whether these patients were prediabetic, it seems prudent, particularly in the young, to leave some margin of protection for the surgeon's estimate of what constitutes an 80% resection in a particular gland. When a gland lacks an uncinate process there is a marked decrease in volume of the head of the pancreas. The surgeon may not recognize this normal variation and assume a resection of the neck of the gland is removing 60% to 65% of the gland when it is more likely, in the congenital absence of the uncinate, 70% to 80% of the gland is being removed.

Although definitive therapy of the pancreatic injury is an important goal in pancreatic injury, the first priority is to save the patient's life. In the event the patient's condition is precarious from associated injuries and operative time needs to be minimized, the pancreatic ductal disruption can be managed by sump drainage.[51,53,112,115] Creation of a controlled fistula will prevent loculated collections that otherwise could culminate in pseudocyst or abscess formation.

3. Most duodenal injuries (85%) can be managed by debridement and simple closure.[55,70,108,114] However, those few patients with 75% circumferential crush injuries, large

lacerations with loss of tissue, or devascularization, of a large segment of duodenum require an operative solution tailored to the anatomy of the injury.[108] No one operation for duodenal repair is suitable for all duodenal injuries. Therefore, the trauma surgeon, to do best by the patient, must be familiar with those operative procedures most appropriate for injuries of different size and shape in a variety of duodenal locations, as well as take into account the patient's general condition from associated injuries or preexisting illness.[21,23,81,108,114]

4. In an injury of the common duct and duodenum in association with a pancreatic ductal disruption, there is potential for much mischief from the devastation created by uncontrolled loss of a combination of gastric, duodenal, pancreatic, and biliary secretions, which may lead to fluid and electrolyte disorders, dehydration, digestion of skin, intraabdominal collections, abscesses, and sepsis. Therefore, it is essential that lack of intestinal and ductal integrity be treated by pancreaticoduodenectomy. If the patient is judged by the operating surgeon to be unable to tolerate pancreaticoduodenectomy,[1,4,13,16,31,33,41,51,65,73,83,89,99,116,128,131] then diversionary drainage separating the secretions should be implemented.

PANCREATIC INJURY AND ITS OPERATIVE MANAGEMENT

Suburban hospitals receiving auto accident victims tend to report a higher incidence of blunt than penetrating injuries of the pancreas.[4] In trauma centers located in the metropolitan areas, most injuries result from penetrating trauma.[45,115,128]

One factor that contributes to the mortality of patients with pancreatic trauma is the nature of the wounding agent, with shotgun injuries being the most lethal and stab wounds the least (Table 9–2).[51] Likewise, the condition of the patient on arrival in the emergency department and in the operating room is important; if in shock from associated injuries to major vessels of liver or spleen, the patient's mortality is six times higher than for the patient who is normotensive during preoperative and operative management.[51,115,131] The massive tissue destruction associated with shotgun injuries (58% mortality) and the presence of shock are not usually a reflection of the severity of the pancreatic injury, but of the injuries to major vessels or liver and spleen.[36,51,128,131] Sepsis, the second most common cause of death after hemorrhage, is most often seen in patients who are in hemorrhagic shock pre- and postoperative, and those with associated bowel injuries.[44,51,115,131] Factors related to the pancreas that adversely affect survival are the location of the wound in the head of the gland with injury to the major duct and overlooked injuries of the major duct.[4,108,122] We prefer posterior drainage of the pancreas below the 12th rib. When the major pancreatic duct is intact, leakage from tributary ducts will be short-lived and drainage may be expected to subside in 4 to 6 weeks. If a major ductal injury is recognized but the patient's condition is unstable, prohibiting definitive treatment, and the injury is drained, then it is advisable to employ a sump drainage. With injury to the major duct, these controlled fistulae are often persistent and further operative management may be required after the patient is fully recovered from any associated injuries.

Isolated Pancreas Injuries

The junction of the neck and body of the pancreas is the most common site of injury (see Fig. 9–3). The portion of pancreas distal to the neck and body constitutes about 60% to

65% of the mass of the pancreas and can therefore be resected with little immediate or late morbidity from pancreatic exocrine or endocrine insufficiency (Fig. 9–4).[32,132] Distal pancreatic resection is the treatment of choice for any injury involving the neck, body, or tail of the pancreas from either penetrating or blunt trauma (Fig. 9–5).

The pancreas is most often resected with the spleen in continuity. Short gastrics are divided and the attachments between the splenic flexure and the colon and the spleen are severed. The spleen and tail of the pancreas are mobilized and rotated left to right, the splenic artery is divided as it joins the body of the pancreas, and the pancreas is transected at the point of the laceration. Interrupted, interlocking mattress sutures of 2-0 silk on an atraumatic needle has been our standard method of closing the severed distal end of the pancreas. However, stapling using the larger 4.5-mm staples has also been effective in our experience. The main pancreatic duct, if identified, is separately ligated. If the patient is unstable, time should not be spent searching for the main duct, which is 1 to 2 mm in the normal pancreas. In isolated injuries of the body and tail of the pancreas, it is usually possible to preserve the spleen by ligating and dividing the branches of the splenic vein and artery to the tail of the pancreas. The importance of the spleen in immunity and prevention of the overwhelming postsplenectomy sepsis syndrome, particularly in children, is now well recognized. Robey et al.[97] in 1982 reported four cases and cited five other reports in which the spleen had been preserved and the tail of the pancreas resected. Resection of the tail of the pancreas with splenic preservation in trauma is usually more easily accomplished than when being performed for chronic pancreatitis. Splenic preservation is encouraged. Pachter et al. reported it was possible to preserve the spleen in nine consecutive patients with pancreatic injuries requiring distal pancreatectomy.[90] Over an 8-year period we have been able to preserve the spleen in 44% of 32 patients undergoing distal pancreatectomy. Of the 18 patients undergoing distal pancreatectomy and splenectomy, 8 had major injuries to the spleen itself.[132]

However, it should be kept in mind that in adult trauma patients, concern over postsplenectomy sepsis does not justify preserving the spleen if the patient is hemodynamically unstable, requires blood transfusions in attempts to preserve the spleen, or has major associated injuries.[9,68] Beal and Spisso calculated that the risk of hepatitis from blood transfusion would result in 87 deaths/31,000 patients transfused versus 8 deaths from postsplenectomy sepsis/31,000 patients undergoing splenectomy.[9]

Eighty to 95% resection of the distal portion of the pancreas can be carried out in injuries involving the major pancreatic duct in the head of the gland. However, because of the high incidence of pancreatic endocrine and exocrine insufficiency, 80% to 95%

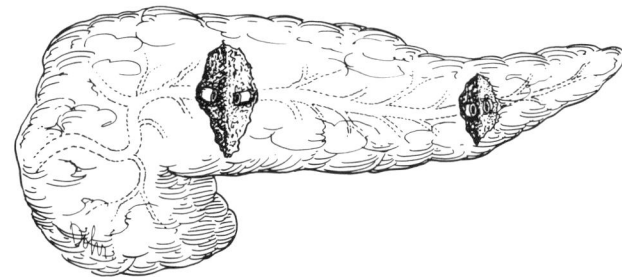

Figure 9–4. Lesions readily amenable to treatment by distal pancreatic resection.

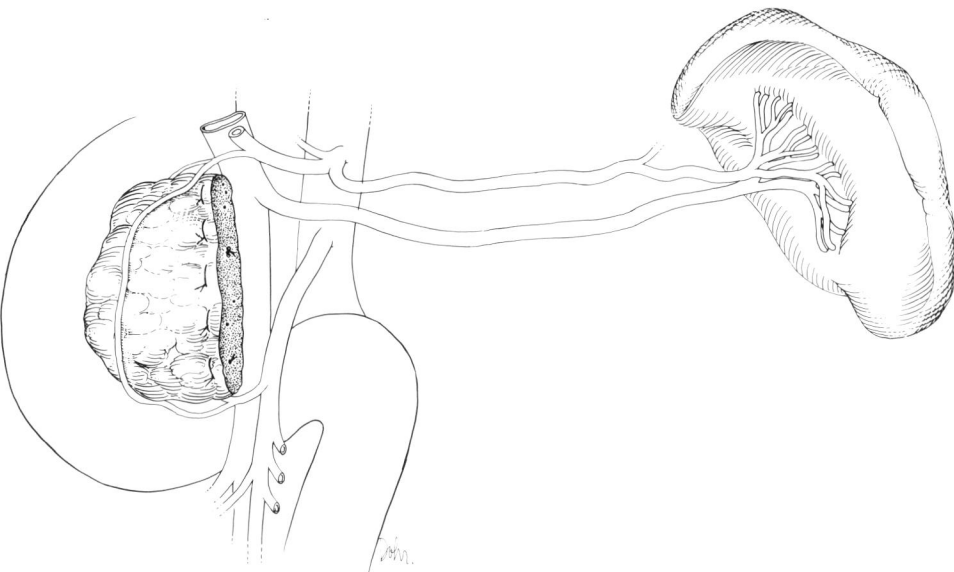

Figure 9–5. An example of extensive distal pancreatic resection (80%) with preservation of the spleen and its blood supply. The preservation of the splenic vein is crucial and the dissection is difficult and indicated only in good-risk patients with isolated pancreatic injury.

resection should be carried out only when the patient is unstable and preferably already a diabetic and a short operation is essential for survival. For the proximal pancreatic ductal fractures, there is a better option than 80% to 95% distal resection, that is, oversewing the proximal severed end of pancreas with interlocking mattress sutures of 2-0 silk and then anastomosing the distal end of the pancreas end-to-side into a Roux-en-Y limb of jejunum in a duct to jejunal mucosa anastomosis (Fig. 9–6). We do not recommend placement of a Roux-en-Y jejunal limb blindly over fresh lacerations and stellate fractures in lieu of a duct to jejunal mucosal anastomosis, nor do we recommend trying to drain the proximal portion of the pancreas into the Roux-en-Y limb as well as the distal segment in a T-type anastomosis. Draining the proximal segment of the pancreas with a Roux-en-Y limb is unnecessary and may compromise the anastomosis of the distal segment of pancreas with a Roux-en-Y limb. There is the additional risk of gastrointestinal contamination from two rather than one suture line. If the duodenum and common bile duct are intact, pancreaticoduodenectomy is not indicated for a major pancreatic ductal injury in the head of the gland. In the occasional patient in whom there has been minimal trauma to the adjacent pancreatic tissue, a primary repair of the fractured duct may be considered.[31,69]

Mortality

In major trauma centers, half the deaths (8% of cases in which the duodenum is injured) occur early from massive hemorrhage and shock due to associated extraduodenal injuries (see Table 9–6). Most of these patients die in the operating room or within 72 hr of injury. The duodenal injury in these instances has little to do with the fatal outcome.[21,48,55,70,103,108,114]

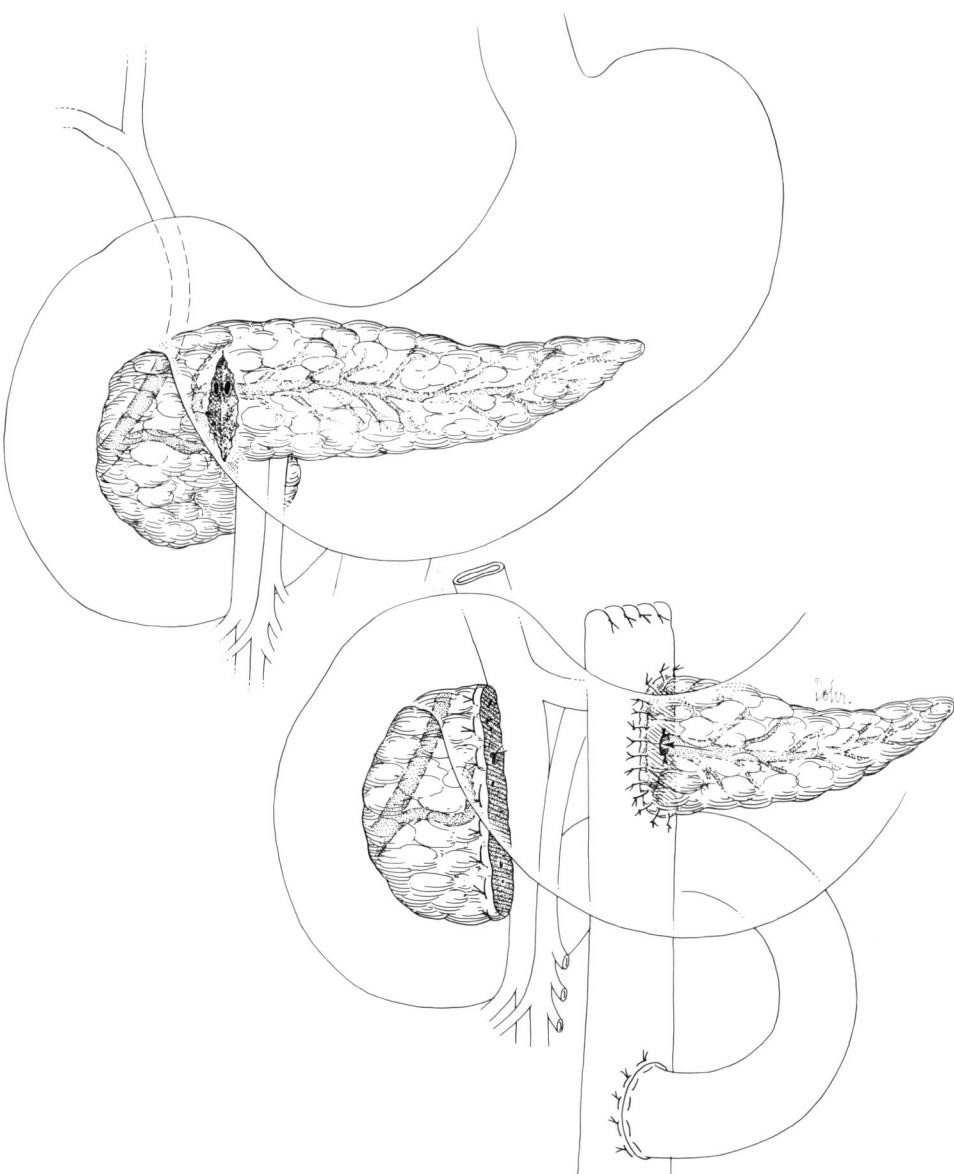

Figure 9–6. In many instances of injury to the head of the pancreas, preservation of the tail of the pancreas may be indicated to prevent diabetes.

Factors that contribute to a fatal outcome in the other 8% of patients include delays in operative treatment owing to failure to diagnose the injury or to recognize it at operation. The operative mortality in these patients, most of whom have had blunt trauma, is 40% to 50% if the delay in operative therapy is 24 hr or longer.[21,67,108] The location of the duodenal wound and the size of the wound are believed to influence the mortality.[108,115] The larger the duodenal wound, the more complex the operation is to reconstitute intestinal continuity. The wounding agent is also important, in that the agent affects the size of the wound: shotgun wounds are the most lethal and stab wounds are the least lethal (Table 9–5).

Penetrating wounds most frequently affect the liver, small and large bowel, pancreas, and stomach. The great vessels are always involved in the early deaths. Blunt trauma more often affects the solid organs, that is, the liver, spleen, pancreas, and kidney.[23] Mortality of duodenal wounds increases as the number of associated injuries increases.

Isolated Duodenal Injuries

The site and presence of duodenal injury may be identified at operation by tracing the missile track or noting the site of active bleeding or hematoma, or by bile staining or crepitation of surrounding tissues. A higher percentage of blunt injuries than penetrating trauma, 46% versus 7%, can be said to be extensive (extensive being defined as involving more than 75% percent of the circumference of the duodenal wall according to Snyder and colleagues) (Fig. 9–7).[108] Fortunately, in most patients with penetrating duodenal injury, the wounds are not extensive and local debridement and duodenal closure in two layers is safe and sufficient therapy.[108,114] The closure of the duodenum should be performed without tension. This may be accomplished by closing the duodenum either in a transverse or vertical direction according to Krauss and Gordon.[58] The mortality associated with duodenotomy is high but is attributed to the condition that prompted duodenotomy.[46] In larger defects, application of a serosal patch may be helpful.

There is controversy over whether tube duodenostomy or gastrostomy is beneficial in these injuries.[67,108,114] Neither Kashuk nor Martin employs tube duodenostomy; Kashuk supports the use of feeding jejunostomy.

The more extensive duodenal wounds require segmental resection or Roux-en-Y duodenojejunostomy (Fig. 9–8). Segmental resection and end-to-end anastomosis with standard two-layer closure is indicated in circumferential crush injuries. This can be accomplished in the first, second, third, or fourth portion of duodenum. To avoid injury to the common duct and ampulla, the distal bile duct can be intubated with a Bakes dilator passed into the duodenum and maintained there during the resection and anastomosis. If a large segment of duodenum has been devitalized and segmental resection performed, it may not be possible to mobilize sufficient duodenum to perform an end-to-end duodenostomy. This problem, particularly if the duodenal injury is distal to the ampulla, lends itself to Roux-en-Y duodenojejunostomy (Fig. 9–9). The jejunum is divided 20 cm distal to the ligament of Treitz. The distal limb of the jejunum is advanced and anastomosed end-to-side to the proximal duodenum. Proximal jejunum is anastomosed end-to-side 30 cm from the site of duodenojejunostomy. The distal duodenum can be oversewn.

Duodenojejunostomy side-to-end has limited applicability except for injuries of the third part of the duodenum along its antimesenteric border (see Fig. 9–9). Occasionally useful is the duodenal patch by Roux-en-Y duodenojejunostomy.

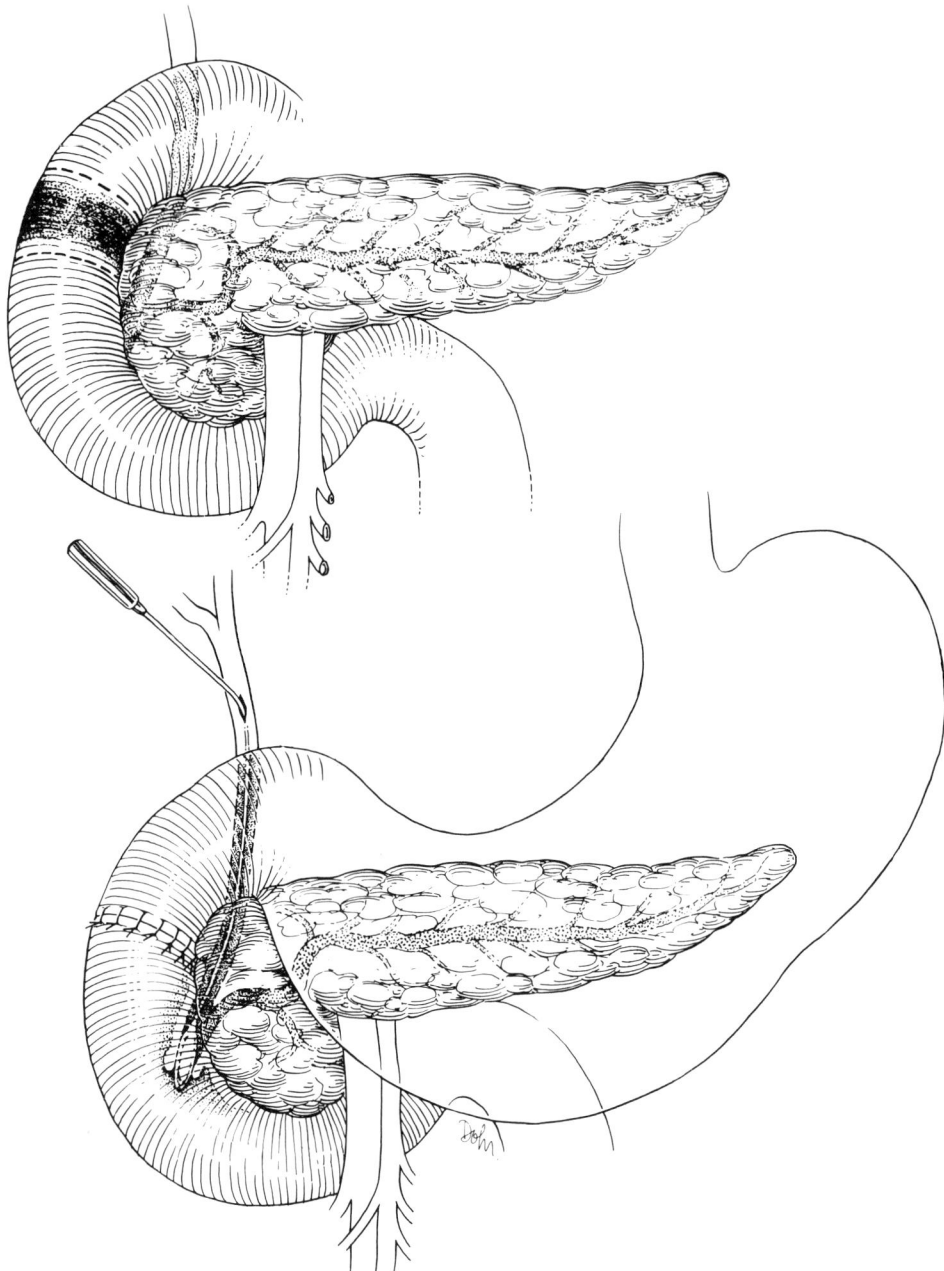

Figure 9–7. Lacerations of the duodenum may be treated by primary suture or by resection and reanastamosis if there is segmental circumferential injury.

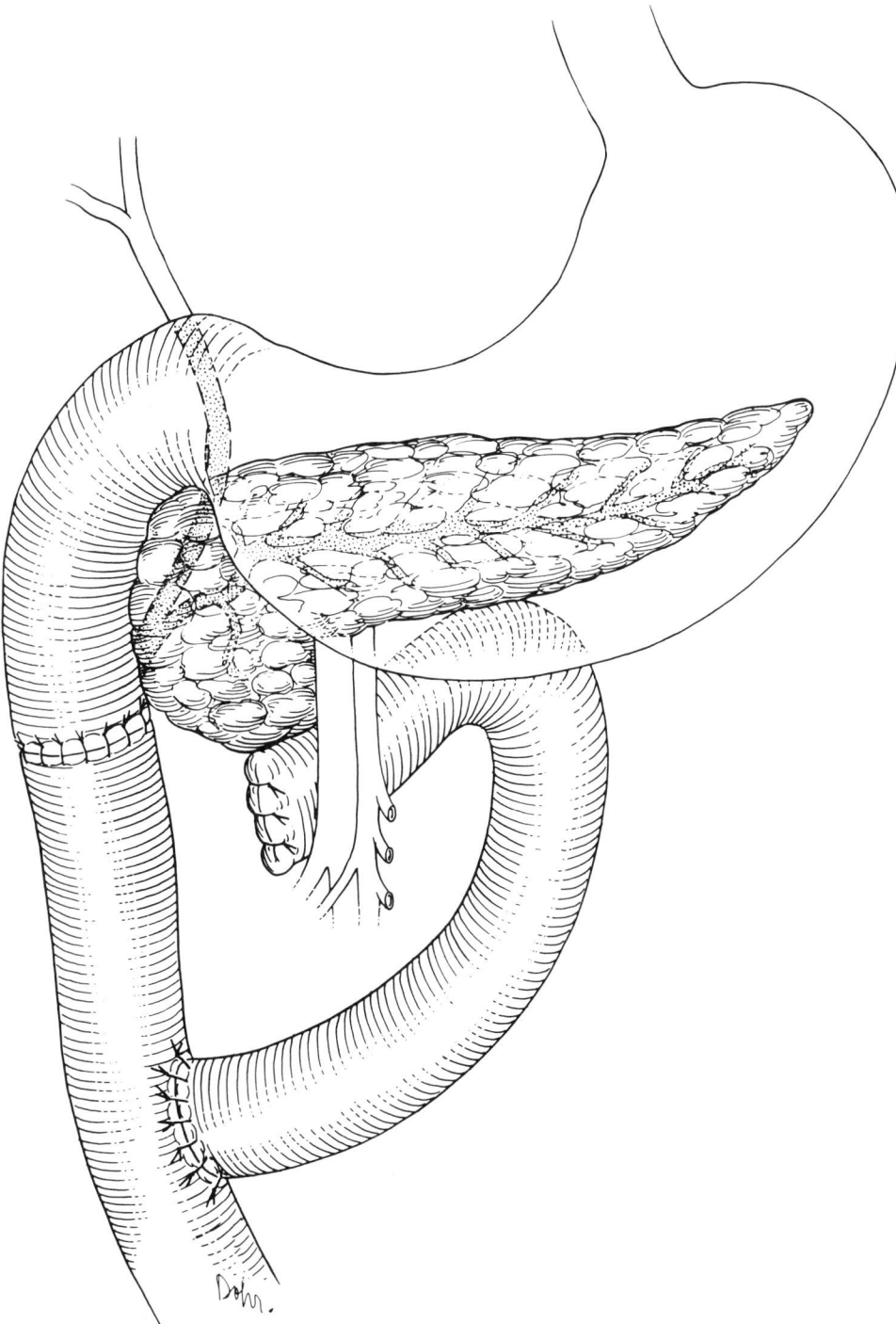

Figure 9–8. Distal duodenal injuries may be treated by resection and duodenal jejunal anastomosis.

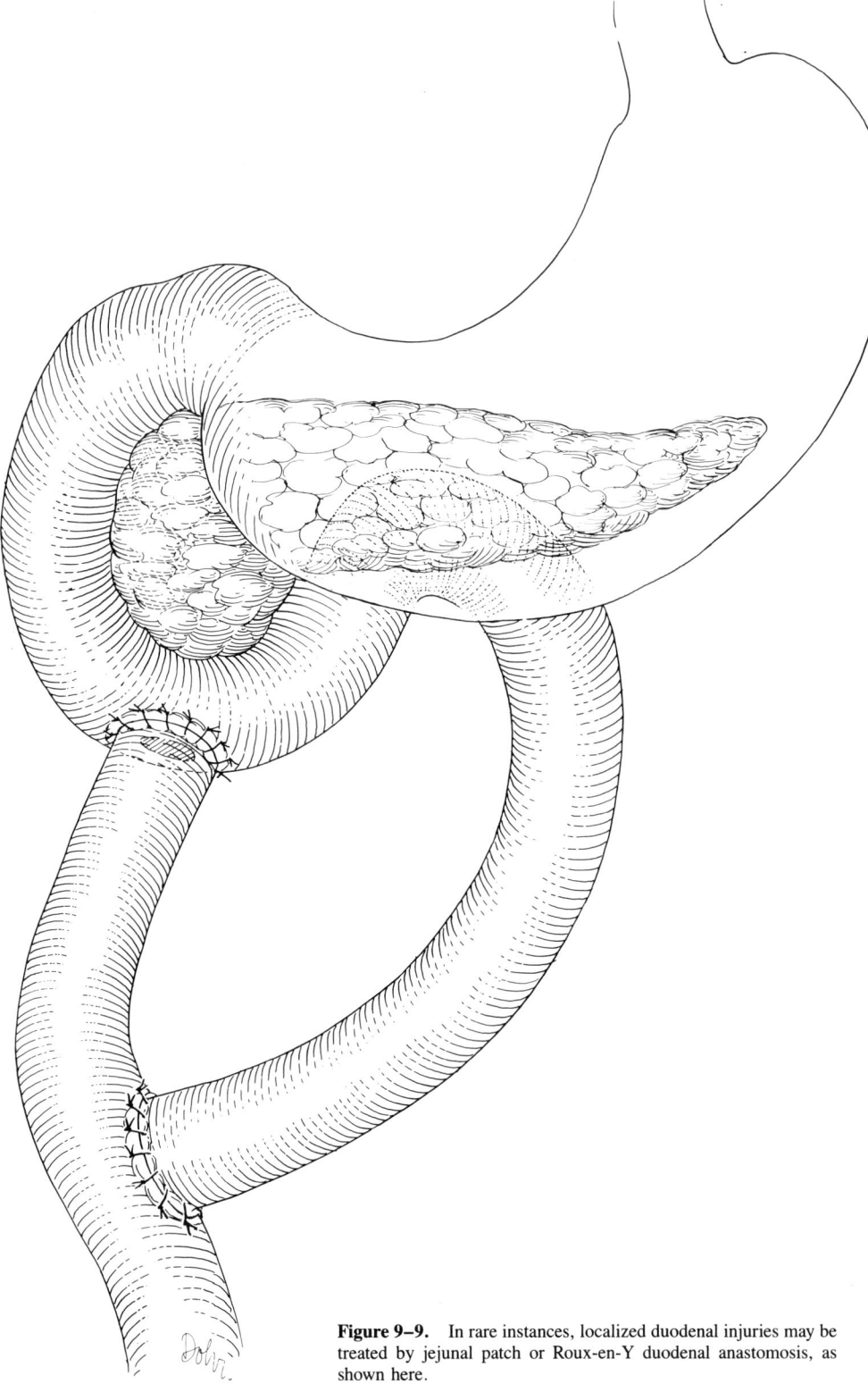

Figure 9–9. In rare instances, localized duodenal injuries may be treated by jejunal patch or Roux-en-Y duodenal anastomosis, as shown here.

Diverticulization Procedure

Patients having more than one duodenal perforation or extensive loss of duodenal tissue (greater than 75% of the circumference) that could compromise the lumen or in whom the agent of injury was a high velocity missile, or in whom there has been a delay in operation that leads to peritonitis, edema, and infection, or in whom the blood supply is compromised may benefit from the diverticulization procedure. The diverticulization procedure converts a lateral fistula, should it develop, to an end fistula. The diverticulization procedure was originally described by Berne but simplified by Graham, Mattox, Vaughan, and Jordan (Fig. 9–10).[7,28] As described by Berne et al., the procedure included a gastrojejunostomy, tube duodenostomy, T-tube biliary drainage, and oversewing the duodenal lacerations.[10] Mortality associated with its use was reported to be 16%.[11] The modified diverticulization or pylorus exclusion procedure described by Graham et al.[36,37] is now widely used and is an important adjunct to the management of complicated duodenal injuries. The stomach is opened at the site for a gastrojejunostomy and the pylorus oversewn through the opening, (Fig. 9–10A). Mortality associated with the Graham diverticulization in severely injured patients in recent reports ranges from 4% to 15%.[55,70]

We do not recommend the diverticulization procedure in patients having associated injuries consisting of disruption of the duct of Wirsung in the head of the pancreas and/or

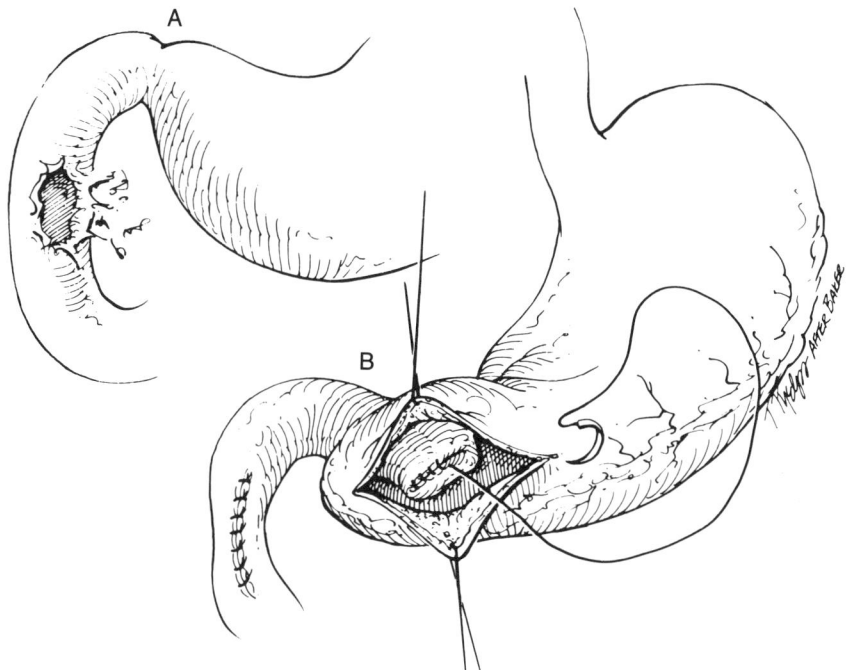

Figure 9–10. A,B: Modified diverticulization procedure described by Graham and Mattox is useful when duodenum closure is difficult. (Figure continued on next page)

146 *Abdominal Trauma*

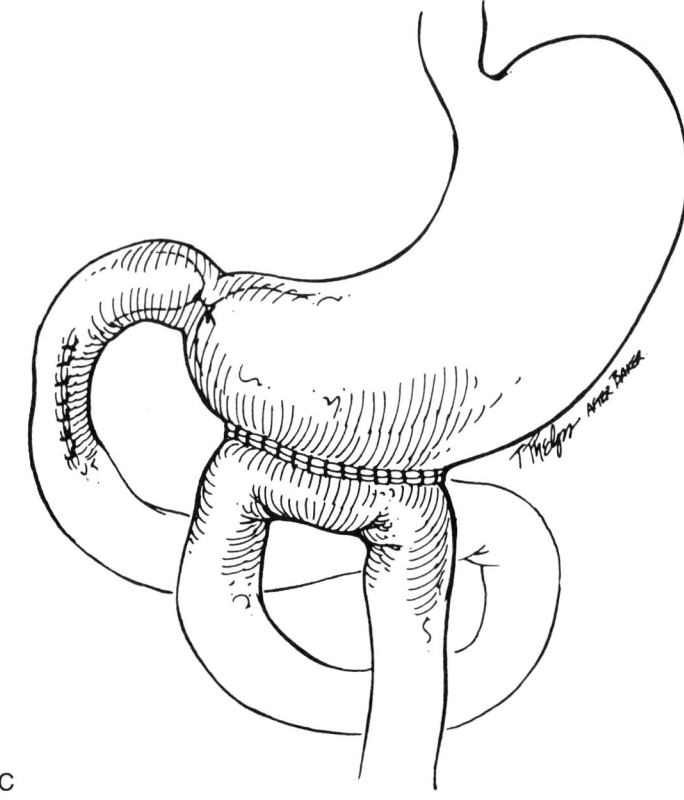

Figure 9–10, Cont. C: Completion of diverticulization procedure with duodenal closure and gastrojejunostomy.

transection of the common bile duct unless accompanied by other operative maneuvers to deal with the divided bile duct or pancreatic duct, problems that are not addressed by diverticulization. There is no substitute for pancreaticoduodenectomy in patients with combined injuries of the major pancreatic duct, common bile duct, and duodenum.

Major Pancreatic Head Ductal Disruptions with Associated Duodenal Laceration

Except under unusual circumstances, neither 80% to 95% distal pancreatectomy nor pancreaticoduodenectomy is indicated.

Segmental resection and end-to-end repair of the duodenum is often possible in the duodenum even in the second portion close to the ampullar of Vater. A Fogarty irrigation catheter may be employed to intubate the ampulla of Vater through the duodenal wound to obtain an on-the-table pancreaticogram or to ascertain the integrity of the pancreatic duct. If the duct is found to be injured in the head of the gland, a Roux-en-Y jejunal limb may be used to drain the distal segment of pancreas. The proximal end of the pancreas is oversewn (Fig. 9–11).

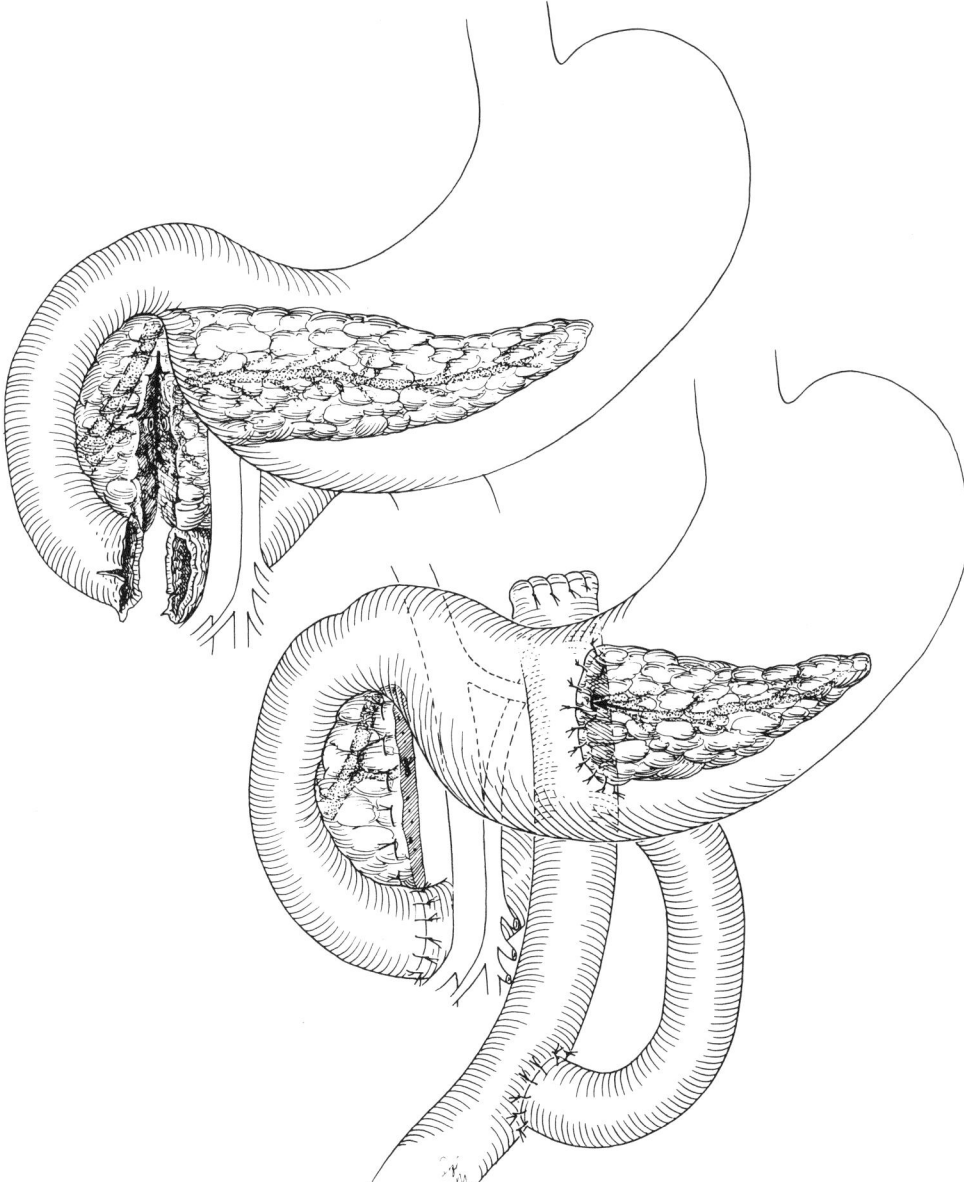

Figure 9–11. Combined duodenal pancreatic ductal injury is treated by resection of the body of the gland, repairing the duodenum and draining the distal pancreas into a Roux-en-Y jejunal limb.

When the duodenum is extensively lacerated but repair is still possible but tenuous and the pancreatic duct is transected in the head of the pancreas, the surgeon is faced with a dilemma. There is no ideal operation that deals with both a major duodenal injury and major pancreatic duct injury. The surgeon must weigh the risk of a less extensive procedure, such as duodenal exclusion or diverticulization, which does not adequately deal with the major pancreatic duct fracture as Jones has noted, versus that of a procedure, pancreaticoduodenectomy, that does deal with the problem but has the disadvantage of requiring a biliary anastomosis when none is required by the injury.[51]

Duodenal diverticulization as described by Berne et al. is effective in the management of duodenal laceration, as it diverts gastric and biliary secretions from the duodenum.[10] Likewise, temporary pyloric exclusion, described by Graham and colleagues, which includes sewing the pylorus shut with absorbable suture, is an effective method for dealing with major duodenal injury.[36] However, neither of these operations provides for management of an associated major ductal injury of the pancreas except by Penrose or sump drainage. Therefore, we must remain skeptical that pyloric exclusion or diverticulization of the duodenum is a procedure with a major role in the management of a combined major duodenal injury and major pancreatic duct fracture, because neither operation addresses the problem of major pancreatic ductal disruption.

Injuries of the pancreas in which the major pancreatic duct remains intact are not associated with serious sequelae, and should not be considered significant injuries. Patients whose duodenal wound was treated definitively but in whom the injury to the major pancreatic duct was treated by suction may require reoperation if the fistula from the distal pancreas has not closed in 3 to 4 months.

Combined Duodenal and Biliary Tract Injuries

These serious injuries fortunately occur in only about 5% of all duodenal injuries.[70] In patients with injury to the duodenum and common duct, it may be possible to perform duodenal closure and an end-to-side choledochojejunostomy to a Roux-en-Y limb of jejunum after injury to the major pancreatic duct has been ruled out by retrograde pancreaticogram (Fig. 9–12). Rarely, avulsion of the ampulla in association with duodenal injury may occur. This injury has also been treated by closure of the duodenum, and placement of the ampulla of Vater end-to-side to a Roux-en-Y jejunal limb. However, more than likely, combined duodenal and biliary tract injuries will require pancreaticoduodenectomy if the duodenal injury is major.[27,62] Pancreaticoduodenectomy is justified in patients with this injury, which has a serious prognosis. Pancreaticoduodenectomy for trauma has a 30% mortality associated with its use, but with other forms of treatment, the mortality is closer to 100%.[51,57,65,121,131,137] The common duct is usually of normal caliber and therefore not as easy to anastomose successfully through an isolated loop of bowel as is the obstructed duct associated with pancreatic tumor or chronic pancreatitis. Cholecystojejunostomy and ligation of the injured common bile duct below the cystic duct combined with diverticulization is one option in these circumstances. Unfortunately, these anastomoses have a failure rate approaching 40% at 1 year when performed for other reasons such as chronic pancreatitis and there is no reason to believe the failure rate would be different when performed for trauma.[2,136] Therefore, cholecystojejunostomy should be considered as an option primarily in patients too unstable to undergo pancreaticoduodenectomy. Pancreaticoduodenectomy can and should be carried out when indicated whenever the patient's condition permits. Although the antrum and pylorus of the stomach are resected in pancreaticoduodenectomy for cancer, it is not necessary in trauma and, as Traverso and Longmire have shown, the antrum and pylorus can be preserved.[124]

The maximal length of common duct should be preserved by carrying the dissection

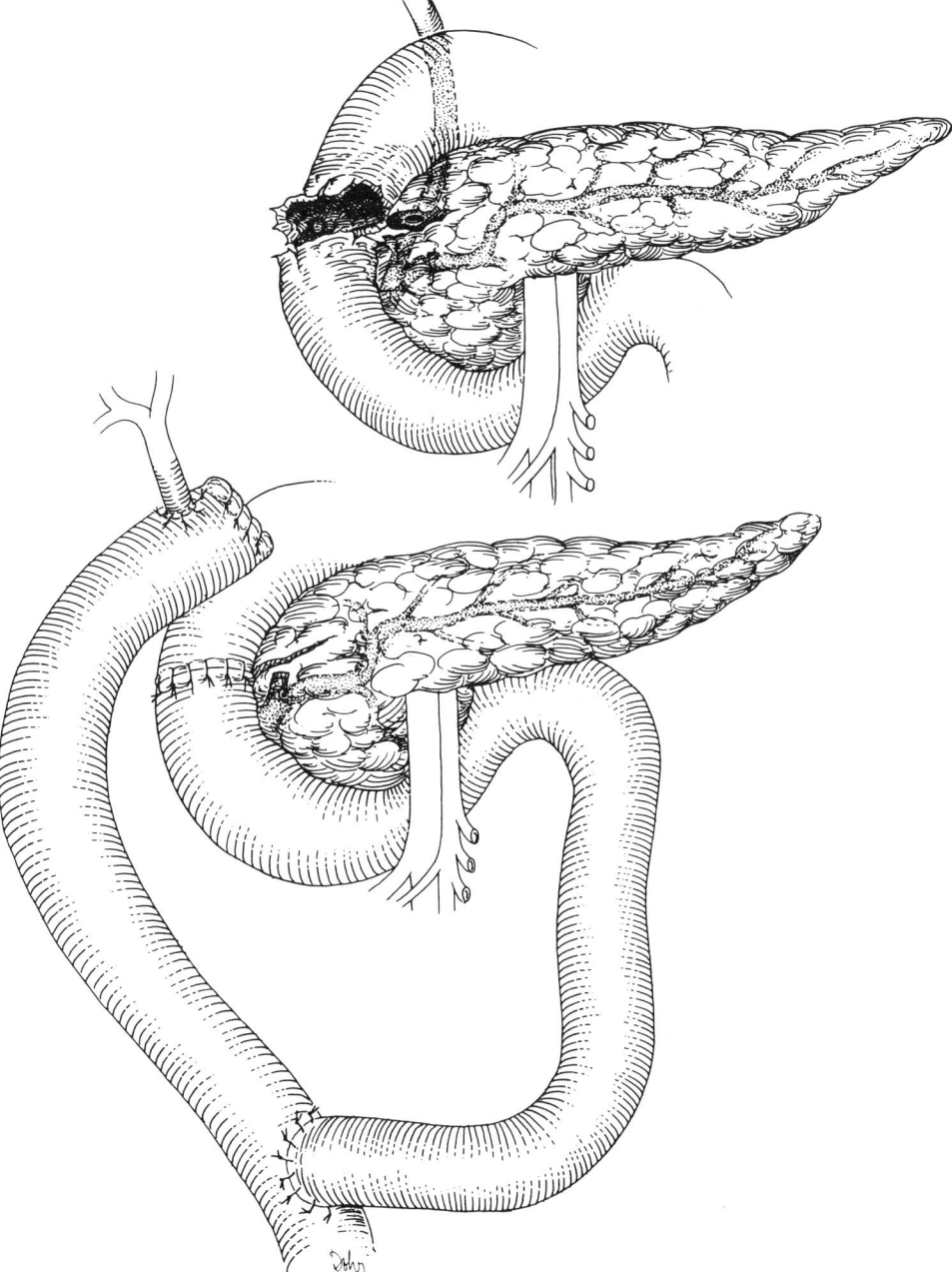

Figure 9–12. The combined duodenal biliary lesion is treated by duodenal repair and choledochojejunostomy using a Roux-en-Y limb.

of the common duct under the duodenum before dividing it. The pancreatic head should be mobilized carefully from the portal vein and the gastroduodenal artery ligated as it passes under the duodenum. The uncinate process can then be mobilized from the mesenteric vessels after the mesocolon is retracted downward and separated from the body of the pancreas and it is divided at the site of the fracture. During the dissection of the uncinate, careful attention must be paid to the possibility of a right hepatic, accessory hepatic, or totally replaced hepatic artery arising from the superior mesenteric artery and transversing the uncinate portion of the head of the pancreas.[73,74,121] The splenic vein is preserved at its junction with the superior mesenteric vein. In freeing the distal segment of pancreas from the splenic vein, numerous small veins entering the pancreas directly from the splenic vein need to be divided and ligated. After removal of the head and uncinate, the distal end of the pancreas is anastomosed end-to-side to the Roux-en-Y jejunal limb in a duct-to-jejunal mucosal–serosal anastomosis performed with 4-0 to 5-0 braided polyester sutures. An end-to-side anastomosis between the common duct and the jejunal limb can then be performed 10 to 15 cm distal to the pancreatic anastomosis using a precise two-layered anastomosis. Twenty to 30 cm farther distal, an end-to-side gastrojejunostomy or pylorojejunostomy can be carried out (Fig. 9–13).

Combined Duodenal, Common Bile Duct, and Major Pancreatic Ductal Injuries

Combined duodenal, common bile duct, and major pancreatic ductal injuries of the head of the pancreas (Fig. 9–14) are fatal if treated by drainage alone and are best managed by a pancreaticoduodenectomy, as recommended by Kerry and Glas and others (Fig. 9–13). The role of pancreatic duodenectomy in trauma to the pancreatic head and duodenum continues to be controversial in some trauma centers. The controversy persists largely because the precise nature of the injury to the pancreatic head is often unknown, i.e., whether the major pancreatic duct is intact, severed, or only partially disrupted.[15,26,48,50] One would expect quite different outcomes and complications depending on the nature of the injury to the major pancreatic duct and how it was treated. Some reports do not mention whether the common bile duct was also injured in patients subjected to pancreaticoduodenectomy. What mortality is associated with pancreaticoduodenectomy is attributable to the nature of the injury, the condition of the patient, and the skill of the operator (Table 9–7). One trauma center reported no deaths in 10 consecutive patients undergoing pancreaticoduodenectomy for combined injuries involving the major pancreatic duct, common bile duct, and duodenum.[87]

In most severe combined pancreatic, duodenal, and biliary tract injuries also involving severe associated injuries to the liver and major vascular structures, it may be necessary to resort to a series of exteriorization procedures as recommended by Owens and Wolfman until the patient is stable enough to restore ductal and enteric continuity of the gastrointestinal tract.[89,134]

POSTOPERATIVE CARE

In patients with pancreatic injuries, the gastrointestinal tract is kept at rest until the ileus has subsided. For major pancreatic injuries, we maintain the patients on nasogastric suction to

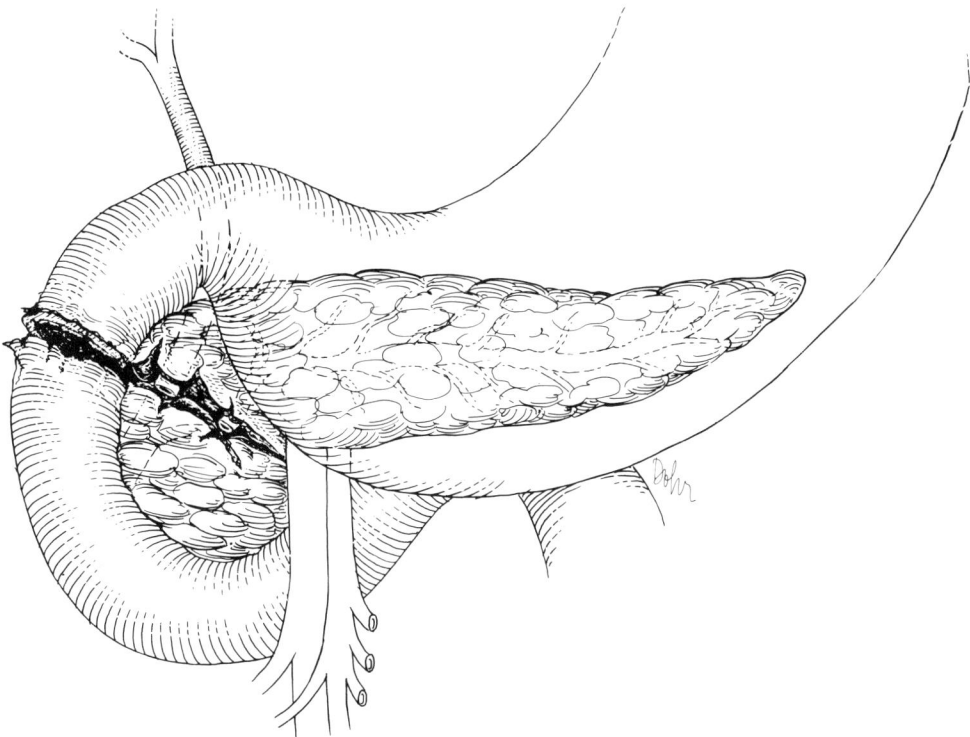

Figure 9–13. A combined duodenal, biliary, and pancreatic ductal injury that is best treated as shown in Fig. 9–14.

avoid acid stimulation of the duodenum and bicarbonate secretion by the pancreas. For duodenal injuries we keep the gastrointestinal tract decompressed by nasogastric tube for an equivalent period of time. The patient is maintained on intravenous fluids. Should there be any overt evidence of complications, as manifest by severe ileus or infection, intravenous hyperalimentation is initiated 4 or 5 days postoperatively. If a duodenal diverticulization or pancreaticoduodenectomy has been performed, hyperalimentation may be initiated as soon postoperatively as the patient is hemodynamically stable.

If, after 5 to 7 days, the patient's condition is benign, nasogastric suction is discontinued. If this is not followed by symptoms and the patient's ileus has subsided, the patient may be started slowly on oral nutrition. Initially, clear liquids are given followed by a regular diet if the former is tolerated. Drains may be left in place until the patient is back on full activity and tolerating a regular diet without overt complications. This can involve the use of drains for 10 days to 2 weeks or even longer if drainage persists. In such cases, drains are often removed on a return visit after hospital discharge. Ordinarily, if drainage has ceased by the fourth or fifth day or none has developed, the drains can be removed.

The concentration of amylase in the drain fluid has been recommended as a guide as to when drains should be advanced. However, we found little correlation between the concentration of amylase in drain fluid at 1 week postinjury when the drain amylase was less than 100,000 units and the development of postoperative complications, e.g., persistence of drainage (fistula) pseudocyst or abscess formation. However, in three patients whose drain

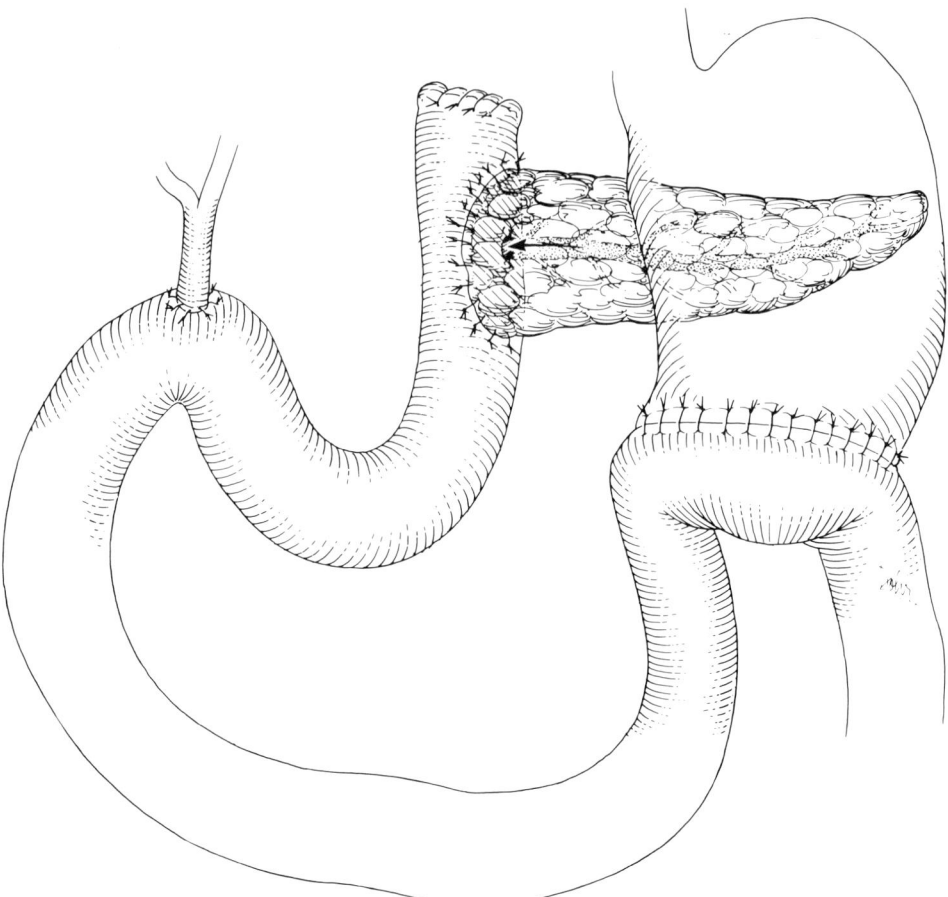

Figure 9–14. A pancreatic duodenal resection followed by reanastomosis of the pancreatic duct, common duct, and gastrojejunostomy.

amylase values exceeded 100,000 units complications developed. These complications consisted of a persistent fistula or abscess. Therefore, even though our experience in patients with drain amylase values exceeding 100,000 units is small, we recommend caution in advancing the drains in such a situation.

The possibility of infection should be anticipated, particularly in penetrating injuries. Preoperative prophylactic antibodies are administered routinely in trauma patients. Currently we are using Cefotetan.

COMPLICATIONS

The complications of pancreatic and duodenal injury are duodenal fistula, duodenal obstruction, pancreatic fistula, pancreatitis, pancreatic abscess, and intraperitoneal abscess and infection, pancreatic pseudocyst, and chronic pancreatitis. Complications most

Table 9-7 Incidence of Mortality and Complications Associated with Pancreatoduodenectomy Peformed for Trauma

AUTHOR	NO.	DEATHS			PANCREATIC COMPLICATIONS
Kashuk[55]	1	0			0
Pororny[95]	1	0			0
Smego[107]	1	0			
Leppaniemi[63]	3	1			2
Oreskovich[87]	10	0	Early	Pancreatitis	2
				Weight loss	2
				DM	1
				Diarrhea	1
				Fistula	1
			Late	Delayed gastric empty	2
				Weight loss	2
				DM	1
				Steatorrhea	1
Moore[78]	1	0			0
Jones[50]	8	3		Insufficiency	1
Wynn[134]	1	0			0
Feliciano[26]					
Whipple	10	6	(2 since 1981)		
Total	3				
McKone[72]	5	0			0
Ivantury[47]	6	2			
Total	50	12*			

*Relating to pancreatoduodenectomy = 8; DM, diabetes mellitus.

frequently associated with pancreatic injury are pancreatic fistulas, the incidence of which is reported to be 3.6% to 35% and pancreatic abscesses, 2.3%. Pancreatic fistulas and pseudocysts are most common after blunt trauma.[128] Abscesses and sepsis are most frequently associated with shock on admission to the hospital from hemorrhage due to associated injuries to major vessels as well as liver and spleen and the presence of colon injuries or contamination created by placement of jejunostomy or gastrostomy tubes.[40,44,51,54,112,114,115,122,128,130,131]

Complications most often noted in association with duodenal injuries are duodenal fistulas, 3.6% to 7%; duodenal obstruction, 1.1% to 1.7%; intraabdominal abscess, 10.9% to 18.4%; recurrent pancreatitis, 2.5% to 14.9%; common bile duct fistula, 1.3%.[108,114] The incidence of duodenal fistulas was lowest when jejunostomy and gastrostomy were employed by Stone et al. (3.6%).[114] However, they also had the highest rate of intraabdominal abscess, 18.4%, which may have resulted from contamination as a result of opening the gastrointestinal tract to perform duodenal decompression.[114] Snyder et al., on the other hand, reported that the adjunctive use of duodenal decompression, when used selectively, was associated with an incidence of duodenal fistula of 9%, two and a half times higher than Stone et al.'s and higher at his own institution than in patients in whom no duodenal decompression was employed (5.6%).[108,114] The incidence of intraabdominal abscess in Snyder et al.'s experience was 10.9%.[108] We recommend, as have Kashuk et al.[55] and Feliciano et al.,[26] the use of feeding jejunostomy in patients with major duodenal and pancreatic injuries. Neither Kashuk, Feliciano, or we have used duodenal tube decompression or gastrostomy.

In patients with combined pancreaticoduodenal injury (in the absence of common duct injury), the combination alone does not increase mortality; however, associated injuries are more common than in either pancreatic or duodenal injuries alone and are more likely to involve the aorta and inferior vena cava.[36,108]

When the common duct is also injured in a pancreaticoduodenal injury or in association with duodenal injury without major pancreatic ductal injury, the complication and mortality rate are higher (Stone et al., 43%; Snyder and Graham, 26%) than in pancreatic or duodenal injuries alone or combined.[36,108,114] The incidence of duodenal, biliary, or pancreatic fistulas has been reported as high as 38% and the mortality rate between 15% and 40%.[114]

These complications occur with greater frequency after pancreatic and duodenal injuries combined with common duct injuries than with any other intraabdominal injuries, and the lethality is secondary only to that after leakage of a colon anastomosis. In these massive combined injuries, there is no substitute for a definitive operation, that is, pancreaticoduodenectomy other than complete separation and diversion of bile, pancreatic, and gastric contents as described by Owens and Wolfman.[89] Simple drainage of these combined injuries is not adequate therapy.[57]

If the pancreas and duodenum are well drained posteriorly, the consequence of duodenal or pancreatic fistula is usually relatively benign. However, if the proximity of the drains to the area of leakage is remote, then there may not be immediate egress of pancreatic or duodenal secretions, resulting in severe complications such as retroperitoneal sepsis. Therefore, if the patient develops evidence of sepsis postoperatively, this is an indication for immediate reoperation and institution of posterior drainage.

Pancreatitis is a complication that results from obstruction of the pancreatic duct and should not occur if the injury to the duct was noted and appropriate operative treatment initiated at the time of initial injury. It is unlikely that edema and hemorrhage in an area adjacent to the duct results in sufficient obstruction to the duct to cause more than a self-limited pancreatitis.

However, in some patients, although an injury to the major pancreatic duct is identified at operation, the surgeon may feel the patient's condition is too unstable, owing to associated injuries, to withstand more than drainage.

Treatment in pancreatitis is initially supportive, maintaining the patient on nothing by mouth, nasogastric suction, and intravenous support, waiting out the complications. Intravenous hyperalimentation should be started once the patient has gone more than 4 or 5 days postinjury with no immediate prospect of taking food by mouth. Pancreatic ductal discontinuity is the cause of pancreatic fistulas after trauma, the most common complication of pancreatic injury, and wholly avoidable if detected and treated at operation.[4,6] If the patient's condition at the time of operation does not permit definitive repair, sump drainage should be instituted to create a controlled fistula. Reoperation will usually be required at a later date to drain any fistula from a major pancreatic duct into a Roux-en-Y limb or resect the distal portion of gland responsible for the fistula secretion. Pancreatic ascites occurs when the ductal discontinuity leads to the pancreatic secretion from the distal segment of pancreas entering freely into the abdominal cavity.[41,92] The whole abdomen, in effect, becomes a pseudocyst.

Pancreatic ductal disruption may also lead to the complications of pancreatic pseudocyst or pancreatic abscess or pancreatitis.[30,44,108,114,124,130] Generally, a well drained pancreas is not susceptible to these complications, even if the ductal injury is overlooked or could not be dealt with because of the patient's condition at the time of initial injury and operation. A pancreatic pseudocyst after trauma is usually associated with blunt injury and results from the accumulation of undrained enzymes secreted from the distal portion of the severed gland.[3,128] A persistent ileus in the absence of overt infection suggests the possibility of a local accumulation of pancreatic enzymes, which has become walled off in the form of a pseudocyst. Ultrasound and CT scans may permit localization of the pseudocyst or abscesses and provide an indication for reoperation. Frequently, the primary manifestation of inflammation around the pancreas is pleural effusion. A collection of fluid in the left pleural space after pancreatic injury is a manifestation of the collection of enzymes dissecting beneath the posterior portion of the diaphragm into the chest. Failure of the patient to respond to conservative therapy is an indication for reoperation and drainage of the subphrenic space or internal drainage of the pancreatic pseudocyst. Occasionally, patients with traumatic pancreatitis, particularly children, will manifest osteolytic lesions that resolve spontaneously over time.[84]

Secondary intraperitoneal infection with abscess formation is not unusual after pancreatic injury.[51,114] An indication for reoperation in this instance is uncontrolled sepsis.

Persistent gastrointestinal obstruction, mechanical or functional, due to altered motility may develop secondary to pancreatitis or inflammation around a duodenal injury.[108] Generally this type of obstruction can be treated conservatively and will resolve spontaneously in 4 or 5 days to a week or two at most. The status of the gastrointestinal tract can be assessed by x-ray contrast studies of the gastrointestinal tract. A few patients with pancreatic injury and ductal transection who have not been initially treated appropriately will go on to develop chronic pancreatitis associated with severe pain.[32] These patients must be treated as are other patients with chronic pancreatitis.[32]

In addition to specific complications related to the pancreas and duodenal injury, other complications such as respiratory failure, renal failure, and, particularly, diffuse sepsis are complications of this major injury. These are treated as described in the previous section.

REFERENCES

1. Anderson CB, Weisz D, Rodger MR, Tucker GL. Combined pancreaticoduodenal trauma. *Am J Surg*. 1973; 125:530–534.
2. Aranha GV, Prinz RA, Freeark RJ, Greenlee HB. The spectrum of biliary tract obstruction from chronic pancreatitis. *Arch Surg*. 1984; 119:595–600.
3. Babb J, Harmon H. Diagnosis and management of pancreatic trauma. *Am Surg*. 1976; 390–394.
4. Bach RD, Frey CF. Diagnosis and treatment of pancreatic trauma. *Am J Surg*. 1971; 121:20–29.
5. Baker RJ, Dippel WF, Freeark RJ, Strohl EL. The surgical significance of trauma to the pancreas. *Arch Surg*. 1963; 86:1038–1044.
6. Baker RJ, Bass RT, Zajtchuk R, Strohl EL. External pancreatic fistula following abdominal injury. *Arch Surg*. 1967; 95:556–566.
7. Balasegarem M, Lumpur K. Surgical management of pancreatic trauma. *Am J Surg*. 1976; 131:536–540.
8. Bass J, DiLorenzo M, Desjardins JG, Grignon A, Ouimet A. Blunt pancreatic injuries in children: the role of percutaneous external drainage on the treatment of pancreatic pseudocysts. *J Pediatr Surg*. 1988; 23: 721–724.
9. Beal SL, Spisso J. The risk of splenorrhaphy. *Arch Surg*. 1988; 123:1158–1163.
10. Berne CJ, Donovan AJ, Hagen WE. Combined duodenal pancreatic trauma. The role of end-to-side gastrojejunostomy. *Arch Surg*. 1968; 96:712–722.
11. Berne, CJ, Donovan AJ, White EJ, Yellin AE. Duodenal "diverticulization" for duodenal and pancreatic injury. *Am J Surg*. 1974; 127:503–507.

12. Berni GA, Bandyk DF, Oreskovich MR, Carrico CJ. Role of intraoperative pancreatography in patients with injury to the pancreas. *Am J Surg.* 1982; 143:602–605.
13. Brawley RK, Cameron JL, Zuidema GD. Severe upper abdominal injury treated by pancreaticoduodenectomy. *Surg Gynecol Obstet.* 1968; 126:516–522.
14. Catell RB, Braasch JW. A technique for exposure of the third and fourth portions of the duodenum. *Surg Gynecol Obstet.* 1960; 111:378–379.
15. Cattell RB. A technique for pancreatoduodenal resection. *Surg Clin North Am.* 1948; 28:761–775.
16. Massive right upper quadrant intra-abdominal injury requiring pancreaticoduodenectomy and partial hepatectomy. *J Trauma.* 1975; 15:714–719.
17. Cleveland HC, Waddell WR. Retroperitoneal rupture of the duodenum due to nonpenetrating trauma. *Surg Clin North Am.* 1963; 43:413–431.
18. Cocke WM Jr, Meyer KK. Retroperitoneal duodenal rupture. Proposed mechanism review of literature and report of a case. *Am J Surg.* 1964; 108:834–839.
19. Cohn I, Hawthorne AR, Frofere AS. Retroperitoneal rupture of the duodenum. *Am J Surg.* 1952; 84:293.
20. Cooper MJ, Williamson RC. Conservative pancreatectomy. *Br J Surg.* 1985; 72:801–803.
21. Corley RD, Norcross WJ, Shoemaker WC. Traumatic injuries to the duodenum: a report of 98 patients. *Ann Surg.* 1975; 181:92–98.
22. Cross KR. Accessory pancreatic ducts. Special reference to the intrapancreatic portion of the common duct. *Arch Pathol.* 1956; 61:434–440.
23. DeMars JJ, Bubrick MP, Hitchcock CR. Duodenal perforation in blunt abdominal trauma. *Surgery.* 1979; 86:632–638.
24. Doublier L, Garron A. Les plaies duodeno-pancreatiques par projectiles. *Lyon Chir.* 1969; 65:842–854.
25. Elman R, Arneson N, Graham EA. Value of blood amylase estimations in the diagnosis of pancreatic disease. *Arch Surg.* 1929; 19:943–967.
26. Feliciano DV, Martin TD, Cruse PA, et al. Management of combined pancreatoduodenal injuries. *Ann Surg.* 1987; 205:673–680.
27. Fish JC, Johnson GL. Rupture of duodenum following blunt trauma: report of a case with avulsion of papilla of Vater. *Ann Surg.* 1965; 162:917–919.
28. Flint LM, McCoy M, Richardson JD, Polk HC Jr. Duodenal injury. Analysis of common misconceptions in diagnosis and treatment. *Ann Surg.* 1980; 191:697–702.
29. Fraser GC. Handlebar injury of the pancreas. *J Pediatr Surg.* 1969; 4:216–219.
30. Freeark RJ, Corley RD, Norcross WJ, Baker RJ. Unusual aspects of pancreatoduodenal trauma. *J Trauma.* 1966; 6:482–492.
31. Freeark RJ, Kane JM, Folk FA, Baker RJ. Traumatic disruption of the head of the pancreas. *Arch Surg.* 1965; 91:5–13.
32. Frey CF, Child CG, Fry W. Pancreatectomy for chronic pancreatic. *Ann Surg.* 1976; 184:403–413.
33. Gibbs BF, Crow JL, Rupnik EJ. Pancreatoduodenectomy for blunt pancreatoduodenal injury. *J Trauma.* 1970; 10:702–705.
34. Glancy KE. Review of pancreatic trauma. *West J Med.* 1989; 151:45–51.
35. Gougeon FW, Legros C, Archambault A, Bessette G, Bastien E. Pancreatic trauma: a new diagnostic approach. *Am J Surg.* 1976; 132:400–402.
36. Graham JM, Mattox KL, Vaughan GD 3d, Jordan GL Jr. Combined pancreaticoduodenal injuries. *J Trauma.* 1979; 19:340–345.
37. Graham JM, Mattox KL, Jordan GL Jr. Traumatic injuries of the pancreas. *Am J Surg.* 1978; 136:744–748.
38. Gray SW, Skandalakis JE. *Embryology for Surgeons*. Philadelphia: WB Saunders; 1972.
39. Grindlinger GA, Vesters R. Transvaginal injury of the duodenum, diaphragm, and lung. *J Trauma.* 1987; 27:575–576.
40. Grosfeld JL, Cooney DR. Pancreatic and gastrointestinal trauma in children. *Pediatr Clin North Am.* 1975; 22:365–377.
41. Halgrimson CG, Trimble C, Gale S, Waddell WR. Pancreaticoduodenectomy for traumatic lesions. *Am J Surg.* 1969; 118:877–882.
42. Hayward SR, Lucas CE, Sugawa C, Ledgerwood AM. Emergent endoscopic retrograde cholangiopancreatography: a highly specific test for acute pancreatic trauma. *Arch Surg.* 1989; 124:745–746.
43. Heiss FW, Shea JA. Association of pancreatitis and varient ductal anatomy, dominant drainage of the duct of Santorini. *Am J Gastroenterol.* 1978; 70:158–162.
44. Heitsch RC, Knutson CO, Fulton RL, Jones CE. Delineation of critical factors in the treatment of pancreatic trauma. *Surgery.* 1976; 80:523–529.
45. Heyse-Moore GH. Blunt pancreatic and pancreaticoduodenal trauma. *Br J Surg.* 1976; 63:226–228.
46. Hutchinson WB. Duodenotomy. *Am J Surg.* 1971; 122:777–780.
47. Ivantury RR, Gaudino J, Ascer E, Nallathambi M, Ramirez-Schon G, Stahl WM. Treatment of penetrating duodenal injuries: primary repair vs. repair with decompressive enterostomy/serosal patch. *J Trauma.* 1985; 25:337–341.

48. Ivantury RR, Nallathambi M, Rao P, Stahl WM. Penetrating pancreatic injuries: analysis of 103 consecutive cases. *Am Surg*. 1990; 56:90–95.
49. Janson KL, Stockinger F. Duodenal hematoma. *Am J Surg*. 1975; 129:304–308.
50. Jones RC. Management of pancreatic trauma. *Am J Surg*. 1984; 150:698–704.
51. Jones RC. Management of pancreatic trauma. *Ann Surg*. 1978; 187:555–564.
52. Jordan GL Jr. Pancreatic trauma. In: Howard JM, Jordan GL Jr, Reber HA, eds. *Surgical Diseases of the Pancreas*. 2nd ed. Philadelphia: Lea & Febiger; 1987:875–897.
53. Jordon GL, Overton R, Werschky LR. Traumatic transection of the pancreas. *South Med J*. 1969;62:90–93.
54. Karl HW, Chandler JG. Mortality and morbidity of pancreatic injury. *Am J Surg*. 1977; 134:549–554.
55. Kashuk JL, Moore EE, Cogbill TH. Management of the intermediate severity duodenal injury. *Surgery*. 1982; 92:758–764.
56. Keeling P, Calthorpe D, Lane B, Collins PG. Blunt injury of the neck of the pancreas: a report of nine patients. *Injury*. 1987; 18:93–95.
57. Kerry RL, Glas WW. Traumatic injuries of the pancreas and duodenum. *Arch Surg*. 1962; 85:813–816.
58. Kraus M, Gordon RE. Alternate techniques of duodenotomy. *Surg Gynecol Obstet*. 1974; 139:417–419.
59. LaLaoude J, Segal P, Evaard C. Les traumatiques du pancreas à propos de 11 observations. *Ann Chir*. 1973; 27:278–384.
60. Lambert MA, Linehan IP, Russell RC. Duodenum-preserving total pancreatectomy for end stage chronic pancreatitis. *Br J Surg*. 1987; 74:35–39.
61. Laustsen J, Jensen KE, Bach-Nielsen P. Closed pancreatic transection treated by Roux-en-Y anastomosis. *Injury*. 19:42–43.
62. Lee D, Zacher J, Vogel TT. Primary repair in transection of duodenum with avulsion of the common duct. *Arch Surg*. 1976; 111:592–593.
63. Leppaniemi A, Haapiainen R, Kiviluoto T, Lempinen M. Pancreatic trauma: acute and late manifestations. *Br J Surg*. 1988; 75:165–167.
64. Letton AH, Wilson JP. Traumatic severance of pancreas treated by Roux-en-Y anastomosis. *Surg Gynecol Obstet*. 1959; 109:473–478.
65. Lowe RJ, Saletta JD, Moss GS. Pancreatoduodenectomy for penetrating pancreatic trauma. *J Trauma*. 1977; 17:732–741.
66. Lucas CE. Diagnosis and treatment of pancreatic and duodenal injury. *Surg Clin North Am*. 1977; 57:49–65.
67. Lucas CE, Ledgerwood AM. Factors influencing outcome after blunt duodenal injury. *J Trauma*. 1975; 15:839–846.
68. Luna GK, Dellinger EP. Nonoperative observation therapy for splenic injuries: a safe therapeutic option? *Am J Surg*. 1987; 153:462–468.
69. Martin LW, Henderson BM, Welsh N. Disruption of the head of the pancreas caused by blunt trauma in children: a report of two cases treated with primary repair of the pancreatic duct. *Surgery*. 1968; 63:697–700.
70. Martin TD, Feliciano DV, Mattox KL, Jordan GL Jr. Severe duodenal injuries. *Arch Surg*. 1983; 118:631–635.
71. McCorkle H, Goldman L. The clinical significance of the serum amylase test in the diagnosis of acute pancreatitis. *Surg Gynecol Obstet*. 1942; 74:439–445.
72. McKone TK, Bursch LR, Scholten DJ. Pancreaticoduodenectomy for trauma: a life-saving procedure. *Am Surg*. 1988; 54:361–364.
73. Michels NA. *Blood Supply and Anatomy of the Upper Abdominal Organs*. Philadelphia: Lippincott; 1955.
74. Michels NA. The hepatic, cystic and retroduodenal arteries and their relation to the biliary ducts. *Ann Surg*. 1951; 133:503–524.
75. Millbourn E. On excretory ducts of pancreas in man, with special reference to their relations to each other, to common bile duct and to duodenum. Radiological and anatomical study. *Acta Anat*. 1950; 9:1–34.
76. Miller RT. Retroperitoneal rupture of the duodenum by blunt force. *Ann Surg*.1916; 64:550–578.
77. Moore EE, Dunn EL, Moore JB, Thompson JS. Penetrating abdominal trauma index. *J Trauma*. 1981; 21:439–445.
78. Moore FA, Moore EE, Moore GE, Millikan JS. Risk of splenic salvage after trauma. *Am J Surg*. 1984; 148:800–805.
79. Moore JB, Moore EE. Changing trends in the management of combined pancreatoduodenal injuries. *World J Surg*. 1984; 8:791–797.
80. Moretz JA III, Campbell DP, Parker DE, William GR. Significance of serum amylase in evaluating pancreatic trauma. *Am J Surg*. 1975; 130:739–741.
81. Morton JR, Jordon GL Jr. Traumatic duodenal injuries. Review of 131 cases. *J Trauma*. 1968; 8:127–139.
82. Naffziger HC, McCorkle HJ. The recognition and management of acute trauma of the pancreas, with particular reference to the use of the serum amylase test. *Ann Surg*. 1943; 118:594–602.
83. Nance FC, DeLoach DH. Pancreaticoduodenectomy following abdominal trauma. *J Trauma*. 1971; 11:577–585.

84. Neuer FS, Roberts FF, McCarthy V. Osteolytic lesions following traumatic pancreatitis. *Am J Dis Child*. 1977; 131:738–740.
85. Nilsson E, Norrby S, Skullman S, Sjodahl R. Pancreatic trauma in a defined population. *Acta Chir Scand*. 1986; 152:647–651.
86. Nowak MM, Baringer DC, Ponsky JL. Pancreatic injuries. Effectiveness of debridement and drainage for nontransecting injuries. *Am Surg*. 1986; 52:599–602.
87. Oreskovich MR, Carrico CJ. Pancreaticoduodenectomy for trauma: a viable option? *Am J Surg*. 1984; 147:618–623.
88. Penetrating wounds of the abdomen; surgical history. In: *The Medical and Surgical History of the War of the Rebellion (1861–1865)*. Prepared under the direction of Surgeon General J. K. Barnes. Washington, Government Printing Office. 1870–88; 2(4):158–161.
89. Owens MP, Wolfman EF Jr. Pancreatic trauma: management and presentation of a new technique. *Surgery*. 1973; 73:881–886.
90. Pachter HL, Hofstetter SR, Liang HG, Hoballah J. Traumatic injuries to the pancreas: the role of distal pancreatectomy with splenic preservation. *J Trauma*. 1989; 29:1352–1355.
91. Pantazelos HH, Kerhulas AA, Byrne JJ. Total pancreaticoduodenectomy for trauma. *Ann Surg*. 1969; 170:1016–1020.
92. Parrish RA, Humphries AL, Moretz WH. Massive pancreatic ascites. *Arch Surg*. 1968; 96:887–891.
93. Pollock AV. Pancreatic trauma and idiopathic retroperitoneal fibrosis: a long term follow up study of 4 patients. *Br J Surg*. 1974; 61:112.
94. Poole LH. Wounds of the pancreas (62 casualties). In: *Surgical History of World War II*. Office of the Surgeon General, Government Printing Office, Washington DC.
95. Pokorny WJ, Brandt ML, Harberg FJ. Major duodenal injuries in children: diagnosis, operative management, and outcome. *J Pediatr Surg*. 1986; 21:613–616.
96. Reyna TM, Tuten HL. Isolated duodenal transection from blunt trauma treated by pyloric exclusion and triple-tube technique. *Milit Med*. 1988; 153:562–563.
97. Robey E, Mullen JT, Schwab CW. Blunt transection of the pancreas treated by distal pancreatectomy, splenic salvage, and hyperalimentation. *Ann Surg*. 1982; 196:695–699.
98. Sako Y, et al. A survey of evacuation, resuscitation, and mortality in a forward surgical hospital. *Surgery*. 1955; 37:602–611.
99. Salyer K, McClelland RN. Pancreatoduodenectomy for trauma. *Arch Surg*. 1967; 95:636–639.
100. Scher K, Scott-Connor C, Jones CW, Wroczynski AF. Methods of splenic preservation and their effect on clearance of pneumococcal bacteremia. *Ann Surg*. 1985; 202:595–599.
101. Schumaker ED. Zur duodenum chirurgie. *Beitr Z Klin Chir*. 1910; 71:482.
102. Sheldon GF, Cohn LH, Blaisdell FW. Surgical treatment of pancreatic trauma. *J Trauma*. 1970; 10:795–800.
103. Shorr RM, Greaney GC, Donovan AJ. Injuries of the duodenum. *Am J Surg*. 1987; 154:93–98.
104. Sims EH, Mandal AK, Schlater T, Fleming AW, Lou MA. Factors affecting outcome in pancreatic trauma. *J Trauma*. 1984; 24:125–128.
105. Skandalakis JE, Gray SW, Rowe JS, Skandalakis LJ. Anatomical complications of pancreatic surgery—Part II. *Cont Surg*. 1979; 15:21–50.
106. Smanio T. Varying relations of the common bile duct with the posterior face of the pancreas in Negroes and white persons. *J Int Coll Surgeons*. 1954; 22:150–173.
107. Smego DR, Richardson JD, Flint LM. Determinants of outcome in pancreatic trauma. *J Trauma*. 1985; 25:771–776.
108. Snyder WH, Weigelt JA, Watkins WL, Beitz DS. The surgical management of duodenal trauma. *Arch Surg*. 1980; 115:422–429.
109. Sorensen JV, Obeid FN, Horst HM, Bivins BA. Penetrating pancreatic injuries 1978–1983. *Am Surg*. 1986; 52:354–358.
110. Stauffer UG, Grob M. Traumatische: Pankreaspseudozystem im Kindesalter. *Helv Paediatr Acta*. 1971; 26:625–635.
111. Steele M, Sheldon GF, Blaisdell FW. Pancreatic injuries. *Arch Surg*. 1973; 106:544–549.
112. Stigall KE, Dorsey JS. Transection of the first portion of jejunum from blast injury in accidental discharge of (2.75-inch aircraft) rocket from an F-15. *Milit Med*. 1989; 154:431–433.
113. Stone HH, Fabian TC. Management of duodenal wounds. *J Trauma*. 1979; 19:334–339.
114. Stone HH, Stowers KB, Shippey SH. Injuries to the pancreas. *Arch Surg*. 1962; 85:525–530.
115. Sturm JT, Quattlebaum FW, Mowlem A, Perry JF Jr. Patterns of injury requiring pancreaticoduodenectomy. *Surg Gynecol Obstet*. 1973; 137:629–632.
116. Tavers B. Rupture of the pancreas. *Lancet*. 1927; 12:384.
117. Taxier M, Sivak MV Jr, Cooperman AM, Sullivan BH Jr. Endoscopic retrograde pancreatography in the evaluation of trauma to the pancreas. *Surg Gynecol Obstet*. 1980; 150:65–68.

118. Thal AP, Wilson RF. A pattern of severe blunt trauma to the region of the pancreas. *Surg Gynecol Obstet.* 1964; 119:773–778.
119. Thomasson B, Linna MI, Viljanto J, Ano AJ. Blunt pancreatic trauma. *Acta Chir Scand.* 1973; 139:48–54.
120. Thompson IM. *On the Arteries and Ducts in the Hepatic Pedicle: A Study in Statistical Human Anatomy.* Berkeley, Calif: University of California Press; 1933.
121. Thompson RJ Jr, Hinshow DB. Pancreatic trauma: review of 87 cases. *Ann Surg.* 1966; 163:153–160.
122. Thomson RG, McFarland JB. Traumatic rupture of the pancreas with complications. *Br J Surg.* 1969; 56:117–120.
123. Traverso LW, Longmire WP Jr. Preservation of the pylorus during pancreaticoduodenectomy. *Surg Gynecol Obstet.* 1978; 146:959–962.
124. Walters RL, Gaspard DJ, Germann TD. Traumatic pancreatitis. *Am J Surg.* 1966; 111:364–368.
125. Walton AJ. *A Textbook of the Surgical Dyspepsias.* London: E Arnold; 1923.
126. Weitzman JJ, Rothschild PD. The surgical management of traumatic rupture of the pancreas due to blunt trauma. *Surg Clin North Am.* 1968; 48:1347–1352.
127. Werschky LR, Jordan GL. Surgical management of traumatic injuries to the pancreas. *Am J Surg.* 1968; 116:768–772.
128. Whalen GF, Robbs JV, Baker LW. Injuries of the pancreas and duodenum: results of a conservative approach. *S Afr J Surg.* 1987; 25:15–18.
129. White PH, Benfield JR. Amylase in the management of pancreatic trauma. *Arch Surg.* 1972; 105:158–163.
130. Wilson RF, Tagett JP, Pucelik JP, Walt AJ. Pancreatic trauma. *J Trauma.* 1967; 7:643–651.
131. Wisner DH, Wold RL, Frey CF. Diagnosis and treatment of pancreatic injuries: factors influencing morbidity and mortality. Unpublished data.
132. Wittingen J, Frey CF. Islet concentration in the head, body, tail and uncinate process of the pancreas. *Ann Surg.* 1974; 179:412–414.
133. Wurtz A, Henriet P, Ribet M. Fistuliarterio veinuse renocave traumatique et plaie duodenopancreatique. *Chirurgie.* 1973; 99:489–493.
134. Wynn M, Hill DM, Miller DR, Waxaman K, Eisner ME, Gazzaniga AB. Management of pancreatic and duodenal trauma. *Am J Surg.* 1985; 150:327–332.
135. Yadegar J. Common duct stricture from chronic pancreatitis. *Arch Surg.* 1980; 115:582–586.
136. Yellin NE, Rosoff L. Pancreatoduodenectomy for combined pancreatoduodenal injuries. *Arch Surg.* 1975; 110:1117–1183.
137. Yeo CK, McNamara J. Retroperitoneal rupture of duodenum with complicating gas gangrene. *Arch Surg.* 1973; 106:856–857.

10
Injuries to the Liver and Extrahepatic Ducts

JOHN RAGSDALE, M.D.
DONALD D. TRUNKEY, M.D.

HISTORY: In his classic treatise "On the Blood Inflammation and Gunshot Wounds," Hunter[1] gave some rather classic description of "wounds that enter the belly." He stated "because the belly contains more parts of very dissimilar uses than any other cavity in the body; each of which will produce symptoms peculiar to itself, and the nature of the wound." He continues "From a wound in the liver there will be pain in the part, of the sickly or depressing kind; and if it is in the right lobe, there will be a delusive pain in the right shoulder, or in the left shoulder, from a wound in the left lobe."

De Chauliac[2] was more specific on the treatment of injuries to the viscera including the liver. He adhered to the principles of Galen and Avicenna. Specifically, de Chauliac recommended "Clysters of sharp black warm wine and a very specific diet." "Let the diet or manner of living be restricted for at least seven days, and let the food be such that it does not engender feces nor superfluous putrefactions, but rather things that consolidate. If the patient's strength is weak, chicken broth may be given to him. If some tragacanth and gum arabic be put in it which will not irritate it would be well."

Larrey[3] may have been one of the first to treat a liver wound successfully. He describes the case: "A young officer of the light infantry, wounded by a ball in the right hypochondrium, the ninth rib being fractured, and the liver injured, during the battle of Dresden, has been cured."

"In the first place, I incised the flap in the integuments occupying the interval of the two wounds. Several splinters of the fractured rib were then detached and removed. With a pair of nippers, I cut off a projecting point of a fragment of this bone, which would have pricked the parts, and impeded the dressing of the wound. I extended the inferior incision over the part from which the ball issued, in a posterior direction, in order to facilitate the escape of fluids. The edges of the wound were then brought together, an opening, however, being left in its lower part, and maintained in their relative positions, by means of a piece of linen, dipped in warm wine containing a large quantity of honey. The injured parts were dressed rarely,

and with the precautions indicated. This treatment was pursued a pretty long time, and with complete success, for the subject of it recovered before this seventieth day."

Larrey recommended to lay open the wound deep to extract foreign body and the use of cups. He admonishes surgeons in the use of blood letting as it is "attended with many ill consequences." He also adheres to many of the principles outlined by Guy de Chauliac and specifically he puts the patient on "a rigid diet, and cooling mucilaginous, and laxative drinks, according to circumstances."

Larrey accurately described the signs and symptoms of shock associated with liver injury and the consequences of injury to an obstruction of the biliary duct. It was not until the introduction of anesthesia, antibiotics, and the understanding of liver anatomy that surgical wounds of the liver could be addressed more definitively.

The liver is the largest organ in the abdomen. It weighs approximately 1500 g and plays an essential role in carbohydrate, protein, and fat metabolism for sustaining life. Because of its size and vulnerability, it is probably the most frequently injured abdominal organ following penetrating and blunt trauma. Many minor injuries are undoubtedly not diagnosed, so that, statistically, the frequency of injury appears second to that involving the spleen.

ANATOMY OF THE LIVER

Repair and resection for treatment of hepatic trauma demands a working knowledge of the anatomy of the liver. The liver has three major surfaces: superior, inferior, and posterior (Fig. 10–1). The superior surface is smooth, rounded, and contiguous with the posterior surface. Both the superior and posterior surfaces rest against the diaphragm. The inferior surface is more complex. The inferior surface contains the gall bladder, hepatic ducts, hepatic arteries, and portal veins. The inferior surface has impressions from the colon (anterior and right), right kidney (right posterior), and stomach (left). The liver is attached to surrounding structures by ligaments, the reflection of parietal peritoneum. The coronary ligament is formed along the superior surface of the right lobe and secures the liver to the diaphragm posteriorly and superiorly. The two leaves of the coronary ligament join at the extreme left to form the triangular ligament. The falciform ligament and ligamentum teres (obliterated umbilical vein) provide anterior attachment of the midportion of the liver to the anterior abdominal wall.

Segmental Anatomy

Morphologically, the liver is described as having two main (right and left) lobes and an accessory (caudate) lobe. The right and left lobes are divided by a plane or major fissure that is not apparent on the external surface. This extends from the midportion of the gall bladder fossa inferiorly to the suprahepatic inferior vena cava superiorly. It forms an angle of about 35° with the vertical plane and 25° with the sagittal plane (Fig. 10–2). This plane is devoid

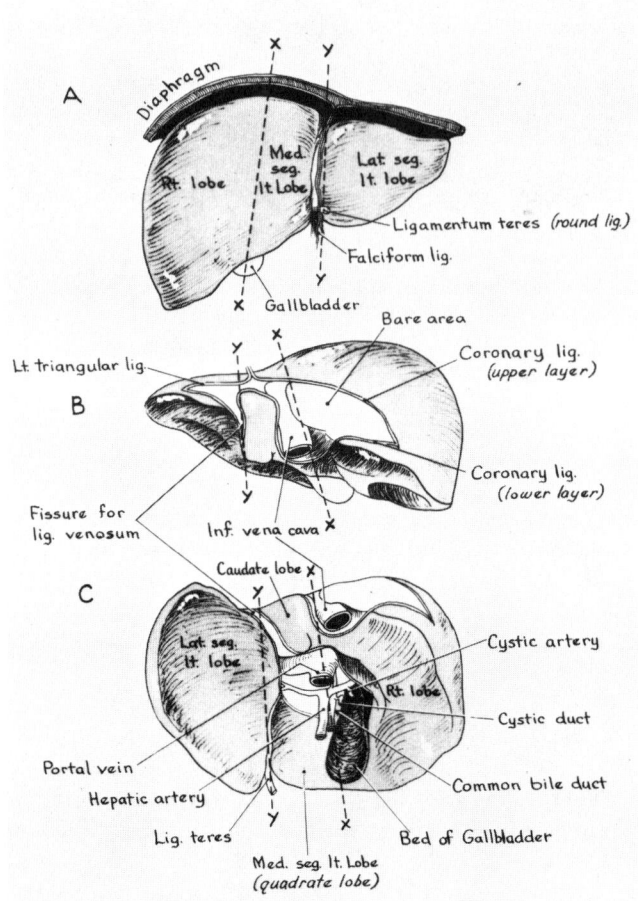

Figure 10–1. Surface anatomy of the liver. **A:** Anterior; **B:** superior, and **C:** interior surfaces of the liver. (From Madding.[37] Reprinted with permission.)

of anatomy except the middle hepatic veins. The quadrate lobe is that portion of the right lobe lying anterior to the transverse hilar fissure, medial to the gall bladder fossa, and lateral to the umbilical fissure. The caudate lobe lies posterior to the transverse liver fissure.

Surgical resection and treatment of traumatic injuries require an understanding of the functional anatomy of the liver. Segmental anatomic resection has been well documented by Bismuth[4] using an anatomic description from Couinaud. Functional anatomy is defined by hepatic segmentation, which is based on the distribution of the portal pedicle and location of hepatic veins (Fig. 10–3). The three main hepatic veins (right, left, and middle) divide the liver into four sections: right posterior lateral, right anterior medial, left anterior, and left posterior. Each of these sectors receives a portal pedicle. The sectors of the right liver can be further divided into two segments each (Fig. 10–4). The anteromedial sector: segment V anteriorly and segment VIII posteriorly; and the posterolateral sector: segment VI anteriorly and segment VII posteriorly. With regard to the left lobar hepatic anatomy, the left lobar

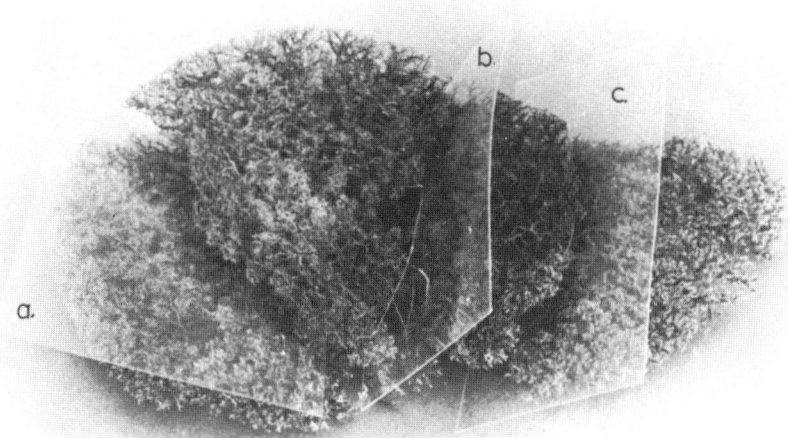

Figure 10–2. Major liver lobes and segments. **A:** Division between the anterior and posterior segments of the right lobe of the liver. **B:** Division between the right and left lobes of the liver. **C:** Division between the medial and lateral segments of the left lobe of the liver.

hepatic vein courses lateral to medial and receives tributaries in a horizontal plane that functionally divides the left lobe into anterior and posterior divisions.

However, from a practical point of view all of the arterial and venous supply and drainage course through the medial portion of the lobe to reach that portion lateral to the umbilical fissure and ligamentum teres. The left lobe is therefore practically divided into medial and lateral segments. From the standpoint of segmental anatomy of Couinaud, the left anterior sector is divided by the umbilical fissure into segment IV, the anterior portion

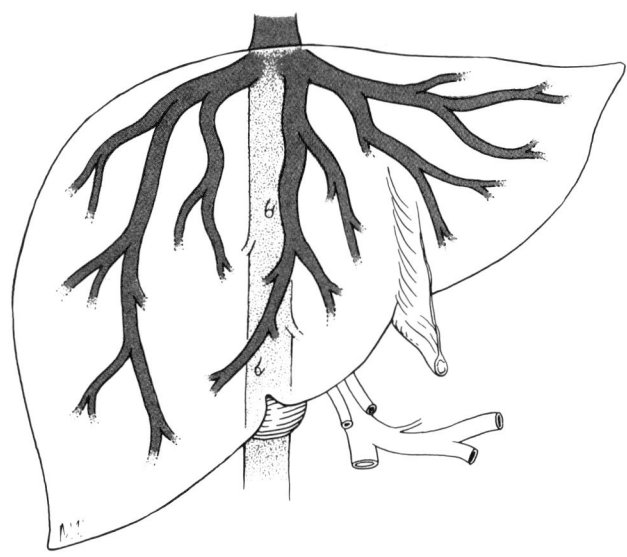

Figure 10–3. Anatomy of the hepatic veins. Knowledge of the location of the middle hepatic vein is critical. It courses between the right and left lobes entering the vena cava separately or, more commonly, joins the left hepatic vein a variable distance from its insertion into the cava.

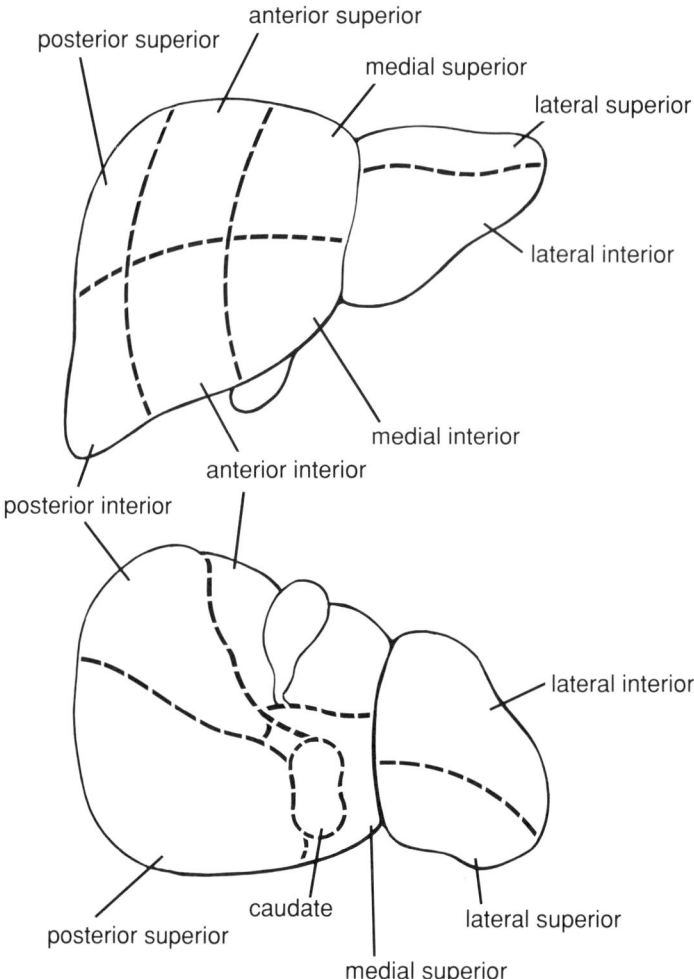

Figure 10–4. The segmental anatomy of the liver.

of the quadrate lobe, and segment III, the anterior portion of the left lobe of the liver. The posterior sector comprises only one segment (II) and lies in the posterior portion of the left lobe. The caudate lobe is considered independently as segment I. Although the segmental anatomy is rarely of value in the trauma setting, it can be used to facilitate the decision to resect damaged or devitalized liver parenchyma.

Hepatic Artery

The hepatic artery supplies 25% of the blood flow to the liver and 50% of the oxygen. In 55% of cases the hepatic arterial supply is exclusively from the celiac trunk.[5] The common hepatic artery is the continuation of the celiac trunk after the left gastric and splenic arterial branches (Fig. 10–5). The common hepatic artery traverses along the upper border of the head of the pancreas then turns to ascend in the lesser omentum. It lies to the left of the common bile duct and anterior to the portal vein. The gastroduodenal artery arises from the distal horizontal position of the common hepatic artery, which continues as the proper hepatic artery. The right gastric artery arises from the proper hepatic artery (40% of cases) or left hepatic artery (40% of cases) most of the time.[5]

The hepatic artery bifurcates in the porta hepatis to give rise to the right and left hepatic arteries. The right hepatic artery usually courses to the right behind the common bile duct. The anterior and posterior segmental arteries of the right lobe take separate origin from the right hepatic artery. The anterior segmental branch courses along the gall bladder fossa in close proximity to the cystic duct. The posterior segmental branch courses along the inferior border of the segmental hepatic duct.

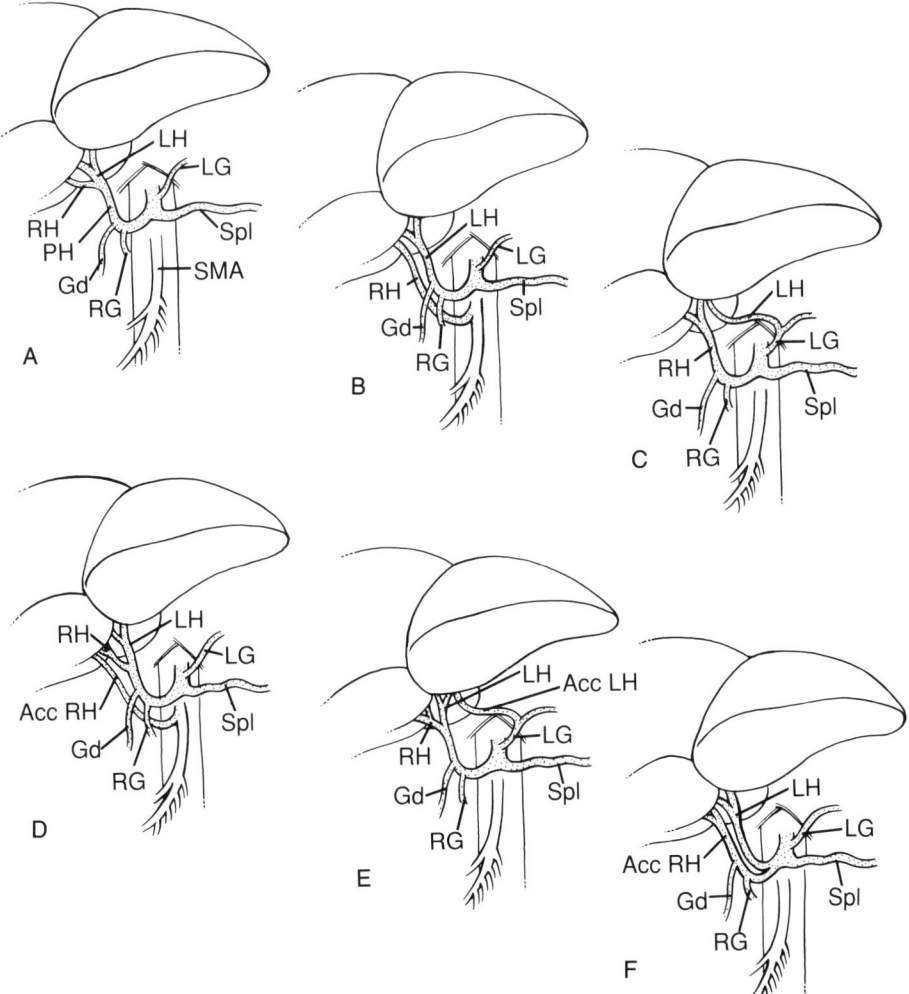

Figure 10–5. Hepatic artery anatomy and its variants. **A:** Standard anatomy. **B–F:** Variants.

The left hepatic artery runs upward and obliquely to the left and divides into its two terminal branches: the medial and lateral segmental arteries. The medial segmental artery descends into the quadrate lobe (segment IV). The lateral segmental artery travels obliquely toward the upper, outer aspect of the lateral segment, where it divides into the superior and inferior branches.

The blood supply to the caudate lobe (segment I) is variable. In approximately 35% of cases the entire blood supply of the caudate lobe comes from the right hepatic artery, and in 12% entirely from the left hepatic artery. In most, however, the blood supply is from both.

Aberrant hepatic arteries occur frequently, in about 40% to 45% of cases[6] (Fig. 10–5B–F). The most frequent anomaly is the left hepatic artery arising from the left gastric artery (25–30%)[7,8] (Fig. 10–5C). This includes a 10% incidence of a totally replaced left hepatic artery and a 15% incidence of an accessory left hepatic artery (Fig. 10–5E).

The right hepatic artery originates from the superior mesenteric artery in 17% of cases; 10% total replacement (Fig. 10–5B), and 7% accessory[7] (Fig. 10–5D). The middle hepatic artery arises from the left or right hepatic arteries with equal frequency.

The cystic artery usually is a branch of the right hepatic artery. It usually reaches the gall bladder behind the common hepatic duct after traversing the cystohepatic triangle to the right of the common hepatic duct. In 85% to 90% of cases there is a single cystic artery.

Portal Vein

The portal vein carries 75% of the blood flow to the liver and 50% of the oxygen. The portal vein is formed by the confluence of the superior mesenteric vein and the splenic vein behind the neck of the pancreas (Fig. 10–6). Approaching the liver within the porta hepatis, the

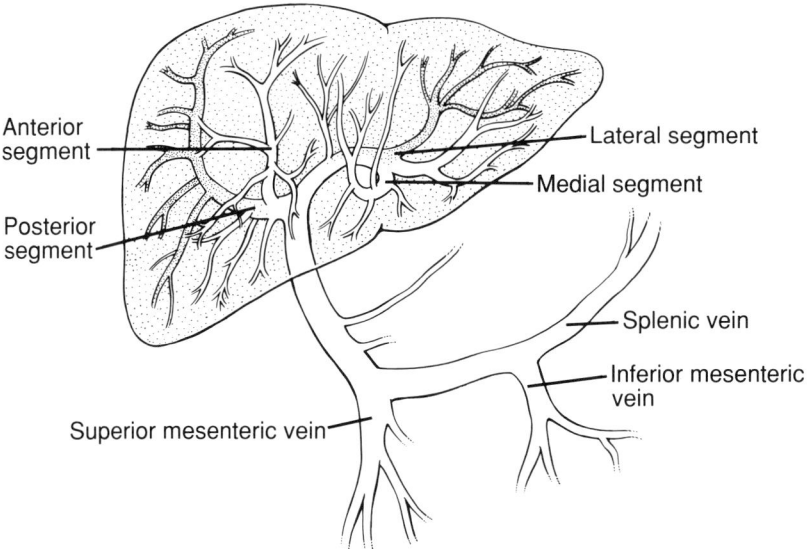

Figure 10–6. Portal vein anatomy. The portal veins along with the hepatic artery and bile ducts occupy the central area of the liver segments.

portal vein lies anterior to the inferior vena cava and posterior of the common bile duct and the hepatic artery. The portal vein is 7 to 10 cm in length and bifurcates into the left and right portal veins.

The portal lobar veins lie posteriorly to the hepatic arteries and bile ducts. The right lobar portal vein is short and divides into anterior and posterior segmental vessels. Each of these segmental vessels further divides into inferior and superior subsegmental branches. The right portal vein sends a branch to the right side of the caudate lobe (segment I).

The left portal vein is longer than the right and courses to the left from the bifurcation. It then turns inferiorly in the liver at the umbilical fossa forming a venous lake at the site of entry of the umbilical vein. The superior and inferior subsegmental veins of the lateral segment (segments II and III) arise from the left side of the umbilical portion of the left portal vein. The medial segmental veins arise from the right side of the umbilical portion of the left portal vein. This is of importance when performing a left lateral segmentectomy (segments II and III) as the umbilical portion of the left portal vein should be left intact.

Hepatic Veins

The venous drainage of the liver is simple. The hepatic veins lie in the planes dividing the segments of the liver and, thus, are intersegmental (Fig. 10–3). There are three major veins: right, middle, and left. The right hepatic vein is the largest and drains the anterior and posterior portions of the right lobe of the liver (segments VI, VII, and VIII). The middle and left hepatic veins frequently (85%) enter the inferior vena cava as a single trunk. The middle hepatic vein drains the superior aspect of the anterior segment of the right lobe (segment V). The left hepatic vein drains the superior aspect of the medial segment (III) and the lateral segments (II and IV) of the left lobe. The caudate lobe (segment I) usually drains directly into the inferior vena cava via multiple small branches.

Bile Ducts

The biliary drainage of the liver follows a segmental and lobar pattern and shares a common pathway with the blood supply (portal triad) (Fig. 10–7). The right hepatic duct is formed by the joining of the anterior and posterior segmental ducts at the porta hepatis. In 30% of cases, one of the two ducts, usually the posterior, crosses the segmental fissure to drain into the left hepatic duct.[9] The left hepatic duct is formed by the confluence of the medial and lateral segment ducts. This is in the left segmental fissure in 50% of cases and to the right of the fissure in 42% of cases. The caudate lobe (segment I) drainage is variable and may drain into either the left or right duct.

The common hepatic duct is formed by the confluence of the right and left hepatic ducts in the transverse fissure of the liver. Its distal end is defined by the junction with the cystic duct and may range from 1 to 7.5 cm in length. The normal diameter is 4 to 6 mm. The common bile duct is the continuation of the common hepatic duct, distal to the cystic duct. It ranges in length from 2 to 7 cm. It has a consistent course and is divided into four portions: supraduodenal, retroduodenal, pancreatic, and intramural. The supraduodenal portion lies between the layers of the hepatic duodenal ligament, anterior to the foramen of Winslow. The retroduodenal portion is between the superior margin of the first portion of the duodenum and the superior edge of the head of the pancreas. The gastroduodenal

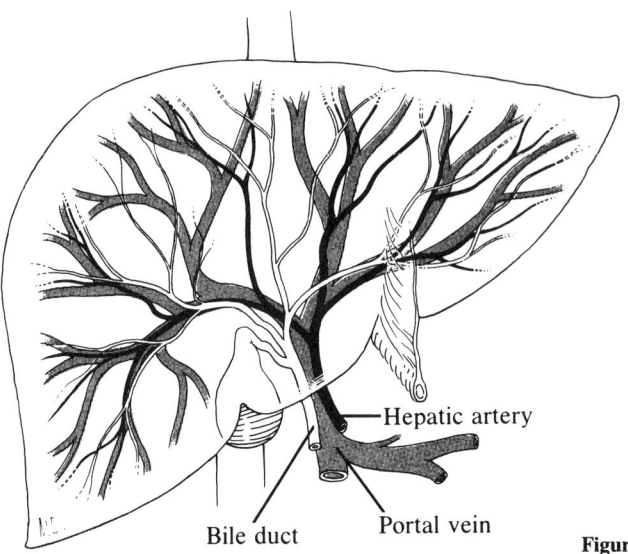

Figure 10–7. Anatomy of the bile ducts.

artery lies to the left and the posterior superior pancreaticoduodenal artery lies anterior to the bile duct. The pancreatic portion of the common bile duct passes from the upper margin of the head of the pancreas obliquely to the right, posterior to the pancreas, to its entrance into the duodenum. The intramural portion of the common bile duct travels an oblique path approximately 1.5 cm long through the duodenal wall. It joins with the main pancreatic duct inferiorly.

PATTERNS OF INJURY

Understanding the anatomy and differences in tissue elasticity helps explain some of the patterns of injury after blunt trauma. The forces from blunt injury are usually direct compressive forces or shear forces. The elastic tissue within arterial blood vessels makes them less susceptible to tearing than any other structures within the liver. Venous and biliary ductal tissue are moderately resistant to shear forces, whereas the liver parenchyma is the least resistant of all. Thus, fractures within the liver parenchyma tend to occur along segmental fissures or directly into the parenchyma. This causes shearing of lateral branches to the major hepatic and portal veins. With severe deceleration injury the origins of the hepatic veins may be ripped from the cava, causing devastating hemorrhage. Similarly, the small branches from the caudate lobe entering directly into the cava are at high risk for shearing with linear tears on the caval surface. Direct compressive forces usually cause tearing between segmental fissures in an anteroposterior sagittal orientation. Horizontal fracture lines into the parenchyma give the characteristic burst pattern to such liver injuries. If the fracture lines are parallel, these have been dubbed "bear claw"–type injuries (Fig. 10–8). Occasionally, there will be a single fracture line across the horizontal plane of

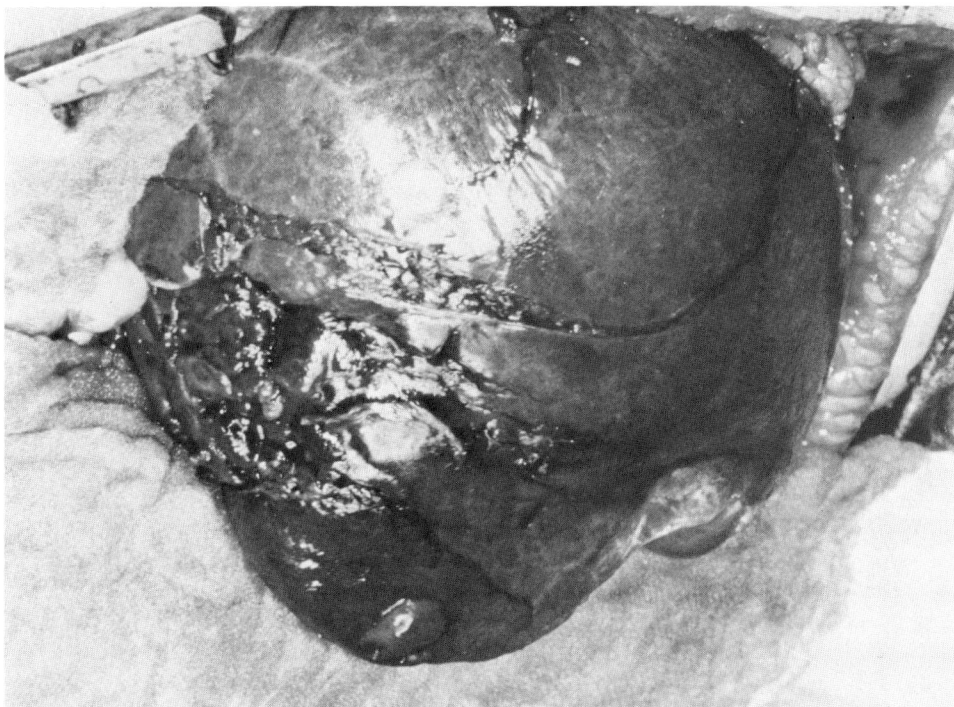

Figure 10–8. "Bear claw" injury of the liver. The lacerations can be superficial or deep.

the liver usually between the anterior and posterior segments. This can cause massive hemorrhage if there is direct extension or continuity with the peritoneal cavity (Fig. 10–9).

DIAGNOSIS AND PREOPERATIVE MANAGEMENT

Abdominal trauma accounts for 13% of all trauma deaths and the liver is the most commonly injured parenchymatous organ. Diagnosis of hepatic trauma preoperatively may be difficult. Any penetrating trauma to the upper abdomen and lower thorax, especially the right upper quadrant, is at risk for damaging the liver. Virtually all penetrating injuries to the abdomen should be explored promptly, especially when they occur in conjunction with hypotension.

The diagnosis of liver injury may be difficult in blunt trauma. Knowledge of the mechanism of injury may be helpful in diagnosing injuries. A history of rapid deceleration may be associated with avulsion of hepatic vein or a retrohepatic vena cava injury. Shoulder harnesses can cause blunt injuries to the liver and rib fractures, which can cause direct laceration of the liver. The initial survey may reveal right lower rib fractures or right upper quadrant ecchymosis as a clue to underlying hepatic injury. Ten percent of patients with significant right lower chest trauma have associated liver injuries.

The initial evaluation and care of the patient should be carried out according to

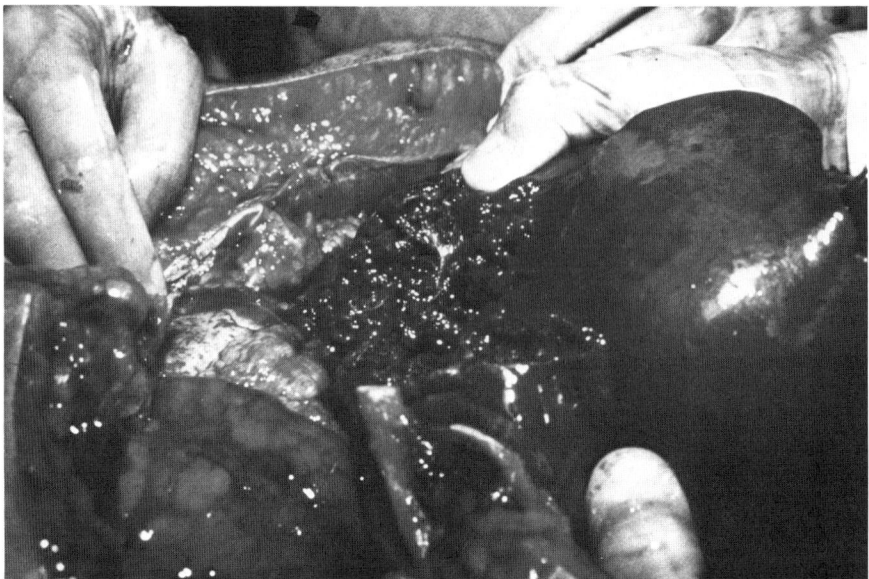

Figure 10–9. Major disruption of the hepatic parenchyma.

Advanced Trauma Life Support (ATLS) guidelines. The airway should be monitored and circulation ensured. Large-bore intravenous lines should be placed and fluid resuscitation initially undertaken with a balanced salt solution. Serial hematocrits should be obtained as massive intraperitoneal hemorrhage is usually associated with a fall in hematocrit. A chest x-ray should be obtained to diagnose a pneumothorax, hemothorax, or possibly a ruptured diaphragm. Evaluation of the trauma patient should also include a general survey to find any evidence of penetrating trauma or external signs of internal injuries. Although these physical signs are important indicators for potential intraabdominal injury, physical exam alone is poor for diagnosing intraabdominal trauma. Physical exam even in an alert patient is accurate in only approximately 50% of cases and carries a 56% false positive rate and 34% to 46% false negative rate.[10,11]

The use of diagnostic peritoneal lavage improves the diagnosis of intraabdominal injury. Diagnostic peritoneal lavage can be performed quickly and is sensitive for diagnosing the presence or absence of intraperitoneal blood. A positive peritoneal lavage is considered an indication for prompt celiotomy. However, because of the sensitivity of diagnostic peritoneal lavage many patients will have inconsequential injuries and a nontherapeutic celiotomy rate of 5% to 25% can be expected. Computerized tomography (CT) is a valuable diagnostic tool in the evaluation of the hemodynamically stable trauma patient (Fig. 10–10). The CT scan is sensitive for intraperitoneal fluid and organ specific for injury compared to peritoneal lavage. CT can demonstrate liver and spleen injuries and can fairly closely quantitate the amount of intraperitoneal blood.[12] There has been some success with the grading of organ injuries as a predictor of the need for surgical intervention. CT cannot, however, detect patients with active bleeding and in need of surgery to control hemorrhage. In the stable patient it may be necessary to repeat the CT scan or perform celiotomy based on the amount of intraperitoneal blood.

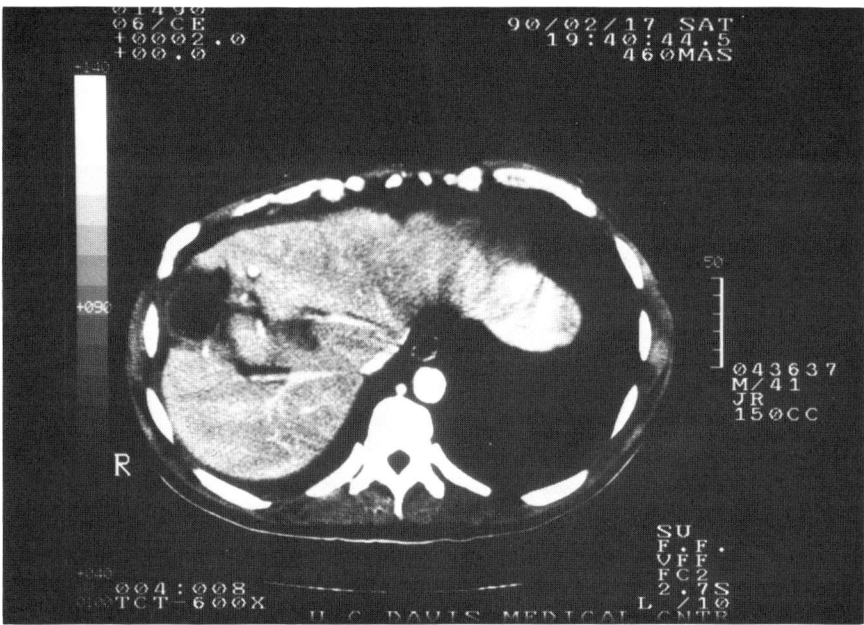

Figure 10–10. CT scan of the liver reveals major hepatic parenchymal disruption.

Based on CT examination an anatomic classification of liver injuries has been developed by Moore.[13] This classification of liver injuries may be useful in determining the need for surgical intervention. Class I injuries involve avulsion of the capsule or parenchymal fractures <1 cm deep. They occur in 15% of cases. Class II injuries involve parenchymal fractures 1 to 3 cm deep, subcapsular hematoma <10 cm in diameter, or penetrating wound with minimal parenchymal damage and bleeding. These occur with a 55% frequency. Class III injuries consist of deep parenchymal fractures (>3 cm), large subcapsular hematoma (>10 cm), or a central penetrating wound. Class III injuries occur in 25% of cases. Class IV injuries involve a massive control hematoma or lobar tissue destruction and occur in only 3% of cases. Class V injuries are highly lethal and involve extensive bilobar disruption or retrohepatic vena cava injury. These occur with a 2% frequency in patients arriving in the emergency room alive.

TREATMENT OF LIVER INJURIES

Once the diagnosis of hepatic trauma has been made, either at celiotomy or by CT scan, a method of treatment must be chosen based on the probable severity of the injury (Table 10–1). Nonoperative management of hepatic injuries is a possible modality of therapy in the hemodynamically stable patient. CT scan has made it possible to diagnose relatively small liver injuries and quantitate the volume of intraperitoneal blood.[14–16] The factor determining success or failure of nonoperative management is hemodynamic stability and not apparent volume of intraperitoneal blood. However, given a small but quantitative risk of blood

Table 10-1 Classification of Liver Injuries

Class I		
Blunt	Capsular tears, lacerations <1 cm	Bleeding negligible
Penetrating	Minor knife wounds	
	Superficial penetrating gunshot wound	
Class II		
Blunt	Lacerations 1–3 cm	Blood loss <500 cc
Penetrating	Knife and gunshot wound with minimal parenchymal damage or bleeding	Little or no active bleeding at operation
Class III		
Blunt	Subcapsular hematomas <10 cm	Blood loss >500 cc
	Deep or stellate fractures	
Penetrating	Central injuries with major bleeding, gunshot wound with moderate parenchymal damage	
Class IV		
Blunt	Large subcapsular hematomas	1000–2500 cc blood loss
	Extensive parenchymal damage	
Penetrating	Bilobar gunshot wounds with extensive parenchymal damage	
Class V		
Blunt	Crush injuries with bilobar damage	Exsanguinating injuries
	Avulsion hepatic vein injuries	
Penetrating	Explosive injuries from shotgun or high velocity gunshot wounds	

transfusion, surgical control is indicated to control possible ongoing hemorrhage rather than risk the need for transfusion.[15-17]

Class I and II liver injuries are the most likely to respond to nonoperative management (Fig. 10–11). If these are found at the time of celiotomy, they can usually be controlled with temporary gauze packing or high current electrocautery. Topical thrombotic agents such as microfibullor collagen or liquid thrombin are also effective. Suture control of bleeding points in Class I or II injuries is rarely needed.[16] When greater than 500 cc blood loss is associated with a Class II injury it should be carefully investigated even though the bleeding may have stopped. Although further bleeding may be predicted by this investigation it is important to ensure that more extensive parenchymal injury is not present.

Identification of severe parenchymal injury and ensuring hemostasis may prevent secondary bleeding or biliary fistula formation (Fig. 10–12). Occasionally lacerations or injuries in critical areas of anatomy such as the falciform ligament may be difficult to control. In these cases a brief Pringle maneuver may permit better visualization of the bleeding point and allow meticulous suture ligation.

The treatment of Class III, IV, and V injuries is obviously more complex. If the patient has been transiently hypotensive in the prehospital setting or the emergency room or is frankly hypotensive in the operating room, certain precautions should be carried out during the preparation for surgery. The patient is prepped and draped from the midneck to the midthighs anteriorly and from table top to table top laterally. This is optimally done before induction of anesthesia since the administration of a muscle relaxant and use of positive pressure ventilation may result in a significant drop in blood pressure. The use of positive pressure ventilation converts the intrathoracic pressure from negative to positive with a

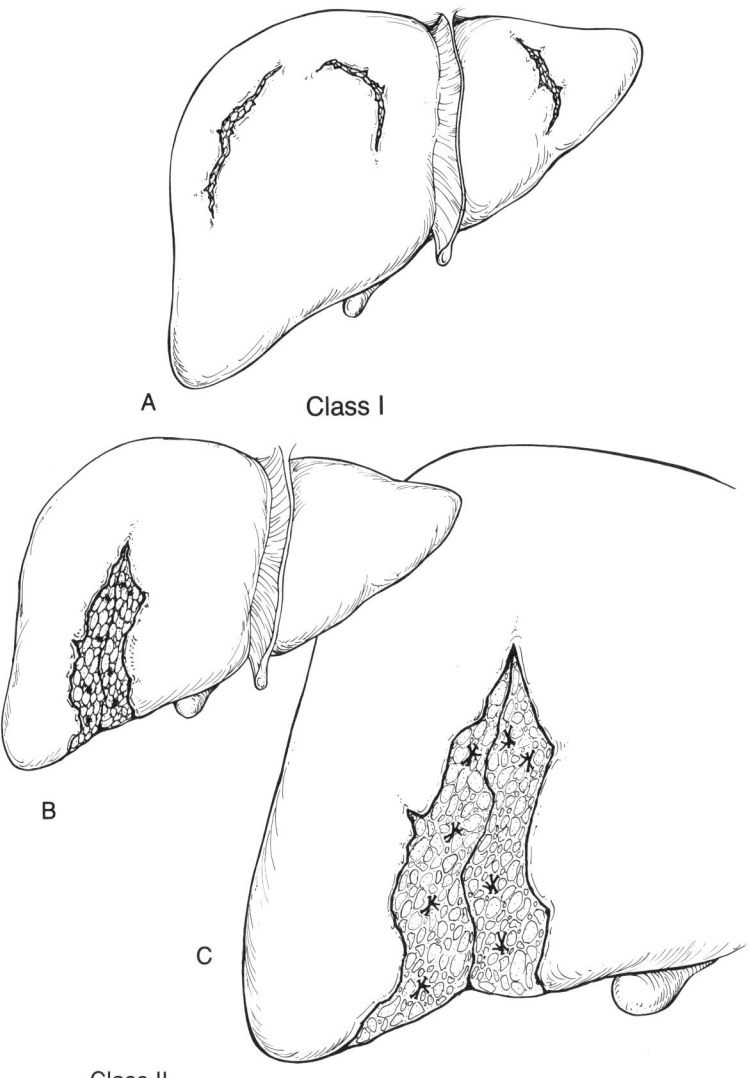

Figure 10–11. Minor liver injuries—Class I and II. **A:** Class I injury; **B:** Class II injury; **C:** Suture ligation of bleeding vessels in Class II injury.

resultant abrupt rise in intraabdominal venous pressure while muscle relaxation causes a decrease in intraabdominal pressure. These two effects combine for a loss of tamponade effect with resultant massive hemorrhage. Sudden deterioration of the patient's condition with the onset of positive pressure ventilation is characteristic of major liver or intraabdominal venous injury.

If there is a large amount of blood within the abdominal cavity, the initial priority is temporary control of hemorrhage. This is done most easily by the application of four quadrant packs. Most catastrophic bleeding from hepatic injury is venous in nature and can

174 Abdominal Trauma

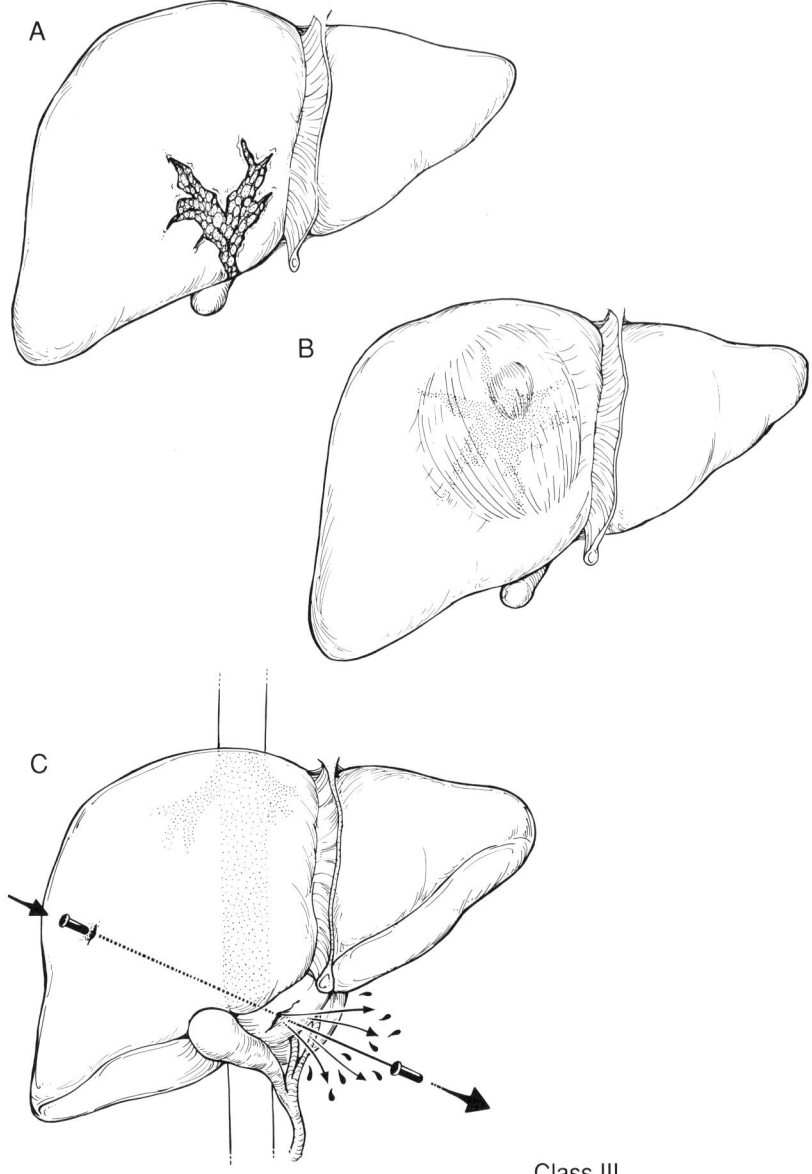

Figure 10–12. Severe parenchymal injury—Class III. **A:** Large stellate laceration. **B:** Subscapular hematoma. **C:** Through-and-through gunshot wound with bleeding.

therefore be controlled by judicious application of liver packs. Sometimes gentle compression of the packs by the surgeon's hand will also aid in stanching the hemorrhage at least on a temporary basis. During this time anesthesia must reestablish normal blood volume; it is also an opportune time to establish more intravenous access lines and other monitoring devices. After hemodynamic stability has been achieved, packs in the two lower abdominal quadrants are removed. If there is concomitant fecal soilage it is appropriate to control this rapidly with bowel clamps or a running chromic cat gut suture. The packs in the left upper quadrant are then removed. If there is an associated spleen injury a decision must be made either to remove it promptly or to clamp the hilum of the spleen temporarily with a vascular clamp to reduce further bleeding. Finally, the packs are removed in the right upper quadrant and the injury to the liver rapidly assessed. It is prudent at this time to enter the gastrohepatic ligament either sharply or bluntly so that a vascular clamp can be placed across the portal triad (Fig. 10–13). If there is a large laceration or penetrating wound of the parenchyma and the Pringle maneuver controls the bleeding, one can assume the bleeding originates either from a portal venous system or hepatic arteries. If the bleeding is not controlled, one should assume that the bleeding is primarily from the hepatic venous system. This can often be confirmed by gently retracting down on the dome of the liver, which will often cause a gush of bleeding from one of the insertions of the hepatic veins or an intrahepatic caval injury. Another means of diagnosing the injury is to have the anesthesiologist temporarily remove the patient from positive pressure ventilation. A cessation or marked decrease in the rate of bleeding confirms a hepatic venous or vena caval injury. If a hepatic venous or intrahepatic caval injury is suspected, packs should be replaced and a decision should be made at that time, before hemodynamic instability or hypothermia, as to what operative technique will be used. This will be discussed later.

If the Pringle maneuver successfully controls the hemorrhage, the parenchymal injury should be further explored by hepatotomy. Hepatotomy can be made by either the finger fracture technique or by using the blunt end of a scalpel handle. Once exposure is complete, bleeding vessels and open bile ducts can be directly suture ligated with fine nonabsorbable sutures. Deep liver sutures or mattress sutures are rarely indicated for control of hemor-

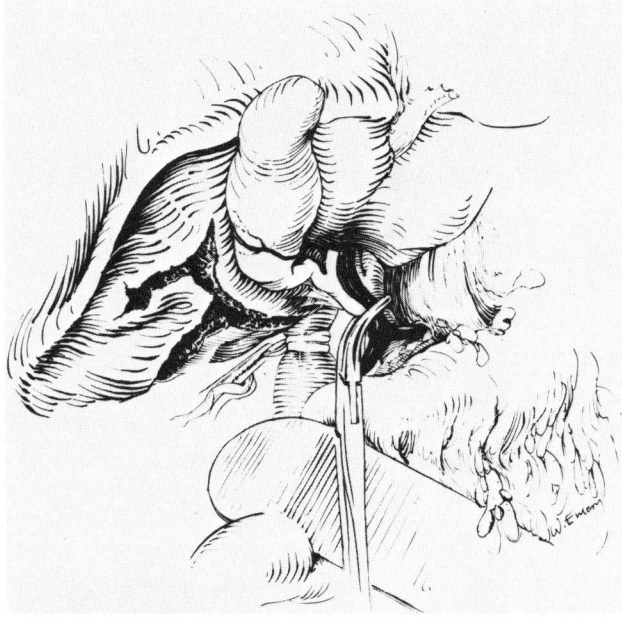

Figure 10–13. Occlusion of the portal triad using a vascular clamp (Pringle maneuver).

rhage. Deep suturing can lead to hepatic necrosis and hematoma formation with possibility of abscess formation and hemobilia as a further complication.

During repair or control of any hepatic injury the importance of the assistant surgeon cannot be overemphasized. Often it is the assistant surgeon by using direct compression of the liver parenchyma with his hands above and below the opposing surfaces that allows the surgeon to visualize and directly ligate the bleeding vessel (Fig. 10–14). A second assistant is also often critical to provide suction (optimally into a cell saver). If a second assistant is not available, the same task can be done by a nurse or operating room technician. It must be emphasized that most (70%) bleeding from liver lacerations that falls into either the Class III or IV category can be controlled by the above described techniques.

Hepatic artery ligation may be of value in a limited number of injuries. The through-and-through wound of the liver is exemplified by stab wounds or low velocity wounds, which injure the hepatic artery with little damage to the liver substance. If the bleeding is brisk and is controlled by the Pringle maneuver, dissection and control of the hepatic artery will confirm that this is the source of the hemorrhage. The appropriate lobar artery should not be ligated until it is established that this is the source of hemorrhage. The right hepatic artery may be the source of the medial segmental artery to the left lobe or the vessel assumed to be the left lobar artery may in fact be the right lobar artery, with the left lobar artery coming into the liver through the falciform ligament (see the section on anatomic

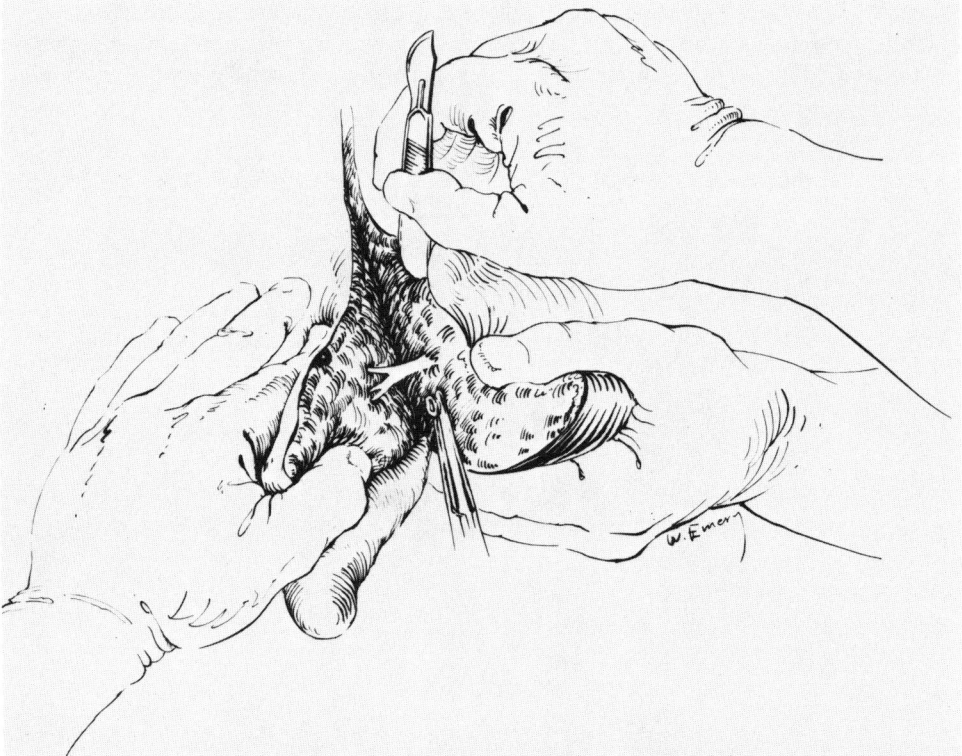

Figure 10–14. Compression of the liver during resection controls bleeding so definitive ligation of bleeding points can be identified and managed.

variations). In these circumstances of major hepatic arterial bleeding with minimal disruption of liver substance, hepatic artery ligation has constituted a major advance. Mortality and morbidity manifest by jaundice, and liver dysfunction have occurred primarily in those cases in which it is necessary to ligate the proper hepatic artery or in those cases in which the attachments of the liver were mobilized before making the decision to treat the bleeding with ligation. The surgeon dealing with the liver trauma should be fully familiar with the anatomical variables, since this is the key to successful operative treatment.

Class IV and V injuries account for most of the deaths caused by liver trauma. In a few cases it may be necessary to perform hepatic vascular isolation in order to resect the injured parenchyma or repair the torn vessel. This is most often necessary when there is a major hepatic venous injury or an injury to the retrohepatic vena cava.

Hepatic vascular isolation can be accomplished by three methods:[17-23] Heaney maneuver,[21] atrial–caval shunting,[17,18,23] and veno–venous bypass.[19,22] The Heaney maneuver is performed by clamping both the supra- and infrahepatic inferior vena cava while simultaneously applying the Pringle maneuver. Repair of the retrohepatic venous injuries can then be performed. It is crucial during the Heaney maneuver that central pressures are monitored and fluid replacement given cautiously to avoid over- or underloading the patient with the inferior vena cava clamped. We have found that almost 50% of the patients undergoing liver transplant tolerate the Heaney maneuver without hemodynamic instability.[21] However, the hypovolemic patient will usually develop profound hypotension or cardiac arrest, giving this technique limited application in the trauma setting.

Vascular isolation with atrial caval shunting[17,18,23] is carried out initially by extending this midline laparotomy incision into a median sternotomy. This can be accomplished with either a power saw or a Leibsche knife. The pericardium is opened and intrapericardiac inferior vena cava isolated with an umbilical tape. The suprarenal vena cava is also isolated with an umbilical tape. An atrial caval shunt is then fashioned from a 32 to 38 F thoracostomy tube. A purse string suture is placed in the right atrial appendage and the appendage clamped with a Satinsky clamp. The right atrial appendage is opened and the chest tube placed into the right atrium and directed down the inferior vena cava as the Satinsky clamp is removed. The tube should be inserted thoracic end first, with a hand placed above the intrapericardiac vena cava to direct the shunt into the distal vena cava and not into one of the hepatic veins. All of the side holes in the tube should be below the renal veins. The distal portion of the tube should be clamped and temporarily withdrawn 3 to 4 inches and a second clamp placed 3 to 4 inches from the first. Two side holes are then quickly cut, the second clamp removed, and the tube reinserted. The tube is inserted to a level such that the newly cut holes are in the right atrium and the distal side holes remain below the renal veins. The purse string suture in the atrial appendage is then tied and umbilical tape around the intrapericardial inferior vena cava and suprarenal vena cava closed around the shunt with Rummel tourniquets (Fig. 10–15). The porta hepatis is also clamped (Pringle maneuver) to provide complete vascular isolation. The liver can then be mobilized and repair of veins or resection of liver carried out. Even when hepatic vascular isolation is accomplished, mortality remains at 50% to 80% in experienced hands.[17]

A third method of hepatic vascular isolation is the use of veno–venous bypass using a centrifugal pump (Fig. 10–16). Initially described by Griffith et al.[19] and Shaw et al.[22] for use in liver transplantation, a similar system can be used in liver trauma instead of the atrial-caval shunt. The inferior vena cava can be accessed by cannulating the femoral vein in the groin. The inflow cannulation site is via cutdown on the axillary or jugular vein. A

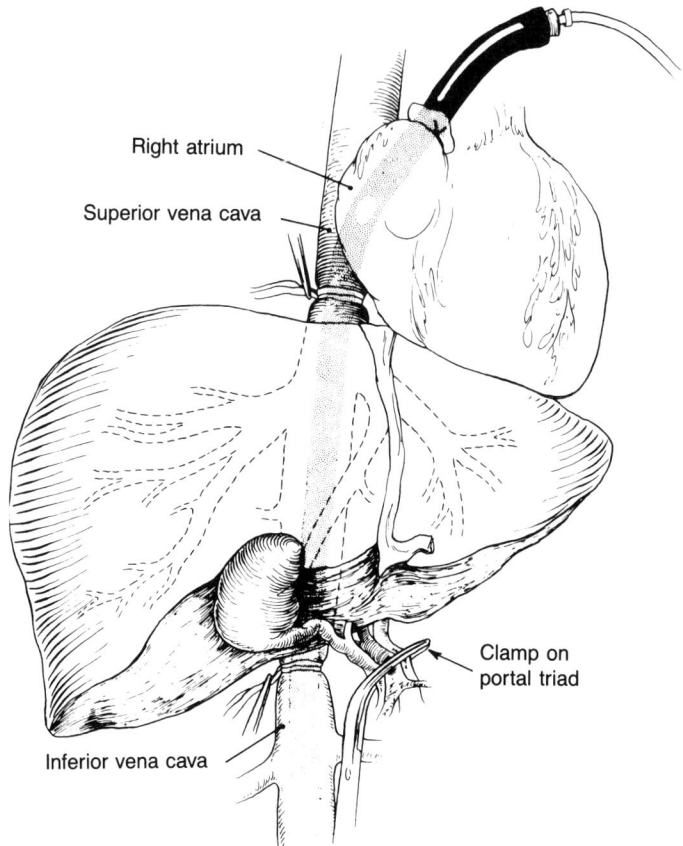

Figure 10–15. View shows a #36 French catheter inserted through right atrial appendage into the inferior vena cava. The tip of the catheter lies just below the level of the renal veins. The side hole of the catheter, 20 cm from the tip, lies at the level of the right atrium. The proximal end of the catheter is connected to an infusion line as depicted. For more rapid infusion, a "Y" connector is provided.

centrifugal pump is used to assist flow. Hepatic vascular inflow occlusion can then be accomplished by clamping the suprahepatic vena cava at the diaphragm, suprarenal vena cava, and porta hepatis. This method eliminates the need to open the chest and avoids the risk of placing the atrial caval shunt through a hole in the retrohepatic vena cava while still maintaining venous return from the inferior vena cava.

Hepatic Resection

Hepatic resection including debridement is indicated in 5% to 15% of cases. Even in experienced centers mortality associated with resection for trauma approaches 50%. Absolute indications for liver resection and debridement include dead or devitalized tissue, intraparenchymal injury to large bile ducts, and inaccessible bleeding. Debridement is usually nonanatomic removal of devitalized tissue with the injury (Fig. 10–17). Anatomic resection in trauma is limited to right lobectomy, left lobectomy, and left lateral segmentectomy. The type and extent of resection are usually determined by the nature of the injury.

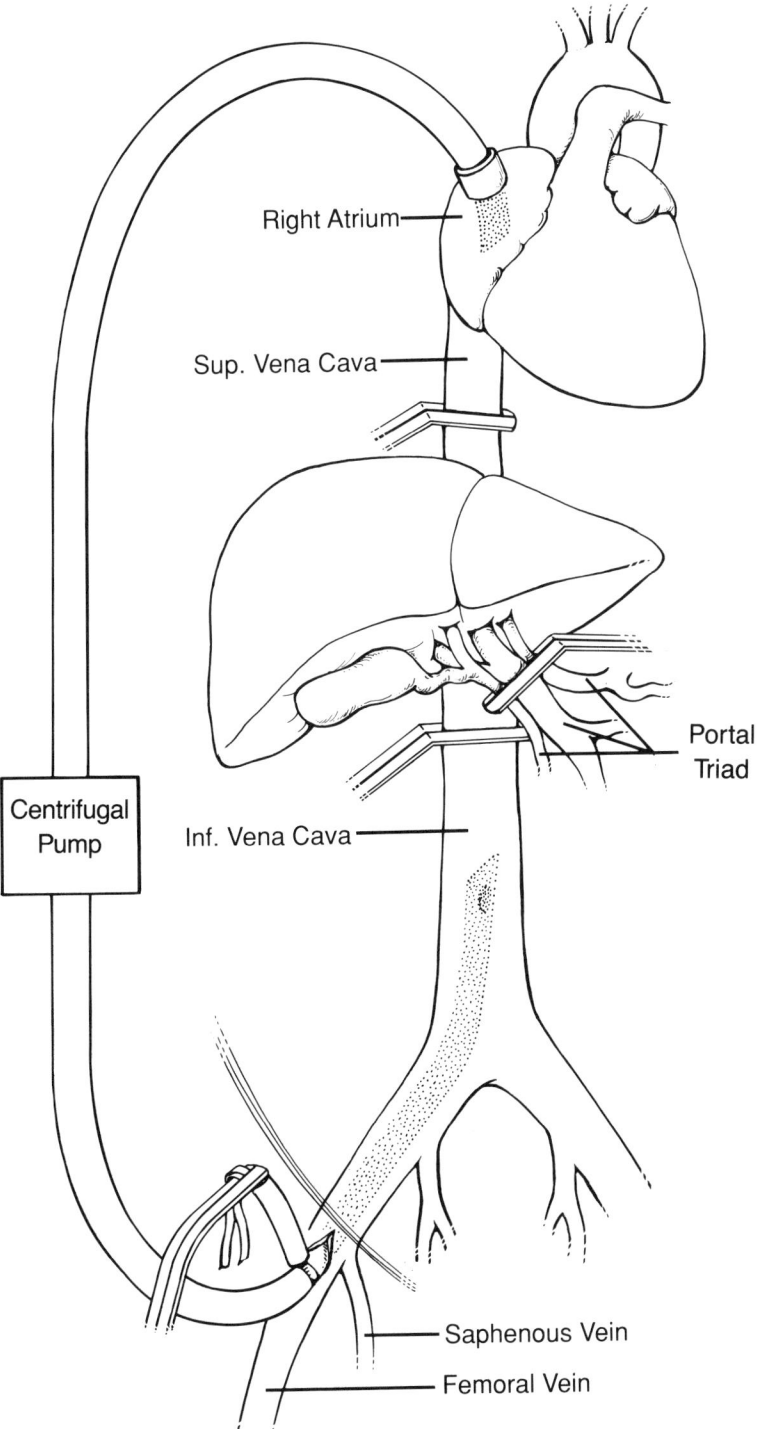

Figure 10–16. Utilization of a venous shunt and centrifugal pump to decompress the vena cava during repair of the hepatic veins.

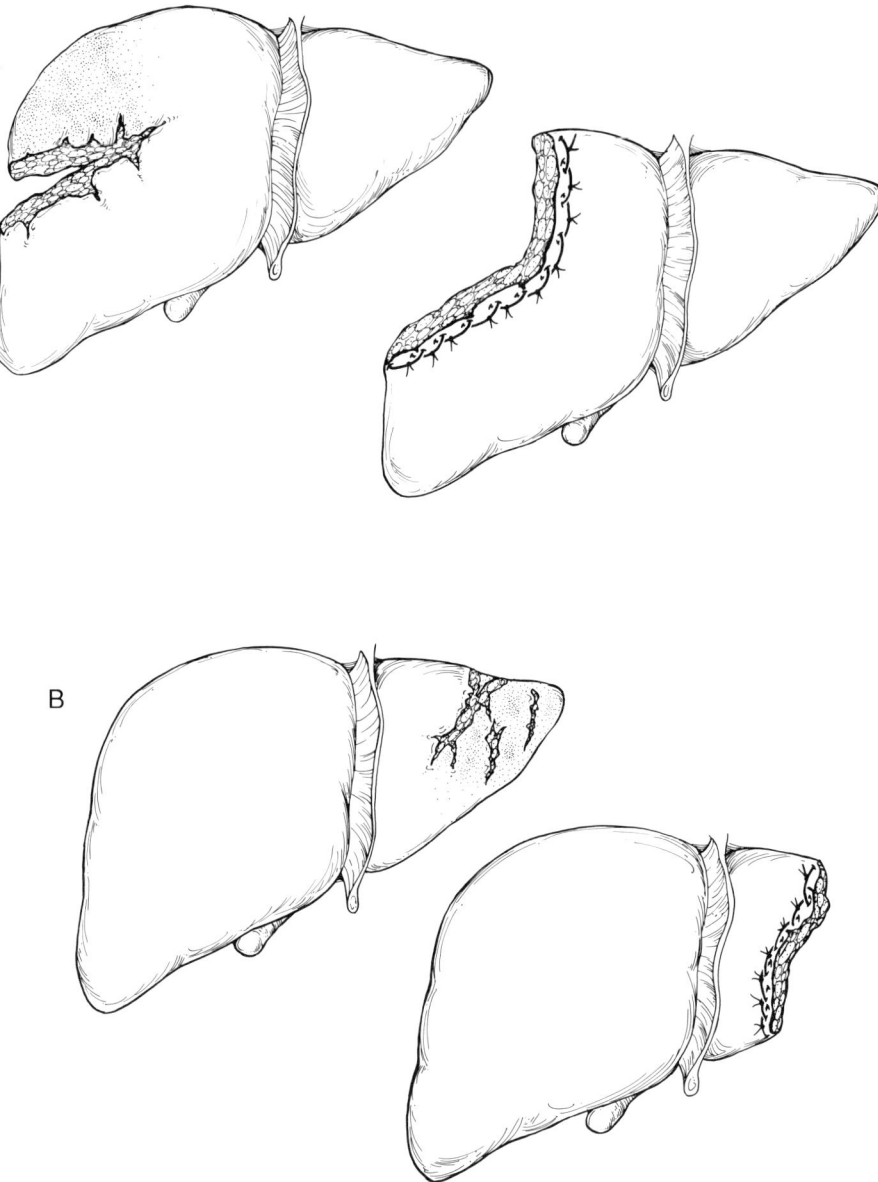

Figure 10–17. Indications for liver resection are primarily related to devitalization of liver tissue. The resection should be carried out so as to result in the minimal cross section of raw tissue (**A**, **B**).

To carry out hepatic resection, the liver must first be mobilized by dividing its ligamentous attachments. To perform a right lobectomy both leaves of the coronary ligament need to be divided. Access for left lobe resection is enhanced by division of the triangular ligament. There are techniques useful in all forms of resectional debridement. After the capsule of the liver is incised the liver parenchyma is readily dissected with the blunt end of a scalpel handle. Blood loss is minimized by compression of the liver between the assistant's hands. As vessels and bile ducts are encountered they can be individually ligated with either clips or suture ligatures; however, the authors prefer ligatures. Small vessels and parenchymal ooze can be controlled with electrocautery or the Argon beam coagulator.

Nonanatomic resection should be carried out for debridement of devitalized tissue that does not fall within a standard anatomical region. Resection should be limited to devitalized tissue. In this instance, however, a knowledge of segmental anatomy is useful in avoiding major hepatic veins and preventing devascularization of additional liver parenchyma. Bleeding vessels should be controlled with either clips or suture ligation. Care should be taken to avoid injury to large vascular structures during nonanatomic resection. Raw surfaces left after resection can be covered with omentum to facilitate hemostasis.[20]

Left lateral segmentectomy consists of resection of the liver that lies to the left of the falciform ligament. The line of resection should be carried out to the left of the falciform ligament. Care should be taken not to ligate vessels that may be supplying the medial segment (segment IV) of the left lobe. This means avoiding the portal vein at the site of insertion of the obliterated umbilical vein. Hemostasis during the resection can be maintained quite well by compression of the medial segment. After resection, the raw surface can be covered by mobilizing the falciform ligament and reflecting it over the raw area.[20]

When the medial segment of the left lobe of the liver (segment IV) is severely damaged, left hepatic lobectomy is indicated (Fig. 10–17). Medial segmentectomy, although a viable option in an elective setting, is time consuming and associated injuries make this a poor choice in the trauma patient. The line of resection for a left lobectomy should be carried out to the left of the gall bladder fossa. It is absolutely necessary to identify the middle hepatic vein during resection as it drains the superior segment of the right lobe and commonly drains into the left hepatic vein. The left hepatic vein should be ligated and divided proximal to the junction with the middle hepatic vein. The left portal vein should not be ligated until it is well exposed within the hilum as it may give off a branch to the anterior segment of the right lobe (Fig. 10–18). Care should also be taken when dividing the left hepatic duct as a segmental hepatic duct from the right frequently crosses the segmental fissure to drain into the left hepatic duct. The left hepatic artery supplies only the left side and can be readily ligated.

In performing a right hepatic lobectomy the line of resection should be carried to the left of the gall bladder fissure (Fig. 10–19). The middle hepatic vein should be divided early and proximally to avoid injury to the left hepatic vein. The dissection should then be carried toward the vena cava to the right of the middle hepatic vein. The right hepatic artery and portal vein can be dissected early in the resection and ligated to decrease blood loss. Care should be taken to avoid damage to the occasional branch of the hepatic artery, which may supply the medial segment of the left lobe. Division of hepatic parenchyma and ligation of small vessels and bile ducts are as previously described.

Occasionally attempts to repair or resect the liver must be abandoned. Massive bleeding, transfusion, and hypothermia all contribute to severe coagulopathy, which can

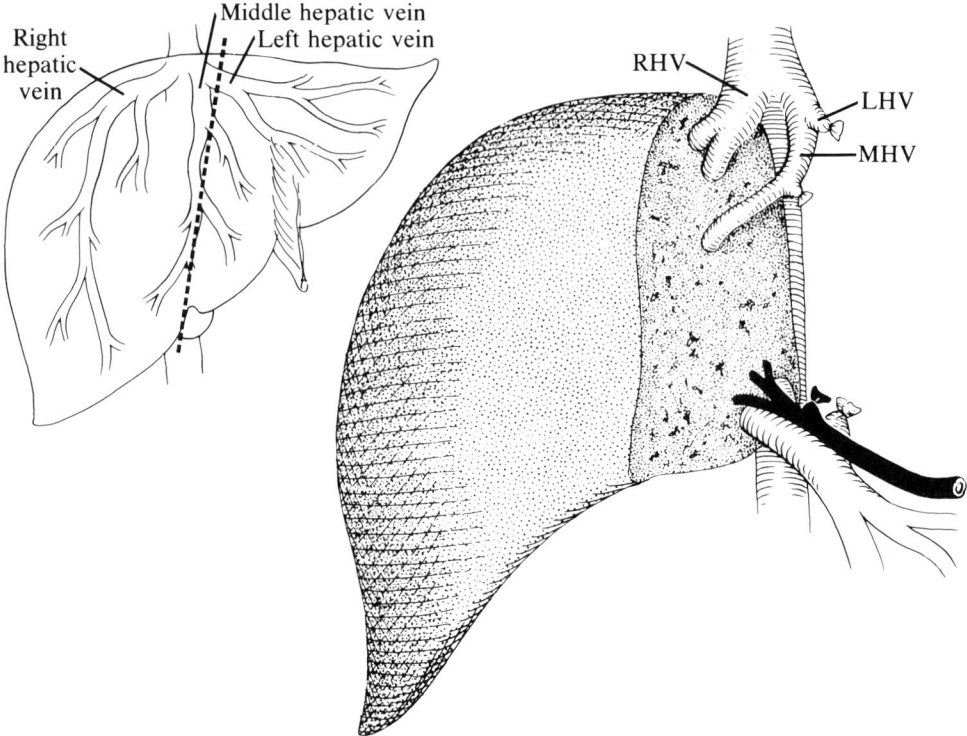

Figure 10–18. Left hepatic lobectomy.

make surgical repair impossible. In 3% to 5% of patients control of hemorrhage with packing of the liver should be performed, the abdomen closed, and the patient transported to the intensive care unit for resuscitation, reversal of the coagulopathy, and warming. Pack removal is then accomplished at 24 to 72 hr. Patients undergoing packing of their liver have a >40% mortality rate and suffer multiple complications because of the severity of their injuries. Proper packing does not involve simply stuffing laparotomy sponges around the liver. Although some have advocated placement of plastic between the gauze packs and the liver, use of omentum, a sheet of gel foam, or plain gauze is equally effective. For large lacerations of the liver the goal is to pack the perihepatic region in such a way as to provide closure and compression of the injury. Packs can be placed in the right retrohepatic space to roll the right lobe anteriorly and close any laceration. Packs can also be placed between the liver and the rib cage to provide posterior compression to control retrohepatic caval or posterior liver injuries. The key is to compress the liver without occluding the inferior vena cava. It is crucial that the anesthesiologist report arterial and central venous pressures when the packs are being placed. If pressures drop, it may be necessary to remove or rearrange the packs to prevent occlusion of the inferior vena cava. When the patient's coagulopathy is controlled and hypothermia reversed, the patient can be returned to the operating room for removal of packs.

Return to the operating room can then be undertaken in a more controlled environment and with a full complement of personnel, which may not be available in the acute trauma

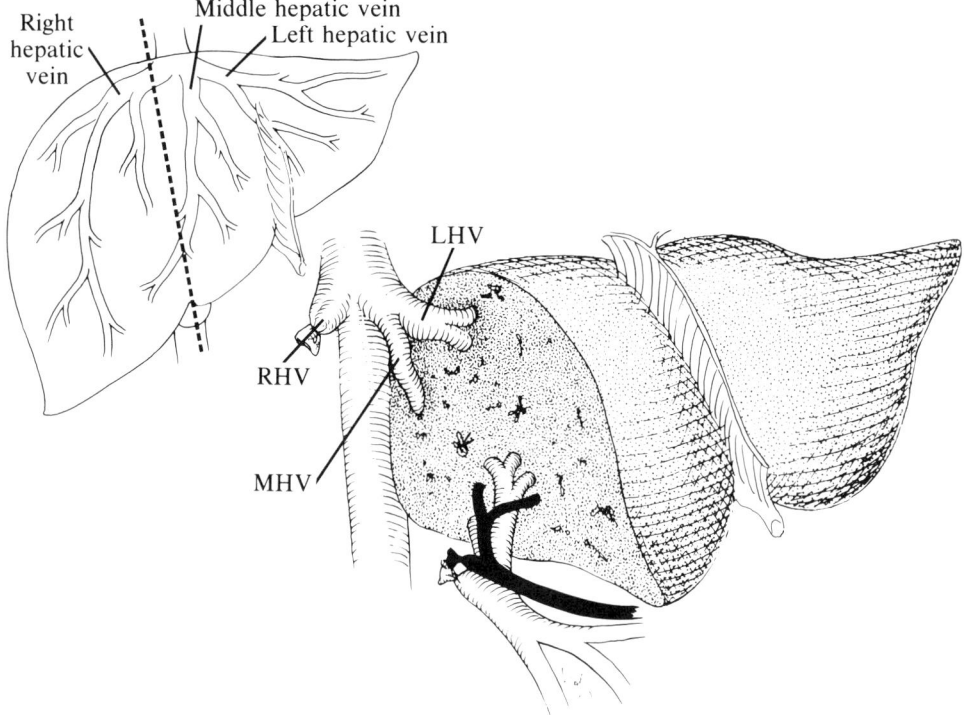

Figure 10–19. Right hepatic lobectomy.

setting. The surgical team should be prepared for massive blood loss. They should also be prepared to perform an atrial–caval shunt or veno–venous bypass to facilitate hepatic vascular isolation for repair of injuries. Another option after packing is to transport the patient to a different center that has additional resources.

Liver transplantation has been performed after hepatic trauma has caused massive parenchymal destruction. There have been three reported cases of transplantation after severe hepatic trauma with two successes.[24,25] The indication for liver transplantation secondary to trauma is severe devascularization with minimal to no associated injuries, especially head injuries. When transplantation is being considered for hepatic trauma the patient should be referred to a transplant center early as organ availability is unpredictable.

Whether or not to drain a liver injury is controversial, especially when dealing with Class I and II injuries. There is little evidence to support drainage in those relatively mild injuries, and the drain may contribute to infection and abscess formation. However, when the preoperative blood loss exceeds 500 to 1000 cc there is an increased probability that a major bile duct and a blood vessel have been injured. These more severe injuries should be drained with closed suction drains to diminish fluid collection and control biliary leak. If hemostasis is not complete, suction drains may not be adequate and dependent open drainage is appropriate (Fig. 10–20). These drains can be contained by a sterile colostomy bag to decrease contamination. Drains should be placed in the region of the injury as well as posterior to provide dependent drainage of fluid collections.

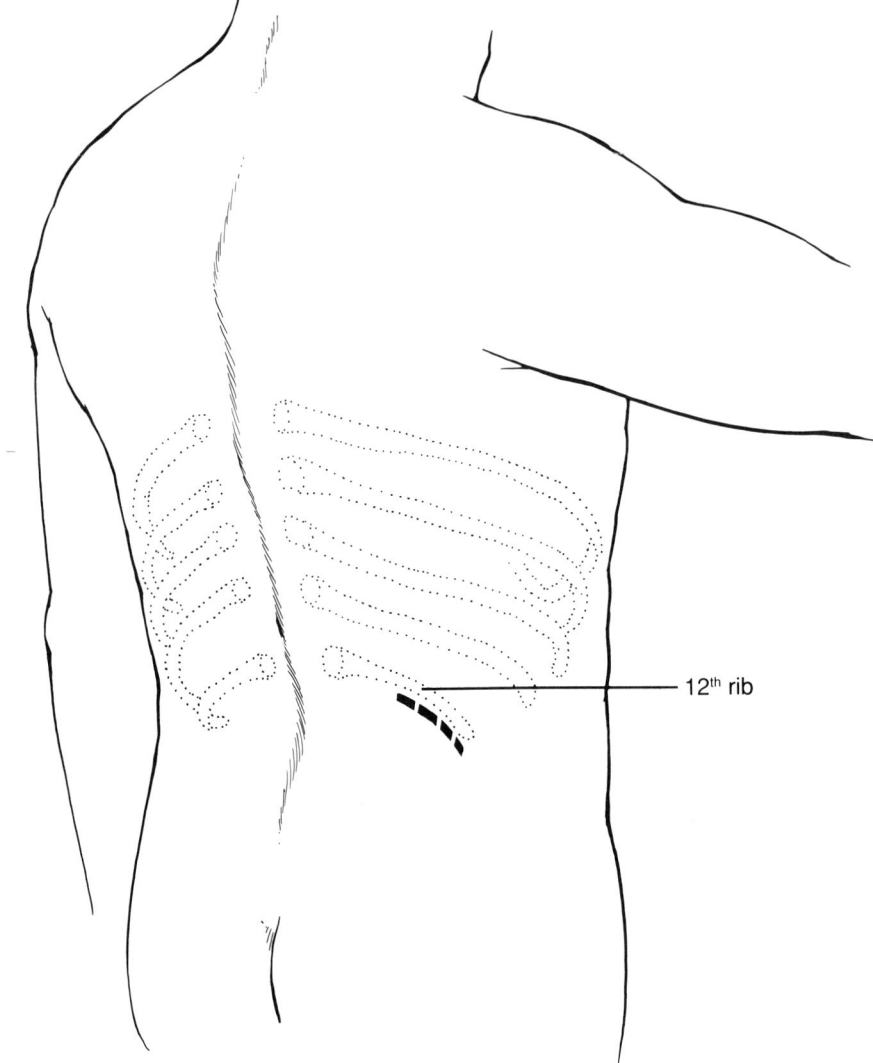

Figure 10–20. Dependent posterior drainage should be used to drain liver bleeding. The incision is best made below the tip of the 12th rib and should be long enough to admit three fingers comfortably.

TREATMENT OF INJURIES TO THE PORTA HEPATIS

Injuries to the porta hepatis are difficult to manage and carry significant morbidity and mortality. Control of hemorrhage is the first priority. Injuries to the porta hepatis are associated with multiple other organ injuries, such as duodenum, pancreas, and vascular, which contribute to the high mortality.

Portal vein injuries have a mortality rate of 54% to 71%. The key to successful management is appropriate wide exposure (see Chapter 19). We favor an extended Kocher maneuver, which entails taking down the entire right colon and mobilizing it toward the midline along with the duodenum. This exposes the portal vein and a significant portion of the inferior vena cava and aorta, which may also be injured. In certain instances it may be necessary to expose the most proximal portion of the portal vein at the junction of the splenic rim and superior mesenteric vein by dividing the neck of the pancreas. After the portal injury has been treated a distal pancreatectomy can be performed. Although ligation can be carried out, sequelae such as mesenteric vein thrombosis or late ammonia intoxication can be catastrophic and therefore every attempt should be made to repair the portal vein injury. Repair can be carried out by direct suture repair or lateral repair.[26] In instances where vein has been lost or destroyed, it may be necessary to place a patch or interposition graft of saphenous or jugular vein to reestablish flow. In the case of associated splenic injury, the splenic vein may be used for the repair after splenectomy.

Injuries to the hepatic artery also create difficult management problems. Although the hepatic artery carries only 25% of blood flow to the liver, it carries 50% of the oxygen supply. Many authors advocate direct ligation of the hepatic artery when the injury is to the common hepatic artery. We prefer to perform repair of the hepatic artery whenever possible. The artery can be dissected free, the damaged area resected, and primary anastomosis performed. When necessary, a saphenous vein or internal iliac artery interposition graft can be used to provide repair without tension. In very proximal injuries the proximal end of the vascular graft can be directly anastomosed to the aorta. We would make a special effort to repair injuries of the proper hepatic artery since collateral flow is less adequate than with common hepatic artery injuries. However, even the proper hepatic artery can be ligated if portal venous flow is intact and lobar hepatic arteries, unless large, can be safely ligated.

Injuries to the extrahepatic biliary tree are usually associated with penetrating trauma, although blunt trauma can cause stretch or avulsion injuries. Gall bladder injuries are the simplest to care for: it should be removed. When the injury is to the bile ducts repair can be tedious. The bile ducts should be meticulously dissected and exposed. Small lacerations can be directly sutured. For moderate injuries the ducts must be debrided before suture repair. Repair should be performed over a T-tube to provide drainage. For proximal common bile duct injuries biliary drainage can be accomplished via Roux-en-Y to either the common hepatic duct or the gall bladder. The Roux-en-Y choledochojejunostomy can be difficult to perform with a normal-sized common bile duct, as is the case in most trauma patients. To make this anastomosis technically easier a modification of the vascular Carrel patch has been described.[27] A 1-cm length of cystic duct is preserved after cholecystectomy and the side wall opened onto the common bile duct remnant. This patch of bile duct is then used to anastomose in an end-to-side fashion to the Roux limb. A Roux-en-Y can also be brought to the right or left hepatic duct to provide drainage. In the unstable patient or when other catastrophic injuries are present, the most appropriate management is simple biliary drainage. This can be accomplished either by placing catheters in the right and left hepatic ducts or a T-tube in the common bile duct and bringing them out of the abdomen laterally. Delayed reconstruction of the biliary system can be accomplished after the patient recovers from other injuries.

Upon accomplishment of hemostasis, the raw surface of the liver should be covered with tissue, as appropriate. The omentum is the optimal tissue and is readily available. It is swung upward, placed over the raw liver surface, and fixed with a few sutures to the liver capsule. In the absence of omentum, the falciform ligament, salvaged portions of liver capsule, or peritoneal grafts may be used.

We do not drain the common duct with a T-tube as a matter of routine. Occasionally, in complex injuries when there has been biliary damage, or when it seems appropriate to monitor the status of bile ducts postoperatively, a small T-tube can be left in the common duct. However, it has been found that the complications associated with a T-tube placement outweigh its advantages.

As a matter of policy, whenever the status of the liver is unclear or questionable on completion of operation, we have no hesitancy about reoperating on a planned basis, 24 hr later. This includes situations where there is any question of viability, in which hemostasis has been incomplete, or external drainage has not been entirely satisfactory. We believe that by so doing subhepatic and subphrenic collections of blood may be identified, devitalized segments responsible for subsequent sepsis and mortality can be located, and unsuspected biliary leaks can be managed and drained appropriately when the patient is hemodynamically stable.

POSTOPERATIVE MANAGEMENT

The immediate operative problem relating to liver surgery is the development of a bleeding syndrome. This is most apt to result when vascular control has required temporary occlusion of the hepatic circulation or when the hepatic resection is completed. Diffuse oozing from all raw surfaces of the liver may represent a consumptive coagulopathy and results from the combination of shock, extensive tissue trauma, and massive transfusions. Treatment of this syndrome requires maintenance of vascular volume using fresh blood. When blood loss exceeds 5 units, as it usually does in cases requiring liver resection, an acquired platelet functional defect is likely. The anesthesiologist should be encouraged to request 6 to 10 units of platelet packs. These should be administered at the completion of hepatic resection or before peritoneal closure. These patients are often hypothermic and warming is appropriate if the temperature is under 35°.

Immediate postoperative management includes careful monitoring of cardiovascular function, including urine output and peripheral perfusion. Maintenance of blood volume to insure good splanchnic and portal blood flow is important; hematocrit should be obtained immediately after operation and every 4 hr if the patient is at all unstable. With major liver resections, blood glucose level should be monitored and hypertonic glucose administered in quantities of 1 liter of 10% dextrose solution per 24 hr.

Platelet count and function, prothrombin time, and partial thromboplastin time should be monitored several times daily. Platelet transfusion and fresh frozen plasma should be administered to correct any deficiencies. Antibiotics are not used routinely unless there has been associated hollow viscus injury or severe shock in these instances; broad spectrum coverage started in the operating room is continued postoperatively for 24 to 48 hr. Wound drainage should be cultured every 2 to 3 days and blood cultures should be obtained if fever spikes occur. Antacids and/or cimetadine should be administered prophylactically to prevent stress ulceration and bleeding. Intravenous hyperalimentation is initiated within 4 to 5 days if the patient is not ready to resume diet by this time.

COMPLICATIONS

Postoperative pulmonary failure is frequent after major trauma. Tissue trauma, large volume fluid resuscitation, and associated injuries (i.e., rib fractures) contribute to pulmonary failure. The patient should be managed with endotracheal intubation and positive pressure ventilation until hemodynamically stable. The patient should be extubated as soon as possible, but with the knowledge that reintubation may be necessary.

Jaundice occurs frequently after liver trauma. This may be a sign of severe hepatic dysfunction, but usually is related to resorption of hematomas, breakdown of transfused red cells, and mild hepatic dysfunction from central lobular necrosis secondary to shock. Hepatic function returns to normal promptly, although elevated bilirubin levels in the serum may persist for weeks.

Bile leaks and fistulas usually can be detected when the perihepatic area has been drained. Unless these leaks are from a major bile duct they will usually close spontaneously.

Hematobilia is an uncommon complication occurring in 1% of complex injuries. The typical presentation is days to weeks after the injury and can be manifest by melena, upper gastrointestinal bleeding, hypotension, or biliary colic. The diagnosis is confirmed by visualizing blood coming from the ampulla at upper gastrointestinal endoscopy. Treatment is preferentially by percutaneous transvascular selective embolization of the involved artery, but reoperation may be necessary.

Sepsis after hepatic trauma occurs in 7% to 12% of patients and is related to intraabdominal abscess, pneumonia, acalculous cholecystitis, and ischemic bowel. Risk factors associated with intraabdominal abscess postoperatively include associated splenectomy, liver packing to control hemorrhage, Class IV or V injury, large transfusion requirement, and colon injury. Subphrenic and subhepatic abscesses are usually marked by fever 4 to 7 days postoperatively. Pleural effusion may be noted on chest x-ray. Diagnosis can be made by either ultrasound or CT scan. Treatment includes drainage percutaneously or surgically and specific antibiotics. Prophylactic antibiotics are not recommended postoperatively unless there is an associated bowel injury.

RESULTS

Despite these advances, injuries to the liver often still result in mortality. Although overall mortality was 50% to 60% in the pre-1940 era, it has stabilized at about 15% today in those patients with injuries severe enough to require operative treatments. The mortality average from blunt trauma is 25% and from penetrating injury it is 5%. The mortality in penetrating wounds depends largely on the type of weapon used. In stab wounds from knives or in low velocity gunshot wounds the primary problem relates to obtaining hemostasis, and complications are low. Often these injuries are singular and recovery is uneventful. However, in high velocity gunshot wounds or shotgun wounds, extensive parenchymal damage usually results, which necessitates extensive debridement of formal hepatic lobectomy. The mortality rate from these latter injuries is high, at about 50%, and the incidence of associated injuries is in the range of 75% to 80%. Associated injuries involving the gastrointestinal tract are particularly lethal because they often result in death from sepsis or multiple organ failure.

Hepatic trauma from blunt injury is more serious than from penetrating injuries. Thirty-one percent in Morton and colleagues' report on blunt trauma died, whereas in their series on penetrating injuries, the mortality rate was only 3% from stab wounds and 15% from gunshot wounds.[28] Despite the large size of the liver, it lies under and is protected by the right lower rib cage. However, if the force of injury is great, the liver is often crushed under the ribs. In a study by Trollope on primates it was noted that the force necessary to create a liver injury appears to be less when transmitted directly onto the liver than directly against the abdominal wall over the liver.[29]

With blunt trauma to the liver, the liver may fracture in several patterns. It will often have multiple linear lacerations with a gross picture of a "bear claw" injury. If the trauma is more severe, there may be devastating pulverization of the parenchyma, with the manifestation of a stellate fracture of the capsule. Complicated to manage and fortunately less commonly encountered are the large, transverse tears across both the right and left lobes of the liver. Technical difficulties in controlling hemorrhage from this type of injury are formidable, and if associated injuries of the hepatic veins or inferior vena cava exist, the salvage rate will be small.

In addition to direct impact on the liver, with a sudden deceleration of the type associated with motor vehicle collisions or falls from heights, sheer force plays a major role in the avulsion of the liver and hepatic veins from their attachments to the diaphragm and the inferior vena cava.

Death from hepatic injury is usually caused by uncontrollable hemorrhage. With improvement in transportation and resuscitation, there has been an increasing number of patients arriving at the hospital alive. It is reported that approximately 50% of patients with major injuries now survive to arrive at the hospital. Moulton et al. reported on a recent pediatric trauma series. Thirty-eight of 144 patients with liver injuries died in the field or failed to respond to initial resuscitation efforts.[30] Frey and associates reported that, if patients had a systolic blood pressure of less than 80 mm Hg, the mortality rate was 80%.[31] No deaths occurred in patients who on arrival to the emergency room were not in shock.

Most patients with liver injury have an uncomplicated course. In penetrating injuries, the mortality ranges between 3% and 15%. In blunt trauma, especially from motor vehicle accidents, the outcome is more serious, with an overall mortality rate of 20% to 40%. In the 10% of liver injuries where major resection is necessary for the management of the injury, the mortality rate is 50% to 60%. The advent of caval shunting has permitted treatment of supravenal and hepatic vein injuries, which previously were lethal—mortality rates in these patients, however, still range between 50% and 90%.[32-35] Studies on long-term survivors after liver trauma showed no sequelae from the damaged liver with or without major resection. Clinical tests noted no compromise of hepatic function and it is apparent that liver regeneration will occur if the patient survives the initial postinjury period.[36]

REFERENCES

1. Hunter J. *A Treatise on the Blood, Inflammation and Gunshot Wounds. The Classics of Surgery Library.* Birmingham: Gryphon Editions; 1985.
2. de Chauliac G. *On Wounds and Fractures. The Classics of Surgery Library.* Birmingham: Gryphon Editions; 1987.
3. Larrey DJ. *Surgical Memoirs of the Campaigns of Russia, Germany, and France.* (Mercer JC, Trans.) Philadelphia: Carey and Lea; 1832.
4. Bismuth H. Surgical anatomy and anatomical surgery of the liver. *World J Surg.* 1982; 6:3–9.
5. Michels NA. *Blood Supply and Anatomy of the Upper Abdominal Organs.* Philadelphia: Lippincott; 1955.
6. Suzuki T, Nakayasu A, Kavabe K, Takeda H, Honjo J. Surgical significance of anatomic variations of the hepatic artery. *Am J Surg.* 1971; 122:505.
7. Michels NA. Newer anatomy of the liver and variant blood supply and collateral circulation. *Am J Surg.* 1966; 112:337.

8. Vandamme JPJ, Bonte J. The branches of the celiac trunk. *Acta Anat.* 1985; 122:110.
9. Healey JE Jr, Schrey PC. Anatomy of the biliary ducts within the human liver: analysis of the prevailing pattern of branchings and the major variations of the bile ducts. *Arch Surg.* 1953; 66:599.
10. Olsen WR, Hildreth DH. Abdominal paracentesis and peritoneal lavage in blunt abdominal trauma. *J Trauma.* 1971; 11:824–829.
11. Bivins BA, Sachatello SR, Daugherty ME, Ernst CB, Griffen WO. Diagnostic peritoneal lavage is superior to clinical evaluation in blunt abdominal trauma. *Am Surg.* 1978; 44:637–644.
12. Federle MP, Goldberg HI, Kaiser JA, Moss AA, Jeffrey RB Jr, Mall JC. Evaluation of abdominal trauma by computed tomography. *Radiology.* 1981; 138:637–644.
13. Moore EE. Critical decisions in the management of hepatic trauma. *Am J Surg.* 1984; 148:712–716.
14. Frederico JA, Horner WR, Clark DE, Isler RJ. Blunt hepatic trauma: nonoperative management in adults. *Arch Surg.* 1990; 125:905–909.
15. Luna GK, Dellinger CP. Non-operative observation therapy for splenic injuries: a safe therapeutic option? *Am J Surg.* 1987; 153:462–468.
16. Lucas CE, Ledgerwood AM. Prospective evaluation of hemostatic techniques for liver injuries. *J Trauma.* 1976; 16:442–451.
17. Burch JM, Feliciano DV, Mattox KL. The atriocaval shunt: facts and fiction. *Ann Surg.* 1988; 207:555–568.
18. Kudsk KA, Sheldon GF, Lim Jr RC. Atrial caval shunting (ACS) after trauma. *J Trauma.* 1982; 22:81–85.
19. Griffith BP, Shaw BW Jr, Hardesty RL, Iwatsuki S, Bahnson HT, Starzl TE. Venovenous bypass without systemic anticoagulation for transplantation of the human liver. *Surg Gynecol Obstet.* 1985; 160:270–272.
20. Doerr RJ, Luchette FA, Gundlach TE, Hess-Cappacing H, Pons P. Further clinical applications at the falciform ligament. *Surg Gynecol Obstet.* 1990; 170:167–168.
21. Heaney J, Scanton W, Halbert D, et al. An improved technique for vascular isolation at the liver: experimental study and case reports. *Ann Surg.* 1966; 163:237–241.
22. Shaw BW, et al. Venous bypass in clinical liver transplantation. *Ann Surg.* 1984; 200(4):524–534.
23. Schrock T, Blaisdell FW, Mathewson Jr C. Management of blunt trauma to the liver and hepatic veins. *Arch Surg.* 1968; 96:698–704.
24. Equivel CD, Bernardas A, MaKowka L, Imatsuki S, Gordon RD, Starzl TE. Liver replacement after massive hepatic trauma. *J Trauma.* 1987; 27(7):800–802.
25. Angstadt J, Jarrell B, Moritz M, et al. Surgical management of severe liver trauma: a role for liver transplantation. *J Trauma.* 1989; 29(5):606–608.
26. Peterson SR, Sheldon GF, Lim RC Jr. Management of portal vein injuries. *J Trauma.* 1979; 19:616–620.
27. Mavroudis C, Trunkey DD. Choledochoplasty for choledochojejunostomy: variations on a theme by Carrel. *Am J Surg.* 1987; 142:305.
28. Morton JR, Roys GD, Bricker DL. Treatment of liver injuries. *Surgery, Gynecology & Obstetrics.* 1972; 134:298.
29. Trollope ML. The mechanism of injury in blunt abdominal trauma. *J Trauma.* 1973; 13:962.
30. Moulton SL, Lynch FP, Canty TG, Collins DL, Hoyt DB. Hepatic vein and retrohepatic vena caval injuries in children: sternectomy first. *Arch Surg.* In press.
31. Frey CF. A fifteen-year experience with automotive hepatic trauma. *J Trauma.* 1973; 13:1039.
32. Beal SL, Ward RE. Successful atriocaval shunting in the management of retrohepatic venous injuries. *Am J Surg.* 1989; 158:409.
33. Buechter KJ, Gomez GA, Zeppa R. A new technique for exposure of injury at the confluence of the retrohepatic veins and the retrohepatic vena cava. *J Trauma.* 1990; 30:329.
34. Pachter H, Spencer FC, Hofstetter S, et al. The management of juxta hepatic venous injuries without an atriocaval shunt. *Surgery.* 1986; 99:569.
35. Kuds KA, Sheldon GF, Lim RC Jr. Atriocaval shunting after trauma. *J Trauma.* 1982; 22:81.
36. Lim RC Jr, Guiliano AE, Trunkey DD. Postoperative treatment of patients after liver resection for trauma. *Arch Surg.* 1977; 112:429.
37. Madding, K. *Trauma to the Liver.* Philadelphia: WB Saunders; 1971.

ced laparotomy for suspected intraabdominal injury, and "the abstention-

11
Small Bowel and Mesentery

MICHAEL SMITH, M.D.
NORMAN CHRISTENSEN, M.D.

HISTORY: *In 1275, Guillaume de Salicet of Italy described the simple suture of an intestinal wound.[1] The patient recovered. Before his death in 1460, Leonard Bertapaglia of Italy discussed the suture of intestinal wounds, declaring that complete transverse section of the bowel was incurable, but if the wound was partial or longitudinal or if it was in the small rather than the large intestine, it should be stitched.[1] In 1720, Sachenus repaired a subparietal rupture of the small bowel and in 1730 Ramdorh successfully sutured a completely divided small bowel.[2]*

In the latter half of the 19th century and the early part of the 20th century, there was a vigorous and continuing argument by military surgeons as to whether or not the abdomen should be explored if it was thought that the contents had been injured. During the American Civil War (1861–1865) there were isolated reports of suture of small bowel injuries but this was limited to eviscerated bowel before its restoration to the abdominal cavity[3] (Fig. 11–1). In 1881, Marian Sims, the American surgeon, urged laparotomy for gunshot wounds of the abdomen, but the results were poor.[4] Military surgeons were divided into two camps: "the interventionists," who advocated laparotomy for suspected intraabdominal injury, and "the abstentionists," who favored no operation even if it was known that intraabdominal injury had occurred. Intervention was practiced in the Sino–Japanese War, the Spanish–American War, and the Tirah campaign, but the results were dismal, and laparotomy for suspected injury was prohibited or ordered stopped by the various medical departments of the involved nations. During the South African War of 1899–1901, laparotomy for suspected perforating wounds of the intestine was tried again, but again results were disastrous and laparotomy was discontinued during the latter stages of the war. The Russians entered the Russo–Japanese War of 1904–1905 with a policy of nonintervention, but changed their policy when it was shown by a female surgeon, Princess Gedroitz, that excellent results much superior to those of nonintervention could be obtained if surgery was performed promptly. Gedroitz operated in a railway carriage unit close enough to the battlefront so that casualties could be treated within 3 to 4 hours of wounding.[4]

The poor results of laparotomy during the Boer War had such a powerful effect on the British that they entered World War I with a policy of

Small Bowel and Mesentery 191

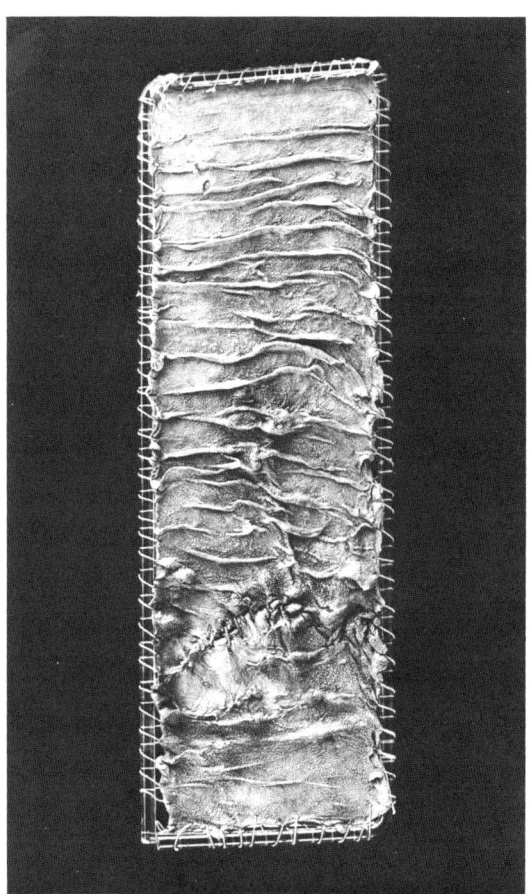

Figure 11–1. Autopsy specimen showing a segment of bowel that was repaired during the Civil War; although the repair appears intact, the end result was obviously unsuccessful.

not operating on combat casualties with wounds of the abdomen even when it was apparent that intraabdominal injury had occurred. Bailey describes the mortality during the first phase of the war as "appalling." By 1915, it had become recognized that prompt surgical intervention was necessary and measures were taken to provide the organization and facilities so that this could be done.[4] But, despite the knowledge that abdominal injuries should be operated on promptly, operation was still not the general rule when the war ended, according to Major General S. B. Hays, former Surgeon General of the United States Army.[5]

The statistics show that small intestinal injuries were lethal in World War I.[4] In British troops, the fatality rate when injury was restricted to the small intestine was 65.9%. A similar fatality rate of between 70% and 80% was found in American troops with the same injury. Lessons learned in World War I and in the Spanish Civil War of 1936–1938, plus the accumulation of civilian experience, resulted in the policy of operating as promptly as possible on patients with abdominal injuries in World War II. In World War

II, the mortality rate of U.S. soldiers with univisceral jejuno–ileal injuries was 13.9%.[5] For multivisceral injuries, the mortality rate was 36.3%. Better anesthesia, improved facilities, prompt evacuation, and an enhanced understanding of the nature of traumatic shock were responsible for the improved outcome.

Injuries to the small bowel and mesentery, if suspected, are generally easy to recognize and straightforward to treat. Shock and a program for resuscitation of the injured patient were some of the factors leading to improvement in outcome. During the Korean and Vietnam conflicts, the overall mortality rate for isolated combat injuries of the small bowel dropped to negligible levels.[6,7] The high morbidity and mortality that follow large bowel injuries are not seen with injury of the small bowel. Leakage from suture lines is unusual. In World War II, the leakage rate in 1168 patients was 1.02%.[5] The rate in civilian practice is also correspondingly low when the injuries are recognized and treated promptly.

ANATOMY

The small bowel distal to the duodenum consists of the jejunum and the ileum with a combined length of about 260 cm, about 1½ times body height. The jejunum is approximately 105 cm long. The mesentery is fan-shaped, with its dorsal root attached to the posterior abdominal wall from the duodenal–jejunal junction to the right sacroiliac joint. It crosses the third portion of the duodenum, the aorta, the inferior vena cava, the right gonadal vessels, and the right ureter. Although typical ileum can be distinguished from typical jejunum, there is no clear-cut dividing line between the two (Fig. 11–2). The jejunum is thicker, owing to more prominent mucosal folds, and has a larger diameter than the ileum. The mesenteric circulation of the jejunum is less complex and contains fewer arcades and longer vasa recti than the ileum. The vasa recti are the vertical vessels that lead from the arcades to the bowel. There is more fat in the ileomesentery so that the spaces between the vasa recti and the arcades are less translucent than they are in the jejunum.

The arterial supply to the small bowel is provided by the superior mesenteric artery, which emerges from under the pancreas, runs over the uncinate process of the pancreas to enter the root of the mesentery, and ends in the ileocolic branch (Fig. 11–3). In its course, it gives off the right colic and middle colic branches and numerous intestinal branches. The intestinal branches form loops or arcades within the mesentery and assure excellent collateral blood supply.

The superior mesenteric vein corresponds to the superior mesenteric artery and receives branches from the colon and small intestine before passing under the pancreas to join the inferior mesenteric vein and splenic vein to form the portal vein.

Additional components of the mesentery, besides the fat, are the lymphatics (which run parallel to the arteries), the veins, and the lymph nodes. There are no major blood vessels communicating between the root of the mesentery and the retroperitoneum, thus making it possible to mobilize the entire small bowel and right colon mesentery up to the inferior surface of the pancreas.

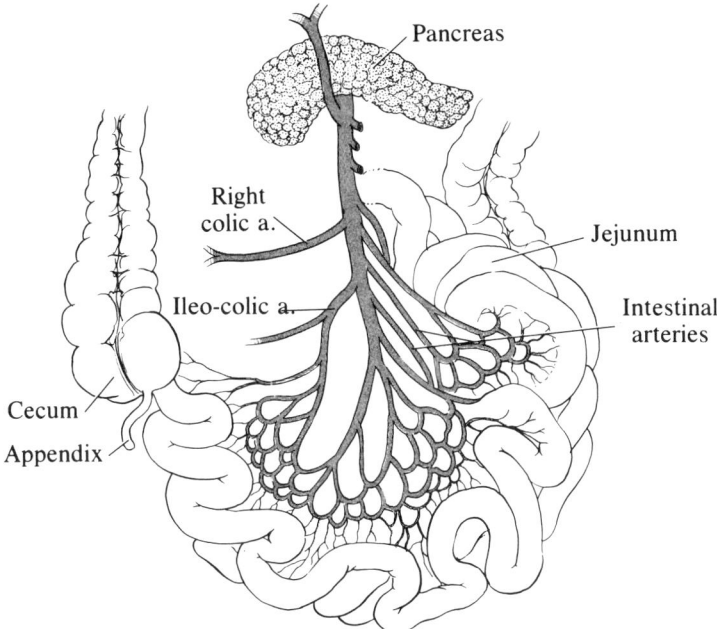

Figure 11-2. Jejunum and ilium showing typical arcades.

MECHANISM OF INJURY

The small intestine may be injured by either penetrating or blunt trauma. Because much of the volume of the abdominal cavity is occupied by the small bowel, one should be concerned that the small bowel has been damaged in cases of penetrating trauma. Stab wounds from knives, shards of glass, or other sharp penetrating objects produce injury to the small bowel far more frequently than any other organ. These are relatively simple problems because unless there have been corresponding mesenteric injury and damage to the circulation, simple repair is all that is necessary.

Gunshot wounds constitute another major cause of injury. The resulting wounds can vary from simple perforating injuries as seen with low caliber hand guns to devastating devitalizing injuries as would occur with close range shotgun injuries or high velocity rifle injuries. They can tax the judgment of even the most experienced surgeon but inevitably require resection to obviously viable bowel.

The mechanisms of injury in blunt trauma are more varied and sometimes less obvious. They include:

1. crushing or lacerating the bowel between the spine and a firm object such as a seat belt, steering wheel, boot, or hoof
2. application of a shearing force at fixed points by sudden deceleration so that the bowel may be torn from its attachment or the mesentery avulsed from its attachment or the mesentery avulsed from its root or from the bowel
3. rupture of the bowel owing to a sudden increase in intraluminal pressure.

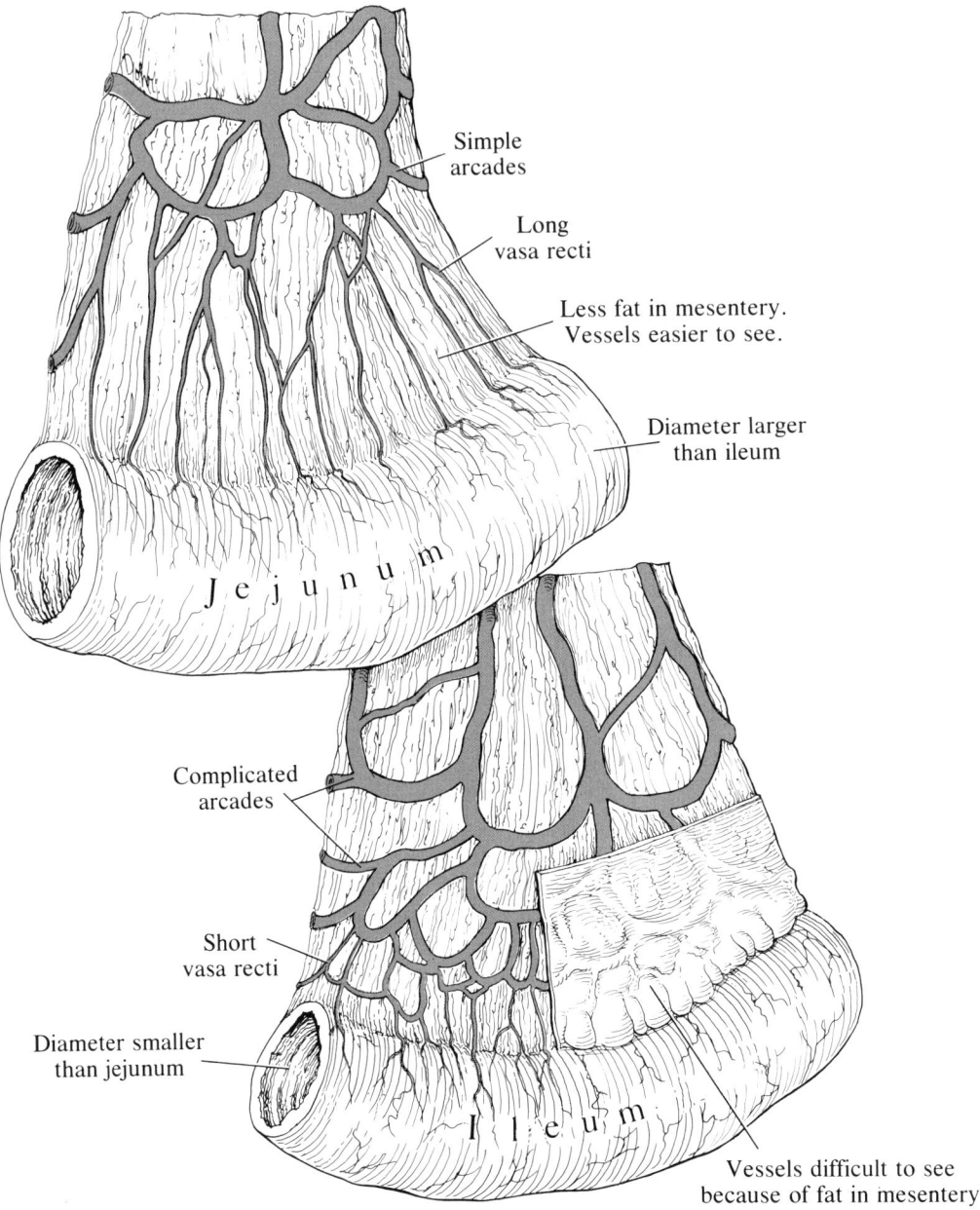

Figure 11-3. Arterial supply to the ileum and jejunum.

Laboratory investigations have shown that rupture of the bowel rarely occurs as a result of increase in intraluminal pressure alone.[6] It is probably necessary that the bowel be obstructed at two places so as to produce a closed loop if rupture is to follow a sudden increase in external or internal pressure.

Underwater blast injuries were noted during World War II. Multiple blowout injuries of both the large and small bowel were seen in sailors who were in the water near their sinking ships when depth charges exploded near them.[6]

Although seat belt usage has been shown clearly to decrease injury and death after motor vehicle accidents,[8] there has been an increase in reports relating the use of seat belts with small bowel injury.[9,10] This association has been seen with both lap belts as well as three-point (lap and shoulder harness) restraints. It has been postulated that many of these injuries are due to improper use of the seat belt. This can be due to loosening of the seat belt, improper seated position, and probably most commonly improper position of the seat belt. If the lap portion of the seat belt is not properly placed over the pelvis, then the significant increased load that occurs during a crash is transmitted to the soft tissues of the abdomen[11] (Fig. 11–4). Also, with isolated lap belt usage, vertebral as well as visceral injuries can occur. This is particularly a problem with children,[12] who are likely to be back-seat passengers where only lap belts are present. Also, the likelihood of improperly fitted belts is higher in children. The increased incidence of spine injuries with lap belt use has also

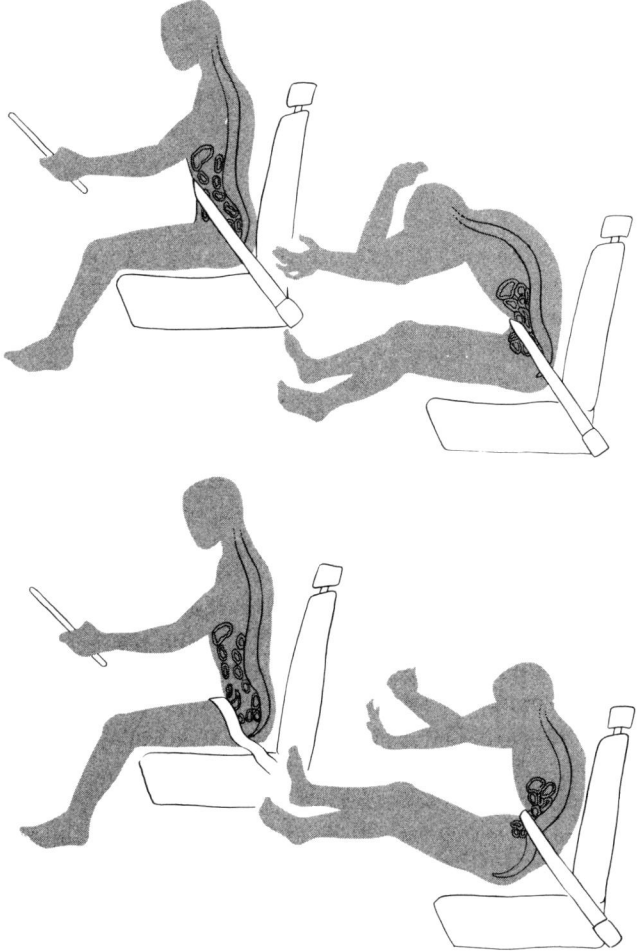

Figure 11–4. Abdominal injuries resulting from improperly used seat belts.

been described in adults.[13] Significant delays in diagnosis have been reported in these patients.

It has been suggested that seat belt–induced small bowel injuries can be divided into three groups.[10] Group 1 injuries are transections of the bowel, generally in the proximal jejunum, and are felt to be deceleration injuries. These injuries can be associated with other deceleration injuries in the abdomen, such as radial mesenteric tears and transverse colon and splenic flexure injuries.

Group 2 injuries are shearing or crushing injuries, usually in the terminal ileum, and are associated with devascularization of the bowel from mesenteric tears. Serosal avulsion injuries are also common. These injuries are associated with cecal, aortic, and caval injuries, as well as lumbar spine injuries.

Group 3 injuries are "blowout" perforations, usually on the antimesenteric border and are primarily due to transmitted pressure to a functionally closed loop of bowel causing acute increase in intraluminal pressure. There is no specific pattern of associated injuries with this group. The larger the lumen of the bowel, the less pressure is needed to rupture it so one would expect to see a higher incidence of Group 3 injuries in patients who are postprandial or have pathological conditions of the bowel causing relative obstruction, such as Crohn's disease.

Clearly, it is important to obtain as much history as possible from patients or field personnel regarding belt usage. Also, if patients demonstrate any external signs of seatbelt trauma, especially ecchymosis or abrasions over the lower abdomen, then one's index of suspicion for the presence of small bowel injury should be raised considerably.

DIAGNOSIS

Although it is often obvious that intraabdominal injury has occurred, clinical findings following both penetrating and blunt trauma to the small intestine may be minimal at first. This is because much of the small bowel content has an almost neutral pH and is relatively sterile, resulting in a minimal inflammatory response.[14,15] For this reason, a high index of suspicion is necessary when evaluating patients with potential small bowel injury.

Perforations of the small bowel may be recognized by signs of peritoneal irritation: tenderness, rebound tenderness, guarding, and a reluctance of the patient to change position.

Small bowel injury after blunt trauma may be difficult to diagnose and must be considered, even if initial signs of intraabdominal injury are absent. In patients wearing lap-type seat belts, combined visceral and lumbar spine injuries may occur and the resultant peritoneal signs may be erroneously ascribed to the lumbar spine injury.[13]

Signs of pure mesenteric injury, if initially present, will be those associated with blood loss and intraabdominal bleeding: hypotension, abdominal distension and tenderness, shoulder pain, and a falling hematocrit. At times, peritoneal blood will not cause many signs or symptoms. Even large amounts of blood can be present in the peritoneal cavity without causing peritoneal signs if the blood is unclotted or in a relatively insensitive area such as the pelvis. Conversely, small amounts of clotted blood may cause striking physical findings on abdominal examination. If there is evidence of bleeding somewhere and the site is not obvious, the most likely place is in the abdominal cavity.

If devascularization of the small bowel occurs as a result of mesenteric injury, it may be recognized by increasing tenderness, pain, and manifestations of obstruction in the devascularized segment. In rare instances, a traumatic laceration of the mesentery may be the site of internal herniation of small bowel with obstruction.

Laboratory work will provide little direct help in making a diagnosis, but a progressive increase in the white blood count after abdominal injury, in the absence of other reasons for its increase, is indirect evidence of intestinal injury. Also, a rising amylase may be indicative of a small bowel injury. However, laboratory findings are nonspecific and cannot be relied on to make the diagnosis of small bowel injury.

The radiographic findings in patients with small bowel injury are limited. Because the small bowel normally contains little gas, pneumoperitoneum is an infrequent finding. Also, in trauma patients it is often impossible to position the patients to obtain an optimal plain film examination.[16] The major indications for plain abdominal x-rays are to localize foreign bodies when the trajectory is in question or to look for associated bony or visceral injuries such as colon or stomach (which have a higher, but still limited, yield on plain films).

The usefulness of a computed tomography (CT) scan in evaluating small bowel injury is unclear. Some authors have found it helpful and have identified findings such as thickened bowel wall or mesentery, peritoneal fluid, and free air as being present on CT with small bowel injury.[17] Possibly as experience increases, CT will establish a role in bowel trauma that it currently does not have. However, small bowel injury should not be ruled out on the absence of findings on CT scan.[16,18]

Peritoneal lavage may be used in the evaluation of patients with potential small bowel injury but is more sensitive for picking up associated injuries such as solid viscus injuries with concomitant bleeding. Mesenteric injuries of the small bowel will usually have enough bleeding associated with them to be identified by peritoneal lavage. Since the inflammatory peritoneal response is generally slow to develop with isolated small bowel injury, the white blood cell count may not be elevated if peritoneal lavage is performed as early as an hour or two after small bowel injury. Clearly, if one retrieves food particles or bile from the lavage, this is indicative of the need for surgical exploration. Other biochemical parameters such as amylase have been measured on lavage fluid[19]; however, it has not been used by us.

PREOPERATIVE PREPARATION

Preoperative preparation for the patient with small bowel injury is generally the same as any trauma patient needing operative intervention and is well described elsewhere in this book. The basic principles of resuscitation and overall assessment should be carried out as the patient is prepared for surgery.

Patients who are at risk for bowel injury should have a nasogastric tube placed and receive antibiotics when that risk is identified. This would be any patient with penetrating trauma who merits operative exploration and those patients with blunt trauma felt to be at risk for bowel injury because of mechanism of injury or physical findings. Currently, a third generation cephalosporin with good anaerobic coverage would be considered the antibiotic of choice. The anaerobic coverage is desirable not only for small bowel contamination but also because of the frequent association of colon injuries with small bowel injuries. Intravenous fluids should be initiated whenever the possibility of any serious injury is recognized. Urine output should be established in excess of 50 cc an hour or fraction thereof by the adjustment of the infusion rate.

The hematocrit should be assessed serially if there is any delay getting the patient to the operating room. A blood specimen should be sent to the Blood Bank for type and screen or appropriate units ordered should the patient be at all unstable. The abdomen should be shaved and prepped bed-line to bed-line and nipples to pubic should an ostomy or dependent drainage be required.

OPERATIVE EXPLORATION

Exploratory laparotomy to treat recognized injury of the intestinal tract is mandatory. There is some controversy, however, regarding the management of patients with penetrating wounds who do not show evidence of visceral injury. This matter is discussed elsewhere in this book. The central point is that prompt recognition of small intestinal injury is necessary to reduce morbidity and mortality. The peritoneal cavity can handle even gross contamination, provided the contamination is not continuous or repeated. Primary mortality from small bowel and mesentery injury alone comes only when there is undue delay in recognition, which allows established peritonitis to develop or gangrene to supervene because of damage to the blood supply. It is probable that when small bowel injuries are treated promptly, the mortality from isolated injury will be minimal and related to devitalization of the impaired bowel or missed associated bowel laceration or other injuries.

The optimal time for definitive treatment is within 6 to 8 hr of wounding. After this, peritonitis can be well established with bacterial invasion of intraabdominal tissues. At this point, removing surface contamination will not suffice to remove the threat of continuing intraabdominal or retroperitoneal invasive infection; secondary breakdown of bowel closure sites and anastomoses is more likely a result.

The abdomen should be opened through a generous midline incision extending from the xiphoid to below the umbilicus.

Exploration should be rapid and systematic. The first priority is to locate and control hemorrhage. The second is to locate any colon injury so that fecal contamination can be controlled until definitive therapy is carried out. The third priority is to identify injuries to the small bowel, including the duodenum, stomach, pancreas, extrahepatic biliary tract, and urinary tract. A thorough examination of all organs should be routine to avoid overlooking an injury remote from where the surgeon expects to find it. The assessment and treatment of injuries to organs other than the small intestine are discussed elsewhere in this book.

After control of hemorrhage and a thorough examination of the large bowel with control of fecal spillage, if it is present, the small intestine should be eviscerated onto the abdominal wall, the mesentery spread out, and the bowel and its mesentery examined in their entirety from the ligament of Treitz to the ileocecal junction, first on one side and then on the other.

Active bleeding from the mesentery takes first priority and should be secured before the small bowel is examined or perforations treated. The surgeon should count the number of perforations. When one perforation is found in a penetrating injury, the presumption is that there is a second. An odd number of perforations must be explained; failure to do so may mean missing another perforation. Usually the missed wound will lie on the mesenteric side of the bowel. Any hemorrhage in the mesentery adjacent to the bowel implies a perforation. In this circumstance the mesentery should be cleared away sufficiently to establish the exact location of the bowel injury. When the initial exploration has been done in haste (because of multiple injuries or vigorous intraperitoneal bleeding), small perforations may easily be missed. Therefore, before closure of the abdomen, a final careful reexamination of the bowel should be made from the ligament of Treitz to the ileocecal junction.

OPERATIVE TREATMENT

Lacerations and hematomas in the mesentery should be investigated (Fig. 11–5). Meticulous hemostasis is obtained by clamping the ends of the divided vessels in such a manner that additional vessels are not injured. Large hematomas at the base of the mesentery should be explored, since the superior mesenteric artery or one of its major branches may be

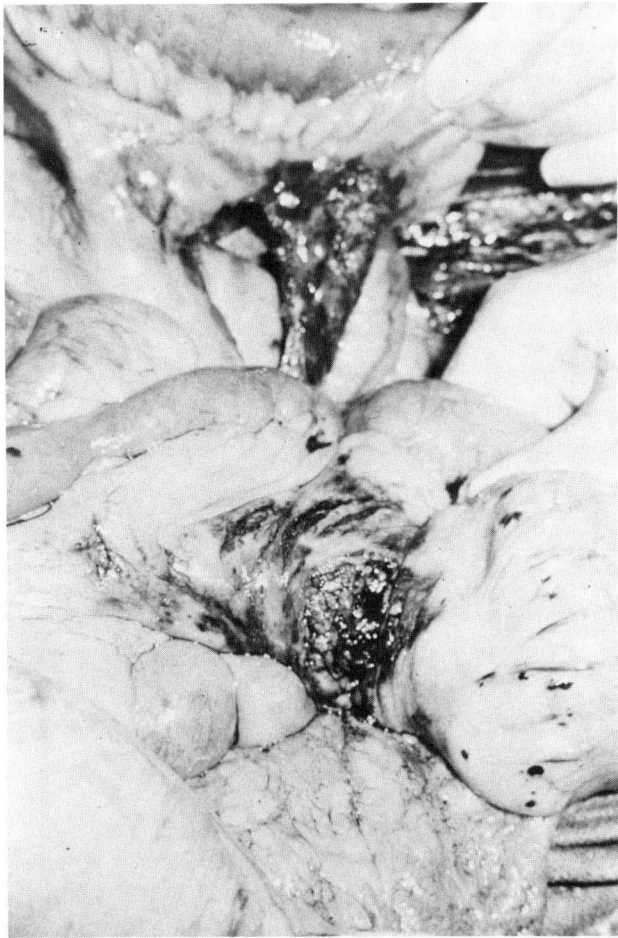

Figure 11–5. Lacerations and hematomas in the mesentery.

involved. To facilitate exposure of the superior mesenteric artery and veins, as well as the dorsal side of the small bowel mesentery, the right colon is mobilized by incising its lateral attachments. Then the right colon and small bowel mesentery containing the superior mesenteric vessels are raised. This exposes the mesenteric vessels as they pass over not only the uncinate process of the pancreas but also the third and fourth portions of the duodenum and the head of the pancreas[20] (Fig. 11–6). Hemorrhage can generally be controlled by pressure.

An alternative approach to the mesenteric vessels distal to their emergence from under the pancreas is to use the left-sided transmesenteric approach (Fig. 11–7). Proximal vascular control can be obtained rapidly at the base of the mesocolon by dividing the peritoneum just under the duodenum as it emerges from under the ligament of Treitz. The index finger can be inserted in the areolar plane between the aorta and the duodenum and base of the mesentery. Digital pressure or the application of a soft vascular clamp across the root of the mesentery should provide control of all mesenteric arterial venous bleeding.

The artery and vein can then be dissected in a dry field after evacuating the mesenteric hematoma. The artery lies to the left and posterior to the vein at the base of the mesentery. Control of bleeding digitally or by occluding vascular clamp as just described should be used when bleeding is present in the mesentery. Blind clamping of mesenteric bleeding risks injury of the truncal artery and vein with resultant impairment of viability of major segments of bowel.

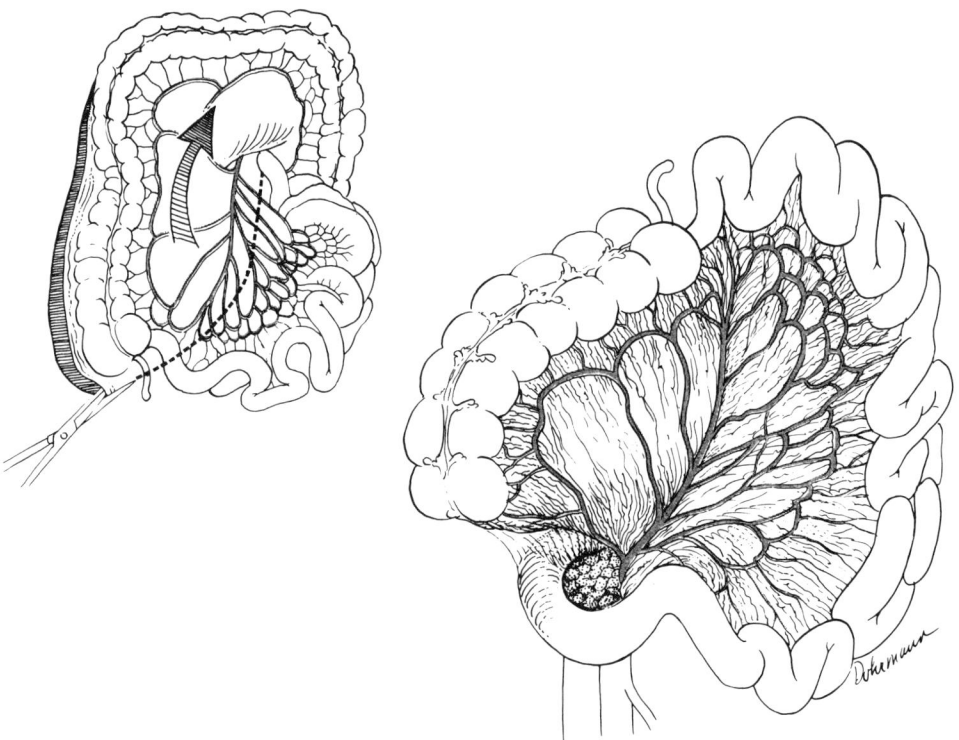

Figure 11–6. The right colon is mobilized and the right colon and small bowel mesentery are raised. The mesenteric vessels can then be exposed from the dorsal surface of the mesentery.

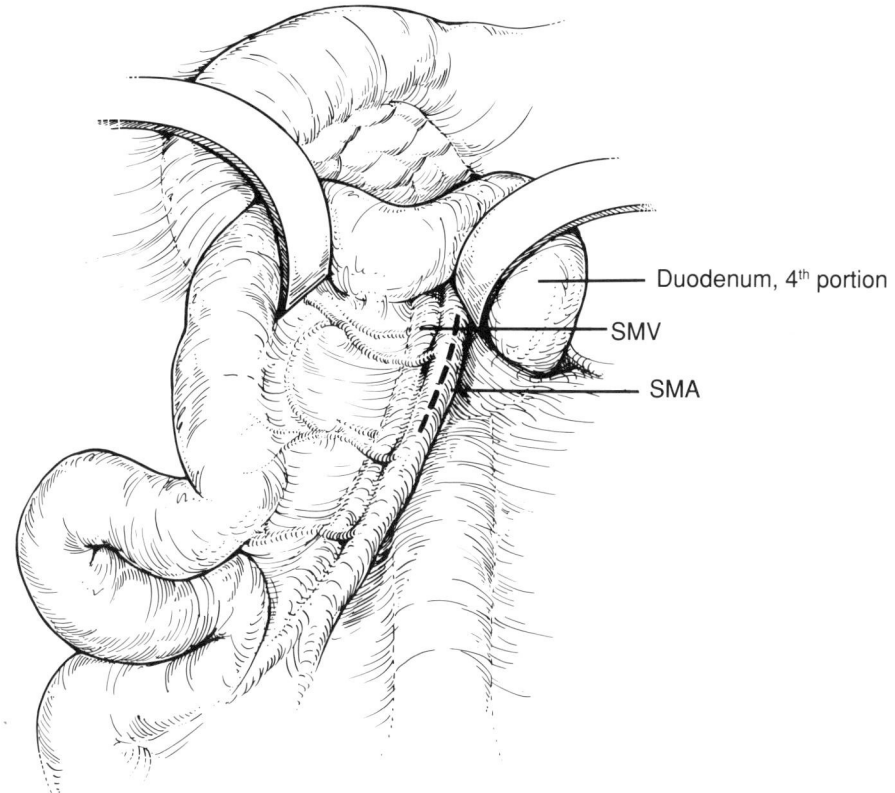

Figure 11–7. The mesenteric artery and vein can be dissected anteriorly from the left. The artery lies to the left and slightly posterior to the vein; with careful dissection 2 cm of artery can be exposed and encircled.

After evacuating the hematoma, small bleeding vessels may be ligated. If there is a major injury to the proximal portion of the superior mesenteric artery or vein, meticulous debridement and repair are indicated (Fig. 11–8). A segment of inferior mesenteric vein or saphenous vein may be used as a patch or replacement when a portion of the wall of either the superior mesenteric artery or vein is missing. When the injury involves the distal portion of the mesenteric artery or vein and the viability of the bowel is questionable, the bowel should be resected and anastomosed and the injured artery or vein ligated rather than repaired. To avoid further injury to blood vessels, defects of the mesentery should be closed by continuous or interrupted sutures placed with care through the peritoneal covering of the mesentery alone. After completion of mesenteric closure, viability of the adjacent small bowel should once again be verified.

Simple perforations and relatively short lacerations of the small bowel may be closed with a single layer of seromuscular nonabsorbable sutures. It makes no difference whether lacerations of the bowel are closed transversely or longitudinally as long as the lumen is not narrowed. Larger wounds, multiple perforations in short segments of the bowel, and devascularized segments of the bowel are indications for resection and anastomosis.

Resection and anastomosis generally should be done when the length of a laceration equals or exceeds 50% of the bowel diameter or when the total length of multiple lacerations

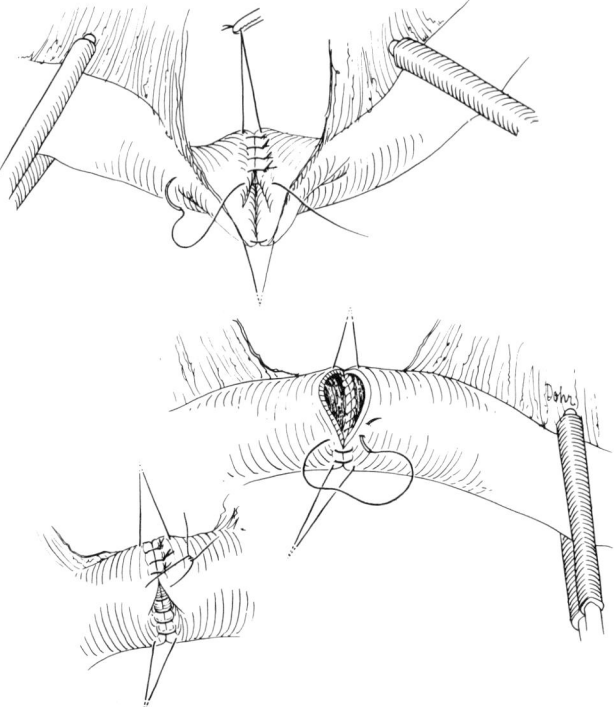

Figure 11-8. A double-layer open anastomosis.

in a short segment of bowel equals or exceeds 50% of the bowel diameter. Individual judgment can be used to increase these limits but if any question exists it is far better to resect than to close primarily and run the risk of the repair breaking as a result of attempting to approximate injured bowel.

All damaged or marginally damaged bowel should be removed. Ragged wounds or wounds made by high velocity missiles must be thoroughly debrided. Often by the time debridement is completed, the defect in the bowel will be so large that resection and anastomosis are necessary. Time can be saved if the surgeon appreciates the extent of injury and goes directly to resection and anastomosis of the injured segment, omitting debridement.

Evidence of compromise of the blood supply to the bowel from an associated mesenteric laceration is a clear indication for performing resection and anastomosis since resection is well tolerated and failure to recognize devitalized bowel can lead to perforation and death. If the bowel has a normal appearance and responds to pinching with peristalsis, it is viable. The mucosa is much more active metabolically than the rest of the bowel. Therefore, if the bowel is dusky on the outside, the mucosa is probably dead or dying and resection is indicated. Hypovolemia with resultant poor perfusion of the bowel often makes evaluation difficult. Therefore, it is important to restore blood volume when trying to determine viability of the bowel. Pulsations in the small vessels of the arcade should be seen or palpated since their presence indicates the bowel is probably viable. If there is any question about viability, the segment of bowel should be resected.

For practical purposes, all but 50 cm of the small bowel may be removed with minimal resultant disability, particularly if distal ileum can be preserved. If resection is required, it should be carried back to where the bowel wall, including the mucosa, bleeds. Depending on the surgeon's preference, the anastomosis can be performed using an open or closed technique with a single- or double-layer closure or with staples. Open anastomosis has the advantage of allowing inspection of the mucosa to determine viability. Noncrushing clamps may be applied proximal and distal to the anastomosis to prevent further contamination through leakage of intestinal content during the anastomosis. A single-layer anastomosis is adequate since there is no evidence to indicate that a two-layer heals better than a one-layer anastomosis.

A single-layer closed anastomosis has the advantage that the risk of contamination is lessened. Its disadvantage is that bleeding is more likely and if technique is not meticulous, inadvertent suture of the opposite wall may obstruct the lumen.

Although bleeding from the suture line in small intestinal anastomosis is rare, if the patient is hypotensive at the time of anastomosis or disseminated intravascular clotting, a two-layer anastomosis should be considered, using the continuous inner layer for hemostasis. This can decrease the risk of bleeding at the suture line as blood pressure later rises.

The double-layer open anastomosis is performed by laying a continuous suture of fine absorbable material followed by an outer layer of fine interrupted seromuscular nonabsorbable sutures (Fig. 11–8).

In emergency circumstances a single-layer open or closed anastomosis is a simpler alternative. A single-layer anastomosis can be performed with interrupted seromuscular, nonabsorbable sutures (Fig. 11–9).

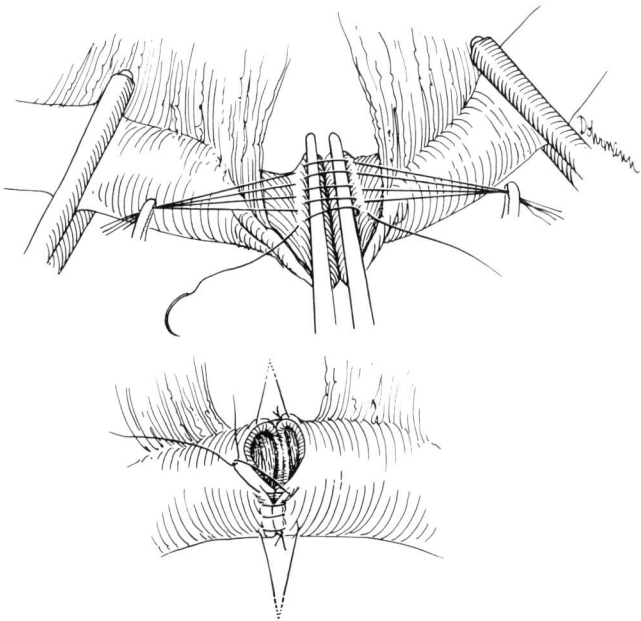

Figure 11–9. A single-layer open anastomosis.

A closed one-layer anastomosis can be carried out by placing Lembert sutures over the occluding clamps and pulling up on the sutures as the clamps are removed, so as to avoid leakage. With tension maintained on the sutures, they are then tied serially (Fig. 11-10).

The peritoneal cavity should be generously irrigated with several liters of saline. All blood clots and any contamination from the gastrointestinal tract should be removed. It is important to aspirate the irrigant out of the peritoneal cavity completely and control any residual bleeding. There is no indication for drains in isolated small bowel injury regardless of the degree of contamination. Drains may be indicated for other associated injuries. If contamination is extensive, the skin and subcutaneous tissue should be left open, to be closed at a later date, whereas if contamination is minimal, the skin and subcutaneous tissue may be closed.

Patients with multiple associated injuries will frequently be unstable. This is particularly true if there is associated liver or abdominal vascular injury. Patients in this situation will frequently develop a coagulopathy, which will make definitive control of bleeding difficult. If it becomes necessary to pack the liver or pelvis because of ongoing bleeding and coagulopathy, it is clearly not advisable to spend a great deal of time doing bowel anastomosis. In this situation it may be prudent to resect the areas of seriously injured bowel rapidly and close the ends of the bowel with surgical staplers, which can be done more quickly. The abdomen can then be closed and the patient taken to the intensive care unit for further resuscitation, warming, and reversal of coagulopathy. When the patient is returned to the operating room for pack removal and definitive control of bleeding, the staple lines can be revised and the bowel anastomosed by hand or the stapled anastomoses can be completed using standard stapling techniques.

POSTOPERATIVE CARE

When there is doubt about hemostasis or viability of the bowel, reexploration within 24 hr is mandatory (Fig. 11-11). Patients can tolerate repeated laparotomy well but they do not tolerate bowel disruption or leakage since these complications invariably lead to a fatal outcome. If the status of the repair of the mesenteric vessels is questionable, thrombosis is a possibility. A second look permits removal of any residual peritoneal blood and resection of marginal-appearing segments of the bowel back to bleeding mucosa. This allows for a maximal amount of bowel to be salvaged and minimizes the risk of leakage, disruption, or fistula formation.

If penetration of the intestine has occurred and established infection has not developed, the antibiotic started preoperatively is continued for two to three doses postoperatively. Longer doses of antibiotics do not reduce the incidence of either peritoneal or wound infection.[21]

Intravenous fluids are continued for several days until there is evidence of return of bowel function. Large amounts of fluid can be sequestered in the bowel wall as well as in the lumen after significant injury. It is important to anticipate this increased fluid requirement postoperatively and assure that the patient's volume status is adequate. Also, it is important to be aware than when this extravascular fluid is mobilized several days postoperatively some patients may develop pulmonary congestive problems. This is generally limited to older patients with preexisting underlying cardiovascular or respiratory compromise.

In uncomplicated cases, one can generally expect bowel function to return in 3 to 5

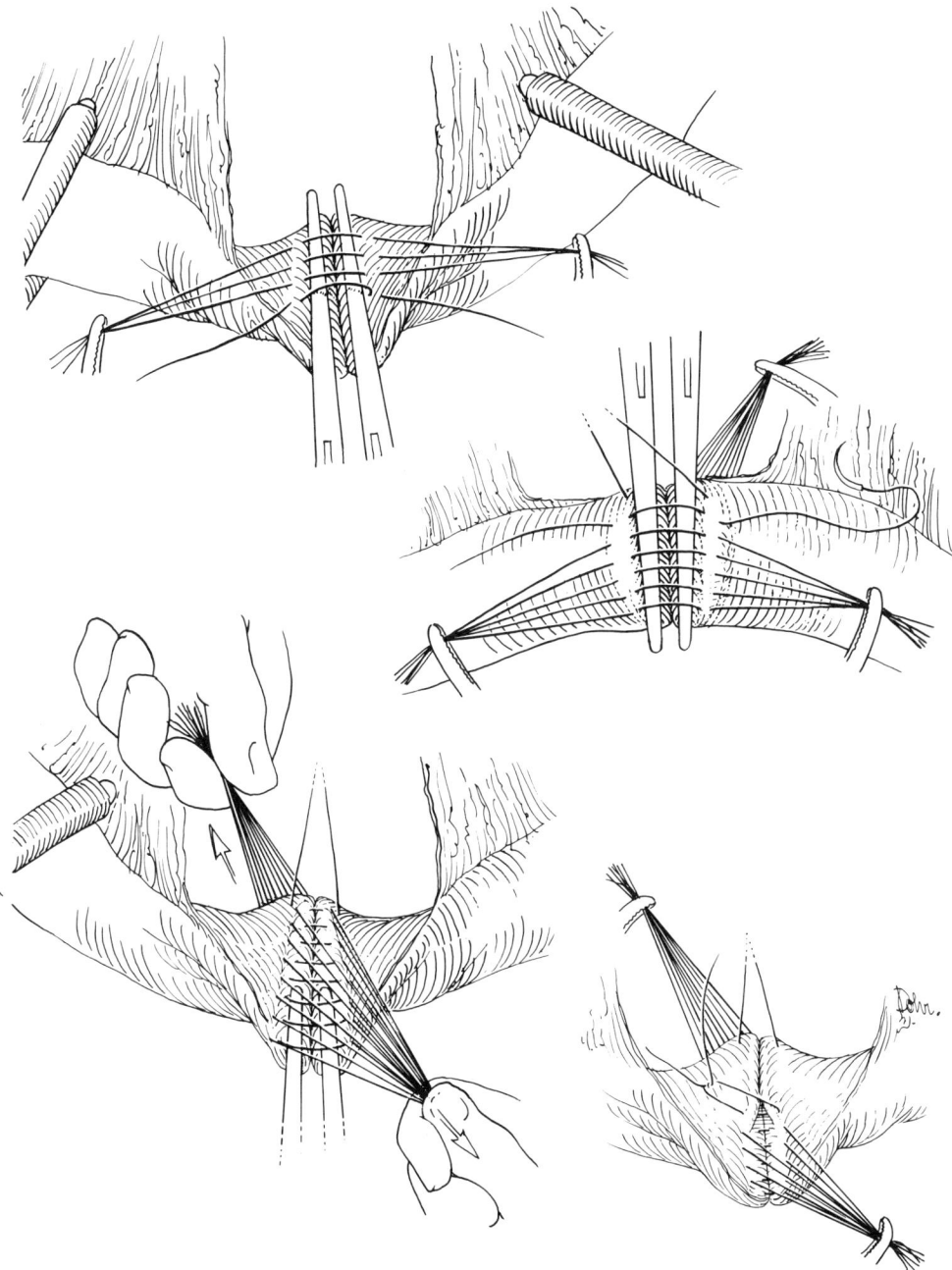

Figure 11–10. A single-layer closed anastomosis.

206 *Abdominal Trauma*

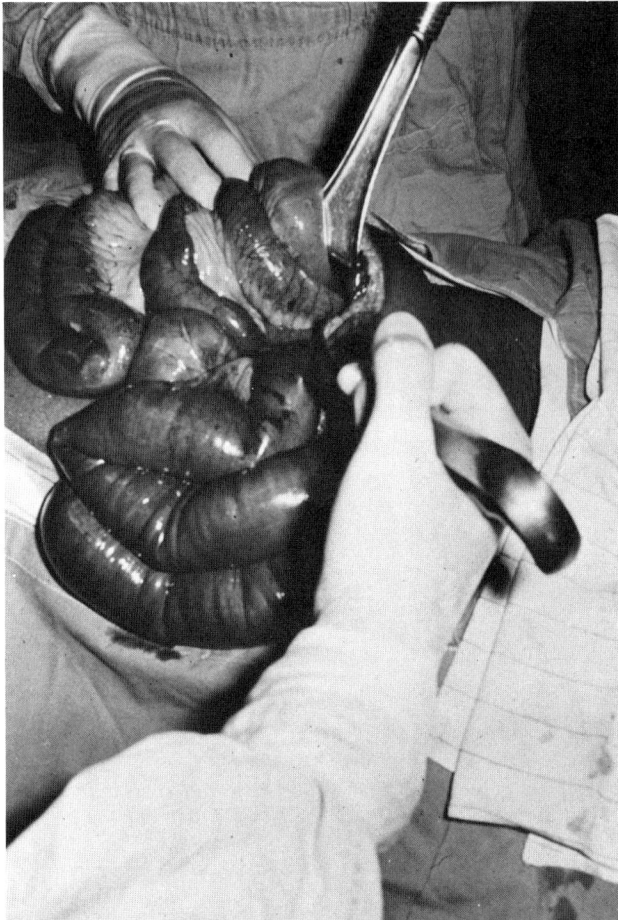

Figure 11–11. Reexploration within 24 hrs. Bowel necrosis is evident.

days. It is advisable to continue nasogastric suction until the ileus resolves. Patients with an uncomplicated course will regain bowel function rapidly enough that nutrition should not become a problem. However, if the patient develops complications or normal bowel function has not developed by 5 days, nutritional support should be initiated. This will generally need to be by total parenteral nutrition (TPN) if there is significant bowel dysfunction after small bowel injury.

COMPLICATIONS

Complications include postoperative bleeding, wound and intraperitoneal infections, suture line leaks, fistula formation, and ischemia of the bowel leading to obstruction or progressing to necrosis with perforation.

Postoperative bleeding may occur into the peritoneal cavity or into the bowel lumen from the suture line. If signs of hypovolemia develop, with or without an initial fall in the hematocrit, bleeding must be suspected, and if stabilization does not occur promptly, reoperation should be performed. If the bleeding is found to be into the gastrointestinal tract, the anastomosis and the small areas of intestinal closure should be taken down, inspected, bleeding controlled, and the closure redone.

Infection of contaminated wounds may often be avoided by closing the fascia but leaving the skin and subcutaneous tissue open. If it looks healthy, the wound may then be closed 4 or more days later with plastic tape strips or sutures (so-called delayed primary closure). Wound infections usually are not evident until the forth or fifth postoperative day and usually require that the closed wound be opened widely. If peritoneal toilet has been good and hemostasis maintained, intraperitoneal infection is rare unless intestinal leakage develops. If a postoperative peritoneal leak occurs, contamination may result with development of intraabdominal abscesses in the pelvis, subphrenic or subhepatic spaces, either lateral gutter or between bowel loops.

Continued unrecognized or untreated leakage of the anastomosis is usually catastrophic, leading to either prolonged morbidity or death from sepsis. The peritoneal cavity can handle contamination if the source of contamination is controlled, but it handles continued contamination poorly. Reoperation is mandatory when acute leakage from the anastomosis is suspected. When detected acutely, the anastomosis should be exteriorized or converted to a proximal "ostomy" and distal mucous fistula. A chronic leak may manifest itself by systemic signs of infection, abscess formation, or fistula formation through the wound. If a fistula develops, it is generally best handled conservatively while the patient is proximally decompressed and nourished intravenously with TPN. An abscess is best treated by dependent drainage, and a fistula accepted. Generalized peritonitis with no localization of the infection requires exteriorization of the leaking bowel. This should be exceedingly uncommon.

Intraabdominal sepsis, whether due to initial contamination or to secondary infection from an anastomotic leak, generally becomes manifest sometime between the fifth and tenth postoperative day. Often, obvious clinical findings may not be present initially and the only clues may be a slowly rising temperature, an increase in pulse rate, and an increase in white blood cell count. Diagnosis may be difficult, even for the most experienced surgeon. The patient should be examined frequently since the change in findings may be much more helpful in reaching a correct diagnosis than are the findings at any single examination. If there is any question, reoperation is indicated since patients tolerate reoperation far better than delay in recognition of bowel leakage. If the patient has received antibiotics for longer than 1 or 2 days after surgery, the antibiotics may mask the signs of developing sepsis.

Ischemia of the bowel is difficult to diagnose and usually, when it is recognized, the patient has reached the point of clinical catastrophe. A high index of suspicion with early reoperation is the key to avoiding serious consequences. Ischemia may be suspected when there is unremitting severe abdominal pain, abdominal distention, a rising temperature, a rising white blood cell count, or signs of systemic sepsis. The patient appears toxic and seems sick out of proportion to the local findings. Signs of ischemia may be similar to those seen in intraabdominal sepsis. An ischemic segment of bowel releases products of devitalized tissue into the mesenteric circulation, which initiates venous thrombosis and extension of the ischemic process to involve previously viable loops of adjacent bowel.

Delay in recognition of a major ischemic loop can be associated with death of most of the bowel.

REFERENCES

1. Malgaine JF. In: Hamby WB, ed. *Surgery and Ambrose Paré*. Norman: University of Oklahoma Press, 1965.
2. Cerise EJ, Scully JH Jr. Blunt trauma to the small intestine. *J Trauma*. 1970; 10:46–50.
3. Barnes JK. *The Medical and Surgical History of the War of the Rebellion*. Vol. II, Part II.
4. Bailey H, ed. *Surgery of Modern Warfare*. Vol. II, 3rd ed. Baltimore: Williams & Wilkins; 1944.
5. *Surgery in World War II, Vol. II, General Surgery*. Office of the Surgeon General, Department of the Army, Washington, DC; 1955.
6. Williams RD, Sargent FT. The mechanism of intestinal injury in trauma. *J Trauma*. 1963; 3:288–294.
7. Mathewson C Jr, Chief of Surgery, 59th Evacuation Hospital, U.S. Army: personal communication.
8. Evans L. Fatality risk reduction from safety belt use. *J Trauma*. 1987; 27:746–749.
9. Zacheis HG, Condon RE. Seat belts and intra-abdominal trauma: Report of two unusual cases. *J Trauma*. 1972; 12:85–90.
10. Christophi C, McDermott FT, McVey I, Hughes ESR. Seat belt–induced trauma to the small bowel. *World J Surg*. 1985; 9:794–797.
11. Sato TB. Effects of seat belts and injuries resulting from improper use. *J Trauma*. 1987; 27(7):754–758.
12. Newman K, Eichelberger MR, Bowman LM, et al. The lap belt complex: Intestinal and lumbar spine injury in children. *J Trauma*. 1989; 29:1035. Abstract.
13. Ritchie WP Jr, Ersek RA, Bunch WL, Simmons RL. Combined visceral and vertebral injuries from lay type belts. *Surg Gynecol Obstet*. 1970; 131:431–435.
14. Thadepalli H, Lou MA, Bach VT, Matsui TK, Mandal AK. Microflora of the human small intestine. *Am J Surg*. 1979; 138:845–850.
15. Drasar BS, Shiner M, McLeod GM. Studies on the intestinal flora. I. The bacterial flora of the gastrointestinal tract in healthy and achlorhydric persons. *Gastroenterology*. 1969; 56:71–79.
16. Rosenberger A, Adler OB, Troupin RH. *Trauma Imaging in the Thorax and Abdomen*. Chicago: Year Book Medical Publishers; 1987.
17. Donohue JH, Federle MP, Griffiths BG, Trunkey DD. Computed tomography in the diagnosis of blunt intestinal and mesenteric injuries. *J Trauma*. 1987; 27:11–17.
18. Rehm CA, Sherman R, Hinz TW. The role of CT scan in the evaluation for laparotomy in patients with stab wounds of the abdomen. *J Trauma*. 1989; 29:446–450.
19. Root HD, Keizer PJ, Perry JF Jr. The clinical and experimental aspects of peritoneal response to injury. *Arch Surg*. 1967; 95:531–537.
20. Cattell RB, Braasch JW. A technique for the exposure of the third and fourth portions of the duodenum. *Surg Gynecol Obstet*. 1960; 111:379.
21. Stone HH, Haney BB, Kolb LD, Geheber CE, Hooper CA. Prophylactic and preventative antibiotic therapy. *Ann Surg*. 1979; 189:691–699.

12
Trauma to the Colon and Rectum

E. JOHN HARRIS, JR., M.D.
DONALD D. TRUNKEY, M.D.

HISTORY: Historically, King William, the Conqueror of England, was one of the unfortunate victims of blunt abdominal trauma. In 1087, he was faced with a revolt of his son, Robert, and the treason of his half-brother, Odo. King Phillip of France was in open rebellion. William and his army crossed the channel and attacked the French with a viciousness that he had not previously displayed. With a large force, he harried the countryside up to Mantes and fell upon the city in a surprise attack, during which terrible destruction ensued. The city was so completely burned that today it is hard to find traces of 11th century buildings in the town. As the king rode through the burning streets, his horse, frightened by burning embers, threw the corpulent king against the high pommel of the saddle with such force that he was lethally ruptured. He was taken initially to the Priory of Saint-Gervais, where he lived an additional 3 weeks with great suffering and then died of intraabdominal sepsis on September 8, 1087. His body was removed to Caen where the final insult occurred. The attendants, who were trying to force his body into the stone coffin, ruptured the abdomen and an incredible stench filled the church. The tomb was destroyed in 1562 by the Calvinists. Only a single thigh bone survived as a remnant of the king, but this too was lost during the revolutionary riots of 1793. Today a simple stone slab is all that marks the grave of William the Conqueror.

For the most part, management policies for colon and rectal injuries have evolved as a result of the large therapeutic experience provided by our world's history of military conflict (Table 12–1). For nearly 20 centuries, from the first recordings of military conflict through the end of the American Civil War, colonic injury was associated with a nearly 100% mortality.[1]

Nonoperative therapy remained the standard of therapy for penetrating colonic injuries through the outbreak of World War I. As the war progressed, elective abdominal surgery was being performed regularly by Leriche,[2] and others, with acceptable mortality rates observed. In 1917, Wallace described the first large series implementing this operative approach emergently. His experience identified an operative mortality of 55% for emergent celiotomy for the treatment of 1200 gunshot wounds to the abdomen.[3] During World War I the average operative mortality was generally reported as 60%.[4] Exploratory celiotomy for penetrating wounds to the abdomen became mandatory military practice in 1915. This aggressive policy resulted in a dramatic decrease in mortality related to colonic injury, and has remained standard military policy in the United States during subsequent military conflicts.[5]

With the onset of World War II, little change in mortality was observed until 1943, when Ogilvie described his experience with the diverting colostomy, as used by the British surgical team during their North African Desert Campaign.[6] A significant reduction in mortality was attributed to the performance of colostomies, and based on these data, the Surgeon General of the United States issued an order that all colon injuries sustained in battle by U.S. armed forces would be treated with a mandatory colostomy.[7] This philosophy, along with generalized improvements in medical care, led to a fall in the mortality rates to 30% by the end of World War II.[8] Colostomy or exteriorization of the injured colon became routine throughout the United States in the 1940s, yet at this same time several groups were reporting low mortality rates with primary repair of the colon.[9,10]

With the Korean and then the Vietnam wars came improvements in antibiotics, blood products, resuscitation, and rapid evacuation, all facilitating earlier operations for penetrating colonic trauma. By the end of the Korean War the mortality for colonic injuries had decreased to 16%.[11]

In the early 1950s, the civilian use of primary closure of the injured colon was described by Woodhall and Ochnser.[12] Primary repair without exteriorization or diverting colostomy was possible in 40% of their patients. Their personal mortality rate for colonic injuries fell from 23% for exteriorization or colostomy to 9% for primary repair.

The mortality from colonic injury today has generally been reported to be 10% to 15%, with most of the fatalities associated with multiple organ trauma.[13–15] Hemorrhage- and transfusion-induced coagulopathies resulting from associated vascular and solid organ injuries account for the majority of early mortality resulting from colonic injury.

ETIOLOGY AND INCIDENCE

Injuries to the colon and rectum are among the most lethal injuries a trauma surgeon encounters within the abdomen. Owing to the anatomical location of the colon within all four quadrants of the abdomen, the colon is at risk in almost all patients with an abdominal wound. Because of the diversity of the native microbiological flora of the colon, polymicrobial sepsis is an ever-present risk with colorectal trauma. Mortality is usually delayed,

Table 12–1 Mortality from Colon Injuries

Civil War	90%
Spanish American War	65%
World War I	60%
World War II	30%
Korean War	15%
Vietnam War	13%

From Haygood and Polk.[70] Reprinted with permission.

and is directly related to septic complications in those patients whose injury breaks the integrity of the colorectal wall.

Injuries to the hollow viscera are more commonly the result of penetrating rather than blunt trauma. Approximately 85% to 96% of civilian colon injuries are caused by low or medium velocity gunshot wounds and stab wounds, with blunt trauma accounting for the rest.[16,17] The incidence of colonic injury from abdominal gunshot wounds varies between 25% and 30% in most series, placing colonic injury second behind the small bowel in the frequency of this injury. Colonic injury ranks third behind liver and small bowel injuries among abdominal stab wound injuries, with an incidence of 5% in this population.[18]

In more general terms, stabbing is responsible for 25% and firearms, predominantly low velocity weapons, for 75% of colonic injuries from penetrating trauma, although there is some regional variance in these statistics.[19] Blunt trauma to the colon is rare. Muscular wall contusions are the most common injury, with full thickness tears uncommon. Blunt trauma is most frequently associated with motor vehicle accidents, pedestrian accidents, assaults, and falls. Delayed colonic wall rupture is seen with blunt trauma, and although uncommon, this injury is associated with high morbidity.[20] Iatrogenic colonic trauma, mostly perforation during colonoscopy, barium enema, or therapeutic enema, is relatively uncommon.[21]

In civilian practice, extraperitoneal rectal injuries represent from 3% to 10% of the total number of injuries to the colon.[18] Foreign bodies introduced during erotic sexual activity are a frequently reported cause of rectal perforation.[22] Rectal lacerations are an often overlooked injury associated with compound pelvic fractures.[20,23,24]

ANATOMIC AND PHYSIOLOGIC CONSIDERATIONS

The colon may be divided into three segments by virtue of its varied blood supply: the right colon, the left colon, and the rectum (Fig. 12–1). The right colon is derived from the midgut and includes the proximal transverse colon. The transverse colon is pendant on a variable amount of mesentery and may extend into the pelvis when one is upright. The blood supply of this area is via the superior mesenteric artery, with collateral circulation from the inferior mesenteric artery by way of the marginal artery of Drummond (Fig. 12–2).

The left colon is derived from the hindgut and extends from the splenic flexure to the peritoneal reflection on the upper rectum. The blood supply of this area is mostly from the inferior mesenteric artery, although a variable contribution from the superior mesenteric artery via the marginal artery is present. This variable influence of collateral blood flow on the left colon theoretically renders this segment at risk for ischemic necrosis as a result of hemorrhagic shock as the left colon endures quantitatively less blood flow than the right colon. Paradoxically, clinical experience has documented a higher incidence of ischemic necrosis in the right colon.[25]

The rectum extends for 12 to 15 cm, with peritoneal investment of the anterior and lateral walls. The anterior pelvic peritoneal reflection is approximately 7 cm above the anal verge. The posterior rectal wall is retroperitoneal from the rectosigmoid junction caudally. The rectum passes through the levator ani muscles to join the anal canal, a 3-cm segment lined by a squamous cell anoderm and innervated somatically. The rectum receives most of its blood flow from the superior hemorrhoidal branches of the inferior mesenteric artery. There are contributions from the middle hemorrhoidal branches of the internal iliac arteries and from the inferior hemorrhoidal branches of the pudendal arteries.

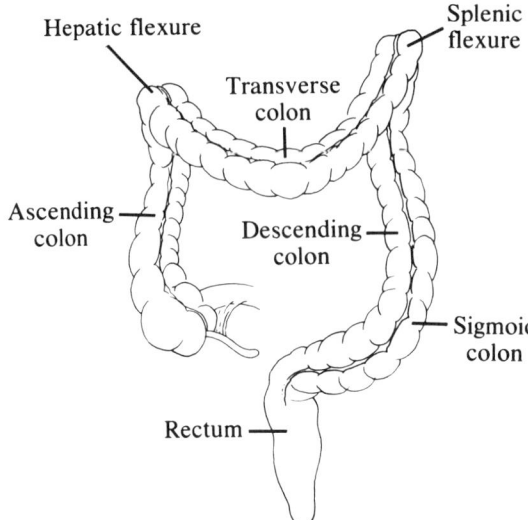

Figure 12–1. Anatomy of the large bowel.

The right colon has a thin wall and a large lumen whereas the left colon is noted to be more muscular with a narrower lumen. The tinea of the colon extend onto the rectum as incomplete longitudinal muscular layers investing only the anterior and posterior surfaces. Functionally, the right colon contains a more liquid stool for this segment of colon serves to absorb and dehydrate the arriving small bowel contents. The left colon serves mainly as a storage vessel with its contents more solid. As the stool becomes more concentrated during its transit toward the left colon, its bacterial content steadily increases, to a point where as much as 60% of its dry weight is composed of bacteria, in a concentration exceeding 10^{11} per ml.[26] *Escherichia coli*, enterococcus, and bacteroides are the predominate flora.

Despite differences in collagen concentration and in the activity levels of collagenase between the left and right colon bowel wall, no difference in suture line dehiscenece between the two sides has been proven to date.[27–29] Multiple reports have failed to define any significant difference in morbidity between injuries to the right versus the left side of the colon when risk factors such as shock time and associated injury severity are taken into account.[30–32]

Therefore, despite known anatomic and physiologic variance between the right and left colon, all trauma to the colon should be managed in a similar manner, with the expectation of similar results for any injured colonic segment.

PATHOPHYSIOLOGY

Stab wounds usually produce clean incised wounds with little adjacent injury to contiguous structures. Repair of stab wounds is usually uncomplicated. Gunshot wounds (GSW) are more complex and depend on the type of gun involved. Military GSW are high velocity and develop a path of destruction. Caution should be employed to assure viability of adjacent tissues. Repair often entails debridement of colon beyond the area of immediate injury.

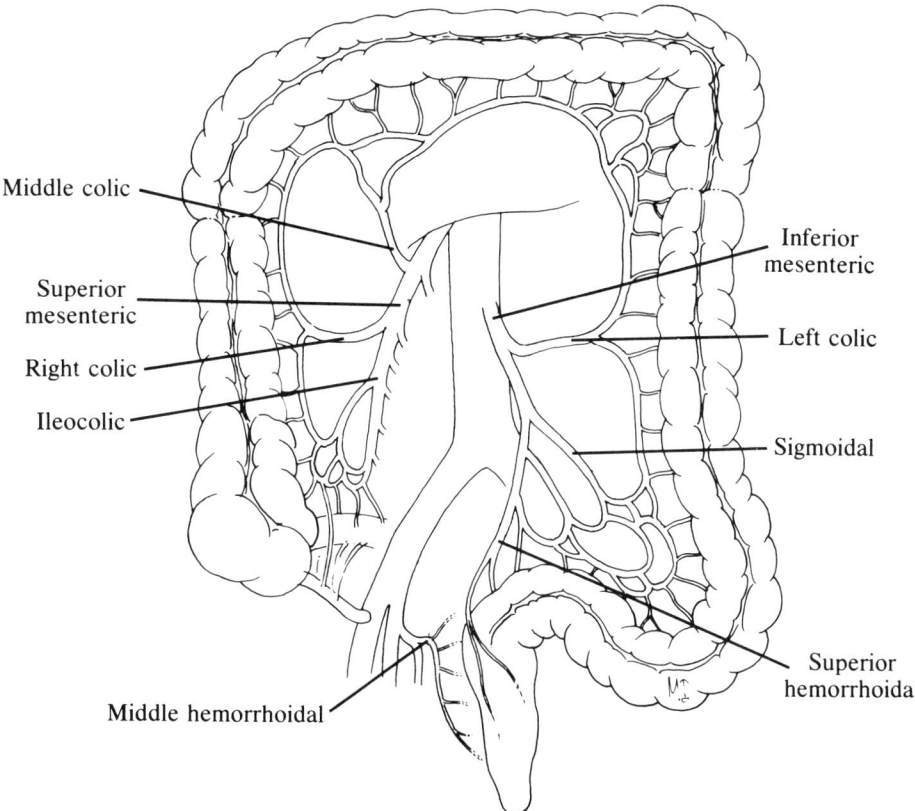

Figure 12–2. Arterial supply of the colon.

Shotgun injuries are also complex for not only is the colon injured, but also adjacent organs and tissues, leading to susceptibility for myonecrosis and sepsis in this macerated area.

Colonic injuries due to blunt trauma are relatively infrequent, representing less than 15% of all colonic trauma.[33] One may identify serosal tears, usually in the ascending or descending colon, often as a result of a malpositioned seatbelt placed above the iliac crests. The tear or even perforation results from the acute compression of the gas-filled viscus.[18] Blunt trauma may also produce intramural hematomas, which are at risk for perforation days or weeks after the initial injury.[34] Avulsion or laceration of the colonic mesentery has also been recognized, producing either acute hemoperitoneum, or more subtly causing bowel ischemia with delayed necrosis, perforation, and peritonitis. The lap seat belt should be worn low on the abdominal wall, at the level of the anterior superior iliac crests where the pelvis is structurally able to dissipate any deceleration forces.

INITIAL ASSESSMENT

Patients arriving in a trauma center with a presumed injury to the large bowel should undergo the same thorough evaluation that is applied to all patients with abdominal trauma.[22] When possible, details surrounding a penetrating traumatic incident should be elicited: the type of weapon or instrument involved and the distance between assailant and victim. Fragmentation of a high velocity missile after penetration is an important phenomenon that increases the magnitude of tissue disruption.[35] Following blunt trauma, the condition of the steering column, the use of restraint devices, ejection from the vehicle, and the length of extrication time are useful historical facts that can be associated with an increased risk for colon injury.

The abdomen, both flanks, back, buttocks, perineum, and genitalia should all be evaluated during the secondary survey for signs of external trauma. In a conscious patient, rebound peritoneal tenderness is usually a delayed sign requiring a significant degree of intraperitoneal contamination by blood or feces. Overall, 15% to 25% of patients with significant intraabdominal injuries lack initial peritoneal signs, and conversely, equivocal physical findings of pain are falsely positive in 30% of patients.[36] Not surprisingly, the vast majority of acute colonic perforations are diagnosed coincidentally at celiotomy for penetrating torso trauma.

It is imperative that one perform a digital rectal examination in every patient with abdominal trauma. If blood is detected on the examining finger or if external signs of rectal injury exist, the patient should undergo anoscopy and sigmoidoscopy.

Local Wound Exploration

Any penetrating wound between the nipples and the groins is capable of injuring the colon, yet not all these wounds require exploratory celiotomy. A suspicion of significant vascular or visceral injury may prompt an emergent celiotomy, especially with a gunshot wound to the abdomen where peritoneal violation is present. Exploratory celiotomy identifies an incidence of visceral injury in this setting exceeding 95%.[37,38] We feel all patients with a gunshot wound to the abdomen should undergo exploratory celiotomy.

Stab wounds to the anterior abdomen violate the peritoneum in two-thirds of cases but produce significant injury in less than one-half of these patients.[5] All patients with an abdominal stab wound and hemodynamic instability or peritoneal irritation should undergo immediate celiotomy after chest x-ray and one shot intravenous pyelogram (IVP). In hemodynamically stable patients, it is important to determine the level of abdominal wall perforation. Unless there is obvious evisceration, the stab wound is explored under local anesthesia in hemodynamically stable patients. The stab wound is extended surgically to facilitate inspection of the underlying fascia. If the anterior fascia is penetrated, we feel exploratory celiotomy is indicated, although others reserve celiotomy only for penetration of the posterior abdominal fascia.[5] Peritoneal lavage can be used to settle the indications for surgery in equivocal cases.[39]

Diagnostic Peritoneal Lavage

Diagnostic peritoneal lavage (DPL), a technique widely employed during the evaluation of abdominal trauma, has little utility in the specific diagnosis of colonic injuries. DPL is used to detect the presence of blood, bacteria, or vegetable matter in the peritoneal cavity. The test is nonspecific for determination of type or extent of organ injury. Diagnosis of a colonic injury is based on the presence of fecal fibers or bacteria in the lavagate, or the finding of elevated white blood cells if lavage is performed less than 3 hr after injury.[40] Most patients with colonic injuries of sufficient severity to render a positive DPL will have enough physical findings warranting early celiotomy.

Computed Tomography

Computerized tomography (CT) is specific and sensitive for the diagnosis of intraabdominal injury. Detection of intraperitoneal and retroperitoneal blood is highly reliable in the evaluation of stable patients with abdominal injuries. We feel patients with blunt abdominal trauma who are hemodynamically stable should be evaluated with contrast-enhanced CT imaging. CT has not been particularly useful in the diagnosis of injuries to hollow organs. Recently, a contrast enhanced CT enema (CECTE) has been described.[41] This technique involves the simultaneous opacification of the gastrointestinal, genitourinary, and vascular systems. The real value of CECTE in colon injuries lies in its ability to detect injury to the retroperitoneal sections of ascending and descending colon. The CECTE has found its major application in stable patients with penetrating trauma to the back and flank,[41] for DPL would not detect these injuries. If a patient presents with hemodynamic stability and a stab wound between the anterior axillary line and the paraspinous muscles, rather than explore, an alternative is to obtain a CECTE. If no injury is detected by this study, the patient can be followed with serial abdominal and laboratory examinations. If the clinical condition of the patient deteriorates, exploratory celiotomy is performed.

OPERATIVE EXPOSURE AND EVALUATION

A midline incision is preferred for exploratory celiotomy after acute traumatic injury. The incision allows for the rapid exposure, evaluation, and repair of virtually all associated intraabdominal injuries. Control of hemorrhage assumes the first priority upon entering the peritoneal cavity, then control of fecal soilage may be temporarily contained with suture ligation or occlusion with noncrushing bowel clamps placed proximal and distal to the injury. Obvious fecal contamination is controlled with aspiration and irrigation of the entire peritoneal cavity. A systematic examination of the abdominal cavity, as previously described (Chapter 4), is then performed.

When necessary, especially with penetrating abdominal trauma posterior to the anterior axillary line, the retroperitoneal segments of the right colon are easily reflected for inspection by incision of the lateral peritoneal reflections (Fig. 12–3). The transverse colon is circumferentially visualized following detachment of the omentum from the colon along the avascular plain of fusion, with reflection of the greater omentum cephalad. Care must be taken with this dissection to avoid inadvertent vascular injury to the transverse mesocolon and the appendices epiploicae, both of which frequently adhere to the omentum.

The splenic flexure is best evaluated without mobilization. If there is evidence of hemorrhage or fecal soilage, or there is a penetrating wound in proximity, the flexure should be mobilized for a thorough evaluation. This dissection is facilitated by the elevation of the omentum off the left transverse colon. The descending colon is then mobilized along its lateral peritoneal reflection, with gentle blunt dissection developing a plane between

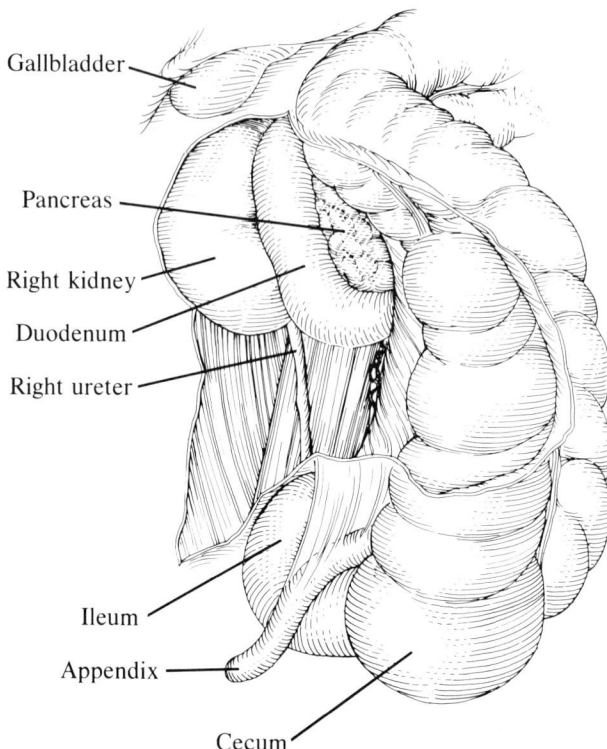

Figure 12–3. Mobilization of the right colon is readily performed by severing the lateral peritoneal attachment. This exposes the duodenum and right kidney.

the mesocolon from Gerota's capsule posteriorly (Fig. 12–4). Gentle traction caudally now identifies the remaining attachment of the splenic flexure to the diaphragm, the left phrenicocolic ligament. The inferior pole of the spleen rests on this ligament, often referred to as the supporting ligament of the spleen. Sharp division of the ligament releases the splenic flexure.

Examination of the colon should extend distally to the peritoneal reflection. As with the flexures and ascending and descending colonic segments, mobilization of the retroperitoneal rectum should proceed only after preoperative observation of the presumed rectal injury. If proctoscopy identifies an injury in this region, mobilization with exploration is then warranted. Entering the deep pelvis to search for an unidentified rectal injury is ill-advised.

INFLUENCE OF ASSOCIATED RISK FACTORS

Over the years, a number of factors have been identified with the development of postoperative complications after surgery for colonic trauma. These retrospectively identified factors have served to influence the decisions a surgeon makes when choosing the type of repair for trauma to the colon and rectum. Recently, the conclusions of this early work have come under renewed scrutiny, and currently there does not appear to be a consensus regarding the significance of any one or group of these factors.[41]

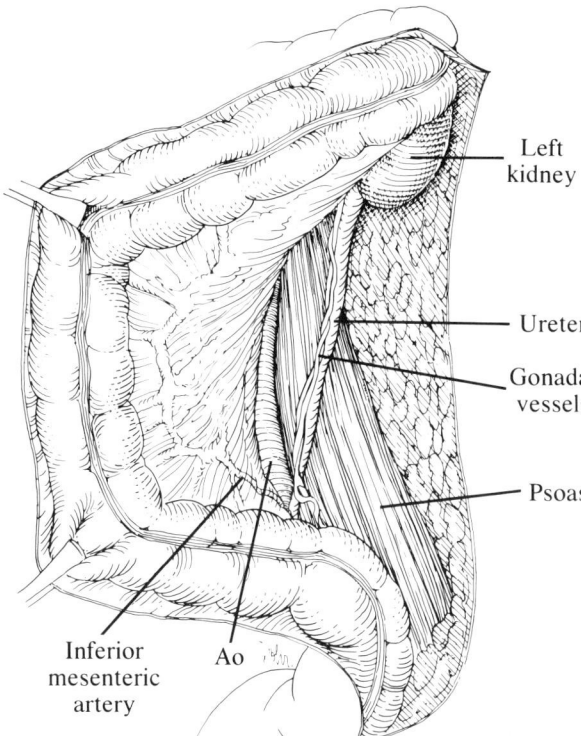

Figure 12–4. Left colon is mobilized by severing the lateral peritoneal attachment and developing the areolar plane behind the mesocolon.

Shock

Traditionally, shock has been a contraindication to primary repair of colonic trauma. Intuitively, one would suspect hypotension promotes bowel ischemia during the physiologic vasoconstriction of the mesenteric blood flow in response to the diminished blood pressure. The ischemic bowel would not necessarily be detected at celiotomy and such bowel involved in an anastomosis would be at risk for anastomotic disruption. Apparently, preoperative hypotension is not as critical as is intraoperative hypotension, with postoperative hypotension associated with the highest mortality risk.[42] A more recent review of similar retrospective data suggested no association between shock and postoperative sepsis.[43] Nelken and Lewis found the presence of shock correlated strongly with the ultimate development of multiple organ failure from sepsis.[41]

Fecal Contamination

Although the degree of fecal contamination is most certainly a significant risk factor for postoperative complications, the quantification is quite subjective and difficult to assess from the literature. Gross contamination has been associated with a significantly higher rate of abscess formation[43] and major complications.[41] Interestingly, several other studies showed a much lower rate of complication and abscess formation in a population of patients classified as grossly contaminated.[13,14] Most authors would agree that minimal fecal contamination would not be a contraindication to primary closure. Disagreement continues over the proper therapy for a patient with gross contamination.

Injury to Repair Interval

Often there is a delay in performing definitive repair in the trauma setting, allowing intraabdominal mixing of blood and feces. The interval length often influences the type of repair performed, although both a correlation[13] and lack of correlation[15] between delay in repair and anastomotic disruption have been reported. Most surgeons would not consider primary repair if the delay interval exceeded 6 to 8 hr.

Blood Transfusions

Although routinely cited as a risk factor for colon injury, blood transfusion is more likely a measure of injury severity. Patients requiring low volume transfusions (zero–four units) usually have acceptable complication rates whereas those patients requiring more than five units of blood transfusion have complication rates from 70% to 80%.[41,43]

ASSESSMENT OF INJURY SEVERITY

Owing to the multiple factors involved in assessing operative risk and postoperative complications, several systems for injury assessment have evolved from retrospective reviews. Organ systems and injury types have been scored and factored into various indices of injury severity.

The penetrating abdominal trauma index (PATI) is used for the assessment of associated intraabdominal injuries and attempts to quantify the magnitude of these injuries.[44] Each organ system receives a complication risk factor that is multiplied by a severity of injury estimate. The complication risk values were estimated from previously reported morbidities associated with the respective organs. The colon and pancreas are assigned the highest risk factor of 5. Injury severity is estimated by a modification of the abbreviated injury score (AIS),[33] with a minimal injury scored as 1 and a maximal injury scored as 5. Colon injury severity has been assessed by the following scale: grade I, serosal injury; grade II, single wall injury with less than 25% mural involvement; grade III, less than 50% mural involvement; grade IV, greater than 50% mural involvement; and grade V, mural injury associated with adjacent blood-supply injury.[45] The PATI has been shown to reliably predict outcome from intraabdominal trauma, with a score < 25 suggesting a favorable outcome.

The injury severity scale (ISS) is a commonly used index that is derived from the AIS,[33] and considers the effect of all injuries sustained. The index is based on the severity of injury to each of six different regions of the body and is calculated by adding the square roots of the three highest scoring regions. The ISS is useful in predicting eventual outcome for multiple trauma victims, but the ISS is nonspecific when tabulating complex intraabdominal injury.[41]

The Flint severity score has gained acceptance for its simplicity, with only three grades of colonic injury as determined in the operating room.[33] The grades are as follows: grade 1, isolated colon injury, minimal contamination, no shock, minimal delay; grade 2, through-and-through perforation, lacerations, moderate contamination; grade 3, severe tissue loss, devascularization, heavy contamination. The Flint scale has been useful in predicting complications from colon trauma, but it has been too restrictive to distinguish complication rates between various treatment options for colon repair.[41,42]

Although not acutely applicable to the practicing trauma surgeon, the injury assessment indices are most useful for the comparison of various published series of abdominal trauma. From these comparisons, trends favoring one repair option for colon injury in certain patients might be defined. For now debates over the best course of treatment persist.

ADJUNCTIVE ANTIBIOTICS

Clearly, true antibiotic prophylaxis in the trauma setting is not possible. Therefore, antibiotic administration in the trauma patient should be viewed as therapeutic rather than prophylactic. Optimally, the adjunctive antibiotics should be given before surgery, usually in the emergency room or trauma resuscitation room. Exogenous contamination from the common aerobic gram positive cocci can be prevented with narrow spectrum agents such as cefazolin. If peritoneal soilage is identified at celiotomy, our practice is to continue the antibiotics for 72 hr, otherwise the antibiotics are discontinued after surgery. Known or suspected disruption of a hollow viscus preoperatively should be treated with broad spectrum antibiotics known to cover gram negative and anaerobic species.[46] Controversy over the specific agents or combination of agents continues to exist, yet most regimens attempt to cover enterobacteriacae, enterococci, and bacteroides. Broad spectrum antibiotic coverage with an aminoglycoside and clindamycin or metronidazole, a second generation cephalosporin, or an extended spectrum penicillin with or without clavulinic acid are currently the agents of choice in patients with colonic injury.[5] We currently prefer to use a single agent, cefoxitin, with little or no nephrotoxicity as our adjunctive antibiotic for known or suspected colonic injury. This regimen (1 g of cefoxitin intravenously every 6 hr for 3 days) has been shown to be equally[47] or more effective[48] than an aminoglycoside combined with clindamycin as an adjunctive antibiotic therapy for traumatic colon injuries.

METHODS OF REPAIR

Primary Repair

There is an ever-growing body of evidence that primary repair of colonic injuries is safe in many clinical settings, specifically in low risk patients (Fig. 12–5). Optimal candidates would include low velocity GSWs and stab wounds of less than 50% of the colonic circumference, remote from the segmental vascular supply. Thorough debridement is critical for the success of this modality, to assure adequate blood flow at the anastomotic site. Both one- and two-layer closures have been successful.[5,42] A transverse closure is preferred to preserve luminal diameter. However, tension on the closure must be avoided so that longitudinal lacerations should be closed longitudinally. Newer stapling techniques

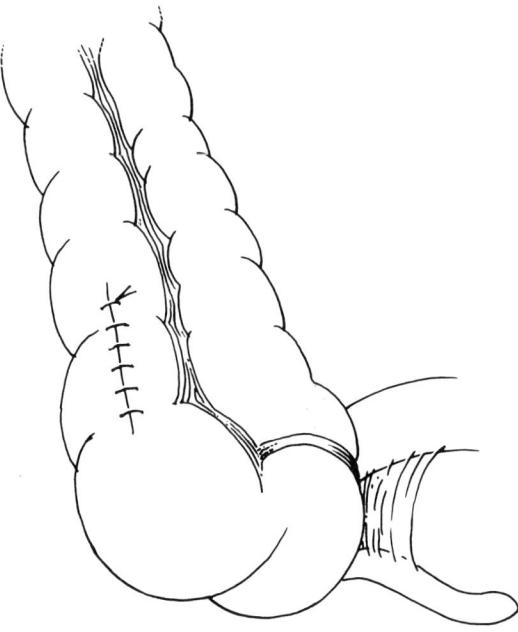

Figure 12–5. Primary suture of the colon.

have also been used with success.[18] Although traditionally the right colon has been deemed more favorable for primary repair than the left colon, recent experience contradicts this thesis, with no difference in outcome between primary repair of these segments.[32,49]

Primary Resection and Anastomosis

In the case of extensive bowel wall disruption or segmental vascular compromise, the involved segment should be resected. This therapy has been used mostly for extensive injury to the right colon.[50] An ileostomy is not without its own morbidity. Several reports have identified a high morbidity when ileostomy is performed in the presence of peritonitis,[33,50] and they recommend ileocolostomy even in the presence of peritonitis (Fig. 12–6). Primary anastomosis in the left colon has had less justification and has been advocated when there are few associated injuries, no shock, and minimal fecal contamination. An ATI of less than 25 has generally been accepted as compared with primary anastomosis.[5,41]

Colostomy Exteriorization

Over the past several decades, the indications for colostomy in the management of colon injuries has declined. Most authors agree that a colostomy is indicated in patients with protracted shock where secondary mesenteric vasoconstriction persists despite adequate volume resuscitation. Less uniformity of opinion favors colostomy in patients with severe

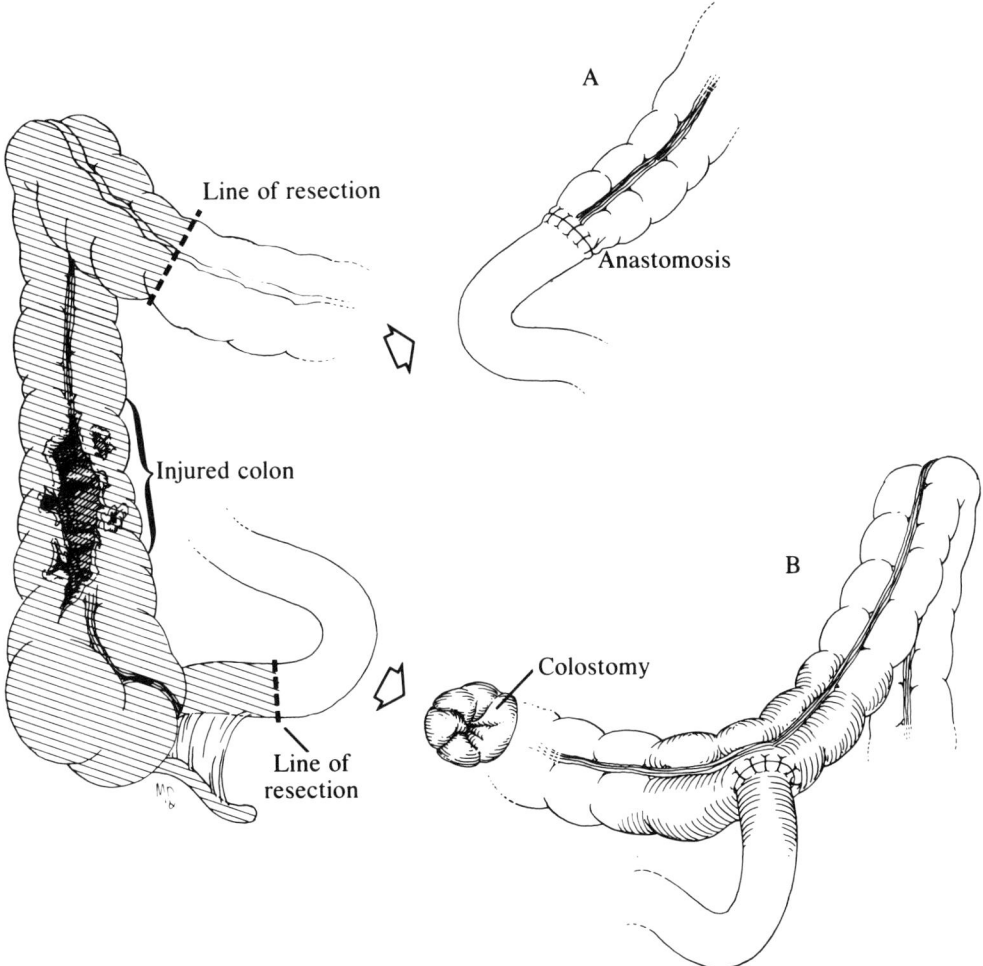

Figure 12–6. **A:** A badly lacerated ascending colon—the shaded area represents the area of resection. **B:** An ileocolic anastomosis has been carried out.

head injury, or in patients expected to have a protracted convalescence, or for patients who present with a large interval of delay from injury to therapy. Although colostomy was initially felt to decrease septic complications, most recent series are reporting higher incidences of intraabdominal septic complications for colostomy patients than for patients treated without colostomy.[13,15,32,39]

When a colostomy is performed, most authors prefer end colostomy and mucous fistula creation for ascending colonic injuries (Fig. 12–7), and end colostomy with Hartman's pouch for descending colonic injuries (Fig. 12–8). Maturation of the colostomy may be deferred for 24 to 28 hr. Some authors advocate anchoring the defunctional limb of colon adjacent to the functional limb to aid in future colostomy closure. Care must be taken in creating a large enough fascial opening for the colostomy to prevent postoperative obstruction.

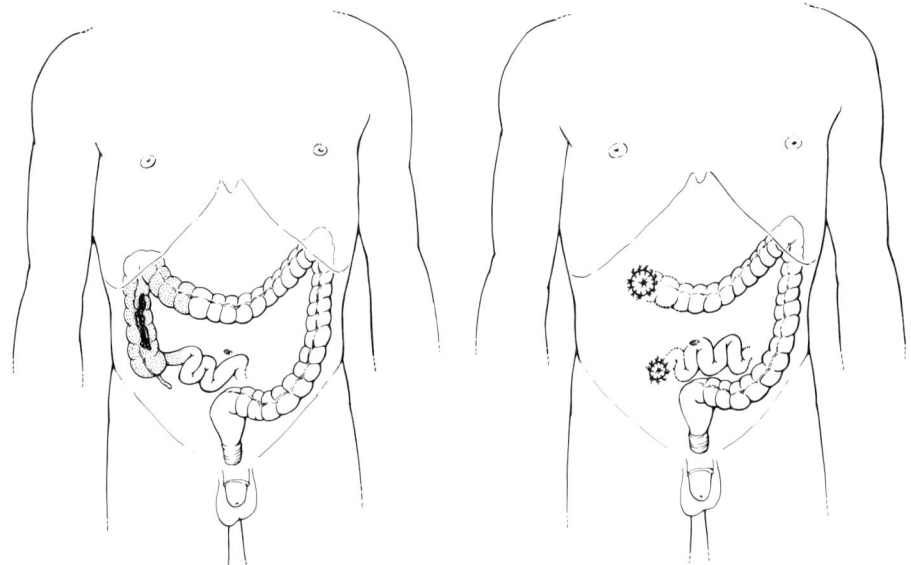

Figure 12–7. Injury to the ascending colon. When there is a gross injury, ileostomy and distal mucous fistula or colostomy may be indicated.

Colostomy closure is associated with a lower complication rate if deferred for at least 6 weeks.[18] The complication rate for colostomy closure in trauma patients is less than that for nontrauma patients.[42] Colostomy closure after colonic injury is a low morbidity procedure with complications identified in less than 5% of patients in several recent 5-year review series.[13,51] Routine preoperative evaluation of the colonic anatomy and standard bowel preparation are indicated.

Exteriorization of Primary Repair

Exteriorized primary repair of the colon, first described by Okies et al.,[52] is a rapid method available for the management of colon injury that obviates the morbidity of mandatory colostomy, yet avoids the risks of primary repair. The injured colon is mobilized sufficiently to permit colostomy formation, then a formal primary repair is made, and the repair site is brought out onto the abdominal wall, and fixed over a rod, Penrose drain, or bridge of fascia (Fig. 12–9). The exteriorized segment is protected in an aseptic moist environment with daily observation of the segment. If a leak is identified, the segment is matured into a loop colostomy. If no leak occurs by 5 to 10 days the segment is returned to the abdomen.[53] Although some have enjoyed successful return of the exteriorized segment in 60% to 70% of their patients,[53,54] others have shown failure rates of 50% to 70%.[18,55,56]

Prograde colonic lavage, as originally described by Dudley et al.,[57] has not been shown to improve the interiorization rate for exteriorized colonic repairs.[58] Prograde colonic lavage, which theoretically reduces the intraluminal volume of enteric organisms thus

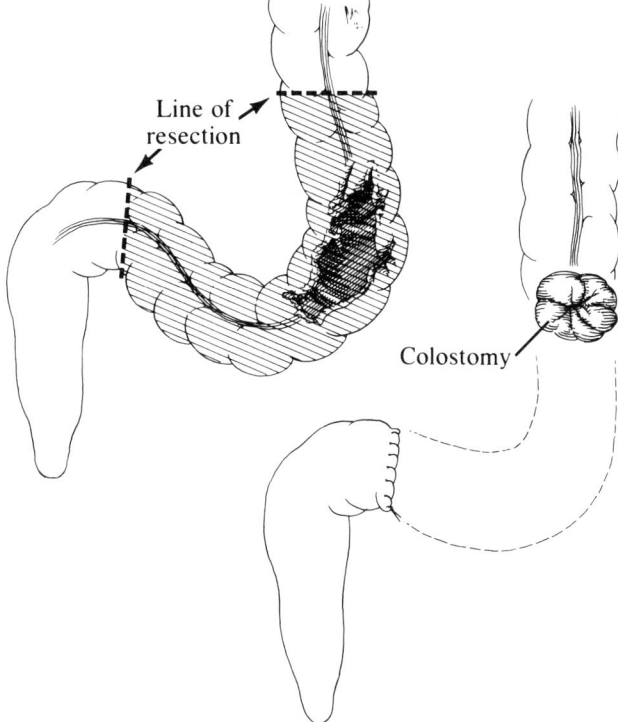

Figure 12–8. Resection of the area of injury with the proximal bowel end brought out as a colostomy. The distal end can be brought out as mucous fistula or closed and left in the abdominal cavity.

decreasing the production of potentially harmful toxins, has not been shown to decrease the mortality from traumatic large bowel injury.[58]

Rectal Injuries

If a rectal injury is suspected, sigmoidoscopy is essential in the evaluation. Minor partial thickness injuries to the rectal wall originating from within the lumen, such as those caused by foreign bodies, require no specific therapy. If a full thickness injury with perforation is identified, diversion, drainage, and debridement if possible are indicated. Establishment of adequate drainage and fecal diversion are the essential components. If the rectal injury is extraperitoneal, drainage is essential, and usually established in the presacral space with exit adjacent to the coccyx, through an incision posterior to the anus. Rectal injuries should be repaired if possible, either from above at the time of diversion of the fecal stream, or if low, from a transanal approach. Proximal fecal diversion is accomplished with a divided sigmoid colostomy with mucous fistula (Fig. 12–10).

Washout of the distal rectosigmoid was introduced during the Vietnam War, where there was a high incidence of septic complications from mostly high velocity GSWs to the

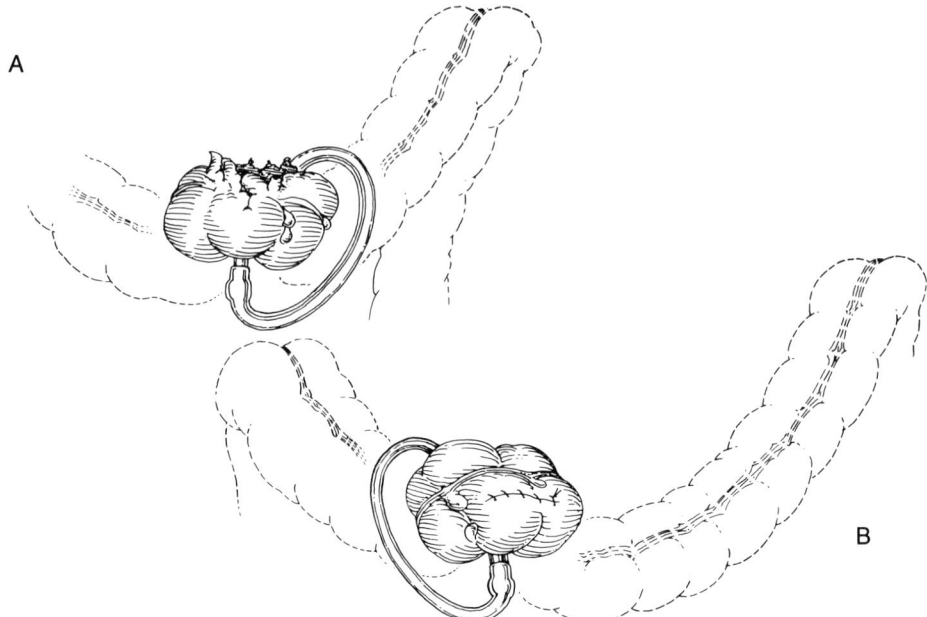

Figure 12-9. **A:** Exteriorization of the area of injury is carried out over a glass rod. **B:** Primary closure is demonstrated.

rectum.[59] This technique, in which the distal segment of bowel is copiously irrigated with saline and/or antibiotic solution, was credited with a reduction in morbidity from 72% to 10% and a reduction in mortality from 22% to 0%.[60] Civilian rectal trauma is low velocity, and although some advocate distal rectal washout,[61] this may be unnecessary for civilian rectal trauma.[62] Irrigation through the proximal colon must be done under low pressure with the sphincter dilated or it may aggravate the contamination through an inaccessible rectal wound.

If no significant leak is apparent at the end of 5 days, the drains are removed. Both Penrose and sump drains have been used with success. If a leak develops, it will usually spontaneously close with time, as long as fecal diversion is maintained.

In conclusion, based on our experience and that of the current literature, which is rapidly expanding, several general conclusions seem plausible. It now seems clear that primary repair of colonic wounds is appropriate in at least some, and in many hands most, patients. Exteriorization of the repaired colonic segment does not seem necessary, and in fact may complicate the patient's course, requiring conversion to colostomy in a distressingly high frequency. Colostomy continues to have a place in the treatment of colonic trauma, particularly with medium and high velocity gunshot wounds. Colostomy closure can be performed safely after recovery from the associated injuries. The difference between injuries to the right and left colon appears to be negligible, and all colonic injury should be treated with similar principles. Rectal injuries require diversion and drainage, and repair when feasible. Distal rectal washout remains unproven in the civilian setting. Wounds are best treated as uniformly contaminated, and most will do well with delayed primary closure.

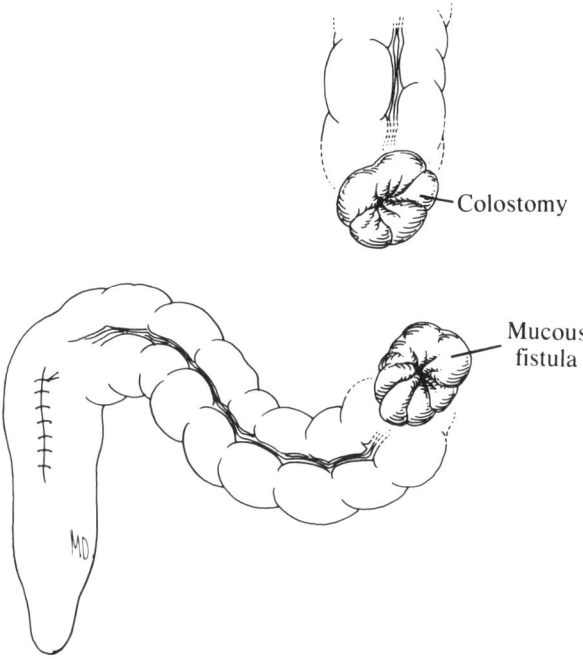

Figure 12–10. Proximal colostomy and mucous fistula defunctionalize the injured bowel, permitting primary closure.

WOUND MANAGEMENT

As with the previous therapeutic options discussed, controversy exists over the question of wound closure: primary versus delayed primary closure versus healing by secondary intention. By definition, all wounds associated with colon injury are contaminated. The most conservative option is to leave the wound open to heal by secondary intention. These wounds will have the lowest complication rates and the eventual scar will be little different than a primarily closed wound.

Delayed primary closure is a middle position, for it prevents wound infection and it speeds the healing process. Delayed primary closure can be performed at the bedside, usually on the fifth postoperative day, if the wound remains clean and uninfected.[63] The closure can be with tape strips or with previously placed sutures.

POSTOPERATIVE CARE

Associated injuries pose the greatest threat to the patient during the first few postoperative days. Maintenance of good circulation and oxygenation is important for healing of colonic wounds and prevention of infection, as well as for protection of other organ systems.[64]

Although necrotizing infections can appear within hours of injury, more commonly the development of such infections is delayed for several days. Antibiotics that were started preoperatively should be continued for 24 to 48 hr, and patients should be watched closely for indications of abdominal or incisional infection. Modern radiographic and nuclear medicine imaging techniques have greatly improved the success of pinpointing the location of intraabdominal abscesses for surgical drainage.

Exteriorized colon should be protected by petrolatum or moist saline dressings. A colostomy is managed by standard methods. If a colostomy has been done, it requires formal surgical closure later. Authorities disagree on the optimal interval from construction to closure of a colostomy, and recommendations vary from 2 weeks to several months.[65,66] It is advisable to wait until the colonic wall is no longer edematous, because edematous colon does not hold sutures and dehiscence is likely. An interval of 6 weeks to 3 months is optimal before attempting closure of a loop colostomy. A few weeks may be enough if the loop is resected and normal colon is anastomosed end-to-end and the patient is young and in good condition. Restoration of continuity in patients with end sigmoid colostomy and a Hartmann closure of the rectum is a major operation that may not be feasible for 3 months or longer.

COMPLICATIONS

The mortality rate from penetrating trauma to the colon and rectum is now below 10%, and some authors report a rate under 5%.[17,21,30,55,67,68] Death within the first 24 hr is due to hemorrhage, head injuries, or other problems not directly related to the perforated bowel. Later deaths, about half of the total mortality, are most commonly due to septic complications. The main correlation of survival is the number of associated injuries: survivors generally have only one or two organ systems injured, and as the number of involved organs increases, so does the mortality rate. If the liver, pancreas, or kidney is injured along with the large bowel, the mortality rate is as high as 30%.[17,53] Shotgun wounds, high velocity missile injuries, and blunt trauma also are fatal more frequently than simple penetrating trauma.

Even among patients who survive trauma to the large bowel, complications are common. The overall morbidity rate is about 50%, and many of these patients have more than one complication. In selected groups, such as those with massive rectal trauma, recovery without complication is exceptional.

Infection is the most important complication, affecting about one-third of patients in most reports. Wound infection was discussed in an earlier section; it occurs in 20% to 40% of primarily closed wounds and 8% to 20% of delayed primary closures. Abdominal abscesses develop in about 20% of patients, and numbers much larger and smaller have been reported. The interval from injury to operation influences the incidence of abdominal abscess importantly: abscesses occur in twice as many patients if operation is delayed beyond 6 hr.

Leakage of a primary sutured perforation or a primary anastomosis is unusual if patients are selected carefully according to the criteria discussed earlier. Recently, colonic suture line dehiscence has been reported in 2% to 5% of patients.[22,68–72] These leaks are all clinically obvious, and the true incidence of leakage must be higher. Fecal fistula develops in approximately 3% of patients. When leakage is suspected, prompt operative intervention with exteriorization or resection of the suture line and colostomy is mandatory.

Early colostomy complications include peristomal herniation, necrosis, retraction, and peristomal infection. These problems are serious and often require reoperation. Later complications of colostomy—hernia, stenosis, and prolapse—are usually just inconveniences and are resolved when the temporary colostomy is closed. Complications of colostomy closure are relatively frequent and include wound infection, anastomotic leakage, and intraperitoneal infection. These complications must be considered in determining total morbidity of trauma of the large bowel.[65-66]

Dehiscence is another serious wound complication; usually it is related to wound infection. Small bowel obstruction and pulmonary, cardiac, and renal complications also occur in these severely injured patients.

REFERENCES

1. Otis GA. *The Medical and Surgical History of the War of the Rebellion, Part II*. Washington, DC: Government Printing Office; 1876.
2. Leriche R. Necessite d'operer systematiquement les plaies de l'abdomen. *Presse Med*. 1915; 28:221–222.
3. Wallace C. A study of 1200 cases of gunshot wounds of the abdomen. *Br Med J*. 1917; 4:679–743.
4. Fraser J, Drummond H. A clinical and experimental study of three hundred perforating wounds of the abdomen. *Br Med J*. 1917; 1:321–325.
5. McEnena OJ, Moore EE, Moore FA. The injured colon. *Postgrad Adv Trauma Surg*. 1990; I-I:1–14.
6. Ogilvie WH. Abdominal wounds in the Western Desert. *Surg Gynecol Obstet*. 1944; 78:225–238.
7. Office of the Surgeon General. Circulation Letter, no. 178. October 23, 1943.
8. Taylor ER, Thompson JE. The early treatment, and results thereof, of injuries to the colon and rectum—with 70 additional cases. *Int Abst Surg*. 1948; 87:105–228.
9. Imes PR. War surgery of the abdomen. *Surg Gynecol Obstet*. 1945; 81:608–616.
10. Gordon-Taylor G. Second thoughts on the abdominal surgery of "total" war. Review of over 1300 cases. *Br J Surg*. 1944; 32:247–258.
11. Zipperman HH. The management of large bowel injuries in the Korean campaign. *US Armed Forces Med J*. 1956; 7:85–91.
12. Woodhall JP, Ochsner A. The management of perforating injuries of the colon and rectum in civilian practice. *Surgery*. 1951; 29:305–320.
13. Burch JM, Brock JC, Gevirtzman L, et al. The injured colon. *Ann Surg*. 1979; 203:701–711.
14. Adkins RB, Zirkle PK, Waterhouse G. Penetrating colon trauma. *J Trauma*. 1984; 24:491–499.
15. Stone HH, Fabian TC. Management of perforating colon trauma; Randomization between primary closure and exteriorization. *Ann Surg*. 1979; 190:430–436.
16. Crass RA. Duodenum, small intestine, and colon. In: Trunkey DD, Lewis FR, eds. *Current Therapy of Trauma*. Toronto: BC Decker; 1986; 2:293–297.
17. Haynes CD, Gunn CH, Martin JD Jr. Colon injuries. *Arch Surg*. 1968; 96:944–948.
18. Nance FC. Injuries to the colon and rectum. In: Mattox KL, Moore EE, Feliciano DV, eds. *Trauma*. Norwalk/San Mateo: Appleton and Lange; 1988; 495–504.
19. Yaw PB, Smith RN, Glover JL. Eight years experience with civilian injuries of the colon. *Surg Gynecol Obstet*. 1977; 145:203–208.
20. Howell HS, Bartizal JF, Freeark RJ. Blunt trauma involving the colon and rectum. *J Trauma*. 1976; 16:624–629.
21. Steele M, Blaisdell FW. Treatment of colon injuries. *J Trauma*. 1977; 17:557–562.
22. Walt AJ. Emergency treatment of wounds of the colon. *Compr Ther*. 1976; 2:60–64.
23. Haas PA, Fox TA Jr. Civilian injuries of the rectum and anus. *Dis Colon Rectum*. 1979; 22:17–24.
24. Wanebo JH, Hunt TK, Mathewson C Jr. Rectal injuries. *J Trauma*. 1969; 9:712–716.
25. Byrd RL, Cunningham MW, Goldman LT. Nonocclusive ischemic colitis secondary to hemorrhagic shock. *Dis Colon Rectum*. 1987; 30:116–118.
26. Sommers HM. Indigenous microbiota in the human. In: Simmons RI, Howard RJ, eds. *Surgical Infectious Diseases*. New York: Appleton-Century-Crofts; 1982: 29–38.
27. Hunt TK, Hawley RK, Dunphy JE. Aetiology of colonic leak. *Proc Soc Med*. 1970; 63(suppl):28–30.
28. Beahrs O. Complications of colon surgery. *Surg Clin North Am*. 1967; 47:983–988.
29. Debas T, Thompson FB. A critical review of colectomy with anastomosis. *Surg Gynecol Obstet*. 1972; 135:747–752.
30. Chilimiadris C, Bopud DR, Carlson LE, et al. A critical review of management of right colon injuries. *J Trauma*. 1971; 11:651–660.
31. Steele M, Blaisdell FW. Treatment of colon injuries. *J Trauma*. 1977; 17:557–562.
32. Thompson JS, Moore EE, Moore JB. Comparison of penetrating injuries of the right and left colon. *Ann Surg*. 1981; 193:414–418.

33. Flint LM, Vitale GC, Richardson JD, et al. The injured colon: relationship of management to complications. *Ann Surg*. 1981; 193:619–623.
34. Shannon EL, Moore EE. Primary repair of the colon: when is it a safe alternative? *Surgery*. 1985; 98:851–860.
35. Fackler ML, Bellamy RF, Malinowski JA. The wound profile illustration of the missile-tissue interaction. *J Trauma*. 1988; 28:S21–S28.
36. Thompson JS, Moore EE, Van Duzer-Moore S, et al. The evolution of abdominal stab wound management. *J Trauma*. 1988; 20:478–484.
37. Lowe RJ, Saletta JD, Read DR, et al. Should laparotomy be mandatory or selective in gunshot wounds of the abdomen? *J Trauma*. 1977; 17:903–907.
38. Moore EE, Moore JB, Van Duzer-Moore S, et al. Mandatory laparotomy for gunshot wounds penetrating the abdomen. *Am J Surg*. 1980; 140:847–851.
39. Mackersie RC, Lewis FR Jr. Local exploration and exploratory laparotomy. In: Dailey RH, Callahan M, eds. *Clinics in Emergency Medicine, Vol. 6: Controversies in Trauma Management*. New York: Churchill Livingstone; 1985.
40. Root HD, Keizer FJ, Perry JF. The clinical and experimental aspects of the peritoneal response to injury. *Arch Surg*. 1967; 95:531–535.
41. Nelken N, Lewis FR. The influence of injury severity on complication rates after primary closure or colostomy for penetrating colon trauma. *Ann Surg*. 1989; 209(4):439–447.
42. Huber PJ, Thal ER. Management of colon injuries. *Surg Clin North Am*. 1990; 70(3):561–573.
43. George SM Jr, Fabian TC, Voeller GR, et al. Primary repair of colon wounds. *Ann Surg*. 1989; 728–734.
44. Moore EE, Dunn EL, Moore JB, et al. Penetrating abdominal trauma index. *J Trauma*. 1981; 21:438–445.
45. Asbun HJ, Irani H, Roe EJ, et al. Intra-abdominal seatbelt injury. *J Trauma*. 1990; 30:189–193.
46. Thadepalli H, Gorbach SL, Broido PW, et al. Abdominal trauma anaerobes, and antibiotics. *Surg Gynecol Obstet*. 1973; 137:270–274.
47. Nichols RL, Smith JW, Klein DB, et al. Risk of infection after penetrating abdominal trauma. *N Engl J Med*. 1984; 311:1065–1070.
48. Jones RC, Thal ER, Johnson RC, et al. Evaluation of antibiotic treatment following penetrating abdominal trauma. *Ann Surg*. 1985; 201:576–579.
49. Ridgeway CA, Frame SB, Rice JC, et al. Primary repair vs. colostomy for the treatment of penetrating colon injuries. *Dis Colon Rectum*. 1989; 32:1046–1049.
50. Garrison RN, Shively EH, Baker C, et al. Evaluation of management of the emergency right hemicolectomy. *J Trauma*. 1979; 19(10):734–739.
51. Crass RA, Salbi F, Trunkey DT. Colostomy closure after colon injury: a low-morbidity procedure. *J Trauma*. 1987; 27:1237–1239.
52. Okies EJ, Bricker DL, Jordan GL, et al. Exteriorized repair of colon injuries. *Am J Surg* 1972; 124:807–811.
53. Kirkpatrick JR, Rajpal SC. The injured colon: therapeutic considerations. *Am J Surg*. 1975; 129:187–191.
54. Nallathambi MN, Ivantury RR, Rohman M, et al. Penetrating colon injuries: exteriorized repair vs. loop colostomy. *J Trauma*. 1987; 27:876–882.
55. Shrock TC, Christensen N. Management of perforating injuries to the colon. *Surg Gynecol Obstet*. 1972; 132:65–68.
56. Thompson JS, Moore EE. Factors affecting the outcome of exteriorized colon repairs. *J Trauma*. 1982; 22(5):403–406.
57. Dudley HAF, Radcliffe AG, McGeehan D. Intraoperative irrigation of the colon to permit primary anastomosis. *Br J Surg*. 1980; 67:80–81.
58. Baker LW, Thomson SR, Chadwick SJD. Colon wound management and prograde colonic lavage in large bowel trauma. *Br J Surg*. 1990; 77:872–876.
59. Armstrong RG, Schmitt HJ, Patterson LT. Combat wounds of the extraperitoneal rectum. *Surgery*. 1973; 74:570–574.
60. Lavenson GS, Cohen A. Management of rectal injuries. *Am J Surg*. 1971; 122:225–230.
61. Shannon FL, Moore EE, Moore FA, et al. Value of distal colon washout in civilian rectal trauma—reducing gut bacterial translocation. *J Trauma*. 1988; 28(7):989–994.
62. Trunkey DD, Hays RJ, Shires GT. Management of rectal trauma. *J Trauma*. 1973; 13:411–415.
63. Kenady DE. Management of abdominal wounds. *Surg Clin North Am*. 1984; 64:803–807.
64. Gilmour DG, et al. The effect of hypovolemia on colonic blood flow in the dog. *Br J Surg*. 1980; 67:82–85.
65. Machiedo GW, Casey KF, Blackwood JM. Colostomy closure following trauma. *Surg Gynecol Obstet*. 1980; 151:58–61.
66. Samhouri F, Grodinsky C, Fox T Jr. The management of colonic and rectal injuries. *Dis Colon Rectum*. 1978; 21:426–430.
67. LoCicero J III, Tajima T, Drapanas T. A half century of experience in the management of colon injuries: changing concepts. *J Trauma*. 1975; 15:575–580.
68. Arango A, Baxter CR, Shires GT. Surgical management of traumatic injuries of the right colon. Twenty years of civilian experience. *Arch Surg*. 1979; 114:703–707.

69. Beall AC Jr, et al. Surgical considerations in the management of civilian colon injuries. *Ann Surg*. 1971; 173:971–975.
70. Haygood FD, Polk HC Jr. Gunshot wounds of the colon. A review of 100 consecutive patients, with emphasis on complications and their causes. *Am J Surg*. 1976; 131:213–218.
71. Josen AS, et al. Primary closure of civilian colorectal wounds. *Ann Surg*. 1972; 176:782–786.
72. Mulherin JL Jr, Sawyers JL. Evaluation of three methods of managing penetrating colon injuries. *J Trauma*. 1975; 15:580–586.
73. Baker SP, O'Neill B, Haddon W Jr, et al. The injury severity score: a method for describing patients with multiple injuries and evaluating emergency care. *J Trauma*. 1974; 14:187–196.

13
Splenic Injury

SANDRA L. BEAL, M.D.
DONALD D. TRUNKEY, M.D.

HISTORY: Aristotle (348–322 BC) concluded that the spleen was not essential to life.[1] The spleen was described as an organ of mystery by the Asclepiad, Galen of Perjamon (130–200 AD).[2] Halevi (1086–1145) wrote that the spleen is called laughing because of its nature to cleanse the blood and spirit from unclean and obscuring matter. In the first century, it was postulated by Pliny that the weight of the spleen hindered the speed of runners and could be removed, but with the complication of the loss of the ability to laugh.[3] The concept of the blood-purifying function of the spleen was reemphasized by Maimonides in the mid-12th century.[4]

A partial splenectomy was reported by Viard in 1590.[2] The first successful splenectomy was performed in 1893 by Reigner in a 14-year-old boy sustaining blunt trauma.[4] Kocher, in 1911, stated, "Injuries of the spleen demand excision of the gland; no evil effects follow its removal, while the danger of hemorrhage is effectually stopped."[2] Animal experiments performed during the 18th to early 20th centuries supported the concept of the nonessential nature of the spleen.[2,5] This was accepted as doctrine and not challenged until 1919 when Morris and Bullock in a review of the subject concluded that the human body, deprived of its spleen, would show an increased susceptibility to infection.[6]

The mortality of clinically recognized splenic injuries in the early 1900s was nearly 100%. Splenectomy for trauma was performed frequently during the early decades of the 20th century with a mortality of 30% to 40%.[7] A nonoperative approach was tried by Bland-Sutton in 1912 with a resultant 90% mortality.[8] Thus, splenectomy became the gold standard of treatment for splenic injury.

Until recently, the spleen has been regarded as little more than a sac of blood with no essential function. As a result, general policy dictated removal should there be any evidence of injury, including minor iatrogenic tears during other surgical procedures. One factor that contributes to the problem is that delayed hemorrhage from the spleen is a well established fact. Although this has been referred to as delayed rupture, we do not know of any established case in which a spleen verified to be intact at laparotomy accounted for secondary hemorrhage. A poll conducted at the Western Surgical Association disclosed that no member of that organization could verify delayed rupture.[9] A similar poll taken of 500 trauma surgeons also failed to elicit a case of delayed rupture.[9] Delayed hemorrhage simply implies that the spleen initially ruptured may not bleed sufficiently to produce clinical signs. Hours, days, or even months later, secondary hemorrhage may occur. This is due to further trauma to the spleen, the expansion of a large hematoma, or continued ongoing slow hemorrhage. The highest incidence of delayed hemorrhage is within the first 24 hr. The incidence of secondary bleeding decreases in geometric fashion with the passage of time.[20]

Fatal sepsis in children after spleen removal was reported by King and Schumacher in 1952.[9] Several reports have since confirmed postsplenectomy sepsis in patients of all ages. A 1.5% incidence of sepsis after splenectomy for trauma and a 2.1% incidence after incidental splenectomy was reported by Singer in 1973.[11] Recently, the incidence of overwhelming postsplenectomy septic death was reported by Luna and Dellinger to be 0.026% in adults and 0.052% in children.[12] This has led to an effort to conserve the injured spleen when possible.

ANATOMY

The spleen is the second largest organ of the reticuloendothelial system and has an average weight of 250 g. It is located in the posterior left upper quadrant of the abdomen, juxtaposed to the 8th, 9th, and 10th ribs. The superior, anterior surface is apposed to the greater curve of the stomach. The hilum of the spleen is in immediate proximity to the tail of the pancreas. Inferiorly, the lower pole is often attached to the splenic flexure of the colon and the greater omentum. The lateral and posterior surface is apposed to the diaphragm and medial surface of the left kidney. The peritoneal attachments of the spleen, the splenophrenic, splenorenal, and splenocolic ligaments, are relatively avascular. The gastrosplenic ligament, which extends from the greater curvature of the body and fundus of the stomach to the spleen, contains the short gastric arteries and veins.

The splenic artery runs transversely from right to left at the superior margin of the pancreas distributing multiple small branches to the pancreas and occasionally to the posterior aspect of the stomach. In 85% of people, the splenic artery bifurcates into two main branches that supply the superior and inferior lobes of the spleen. The lobar arteries divide into cephalic and caudad tributaries creating four anatomic segments. In the remaining 15% of the population, the splenic artery trifurcates, creating six anatomic splenic segments. Each major branch of the splenic artery runs in a transverse plane, perpendicular to the long axis of the spleen, without anastomosing with adjacent vessels. This distribution forms the basis for partial splenectomy (Fig. 13–1).

The splenic vein is formed by the coalescence of polar veins in the splenic hilus. The vein courses inferior to the splenic artery along the dorsal surface of the pancreas. Unlike the arterial anatomy within the spleen, veins in the spleen are highly interconnected and do not follow segmental anatomy.

FUNCTION

Splenic function can be divided into five broad categories, of which four are important to the trauma patient (Table 13–1).[13] The first function is that of filtering; this includes

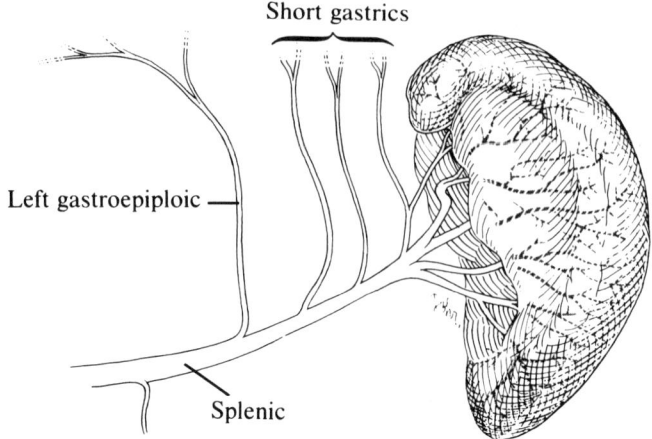

Figure 13–1. Arterial supply of the spleen. Five to six branches take origin proximal to and in the hilum providing segmental circulation to the spleen. The most proximal branch of the splenic artery shown here is the left gastroepiploic followed by the short gastric arteries to the proximal portion of the greater curvature of the stomach.

blood-borne particulate antigens, blood cells, and bacteria. The spleen is an important source of two opsonins, tuftsin and properdin. The spleen is also important in the production of immunoglobulin M (IgM), which is markedly decreased after splenectomy for trauma. It is also an important organ in the regulation of both T and B lymphocytes. The fifth function, hematopoiesis *in utero*, is relatively unimportant to the trauma patient; this function may assume more importance as fetal surgery increases.

The spleen is the primary defense organ when the host is invaded by blood-borne bacteria and has little or no preexisting antibody. This is due to the unique microcirculation of the splenic pulp; arterial blood must pass through the tiny pores between the endothelial cells lining the wall of the venous sinuses in order to enter the venous circulation. This "delays" circulation and allows splenic phagocytes to remove even poorly opsoninized bacteria. Although the liver is the most important organ in removing well opsoninized bacteria from the blood, the spleen, because of this efficient filter, is more effective in removing poorly opsoninized bacteria.

Particular antigens are similarly cleared in this sieving effect and, in addition, initiate IgM antibody response in the germinal center. Red cells are similarly altered or culled as they pass through this splenic sieve. The spleen is capable of removing surface craters, pits from normal red cells, Howell-Jolly bodies, Heinz bodies, or Pappenheimer bodies. As red cells become senescent, they lose enzyme activity and the spleen recognizes this, traps the cells, and destroys them.

Table 13–1 Functions of the Spleen

1. Filter for particulate matter, old red cells
2. Source of opsonins-tuftsin and properdin
3. Source of immunoglobulin IgM
4. Regulation of T and B lymphocytes
5. Source of hematopoiesis *in utero*

Asplenia leads to subnormal levels of tuftsin and properdin. Tuftsin is a tetrapeptide that coats white cells and promotes phagocytosis of particulate matter, bacteria, and aged blood cells. Properdin is an important component of the alternate pathway of complement activation, and subnormal levels will impair the serum opsoninization of encapsulated bacteria such as meningococci and pneumococci.

MECHANISM OF INJURY

The spleen is the most common intraabdominal organ injured in blunt trauma and is a frequently injured organ in penetrating abdominal trauma. The possibility of splenic disruption depends on the injury mechanism, age of patient, and presence of underlying disease. Injuries to the spleen include capsular avulsions, minor parenchymal disruptions, transverse fractures oriented along the planes of the internal vascular architecture, disruption of the hilar vasculature, and massive fragmentation. These injuries have recently been classified by the Trauma Committee of the American College of Surgeons (Table 13–2). There are three basic mechanisms of splenic injury: penetrating, deceleration, and blunt compression trauma. Iatrogenic penetrating injuries have occurred during thoracentesis, closed tube thoracostomy, endoscopic retrograde cholangiopancreatography, colonoscopy, and laparotomy.[14,15] The severity of penetrating splenic injury depends on the wounding instrument and its trajectory. Vascular laceration is common with both arterial and venous hemorrhage.

The spleen is relatively fixed by the splenophrenic, splenorenal, and splenocolic ligaments. In deceleration injury, the mobile stomach and transverse colon can continue to accelerate, producing capsular avulsion and/or tears in the polar and short gastric vessels. With severe deceleration, the spleen may be totally avulsed from its hilar vessels and the retroperitoneum.

Severe blunt injury can also result in diffuse stellate parenchymal disruption that does not parallel the segmental anatomy. There may not only be parenchymal injury but also

Table 13–2 Splenic Injury Scale

GRADE*		INJURY DESCRIPTION
I.	Hematoma	Subcapsular, nonexpanding, <10% surface area
	Laceration	Capsular tear, nonbleeding, <1 cm parenchymal depth
II.	Hematoma	Subcapsular, nonexpanding, 10–50% surface area; intraparenchymal, nonexpanding, <2 cm in diameter
	Laceration	Capsular tear, active bleeding, 1–3 cm parenchymal depth that does not involve a trabecular vessel
III.	Hematoma	Subcapsular, >50% surface area or expanding; ruptured subcapsular hematoma with active bleeding; intraparenchymal hematoma, <2 cm or expanding
	Laceration	>3 cm parenchymal depth or involving trabecular vessels
IV.	Hematoma	Ruptured intraparenchymal hematoma with active bleeding
	Laceration	Laceration involving segmental or hilar vessel producing major devascularization (>25% of spleen)
V.	Laceration	Completely shattered spleen
	Vascular	Hilar vascular injury that devascularizes spleen

*Advance one grade for multiple injuries to the same organ. Based on most accurate assessment at autopsy, laparotomy, or radiologic study.

arterial and venous hilar laceration and hemorrhage. Blunt compression injury often results in fracture of the parenchyma along the direction of the segmental arterial anatomy. This type of primary parenchymal injury causes predominantly venous bleeding. Deep fractures may extend into and lacerate the splenic hilum. The hilum of the spleen is centered on the posterior axillary line, with the spleen lying between and protected by the 8th and 10th ribs. For this reason, rib fractures are commonly found in association with splenic injury. In fact, fractures of the lower ribs are associated with 20% incidence of splenic rupture. In most instances of splenic injury, there is a history of significant trauma to the left lower rib cage and/or upper abdominal quadrant.

Although fractures of the lower ribs are frequently found in adults with blunt splenic injury, in children, because of the flexibility of their rib cage, there may be only minimal chest wall injury despite a major intraabdominal injury. It is important to emphasize (primarily in children) that significant splenic disruption can be present in the complete absence of, or with minimal evidence of, external injury. In children the spleen also is the most commonly injured organ as a result of blunt trauma.[16]

An enlarged or diseased spleen is easily traumatized, and rupture may occur from minimal trauma. Splenomegaly is caused by hematologic disorders, by bacterial and viral infection, and by portal hypertension.[17-19] The splenic capsule may become firm, thickly scarred ("sugar-coated"), and adherent to the diaphragm in elderly persons or those with prior splenic injury, irradiation, or recurrent infarction. During pregnancy the spleen becomes congested, and the splenic capsule thinned and predictably prone to rupture. Recognition of these conditions has diagnostic implications. Patients with an underlying splenic abnormality may have sustained an injury so trivial that it was not remembered by them. However, an enlarged spleen in such a patient is more prone to rupture from blunt trauma than a normal one.

A patient who has sustained multiple injuries has a high likelihood of having an injury to the spleen. In a report on blunt trauma from 1950 to 1960, the spleen was found to be the most commonly injured organ in patients arriving alive at the emergency department.[20] Associated injuries included head injuries (18%), long bone fractures (29%), and rib fractures (37%).[20] Twenty percent of those patients, in addition to the splenic injury, had multiple intraabdominal injuries. In the same report, post mortem examination on patients dead on arrival revealed again that the spleen was the most commonly injured organ. Associated injuries included multiple intraabdominal injuries (40%), head injuries (44%), long bone fractures (45%), and rib fractures (71%).

DIAGNOSIS

The manifestations of the splenic injury can be divided into two distinct categories: (1) the local symptoms of peritoneal irritation in the region of the spleen and (2) the systemic symptoms of acute hemorrhage.

The local manifestations of splenic injury are due to the irritating effect of intraperitoneal blood or adjacent chest and abdominal wall tenderness. Although many signs have been described and attributed to peritoneal irritation secondary to splenic rupture, few have clinical meaning. Fixed dullness in the left flank (Ballance's sign), pain at the top of the left shoulder (Kehr's sign), and pain produced in the neck by pressure over the phrenic nerve (Seagesser's sign) have been of only slight help in diagnosing splenic injury.

Blood per se is a physiological fluid and should be nonirritating. In fact, in the anticoagulated patient intraperitoneal bleeding is not associated with any peritoneal findings, whereas when blood clots it releases many inflammatory enzymes. Thus, if bleeding is rapid, there may be generalized peritoneal signs. If bleeding is slow, all clotting may take place locally, and pain and tenderness be ascribed to rib fractures.

Because the spleen receives 5% of the cardiac output, a laceration through the body of the spleen extending into the splenic pedicle causes continued hemorrhage and results in abdominal distention and shock. A smaller laceration deep into the splenic pulp or capsular avulsion may result in an initial blood loss in the first hour of 500 to 750 ml. If the injury does not involve the major splenic vasculature and is limited to the pulp or capsule, the patient may remain hemodynamically stable. These subclinical hematomas have the potential to expand at a time remote from the injury and account for the phenomenon of "delayed" rupture of the spleen or lead to a chronic splenic cyst.[18]

Peritoneal hemorrhage is usually a diagnosis of exclusion, because overt signs, as indicated, may be absent or attenuated. Assessment of any trauma patient should include a chest x-ray to eliminate the hemithoraces as a significant source of blood loss. Similarly, clinical assessment of the thighs and lower legs will rule out a fracture as the source of hemorrhage. By exclusion, the abdomen then becomes the primary cavity of suspicion for continued blood loss. Thus, serial hematocrits become all important in assessing the patient for ongoing blood loss. In patients with evidence of abdominal trauma, these should be performed every 4 hr. Unexplained, ongoing blood loss then dictates laparotomy.

If the patient is unconscious, paralyzed, uncooperative, has other sources of bleeding, or is lost to physical examination for any reason, peritoneal lavage or an abdominal computed tomography (CT) scan can be helpful (Fig. 13–2). Absolute indications for peritoneal exploration include abdominal tenderness and shock.

Because of the established association between rib fractures and splenic injury, assessment of the possibility of splenic rupture begins with assessment of the integrity of the chest wall. Inspection of the chest wall and abdomen may reveal telltale contusion, abrasion, or penetrating wounds. Posterior penetrating wounds may be overlooked if the patient is not rolled over for complete evaluation. Systematic palpation of the chest wall may exhibit point tenderness over rib fractures. If the patient is able to take a deep breath without discomfort, the likelihood of rib fractures is slight. Conversely, if pleuritic-type pain occurs with respiration and this is referred to the lower ribs, fracture can be assumed despite negative rib x-rays. Furthermore, diaphragmatic irritation secondary to the presence of blood from splenic rupture may closely mimic pleuritic pain. The chest radiograph will be abnormal in as many as half of patients with splenic injury, but none of the findings is specific.[21] In last analysis, diagnosis of splenic injury requires a high degree of suspicion. In doubtful cases, CT scan of the abdomen may provide confirmation.

PREOPERATIVE CARE

Initial resuscitation and evaluation of the acutely injured patient with suspected splenic trauma follows the sequence used for any injured patient. Assuring airway patency and maintaining adequate ventilation are the first priorities. Restoration of intravascular circulating blood volume is the next concern.

The unstable patient requires immediate laparotomy. Blood is not administered to

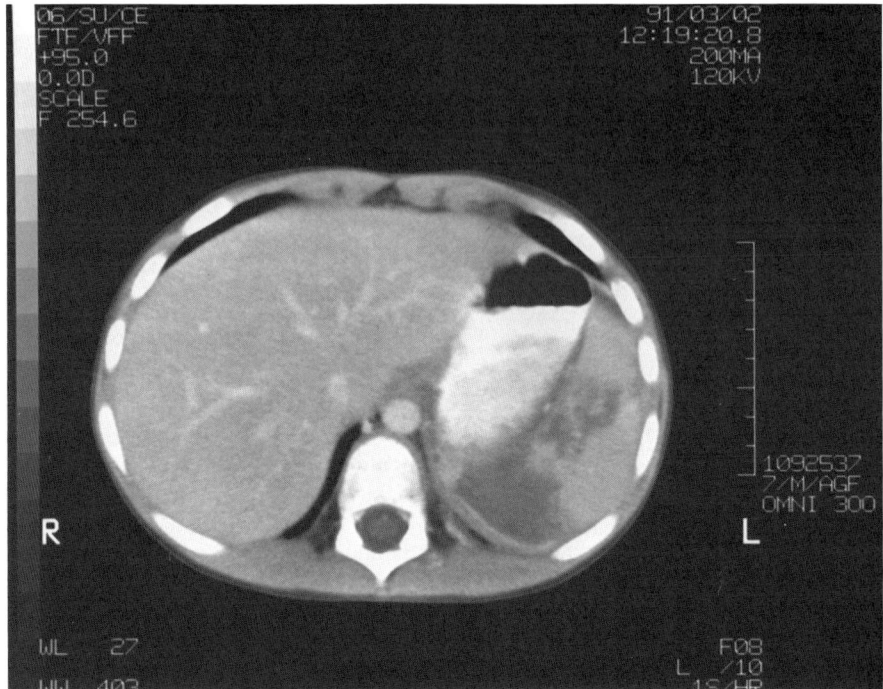

Figure 13–2. CT scan of the spleen. This study demonstrates loss of integrity of the spleen and perisplenic fluid—the combination required for diagnosis.

resuscitate the unstable hypotensive patient. The unstable patient should immediately be transferred to the operating room for definitive control of the ongoing hemorrhage. Blood is given in the operating room where resuscitation, which includes control of hemorrhage as well as volume replacement, can be accomplished.

Most patients with acute blunt splenic trauma will be hemodynamically stable or rapidly stabilized with a relatively small volume of crystalloid infusion. Management of these patients is based primarily on the injury mechanism and age. The stable patient should undergo further evaluation for concomitant injuries, but only so long as he remains stable.

It cannot be overemphasized that overt clinical shock and hypotension do not occur in the overwise healthy adult until the blood volume loss exceeds 30%. This occurs in as many as one-third of patients with acute splenic injury.[22] Delayed recognition of splenic injury is one of the most common causes of preventable death following blunt trauma.

NONOPERATIVE MANAGEMENT

The optimal management of splenic injuries remains controversial. The controversy over operative or nonoperative observation arises because splenectomy, especially in the prepubertal child, carries a small but definite risk of overwhelming postsplenectomy sepsis. Clearly, the spleen should not be removed unnecessarily.

Those who have championed a nonoperative approach recommend operative intervention only if hemodynamic stability cannot be achieved or maintained.[23-28] This approach has been embraced by a significant proportion of those involved in pediatric trauma, and, after diagnosis, further treatment is most often determined by the clinical status of the patient. Patients initially stable hemodynamically are admitted to the intensive care unit for constant observation. The presence of ongoing hemorrhage, as evidenced by a falling hematocrit or an unstable blood pressure, may or may not be managed operatively. In a large percentage of these latter cases, further nonoperative management requires blood transfusions.

Although the safety of blood has improved markedly with the ability to test for non-A, non-B hepatitis and the human immunodeficiency virus,[29-31] transfusion is not risk free and this risk, which is immediate, must be weighed against the risk of overwhelming sepsis should the spleen be removed. Current estimates by blood banking authorities put the risk of death from transfusion at 1:10,000 per unit of blood administered (Table 13–3).[32] These estimates include one of the various forms of viral hepatitis,[33-35] hemolytic transfusion reactions,[36-38] acquired immunodeficiency syndrome (AIDS),[39] and the graft versus host reaction.[40] Moreover, the consequences of these complications, such as chronic hepatitis and AIDS, may not be apparent until decades later.[34,39]

There are also expense and morbidity considerations. Selecting a nonoperative course obliges at least 7 to 14 days of hospitalization, as delayed operations for bleeding occur, on an average, 7 days postinjury. Failed nonoperative management also results in splenectomy four times as often as it does with splenorrhaphy.

From a comprehensive review of 3099 publications in splenectomy literature, Luna and Dellinger calculated the incidence of septic death to be 0.026% in adults and 0.052% in children.[12] He pointed out that a previous estimate of a 1% to 2% incidence of postsplenectomy sepsis appears to be a 10- to 20-fold overestimation of the actual occurrence. The actual incidence, although real, is extremely low.

Even though nonoperative therapy necessitating blood replacement will frequently be successful, the ability to administer transfusions does not substantiate its wisdom. The risks of blood transfusions are significant. Prompt laparotomy and, if absolutely necessary, splenectomy are the safer treatments.[12,41] The belief that spontaneous hemostasis would result in less overall blood loss than operative treatment was first found wrong in 1912 and does not require reconfirmation (see History Section).

The pediatric spleen is easier to mobilize and contains proportionately more smooth muscle and elastica than the adult spleen. The splenic vasculature and the spleen itself are more contractile, enabling easier tamponade or hemorrhage. However, prompt laparotomy

Table 13–3 Blood Transfusion (Mortality Risk 1 Unit Transfusion*)

Hepatitis	1:30,000
Transfusion reaction	1:100,000
AIDS	1:50,000
Host vs. graft	1:20,000
(related donor)	1:400
Total risk approximates	1:10,000

*From Knodell, et al.[32] Reprinted with permission.

will result in quicker and more certain control of bleeding and a much higher rate of splenic salvage and fewer splenectomies.

It has been our experience, as well as others', that attempts to salvage a spleen injured several hours to days previously is less often successful than immediate treatment. The injured spleen is edematous, friable, and congested. It is difficult, if not impossible, to repair. In 80% of children who failed nonoperative therapy, subsequent splenectomy was required.[42]

Another concern with nonoperative management is the lack of definitive evaluation for associated injuries. Trauma-oriented surgeons have documented the importance of the first 60 min after injury and the known increased risks with delays in the management of serious injuries. We and others support a more aggressive diagnostic and operative approach so that all possible injuries are sought.[43–51] A patient with multisystem trauma and potential multiple intraabdominal injuries frequently cannot be distinguished from one with isolated splenic trauma on clinical grounds alone.

There are trivial splenic injuries, superficial lacerations, and capsular tears that are not associated with clinical findings or significant blood loss that can be managed successfully nonoperatively (Table 13–2). However, we believe that all patients with splenic injuries associated with blood loss of a unit or more, whether suspected on clinical grounds, suspected after a positive peritoneal lavage, or suggested by CT, should undergo laparotomy to rule out other associated injuries and to evaluate the spleen itself.[12,52–54] The decision to salvage an injured spleen or to remove it can be made most safely at the time of operation where quantitation of blood loss and assessment of the degree of parenchymal damage can be most safely and accurately accomplished. Exploratory laparotomies do not kill patients. Failure to perform laparotomy and definitively treat injuries is the cause of prolonged morbidity and death in trauma.

OPERATIVE EXPLORATION AND SPLENIC EVALUATION

For rapid access and wide exposure, the midline incision is strongly recommended. Only rarely will transverse or oblique incisions be needed for splenic injuries. The surgeon should always be prepared to extend the midline incision up the sternum or into the left or right chest, if necessary, should other critical problems be found. The chest should therefore always be prepped along with the abdomen before surgery.

After the initial incision has been made (Fig. 13–3A), the surgeon should rule out major vascular injury (see Chapters 19 and 20). After the abdomen is entered, the patient should be eviscerated and blood aspirated from all quadrants of the abdomen, with each quadrant packed to localize bleeding. The presence of clot points to the site of hemorrhage and, with splenic rupture, clot is usually found in the left upper quadrant surrounding the spleen. In the absence of localizing clot, the spleen is probably not injured and may be inadvertently traumatized in an effort to establish that an injury is not present. This is because liquid blood tends to localize in dependent portions of the abdomen, which includes the left subphrenic area.

Once splenic rupture is verified by the presence of clot around the spleen, palpation of the laceration, or visualization of the ongoing hemorrhage, the spleen is mobilized by blunt dissection and the splenophrenic ligament severed posteriorly. With this, the greater

Splenic Injury 239

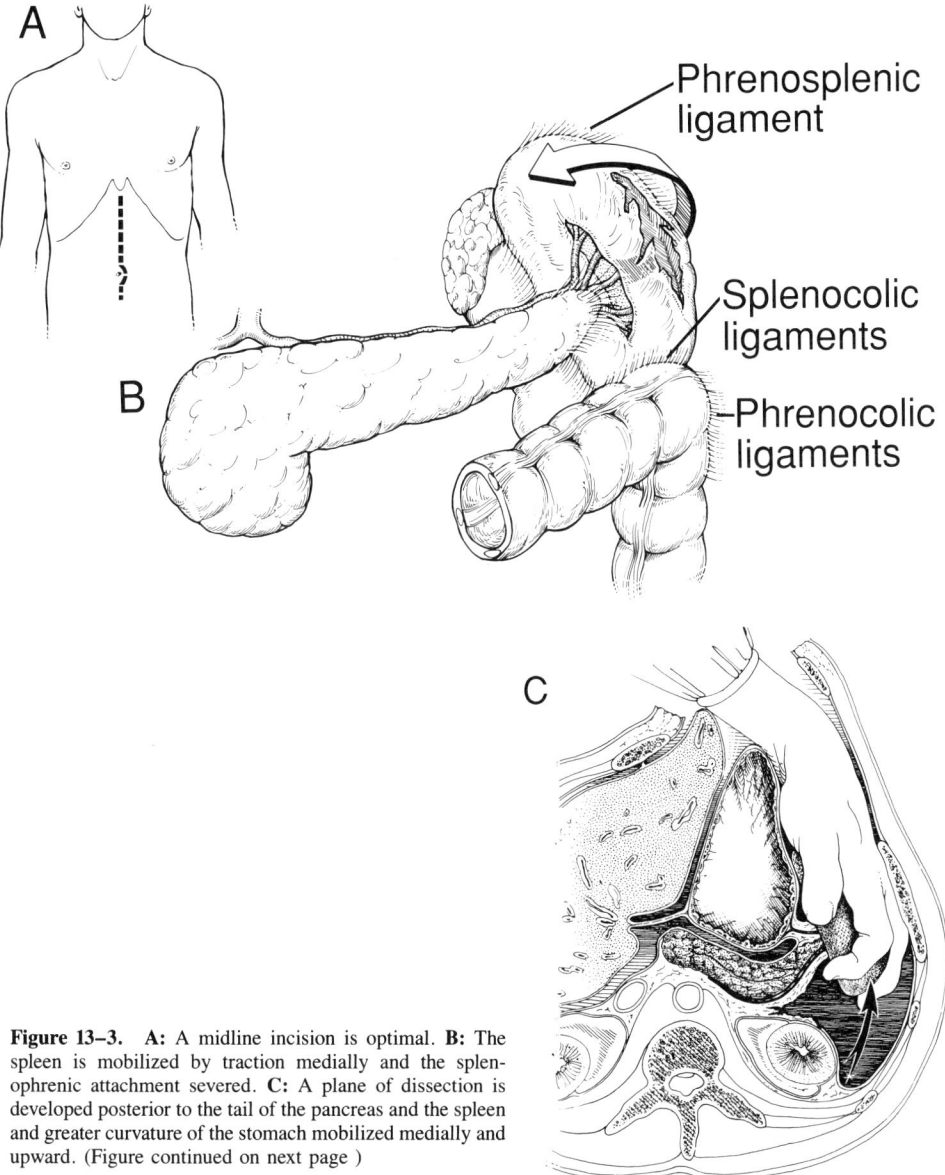

Figure 13–3. **A:** A midline incision is optimal. **B:** The spleen is mobilized by traction medially and the splenophrenic attachment severed. **C:** A plane of dissection is developed posterior to the tail of the pancreas and the spleen and greater curvature of the stomach mobilized medially and upward. (Figure continued on next page.)

curvature of the stomach, the tail of the pancreas, the splenic hilum, and the splenic flexure of the colon can be mobilized medially and into the wound by continued gentle dissection posteriorly (Fig. 13–3B). Severing the lateral attachments of the colon, sharply if necessary, facilitates the exposure. Care should be taken not to injure the pancreas or tear the attachments of the splenic hilum to the greater curvature of the stomach. Exposure and control of splenic hemorrhage is best obtained by full mobilization of the spleen into the

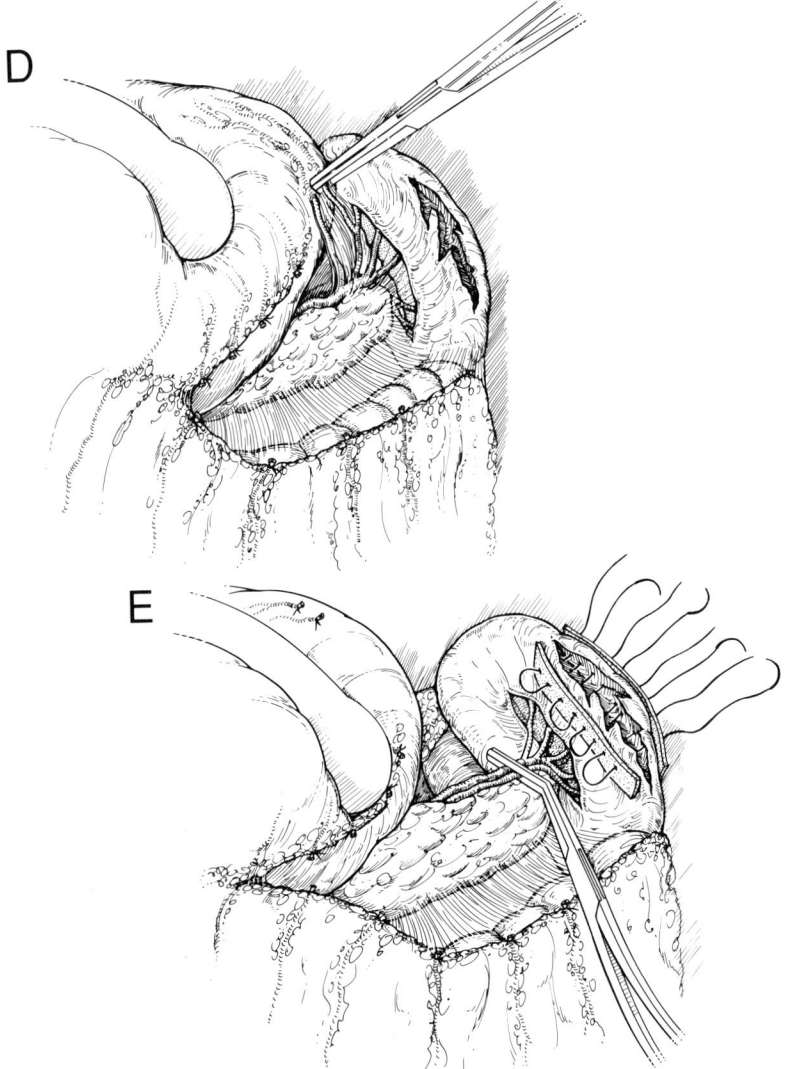

Figure 13–3, cont. **D:** The stomach is mobilized from the spleen by dividing the short gastric vessels and the colon by dividing the splenocolic ligament and the lesser sac entered. **E:** A vascular clamp placed across the splenic hilum provides complete hemostasis for inspection and repair.

midline such that the spleen is in total view of the surgeon. Attempts to control the splenic circulation through the lesser sac or at the hilum before repair or splenectomy are not necessary, for this may aggravate or add to the bleeding.

Splenic injuries vary from small capsular avulsion injuries to the more extensive fragmenting types of injuries. Attempts have been made to classify the severity of splenic trauma; this may or may not be useful.[4] In general, injuries to the costal surface lend themselves to repair more readily than those to the hilar surface. Similarly, horizontal

Table 13–4 Nonoperative Management

1. Minimal or no abdominal findings
2. Hemodynamic stability
3. Minimal laboratory evidence of blood loss
4. Low energy trauma
5. Isolated splenic injury on CT
6. No associated abdominal injuries on CT
7. No hilar involvement/massive disruption on CT

fractures and avulsions of the capsule are easier to control then the larger stellate and fragmenting types of injuries.

Although controversy still exists, there are certain general rules that can now be applied to splenic salvage (Table 13–4). It is prudent to salvage all spleens when possible in both adults and children, particularly if children are below the age of 5 years. Factors that would mitigate against splenic salvage include uncontrollable hemorrhage from the spleen, major hilar avulsion injuries, severe associated injuries requiring considerable time to repair, and fragmenting injuries of such a nature that salvage is impossible.

OPERATIVE TREATMENT

The following guidelines are appropriate for the management of splenic injuries.[13] Using these criteria, approximately one-third of the spleens can be salvaged and two-thirds require splenectomy (Table 13–5). A midline incision is made and the abdominal cavity entered. In the presence of hypovolemic shock or splenic hilar injury, splenectomy is done promptly to control hemorrhage. The spleen should not be salvaged in the multiple organ–injured patient when the time to perform the repair adds to an already lengthy operation or where associated injuries, such as pelvic or femur fracture, can result in ongoing blood loss. If there has been major hemorrhage with more than 2 units of blood in the abdomen, splenectomy is usually indicated.

If blood loss has been less than 500 cc, or bleeding from the spleen has stopped and the conditions described above are not present, the spleen is gently but completely mobilized into the operative field to allow adequate visualization of the entire organ. This is critical to determine accurately the extent and severity of injury.

Table 13–5 Operative Management

OPERATIVE SPLENIC SALVAGE	SPLENECTOMY INDICATED
Blood loss <500 ml (1/3 blood volume in child)	Blood loss >1000 ml
Minimal associated injuries	Associated injuries
No hilar involvement	Hilar involvement
Minimal/moderate splenic disruption	Massive splenic disruption
No coagulopathy	Coagulopathy

A nasogastric tube is passed to decompress the stomach. The spleen is retracted in an anteromedial direction. The lienorenal ligament is incised well away from the lateral margin of the spleen. The sharp dissection is continued across the lienophrenic ligament to the esophagus. With the division of these two ligaments, a plane is developed posterior to the pancreas with blunt finger dissection (Fig. 13–3C). Dissection too close to the spleen can result in avulsion of its posterolateral capsule. The spleen is gradually rotated into the abdominal wound. Resistance inferiorly will necessitate incision of the lienocolic ligament. The splenic artery and vein lie behind the omental bursa. Division of the lienogastric and lienocolic ligaments will be necessary for adequate visualization of the vessel.

With the spleen exposed, the injury can be treated by observation, by packing with microcrystalline collagen or with omentum, by suture of the laceration, by partial splenectomy, or by complete splenectomy. Control of the hilar vessels can be partially obtained manually, the key being to grasp the tail of the pancreas in the thumb and the forefinger. Division of the short gastric vessels between the greater curvature of the stomach and the hilum (Fig. 13–3D) of the spleen facilitates control of bleeding at the hilum. If there is room between the tail of the pancreas and the hilum, a soft vascular clamp (Fogarty type) can be applied to give complete hemostasis (Fig. 13–3E). This is best facilitated by mobilizing and separating the splenic flexure of the colon from the splenic hilum.

Clots are gently removed, actively bleeding vessels ligated or controlled with mattress sutures, and loose, devitalized tissue gently debrided. Minor capsular injuries can be treated with microcrystalline collagen and pressure (Fig. 13–4). Major crushing-type injuries of the spleen are typically encountered in patients presenting with delayed bleeding. Often what is found is a large hematoma involving a deep laceration that when evacuated, leaves an extensive area of denuded, bleeding, raw surface. The spleen can be encased in woven polyglycolic acid mesh. A window is fashioned in the mesh to accommodate the splenic artery and vein (Fig. 13–5A). The spleen is enveloped by approximating the free edges of the mesh with sutures (Fig. 13–5B).

Splenic parenchymal injuries, including those where the hemorrhage has ceased spontaneously, are directly repaired using mattress sutures with buttressing pledgets (Fig. 13–3E). The thicker capsule in children often permits direct suturing (Fig. 13–6) but, in the adult, bolsters are often required. Teflon or Dacron felt or polyglycolic acid mesh can be used for bolsters.

Major splenic fractures may require anatomical resection. Segmental artery ligation produces demarcation at an avascular intersegmental plane (Fig. 13–7A). After identification of the line of resection a vascular clamp placed across the hilum facilitates hemostasis for repair. The ischemic portion of the spleen is then amputated (Fig. 13–7B,C). The cut end of the viable spleen is sutured over pledgets while manual hemostasis is maintained (Fig. 13–7D).

At the completion of splenectomy, it is necessary to recheck the security of the ligatures on the splenic artery and vein. This is best accomplished by locating them in the tail of the pancreas. The greater curvature of the stomach should always be inspected, because this area is the most common source of postoperative bleeding. Frequently, one or two unligated short gastric vessels will be detected, and securing these with ligature and suture insures adequacy of hemostasis. Devascularization of the greater curvature of the stomach is best avoided by meticulous technique rather than by taking gross bites of gastric tissue. In the absence of pancreatic and other associated injuries, the placement of drains is not necessary and may increase the incidence of infection. Irrigation for removal of blood

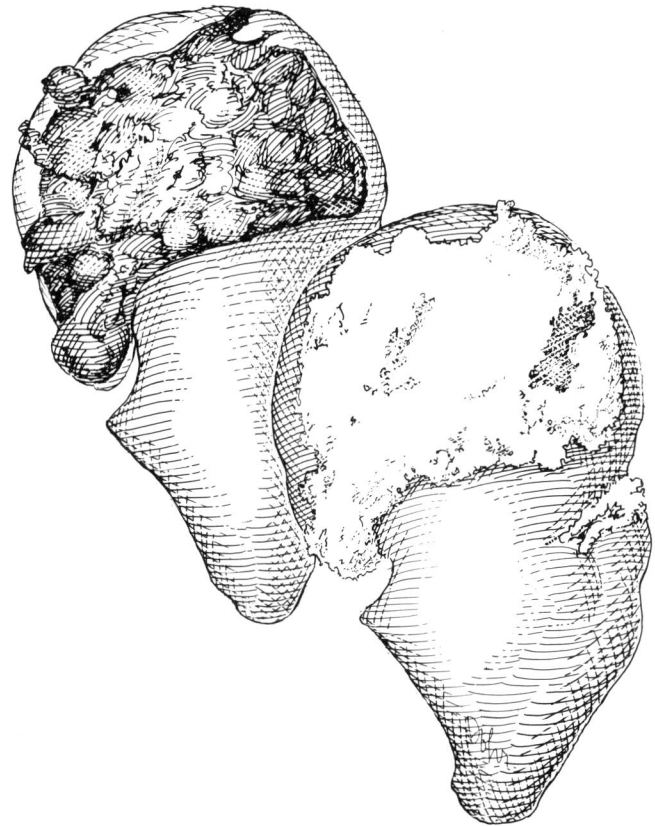

Figure 13–4. Capsular tears or avulsions can be treated with microcrystalline collagen as shown here.

and particulate manner is a useful adjunct. Splenorrhaphy is not complete until hemostasis has been achieved. A "little ooze" at the end of the case is unacceptable. If the spleen continues to ooze slowly after the repair, hemostasis has not been achieved and the repair should be considered unsuccessful and the spleen removed. Meticulously accomplished and using appropriate indications, splenorrhaphy is usually successful. If there is continued blood loss in the postoperative period and the patient's spleen has been repaired, the spleen should be assumed to be the source of blood loss and an immediate reoperation performed.

POSTOPERATIVE CARE

The use of prophylactic antibiotics is probably not warranted in simple noncontaminated injuries but should be used for at least 24 to 48 hr after contaminated and complex injuries. Early mobilization, adequate hydration, and intermittent pneumatic compression are factors that lessen the risk of thrombotic complications. In high-risk cases, heparin anticoagulation may be indicated and started as early as 24 hr postoperatively.

In patients who have undergone splenectomy, the use of polyvalent pneumonococcal

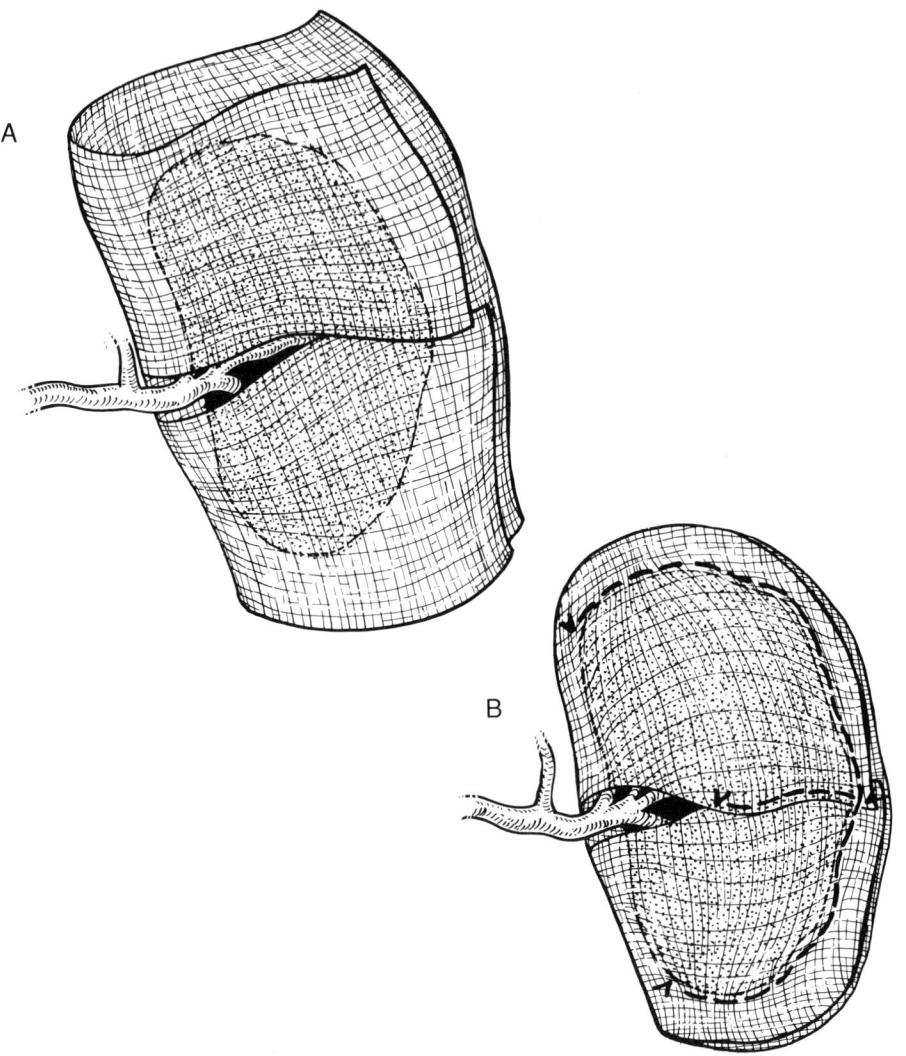

Figure 13–5. **A:** Plastic mesh is slit and laid under the spleen. **B:** The slit and convex surface are sutured so as to compress the spleen.

vaccine is now accepted treatment. However, this vaccine does not encompass all capsule-containing organisms to which the splenic patient is more susceptible and, therefore, does not provide absolute protection against infection. Most reports indicate that susceptibility to infection and overwhelming sepsis lasts for many years. Therefore, in young, susceptible patients, prophylactic, limited spectrum antibiotics such as oral penicillin have been advocated by some. There is universal agreement that the patient should see a physician immediately at the first signs of any upper respiratory illness for antibiotic treatment.

In those patients where splenic salvage has been accomplished, bed rest and inactivity

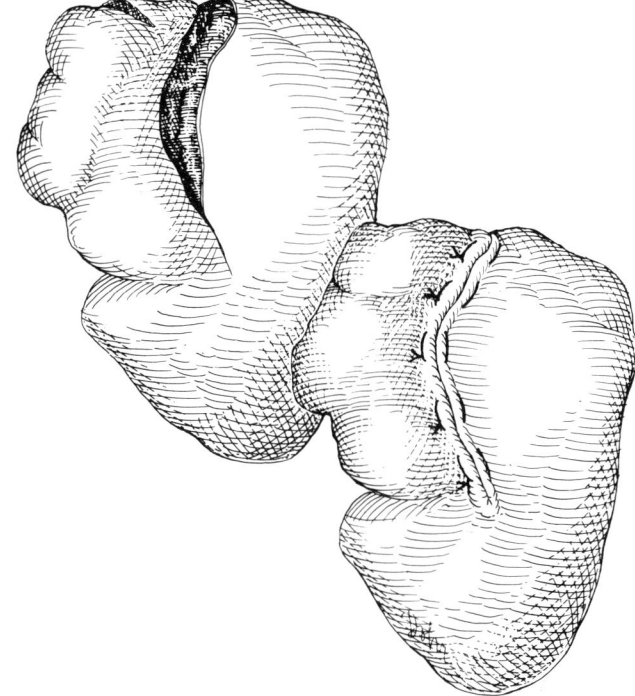

Figure 13–6. Many lacerations of the spleen are amenable to capsular repair using fine monofilament vascular suture.

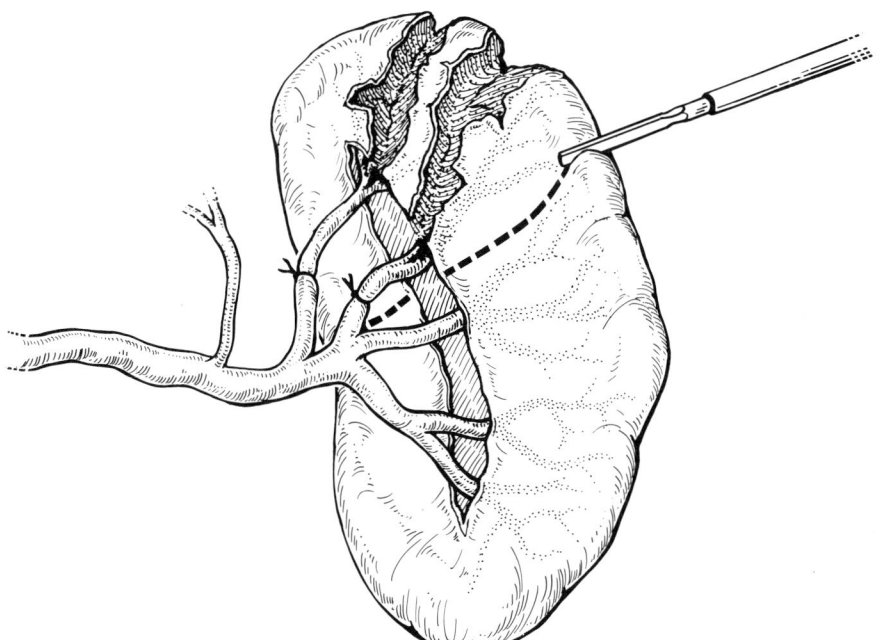

Figure 13–7. **A:** Technique of splenic resection—the remaining hilar branches to the segment to be resected are tied and, using a coagulation unit, the segment resected. (Figure continued on next page)

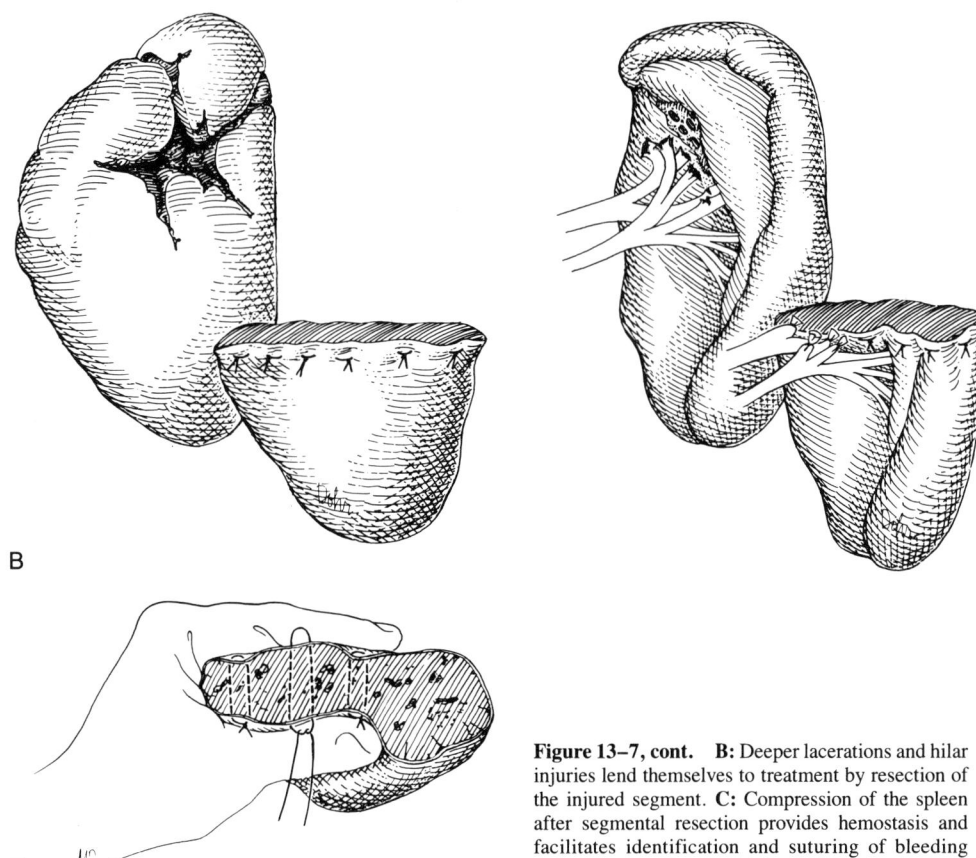

Figure 13-7, cont. B: Deeper lacerations and hilar injuries lend themselves to treatment by resection of the injured segment. **C:** Compression of the spleen after segmental resection provides hemostasis and facilitates identification and suturing of bleeding points and the placement of mattress sutures.

may be a useful adjunct for periods up to 3 weeks after the operation. This may reduce the chances of postoperative hemorrhage and hematoma formation.

COMPLICATIONS

The complications of splenectomy are multiple and are higher than with any other abdominal organ injury (Table 13–6). The most likely initial complication is bleeding from the short gastric vessels, the hilar vessels in the tail of the pancreas, or from the spleen itself in cases of splenorrhaphy. If the patient manifests more than 2 units of ongoing blood loss in the first 24 hr, reoperation should be performed to evaluate and control the source of bleeding. The same aggressive operative approach for postoperative hemorrhage is as appropriate as that for the management of the initial hemorrhage.

Trauma to the pancreas coincident with trauma to the spleen or as a result of splenectomy itself may result in postoperative pancreatitis. If the surgeon is certain that a primary pancreatic duct laceration has not been missed, the treatment is conservative. Pancreatic fistula can occur as late as 7 to 10 days after the initial injury; should morbidity

Table 13-6 Complications of Splenectomy

1. Persistent intraperitoneal bleeding
2. Postoperative pancreatitis
3. Devascularization of the stomach
   Gastric fistula
   Subphrenic abscess
   Peritonitis
4. Thromboembolic complications
   Thrombosis of suprarenal veins
   Thrombosis of deep veins
   Pulmonary embolism
5. Infection
   Acute postoperative
   Catastrophic late
6. Late hemorrhage (splenic salvage)

occur as manifest by fever, impaired diaphragm function, or sepsis, percutaneous catheter drainage or open drainage should be performed.

Rarely, the greater curve of the stomach may be devascularized. This will manifest as a subphrenic abscess or a gastric fistula usually 4 to 7 days after injury. The development of fever, abdominal tenderness, and/or elevation of the white count are the primary initial manifestations. Reoperation is indicated if the problem is suspected. Attempts at direct suture of the stomach are usually unsuccessful, and acceptance of a gastric fistula is necessary. Good posterior drainage should be instituted combined with nasogastric drainage and delayed oral alimentation.

The occurrence of overwhelming postsplenectomy infection has been addressed. More than 80% of cases occur within 2 years of splenectomy. The incidence of left upper quadrant abscess appears much higher after splenic injury than after liver injury, probably because of unsuspected or gastric injury. Splenic abscess can complicate attempts at splenic salvage.[55]

Thromboembolic complications have been a much feared complication of splenectomy. The exact incidence is disputed and difficult to determine. However, we have found in one series that the incidence of thromboembolic complications approached 5%.[56] It is manifest by thrombophlebitis in veins receiving intravenous infusions, clotting in leg veins, or pulmonary manifestations of embolism. Tragic deaths in young patients occasionally have resulted from thromboembolism. In theory, this complication could be prevented by prophylactic anticoagulation, but anticoagulation of the injured postoperative surgical patient is usually contraindicated for at least 24 hr. Less risky forms of prophylaxis consist of intermittent pneumatic leg compression and antiplatelet-aggregating agents such as enteric-coated aspirin or low molecular weight dextran. In high risk patients, the risk of heparin anticoagulation may be acceptable.

Delayed hemorrhage can be a complication of nonoperative treatment of splenic injuries. The sudden onset of bleeding is the result of lysis of a subcapsular clot that had sealed tears in the splenic parenchyma immediately after.[57] In 75% of patients, the hemorrhage occurs within 2 weeks of the injury,[58] but secondary hemorrhage in rare instances can occur months after injury.

REFERENCES

1. Aristotle. *Parts of animals, Book III* (Peck AL, trans). Cambridge, Mass: Harvard University Press; 1955.
2. Sherman R. Perspectives in management of trauma to the spleen: 1978 Presidential Address, American Association for the Surgery of Trauma. *J Trauma.* 1980; 20:1.
3. Reigner O. Ueber einen fall von exstirpation der traumatisach zerrissenen milz. *Berl Klin Wochenschr.* 1893; 30:177.
4. Rosner F. The spleen in the talmud and other early Jewish writing. *Bull Hist Med.* 1972; 46:82–85.
5. Morgenstern L. The surgical inviolability of the spleen: historical evolution of a concept. London: Wellcome Institute of the History of Medicine; 1974:62–68.
6. Morris DH, Bullock SD. The importance of the spleen in resistance to infection. *Ann Surg.* 1919; 70: 513–521.
7. Foster JM Jr, Prey D. Rupture of the spleen: an analysis of twenty cases. *Am J Surg.* 1940; 47:487.
8. Bland-Sutton J. Observation on the surgery of the spleen. *Br J Surg.* 1912; 1:157.
9. Blaisdell FW. In discussion of Olsen WR, Polley TZ. A second look at delayed splenic rupture. *Arch Surg.* 1977; 112:422. Also, American College of Surgeons Trauma Panel 11-22-91.
10. King H, Schumacher HB Jr. Splenic studies number 1 susceptibility to infection after splenectomy is performed in infancy. *Ann Surg.* 1952; 136:239–242.
11. Singer DB. Postsplenectomy sepsis. In: Rosenberg HS, Bolande RP, eds. *Perspectives in Pediatric Pathology.* Chicago: Year Book; 1973:1.
12. Luna GK, Dellinger EP. Non-operative observation therapy for splenic injuries: a safe therapeutic operation? *Am J Surg.* 1987; 153:462–468.
13. Sheldon GF, Croom RD III, Meyer AA. The spleen. In: Sabiston, ed. *Textbook of Surgery.* 14th ed. Philadelphia: WB Saunders; 1991.
14. Trondsen E, Rosseland AR, Moer A, Solheim K. Rupture of the spleen following endoscopic retrograde cholangiopancreatography (ERCP) Case report. *Acta Chir Scand.* 1989; 155(1):75–76.
15. Taylor FC, Frankl HD, Riemer KD. Late presentation of splenic trauma after routine colonoscopy. *Am J Gastroenterol.* 1989; 84(4):442–443.
16. Eichelberger MR, Randolph JG. Progress in pediatric trauma. *World J Surg.* 1985; 9:222–235.
17. Rutkow I. Rupture of the spleen in infectious mononucleosis: a critical review. *Arch Surg.* 1978; 113: 718–720.
18. Hom BL. Rupture of a calcified, non-parasitic splenic cyst after indirect trauma. *J Med Clin, Exp & Theoret.* 1986; 17:241–252.
19. Griffiths JD, Ding JC, Juneja SK, Thomas RJ, Martin JJ. Pathological rapture of the spleen in transforming non-Hodgkin's lymphoma. *Med J Aust.* 1986; 144(3):146–147.
20. Fitzgerald JB, Crawford ES, DeBakey ME. Surgical considerations of nonpenetrating abdominal injuries: an analysis of 200 cases. *Am J Surg.* 1960; 100:22–29.
21. Haertel M, Ryder D. Radiologic investigation of splenic trauma. *Cardiovasc Radiol.* 1979; 2:27.
22. Traub AC, Perry JF Jr. Injuries associated with splenic trauma. *J Trauma.* 1981; 21:840–847.
23. Kakkasseril JS, Stewart D, Cox JA, et al. Changing treatment of pediatric splenic trauma. *Arch Surg.* 1982; 117:758–759.
24. Cohen RC. Blunt splenic trauma in children: a retrospective study of nonoperative management. *Aust Paediatr J.* 1982; 18:211–215.
25. Ein SH, Shandling B, Simpson JS, et al. Nonoperative management of traumatized spleen in children: how and why. *J Pediatr Surg.* 1978; 13:117–119.
26. Howman-Giles R, Gilday DL, Venugopal S. Splenic trauma: nonoperative management and long-term follow-up by scintiscan. *J Pediatr Surg.* 1978; 13:121–126.
27. Douglas GL, Simpson JS. The conservative management of splenic trauma. *J Pediatr Surg.* 1971; 6: 565–570.
28. Eraklin AJ. Spleen and portal circulation. In: Welch KJ, ed. *Complications of Pediatric Surgery.* Philadelphia: WB Saunders; 1982:264–273.
29. Senior JR, Sutnick AI, Goeser E, et al. Reduction of post-transfusion hepatitis by exclusion of Australia antigen from donor blood in an urban public hospital. *Am J Med Sci.* 1974; 267:171–177.
30. Goldfield M, Black HC, Bill J, et al. The consequences of administering blood pretested for HB Ag by third generation techniques: a progress report. *Am J Med Sci.* 1975; 270:335–342.
31. Kuo F, Chou Q, Alter H. An assay for circulating antibodies to a major etiologic virus of non-A, non-B hepatitis. *Science.* 1989; 244:362.
32. Holland P. American Association of Blood Banks, personal communication, 1991.
33. Knodell RG, Conrad ME, Dienstag JL, et al. Etiological spectrum of posttransfusion hepatitis. *Gastroenterology.* 1975; 69:1278–1285.

34. Seeff LB, Wright EC, Zimmerman HJ, et al. Post-transfusion hepatitis, 1973–1975: a Veterans Administration cooperative study. In: Vyas GN, Cohen SN, Schmid R, eds. *Viral Hepatitis*. Philadelphia: Franklin Institute Press; 1978:371–381.
35. Aach RD, Szmuness W, Mosley JW, et al. Serum alanine aminotransferase of donors in relation to the risk of non-A non-B hepatitis in recipients: the transfusion-transmitted virus study. *N Engl J Med*. 1981; 304:989–994.
36. Buntain WL, Gould HR. Splenic trauma in children and techniques of splenic salvage. *World J Surg*. 1985; 9:398–409.
37. Baker RJ, Moinichen SL, Nyhus LM. Transfusion reaction: a reappraisal of surgical incidence and significance. *Ann Surg*. 1969; 169:684–693.
38. McKittrick JE. Banked autologous blood in elective surgery. *Am J Surg*. 1942; 128:137–142.
39. Menitone J. The decreasing risk of transfusion associated with AIDS. *N Engl J Med*. 1989; 321:966.
40. Anderson KC, Goodnough LT, Sayers M. Variation in blood component irradiation practice: implications for prevention of transfusion associated graft versus host disease. *Blood*. 1991; 77:2096.
41. Beal SL, Spisso JM. The risk of splenorrhaphy. *Arch Surg*. 1988; 123:1158–1163.
42. Wesson DE, Filler SG, Ein B, et al. Ruptured spleen-when to operate? *J Pediatr Surg*. 1981; 16:324–326.
43. Eraklis AJ. Spleen and portal circulation. In: Welch KJ, ed. *Complications of Pediatric Surgery*. Philadelphia: WB Saunders; 1982:264–273.
44. Buntain WL, Lynn HB. Splenorrhaphy: changing concepts for the traumatized spleen. *Surgery*. 1979; 86:748–760.
45. Oakes DD. Splenic trauma. *Curr Prob Surg*. 1981; 18:342–404.
46. Morgenstern L, Uyeda RY. Nonoperative management of injuries of the spleen in adults. *Surg Gynecol Obstet*. 1983; 157:513–518.
47. Oakes DD, Charters AC. Changing concepts in the management of splenic trauma. *Surg Gynecol Obstet*. 1984; 153:181–185.
48. Barrett J, Sheaff C, Abuabara S, et al. Splenic preservation in adults after blunt and penetrating trauma. *Am J Surg*. 1983; 145:313–317.
49. Traub AC, Perry JF Jr. Splenic preservation following splenic trauma. *J Trauma*. 1982; 22:496–501.
50. Pachter HL, Hofstetter SR, Spencer FC. Evolving concepts in splenic surgery: splenorrhaphy versus splenectomy and postsplenectomy drainage: experience in 105 patients. *Ann Surg*. 1981; 194:262–269.
51. Millikan JS, Moore EE, Moore GE, et al. Alternatives to splenectomy in adults after trauma: repair, partial resection and reimplantation of splenic tissue. *Am J Surg*. 1982; 144:711–716.
52. Nallathambi MN, Ivantury RR, Wapnir I, Rohman M, Stahl WM. Nonoperative management versus early operation for blunt splenic trauma in adults. *Surg Gynecol Obstet*. 1988; 166:252–257.
53. Barrett J, Feliciano DV, Rypins EB. Letters to the Editor. *Ann Surg*. 1985; 113.
54. Mahon PA, Sutton JE. Nonoperative management of adult splenic injury due to blunt trauma: a warning. *Am J Surg*. 1985; 149:716–720.
55. Shah HR, Cue JI, Boyd CM, Cone JB. Solitary splenic abscess: a new complication of splenic salvage treated by percutaneous drainage. *J Trauma*. 1987; 27(3):337–338.
56. Steele M, Lim RC Jr. Advances in the management of splenic injuries. *Am J Surg*. 1975; 130:159–167.
57. Olsen WR, Polley TZ. A second look at delayed splenic rupture. *Arch Surg*. 1977; 112:422–425.
58. Schwartz SI. Spleen. In: Schwartz SI, ed. *Principles of Surgery*. New York: McGraw-Hill; 1984.

14
The Management of Renal and Ureteral Trauma

PETER R. CARROLL, M.D.
CHRISTOPHER M. DIXON, M.D.
JACK W. McANINCH, M.D.

HISTORY: Ambroise Paré may have been the first to describe a gunshot wound to the kidney.* In his Apology and an Account of His Journeys in Divers' Places *he describes vividly the sieging of the city and chateau of Hesdin. The siege of Emperor Charles was successful and the French surrendered after the accidental explosion of a grenade that burned many soldiers and coincided with the loss of water supplies. Paré, in an attempt to escape torture and death by the Spaniards, disguised himself and accompanied Monsieur de Martigues, who had been wounded. He knew that de Martigues would be held for ransom but he also knew that the wound was fatal. Paré described the wound to his captors, the Spanish surgeons.*

"I commenced to discourse to them how Monsieur de Martigues, looking over the wall to reconnoiter those who were sapping it, received a shot from an arquebus through the body, where presently I was called to dress him. I saw that he cast out blood by his mouth and his wound; moreover, he had difficulty on inspiration and expiration, and cast wind by the said wounds with a whistling, so much that it would blow out a candle; he said he had a very great stabbing pain at the entrance of the wound. I thought and believed that this could be some splinters of bone which pricked the heart when they made their systole and diastole. I put my finger within where I found the entrance of the ball had broken the fourth rib in the middle, and splinters of bone which the said ball had in, and the going forth of it had likewise broken the fifth rib with splinters of bone which had been driven from within, outwards."

He treated the thoracic wound with a tent and dressings containing "yellow of eggs and Venice turpentine, with a little oil of roses." He bled the patient from the basilic vein, and continues his narrative. "Soon after he went to stool, and by his urine and stool evacuated a great quantity of blood." De Martigues grew weak and despite Paré's constant attention became septic.

> "He could lie only on his back, which showed that he had a great quantity of blood diffused in his thorax, which spreading itself along the vertebrae, did not compress the lungs as much as it would lying on his sides or seated. What more shall I say, but that my said Senor de Martigues never had a single hour's rest after he was wounded, and always evacuated bloody urine and stools. These things considered, Monsieur, one can make no other prognosis except that he will die in a few days, to my great grief."

Paré's prognosis was accurate, and despite the treatment of an imposter Spanish surgeon, his patient died a few days later. In retrospect, the patient undoubtedly had a combined wound of the thorax and abdomen with injury to the kidney and colon. Paré did not recognize this; despite his presumed association with Vesalius, he did not understand the anatomy. He described the autopsy as follows:

> "One of the physicians asked which way the blood could pass to be cast out by the urine, being contained in the thorax; I answered him that there was a visible conduit which is the azygos vein, which having nourished all the ribs, its remainder descends under the diaphragm, and on the left side is conjoined with the emulgent vein, which is the way by which the matter of the pleurisy, and pus of empyemas, empties itself manifestly by the urine and stools."*

It was not until 1884 that Weir† recommended nephrectomy for lacerations for contused wounds of the kidney.

Injuries to the ureter are uncommon, yet they were recognized by early wound surgeons and Paré, in his description How to Make Reports, makes the following statement. "When the bladder and ureters are wounded, paine goeth even unto the entralls; departs all about and belonging to the groine are distended, the Urine is bloody that is made, and the same also cometh oftentimes out at the wound."‡ The first successful treatment of an injured ureter was reported by Erichsen¶: "Mr. Stanley has related a remarkable case in which the ureter was ruptured by external violence, and in which the patient recovered; a very large accumulation of fluid forming on the injured side of the abdomen, with considerable circumscribed tumefaction and fluctuation, and which required repeated tapping." Although this success was due to percutaneous drainage of the urinoma, the first successful repair of a ruptured ureter using Van Hook's end-to-side invagination was performed in 1892 by Kelly.**

---

*Packard FR. *The Life and Times of Ambroise Paré*. New York: Paul B Hoeber; 1921:213–222.
†Meade RH. *An Introduction to the History of Surgery*. Philadelphia: WB Saunders; 1968.
‡Keynes G, ed. *The Apology and Treatus of Ambroise Paré*. London: Falcon Educational Books; 1951.
¶Erichsen J. *The Science and Art of Surgery*. Philadelpia: Blanchard and Lea; 1860.
**Leonardo A. *The History of Surgery*. New York: Froben Press; 1943.

RENAL INJURIES

Introduction and Classification

Renal trauma represents the most common genitourinary injury caused by external violence. Renal injuries are usually classified according to their mechanism of injury (blunt or penetrating) and their extent (Fig. 14–1). Major injuries include deep lacerations to the renal corticomedullary junction or into the collecting system. Minor injuries include contusions or superficial lacerations associated with limited retroperitoneal bleeding. Injuries to main or segmental renal arteries and veins are categorized separately because such injuries are more severe and carry a higher likelihood of renal loss and complications.[1]

Approximately 90% of all renal injuries are caused by blunt abdominal trauma resulting from motor vehicle accidents, falls, or personal assault.[2] Most blunt renal injuries are minor, require limited evaluation, and can be managed with surveillance alone. Penetrating renal injuries due to stab or gunshot wounds occur in approximately 6% to 8% of patients who sustain such injuries to the abdomen or flank.[3] In contrast to blunt renal injuries, as many as 70% of penetrating renal injuries can be classified as major or vascular injuries.[4] Patients with penetrating renal injuries require more extensive clinical and radiographic evaluation than do those with blunt renal injuries and often require surgical exploration.

Renal and Perirenal Anatomy

The kidney is a retroperitoneal organ protected by the lower ribs and by several major muscles: the psoas and quadratus lumborum posteriorly, the latissimus dorsi and serratus laterally, and the diaphragm superiorly (Fig. 14–2). The right lobe of the liver and descending colon lie anterior to the right kidney and the duodenum anteromedially. The spleen lies superior and somewhat anterior to the left kidney. The jejunum, pancreas, and stomach lie anteromedially and the splenic flexure of the colon anteriorly. An adrenal gland lies superior and anterior to each kidney.

The renal parenchyma is supported by a tough fibrous capsule, the renal vessels and the renal fascia (Gerota's fascia). The kidneys are surrounded by perirenal adipose tissue and are also enclosed within the renal fascia. Either the renal capsule or renal fascia may contain a hematoma, but when the latter is torn, considerable retroperitoneal bleeding may occur.

A thorough knowledge of vascular anatomy is critical for the trauma surgeon, as it enables confident and expeditious renal exploration and repair. The renal arteries are single vessels in 85% of patients and originate on either side of the abdominal aorta just below the origin of the superior mesenteric artery. The main renal artery divides into four or five segmental arteries.[5] Renal arteries are end arteries, and ligation results in segmental, parenchymal ischemia. The main renal vein is located anterior to the main renal artery. Ligation of segmental veins alone does not result in parenchymal damage, as collateral venous drainage exists. The left renal vein has gonadal and adrenal branches as well as a posterior lumbar branch (commonly).

The retroperitoneum and the region of the kidney may be divided into five compartments.[6] The anterior pararenal space lies between the posterior peritoneum and the anterior

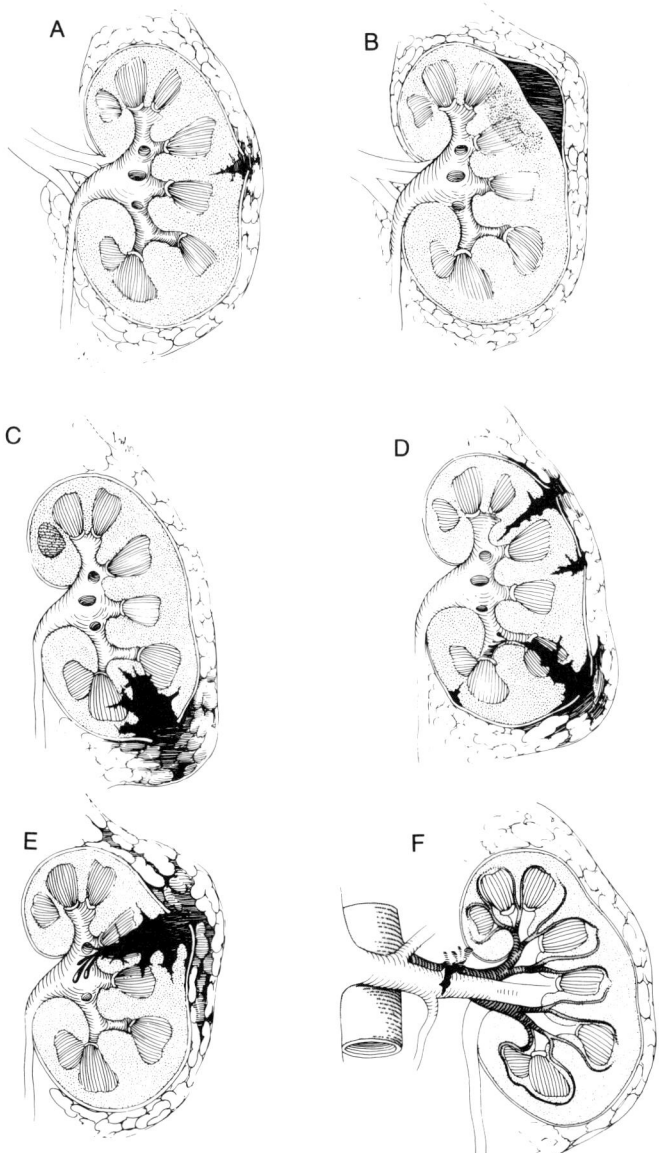

Figure 14–1. Classification of renal injury. **A:** Minor laceration. **B:** Renal contusion. **C:** Major laceration. **D:** Major laceration ("fractured kidney"). **E:** Major laceration (collecting system extension). **F:** Vascular injury.

leaf of Gerota's fascia. Fluid or hematoma in this region usually represents duodenal or pancreatic injury or extensive renal bleeding or urinary extravasation that has penetrated Gerota's fascia. The posterior pararenal space lies between the posterior leaf of Gerota's fascia and the transversalis fascia. Fluid or hematoma accumulation in this region represents injury to either the urinary tract, the spine, the lumbar vessels, or the dorsal vasculature; it may also be an extension of blood from a pelvic injury. Hematoma formation centrally

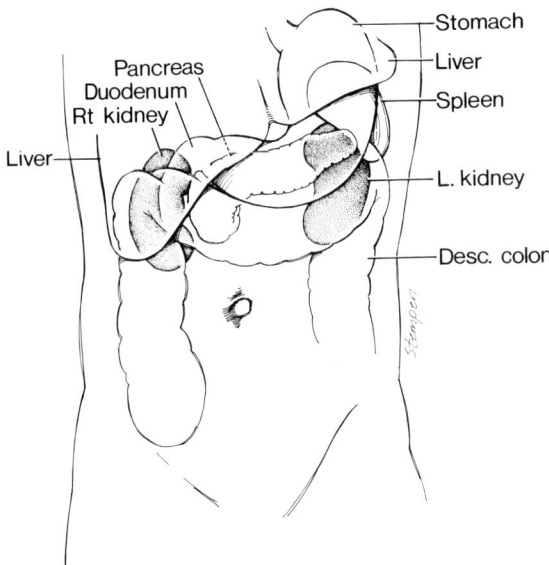

Figure 14–2. Regional anatomy of the kidney. (From Carroll and McAninch.[58] Reprinted with permission.)

most often represents injury to the vena cava or aorta and their branches (the renal artery or vein). Perinephric fluid collections are usually a result of renal or adrenal lacerations and urinary extravasation. Finally, limited renal hemorrhage may be contained by the renal capsule (the subcapsular space).

Detection and Staging

Once renal trauma is detected, its extent must be determined (by staging) (Table 14–1).[7] The staging of renal trauma is a stepwise process that begins with a detailed clinical examination. In selected patients, genitourinary imaging can better define the presence and extent of injury. In a small group of patients, surgical exploration is required to complete the staging process. Accurate staging is of considerable importance, as it allows one to tailor treatment to the extent of renal injury. Patients identified as being at low probability of having sustained major renal injury may be spared the expense and morbidity of radiographic testing. Patients with major renal injury of limited extent, who are hemodynamically stable and who do not require laparotic control of associated injury, may be hospitalized under careful surveillance once careful radiographic staging has determined the extent of their injury. Patients who are found to have extensive injury can undergo a prompt operation to lessen the risk of continued bleeding, secondary surgery, and renal loss.

Clinical staging begins with a careful history, noting the mechanisms of injury, and is followed by a detailed physical examination and limited laboratory testing. Abdominal and flank tenderness are commonly noted, whereas flank ecchymosis and rib fracture are rarer in patients with blunt renal injuries. A palpable flank mass is consistent with significant retroperitoneal bleeding and a major renal or vascular injury. Hematuria is present in most patients with renal injuries. Its degree does not correlate consistently with

Table 14–1 Renal Injury Scale*

GRADE[†]	INJURY DESCRIPTION[‡]	ICD-9[¶]	AIS 85[‖]	AIS 90[**]
I. Contusion	Microscopic or gross hematuria; urologic studies normal			
Hematoma	Subcapsular, nonexpanding without parenchymal laceration	866.01 / 866.11	2	2
II. Hematoma	Nonexpanding perirenal hematoma confined to renal retroperitoneum	866.01 / 866.11	2	2
Laceration	<1.0 cm parenchymal depth of renal cortex without urinary extravasation	866.02 / 866.12	2	2
III. Laceration	>1.0 cm parenchymal depth of renal cortex with collecting system rupture or urinary extravasation	866.02 / 866.12	3	3
IV. Laceration	Parenchymal laceration extending through the renal cortex, medulla, and collecting system		3	4
Vascular	Main renal artery or vein injury with contained hemorrhage		3	4
V. Laceration	Completely shattered kidney	866.03	5	5
Vascular	Avulsion of renal hilum which devascularizes kidney	866.13	5	5

*This classification scheme for acute renal injury has been devised by the Organ Injury Scaling Committee of the American Association for the Surgery of Trauma.
[†]Advance one grade for multiple injuries to the same organ.
[‡]Based on most accurate assessment at autopsy, laparotomy, or radiologic study.
[¶]ICD-9 = ninth edition of the International Classification of Disease.
[‖]AIS 85 = 1985 version of the Abbreviated Injury Score.
[**]AIS 90 = 1990 version of the Abbreviated Injury Score.

the extent of injury. Hematuria may be absent in as many as 40% of patients with renal injuries, including up to 29% of patients with vascular injuries.[8,9] Dipstick urinalysis detects the presence of hematuria but does not seem to predict its extent reliably.[10] Gross hematuria or the presence of shock and microscopic hematuria defines a group of patients with blunt renal injuries who are at increased probability of major renal injury. The likelihood of such injury is approximately 23% in this group of patients.[2,11]

In contrast to blunt renal injuries, penetrating injuries are more likely to be severe. Forty to 60% of such injuries will be classified as major or vascular.[4,12,13] Gunshot wounds are difficult to stage in the basic clinical examination alone, as they are associated with a higher likelihood of associated injury than are stab wounds.[3] Several investigators have managed stab wounds to the flank and back on the basis of clinical examination, wound exploration, and renal imaging.[13–15] However, in our experience the site of the stab wound alone is not a reliable predictor of the extent of renal injury.[4] Therefore, clinical examination must be complemented by radiographic evaluation in all patients with penetrating renal injuries. Such an approach will decrease the incidence of nontherapeutic laparotomy.

Radiographic Staging

Indications for radiographic assessment include pediatric renal injuries, penetrating renal trauma, and blunt renal injuries associated with either gross hematuria or shock and microscopic hematuria.[2,4] These groups of patients are more likely to have incurred major renal injury and cannot be managed on the basis of clinical assessment alone. The objectives of radiographic imaging include injury detection, confirmation of a normal contralateral kidney, and assessment of the extent of renal trauma. Radiographic staging usually begins with an intravenous urogram (IVU) (Fig. 14–3). During initial resuscitation, contrast solution (2 mg/kg for adults) can be injected intravenously, followed by immediate and delayed abdominal radiographs. A hemodynamically stable patient can be transferred to the radiology suite and undergo both urography and nephrotomography, which will improve the staging accuracy of IVU.[16] Although intravenous urography will detect most renal injuries, the films may be inadequate for reliable interpretation.[17-20] Radiographic findings are often nonspecific, showing decreased opacification, irregular cortical margins, or renal displacement. Urinary extravasation and nonfunction, considered to be relatively reliable signs of renal injury, are seen in only 50% and 59% of patients with major renal or renal vascular injuries caused by blunt or penetrating injuries, respectively[4,21] (Fig. 14–4). Additional imaging with computed tomography (CT) is indicated in hemodynamically stable patients who have an indeterminate IVU. CT, readily available at most hospitals, is noninvasive and relatively rapid; it will often detect the presence of associated injury.[22,23] The technique is sensitive and specific and allows selective management of renal injuries (Fig. 14–5).

Arteriography is rarely indicated, as CT will detect renal artery injury.[24,25] Arterial occlusion on CT is manifested as a lack of renal enhancement or excretion, usually in the presence of a normal renal contour, rim enhancement, central hematoma, and abrupt cut-off of an enhancing renal artery (Fig. 14–6). Renal arteriography may be indicated in stable patients with extensive renal lacerations or large retroperitoneal hematomas or in patients

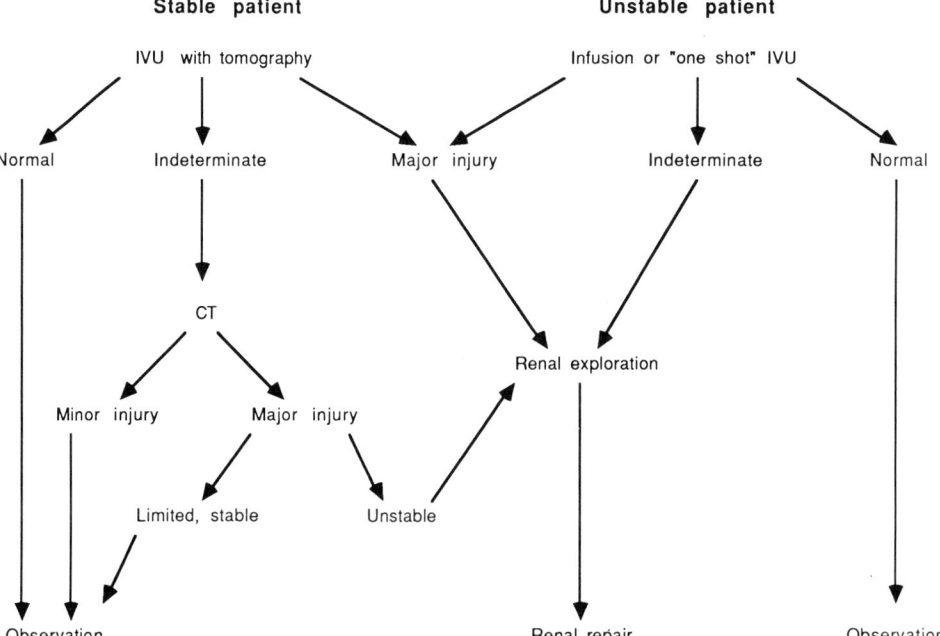

Figure 14–3. Algorithm for radiographic assessment of renal trauma. (From Carroll and McAninch.[7] Reprinted with permission.)

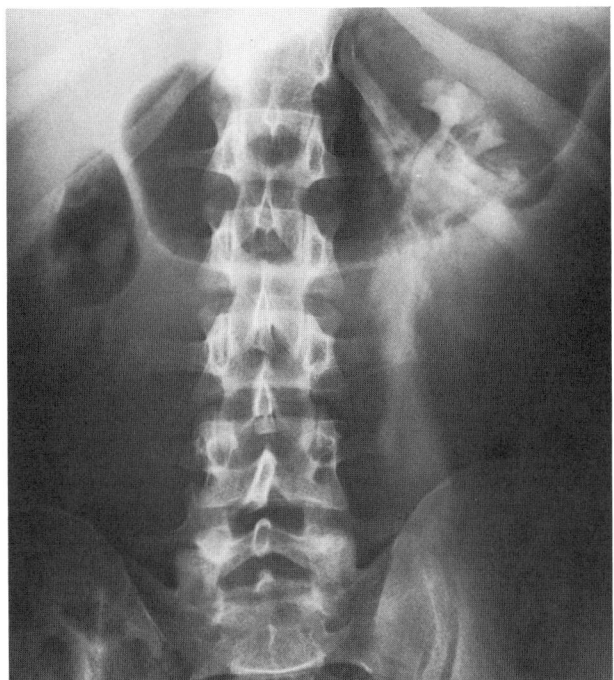

Figure 14-4. Urinary extravasation, after renal trauma, shown on IVU.

with persistent recurrent bleeding after surgery. Patients found to have active arterial bleeding may undergo selective transcatheter embolization.[26,27]

Surgical Staging and Indications for Renal Exploration

Surgical staging is necessary in patients whose injuries are incompletely assessed by clinical or radiographic methods or those in whom these techniques have revealed probable major renal injury. Renal exploration is indicated by an expanding or pulsatile retroperitoneal hematoma.[28] Patients with extensive or persistent urinary extravasation, large segments of nonviable renal tissue, and complete arterial thrombosis are also candidates for renal exploration. Those with minor lacerations or major lacerations associated with limited urinary extravasation or retroperitoneal bleeding who are hemodynamically stable and do not have associated injuries requiring laparotomy are candidates for surveillance alone.

Patients are often transferred to the operating suite for emergency laparotomy due to hemodynamic instability resulting from major abdominal injury. Upon laparotomy, such patients may be discovered to have sustained a renal injury; in this case, if the retroperitoneal hematoma is stable, a limited IVU can be performed in the operating suite.[29] Cases associated with urinary extravasation, nonfunction, or decreased opacification or caliceal distortion should undergo renal exploration.

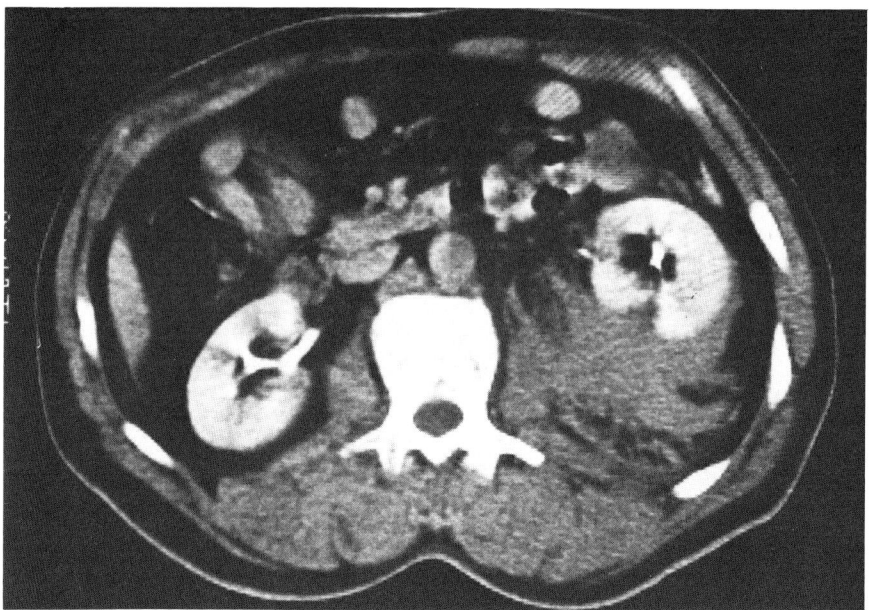

Figure 14-5. CT of a large renal laceration due to blunt abdominal trauma.

Renal Exploration and Reconstructive Techniques

General principles of renal exploration include early vascular control, debridement of nonviable tissue, watertight closure of the renal collecting system, and reapproximation of parenchymal surfaces. With such an orderly approach, renal reconstruction rather than nephrectomy is possible in approximately 78% of patients who undergo renal exploration (Table 14–2).[30] The exact type of reconstructive technique used depends on the mechanism and the site of injury within the kidney.

Renal exploration is best performed through a midline transabdominal incision. This allows for the detection and repair of associated abdominal injuries seen in most patients with renal trauma. The small bowel is positioned superiorly and to the patient's right, exposing the posterior peritoneal surface along the small bowel mesentery. The inferior mesenteric vein is identified, and an incision in the posterior peritoneum is made medial to the vein and over the aorta (Fig. 14–7). Through this incision, either the right or the left renal vasculature can be exposed and controlled. The incision is carried superiorly to the level of the left renal vein as it crosses the aorta. Rarely, the renal vein will be identified posterior to the aorta. The left renal vein is exposed. The left renal artery is identified posteriorly and superiorly to the left renal vein. Medial dissection along the aorta and lateral dissection along the inferior vena cava allows identification of the right renal artery and vein. Soft silicone vessel loops may be placed around the vessels of the injured kidney. Vessel occlusion is usually not necessary at the time of vessel isolation.

Once vascular control has been achieved, the ipsilateral colon can be reflected medially and an incision made along its lateral margin. Any retroperitoneal hematoma can be evacuated and the kidney mobilized, often using blunt dissection alone. If heavy

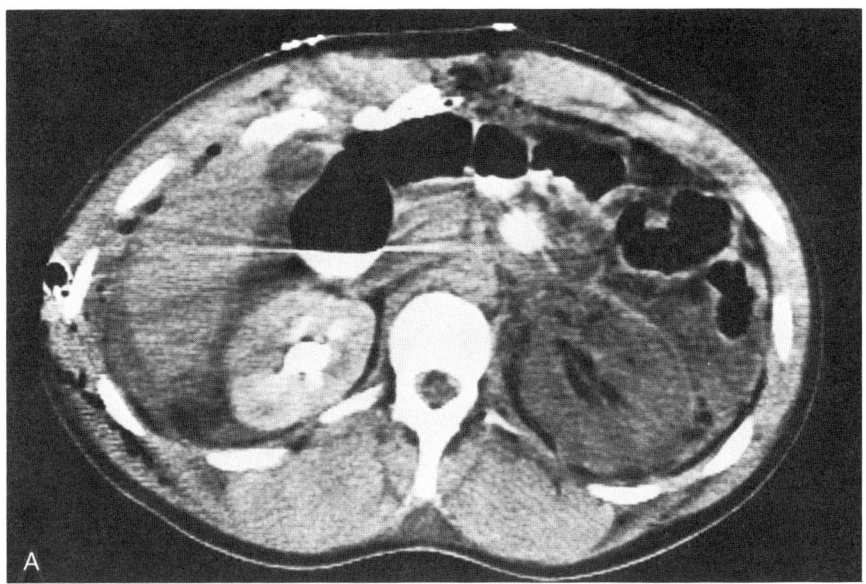

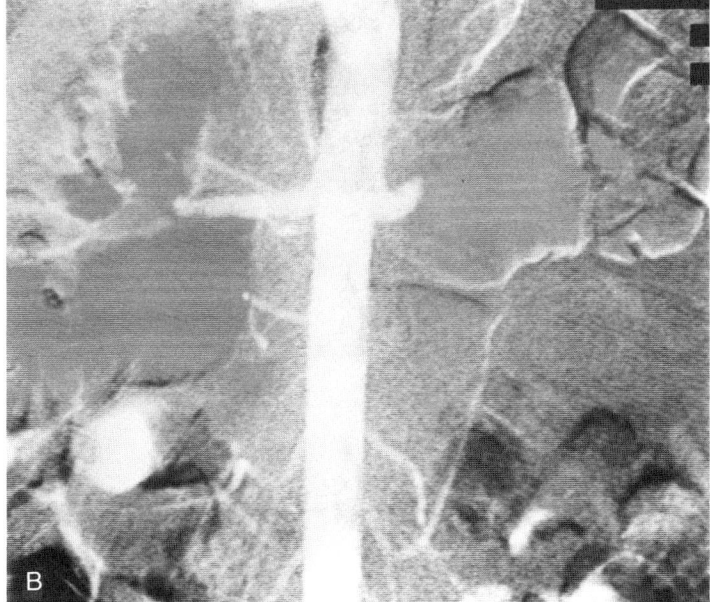

Figure 14–6. **A:** CT showing lack of renal enhancement or excretion as a result of renal artery thrombosis. **B:** Arteriogram showing renal artery thrombosis. (From Carroll and McAninch.[7] Reprinted with permission.)

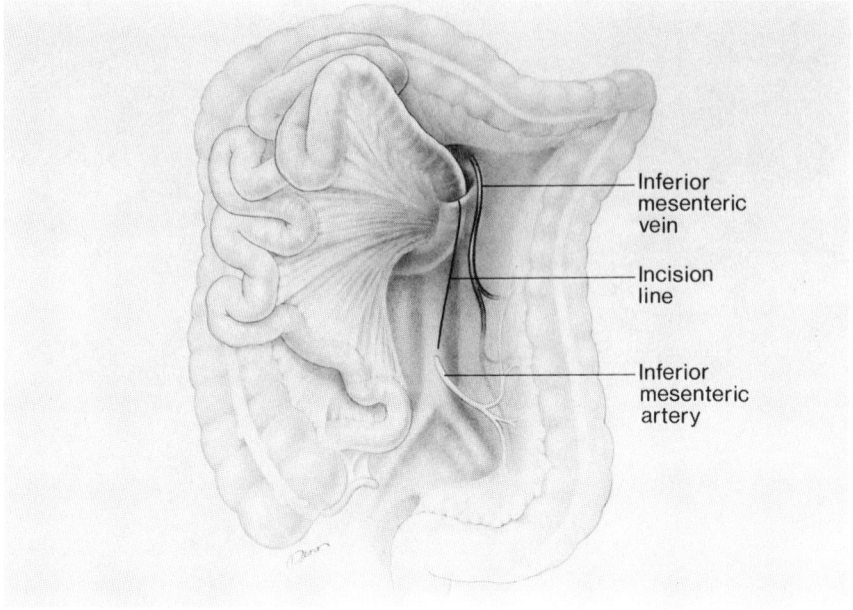

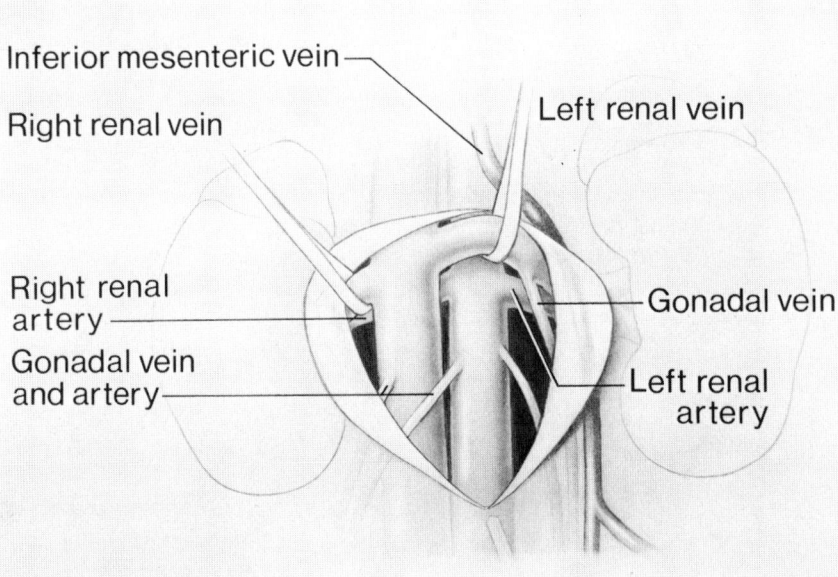

Figure 14–7. Initial approach to the retroperitoneum. **A:** The inferior mesenteric vein is identified, and an incision is made in the posterior peritoneum medial to the vein. **B:** Through this incision, the left and right renal vasculature can be identified.

Table 14-2 Reconstructive Renal Techniques Performed at San Francisco General Hospital

	BLUNT TRAUMA (n = 31) (%)	STAB WOUND (n = 49) (%)	GUNSHOT (n = 53) (%)	TOTAL (n = 133) (%)
Renorrhaphy	11 (35.5)	29 (59.2)	21 (39.6)	61 (45.9)
Partial nephrectomy	4 (12.9)	7 (14.2)	12 (22.7)	23 (17.3)
Nephrectomy	4 (12.9)	4 (8.2)	7 (13.2)	15 (11.3)
Vascular repair only	3 (9.7)	4 (8.2)	4 (7.5)	1 (8.2)
Pelvis repair only	4 (12.9)	1 (2.0)	0	5 (3.7)
Vascular and pelvis only	0	0	1 (1.9)	1 (0.8)
Exploration only	5 (16.1)	4 (8.2)	8 (15.1)	17 (12.8)

From McAninch, et al.[30] Reprinted with permission.

bleeding is encountered, temporary vascular occlusion can be achieved with vascular or Rommel clamps. In approximately 12% of patients, ligation of the renal vasculature is required as part of the nephrectomy. In an additional 12% of patients, temporary occlusion is required for control of renal hemorrhage and renal reconstruction.[31] The time of warm ischemia usually does not exceed 30 min, and renal function is generally well preserved after temporary vascular occlusion and renal reconstruction.

Nephrectomy

Nephrectomy is indicated in those few patients with extensive renal parenchymal or vascular injury not amenable to repair. Such patients are usually severely injured as defined by high transfusion requirement, injury scores, and death and complication rates.[32-34] However, their poor outcome depends more on the extent of associated injury and the development of subsequent multiple organ failure than on the degree of renal injury.

When nephrectomy is indicated, the renal artery should be ligated twice with 2-0 nonabsorbable suture material before ligation of the renal vein. Ligation of the renal vein may be accomplished quickly with 2-0 or 3-0 absorbable suture material or by using a running suture of 5-0 monofilament suture material.

Renorrhaphy

As can be seen in Table 14-2, approximately 45% of patients can be managed with renal debridement and parenchymal reapproximation (renorrhaphy) (Fig. 14-8). Perirenal hematoma should be evacuated and nonviable renal tissue excised. Individual bleeding points can be controlled using figure-eight sutures of 4-0 or 5-0 chromic on a tapered needle. If a collecting system injury is noted, it can be closed using a running suture of 4-0 chromic, ensuring a watertight closure. The closure's adequacy can be tested by occluding the ureter just below the renal pelvis and injecting a small volume of indigo carmine or methylene blue directly into the renal pelvis. The debrided edges of the renal parenchyma can be reapproximated using various methods. If renal capsule is available, interrupted simple or mattress sutures of 2-0 or 3-0 chromic can be placed through the margins of the renal

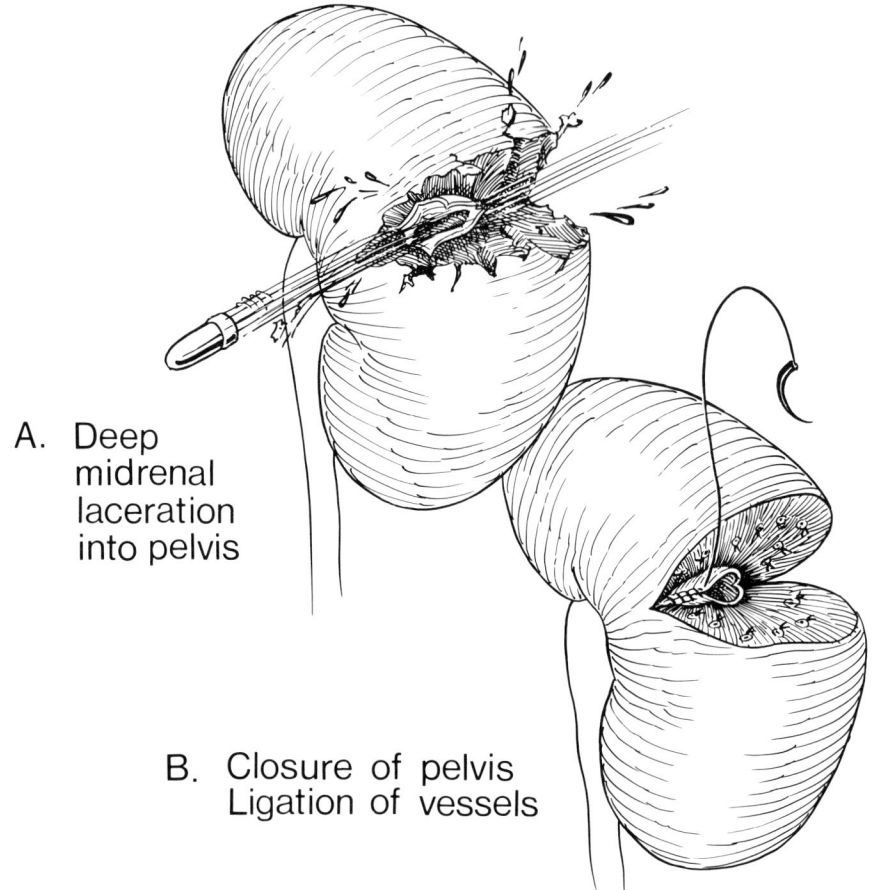

Figure 14–8. Technique of renorrhaphy. **A:** Injury on midportion of kidney. **B:** Debridement, reanastomosis, and closure of the collecting system.

capsule. These sutures can then be tied over bolsters of hemostatic material, vascularized perirenal fat, or omentum. If renal capsule is not available, a pedicle of omentum can be used to cover the parenchymal defect. Rarely, reconstruction will be aided by the use of knitted polyglycolic acid mesh.[35]

Partial Nephrectomy

Partial nephrectomy is most often indicated for deep lacerations of the upper or lower poles of the kidney that result in large sections of devitalized tissue. Evacuation of hematoma, hemostasis, and closure of the collecting system should be performed as described previously (Fig. 14–9). Coverage of the parenchymal defect is particularly important, as the collecting system is often exposed and the parenchymal defect is large. Closure can be carried out using interrupted, capsular sutures placed over bolsters;

The Management of Renal and Ureteral Trauma   263

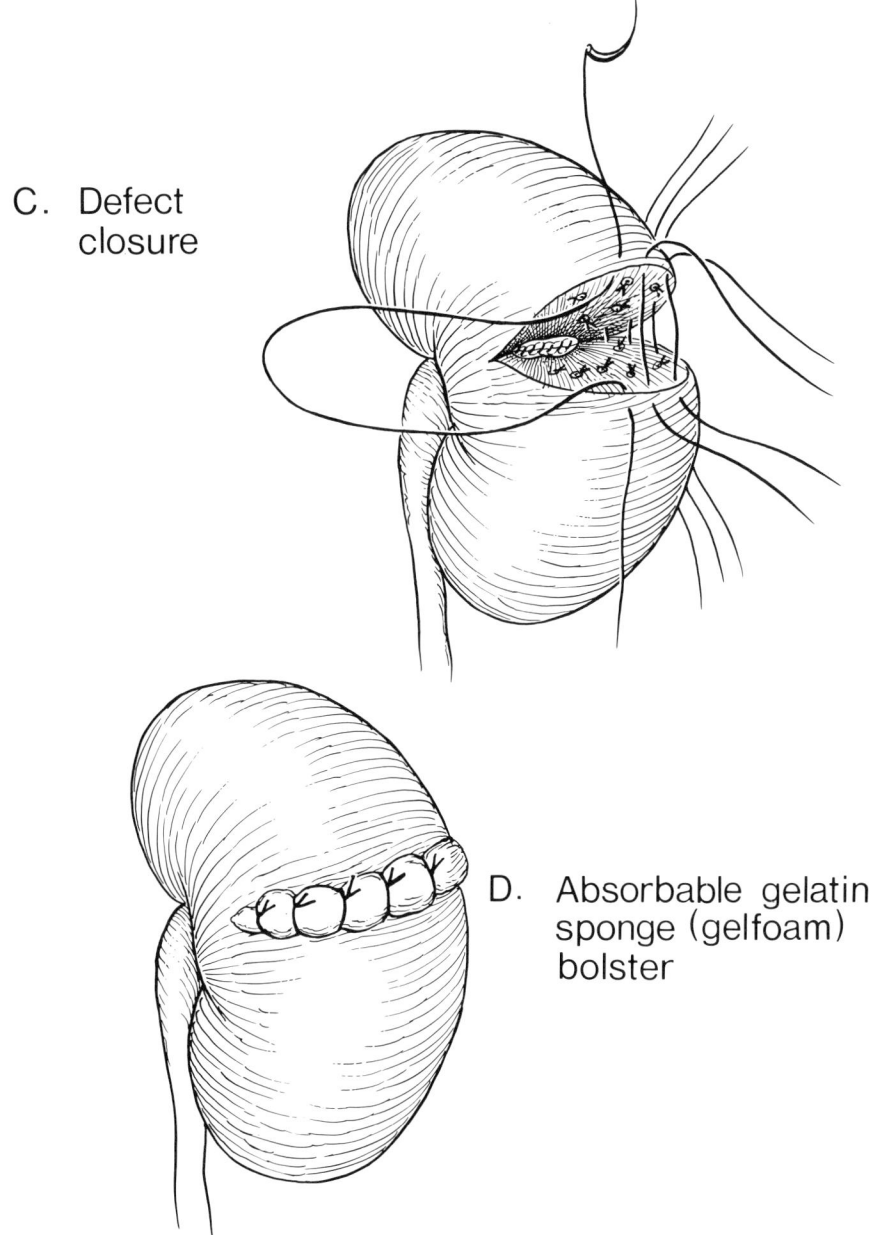

Figure 14–8, cont.   C: Parenchymal edges approximated. D: Capsular sutures placed. (From McAninch.[59] Reprinted with permission.)

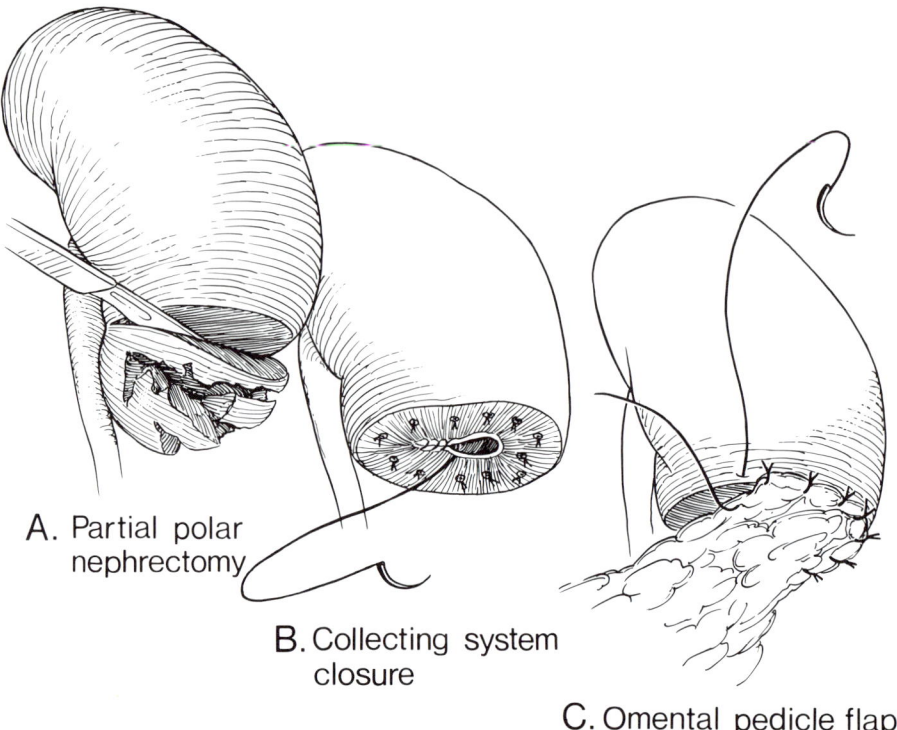

Figure 14–9. Technique of partial nephrectomy. **A:** Sharp removal of nonviable tissue. **B:** Hemostasis obtained and collecting system closed. **C:** Defect covered. (From McAninch.[59] Reprinted with permission.)

however, use of the omentum may be necessary. A pedicle of omentum can be brought through a small incision made in the mesentery of the ipsilateral colon. The omentum can then be sutured in place over the parenchymal defect using interrupted, 3-0 absorbable suture material.

Vascular Injuries

The management of vascular injuries requires special attention as patients with such injuries are at a high risk of renal loss, complications, and death compared to patients with parenchymal injuries alone.[1] Renovascular injuries can occur as a result of both penetrating and blunt abdominal trauma. When caused by blunt trauma, arterial injury may be the result either of rapid deceleration causing stretching of the renal vessel and disruption of the arterial intima or direct trauma to the arterial wall. Injuries to the main renal artery are more likely to require nephrectomy than those to the main vein or segmental vessels (Table 14–3). Segmental arterial injuries can be managed with ligation and excision of devitalized tissue, as previously described. Ligation of segmental veins can be performed, as extensive intrarenal collateral venous drainage exists.

Injuries to the main renal vein are often associated with extensive retroperitoneal bleeding. Because of the shortness of the renal vein on the right and concomitant injury

Table 14–3 Correlation of Type of Vessel Injury,
Outcome, and Extent of Associated Injury

	ARTERY (n = 9) (%)	VEIN (n = 12)* (%)	BOTH (n = 6) (%)	SEGMENTAL VESSELS ONLY (n = 10) (%)
Blunt injury	33	25	33	50
Penetrating injury	67	75	67	50
Transfusion >8950 ml	22	25	83	10
ISS (injury score) >33.3	22	58	67	30
Nephrectomy	56	25	50	0
Creatinine >1.5 mg/dl	56	25	67	0
Major complication	67	50	100	70
Death	0	25	50	10

*Two patients died shortly after arrival in operating room, before repair.
(From Carroll, et al.[1] Reprinted with permission.)

to the vena cava, repair may be difficult. Manual occlusion of the vena cava above and below the renal vein injury will often control bleeding and allow for more precise placement of vascular clamps. Venous lacerations can be closed using running 5-0 monofilament suture material. Complete disruption of the renal vein, most often due to blunt trauma, can be life-threatening, depending on the extent of hemorrhage. Disruption of the left renal vein at the vena cava may be managed with ligation of the renal vein and closure of the vena cava, as left-sided venous runoff is also provided by both gonadal and adrenal branches. If the patient is hemodynamically unstable and reconstruction is difficult, nephrectomy should be considered.

Incomplete injuries to the main renal artery can be repaired with 5-0 monofilament suture material once temporary vascular occlusion has been performed. Complete disruption or arterial thrombosis represents a challenge, as complete restoration of renal function is often difficult to achieve. Attempted repair is indicated in patients with bilateral renal injuries, medical renal disease, and a solitary kidney. Unilateral injury of the main artery associated with a normal contralateral kidney should be considered for repair if the injury is amenable to repair and the kidney is not ischemic. Patients with complete arterial thrombosis associated with renal ischemia or extensive associated injuries may be best served by nephrectomy to avoid the morbidity of extensive surgery, blood loss, and possible postoperative hypertension. Selected patients with complete arterial thrombosis that has been identified preoperatively and is not associated with extensive urinary extravasation or retroperitoneal hemorrhage are candidates for surveillance alone if laparotomy is not indicated for management of associated injuries.

Arterial reconstruction, when indicated, should be performed promptly, as success is related to the timing of revascularization.[36,37] Complete arterial occlusion or disruption requires thrombectomy, debridement, and often segmental excision of the artery.[38,39] Thrombectomy alone, without excision of damaged arterial wall, may lead to recurrent thrombosis. End-to-end reanastomosis of the artery should be considered if it can be performed without tension. If end-to-end reanastomosis is impossible, use of the saphenous vein or a prostatic graft should be considered. Successful use of the inferior mesenteric, hypogastric, or splenic artery and autotransplantation have been reported.[39,40]

Postoperative Care and Complications

Postoperative care of the patient with renal trauma is similar to that of any patient who has undergone major abdominal surgery. The urethral catheter should be removed when the urine has become clear of gross blood. Postoperative drainage of the retroperitoneal space is usually unnecessary but should be considered when there has been extensive repair of the urinary collecting system or when fecal spillage has occurred. Nephrostomy drainage or ureteral stents usually are unnecessary in the absence of renal pelvic or ureteral lacerations. Retroperitoneal drains, when used, can usually be removed within 48 hr. The nature of the drainage, whether urine or lymphatic or peritoneal fluid, can be determined by measuring the fluid's creatinine content. Drainage should continue until urinary extravasation has resolved. Rarely, continued urinary extravasation will require placement of a ureteral stent to facilitate normal renal drainage. The anatomic renal configuration or renal function should be assessed within 3 weeks after repair with IVU, CT, or radionuclide scanning.

Major complications sometimes occur in patients who have sustained major renal injuries,[41] but most often result from associated injury and the development of sepsis or associated organ failure rather than from the renal injury or the method of its repair.[32] Complications resulting from the renal injury or the method of repair occur in less than 10% of patients.[32] Early complications include delayed renal bleeding, persistent urinary extravasation, and perinephric abscess formation. Delayed complications include arteriovenous fistula formation and hypertension, which is uncommon but may occur early or several years after injury and repair.

URETERAL INJURIES

Introduction and Ureteral Anatomy

Ureteral and renal pelvic injuries caused by external violence are rare and account for less than 1% of all urologic trauma. The ureter is divided anatomically into upper, middle, and lower segments. However, for practical purposes, it can be divided into two segments of approximately equal length: the abdominal ureter and the pelvic ureter. The abdominal ureter originates from the renal pelvis and extends along the anterior surface of the psoas muscle. As the ureter descends, it adheres to the posterior peritoneum. Upon entering the pelvis, the ureter crosses the iliac artery at the junction of the internal and external iliac arteries. It then descends posteriorly and inferiorly along the curvature of the pelvis and crosses under the superior vesical artery before entering the bladder. In women, the pelvic ureter lies in the uterosacral ligament and descends inferiorly in a portion of the broad ligament.

The ureteral blood supply is variable and is derived from the aorta, renal, gonadal, iliac, uterine, middle hemorrhoidal, vaginal, and superior vesical arteries. Generally, the abdominal ureter receives blood from branches of the renal artery superiorly and from the aorta medially. The pelvic ureter receives its blood laterally from branches of the iliac arteries. The abundant blood supply to the ureter allows it to be mobilized, transected, and reconstructed safely. However, as the ureter's blood supply courses through its adventitial layers, the surgeon should avoid dissection into this layer as it may lead to ischemic injury.

Mechanisms of Injury

Most ureteral injuries are caused by penetrating trauma.[42-44] Blunt trauma is a rare cause of ureteral injury. These rare cases generally occur in the pediatric age group, are secondary to rapid deceleration, and result in avulsion of the ureter at the ureteropelvic junction.[45,46] Iatrogenic injuries also occur infrequently. Most such injuries occur during gynecologic or colorectal surgery and are localized to the lower ureter.[47,48] Although there are varied mechanisms of ureteral injury, such injuries can be classified as to whether they result in ligation, crush injury, transection (partial and complete), or ischemic injury.

Detection and Staging

Immediate recognition of ureteral injuries is important, as delayed recognition will often result in nephrectomy rather than ureteral repair.[49] The diagnosis of ureteral injury may be difficult as, unlike many other organ injuries, ureteral injuries often present without characteristic clinical signs. A high index of suspicion, rather than characteristic clinical signs or imaging, often allows the surgeon to make the correct diagnosis. Although hematuria of some degree is common in patients with ureteral injuries, hematuria may be absent in 23% to 31% of such patients.[43,44,50,51] Intravenous urography is indicated in any patient with a penetrating injury that has occurred in close proximity to the ureter. Although IVU is generally considered to be sensitive, it may be nonspecific, showing delayed excretion rather than urinary extravasation (Fig. 14-10).[44,52-54] Opacification of the ureter may be poor, as excretion of contrast may be delayed owing to hypotension or concomitant renal injury. In addition, a limited IVU is often performed because of the extent of associated injury and the need for prompt surgical exploration. However, such limited studies are useful in that they establish the presence of a normal contralateral kidney and may localize the side or site of ureteral injury. Retrograde pyelography is perhaps the most sensitive imaging technique for the detection of ureteral injuries. However, many patients will require prompt surgical intervention before such a procedure can be performed. The exact sensitivity of CT for detection of ureteral injuries is unknown, but, like IVU, detection may be limited because of poor opacification of the ureter (Fig. 14-11).

Direct inspection of the ureter will be necessary in those patients determined to have an injury using imaging studies, in those patients in whom imaging is nondiagnostic, and in those patients who could not undergo complete preoperative assessment because of the extent of associated injury. Intraoperative recognition of urinary collecting system injury may be facilitated by intravenous injection of methylene blue or indigo carmine (although this may be unreliable if renal perfusion is decreased because of systemic hypotension or ipsilateral renal injury). In hypotensive patients, methylene blue or indigo blue may be injected directly into the ureter with a 25-gauge needle to assess ureteral integrity. The ureter should be inspected carefully, especially in those patients who have sustained gunshot injuries. Such injuries may result in severe ureteral contusion. In some cases, the ureter may appear to be minimally damaged at the time of intraoperative inspection.[55] However, delayed necrosis of the ureteral wall and urinary extravasation may occur several days after the injury. If a ureter appears severely contused, a segmental resection with debridement and uretero-ureterostomy should be performed. In cases of lesser degrees of ureteral contusion, ureteral stenting alone may suffice.

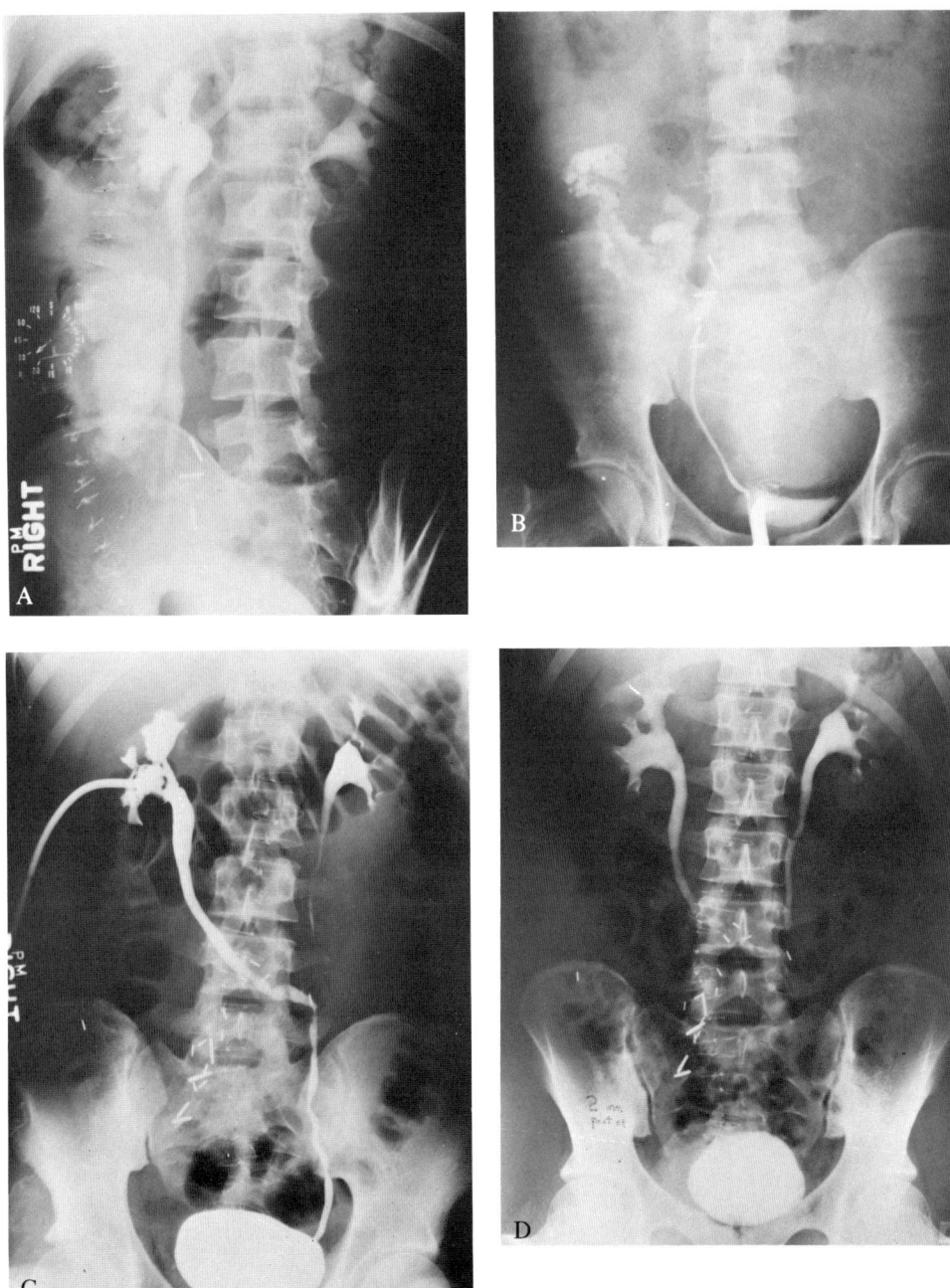

Figure 14–10. **A:** IVU after gunshot wound to right midureter in a 20-year-old man. Mild hydronephrosis with extravasation is noted. **B:** Retrograde pyelogram shows site of injury with extravasation. **C:** Ten days after right-to-left transuretero-ureterostomy showing excellent drainage through the anastomosis. **D:** IVU performed 2 months after repair showing normal excretion of contrast bilaterally.

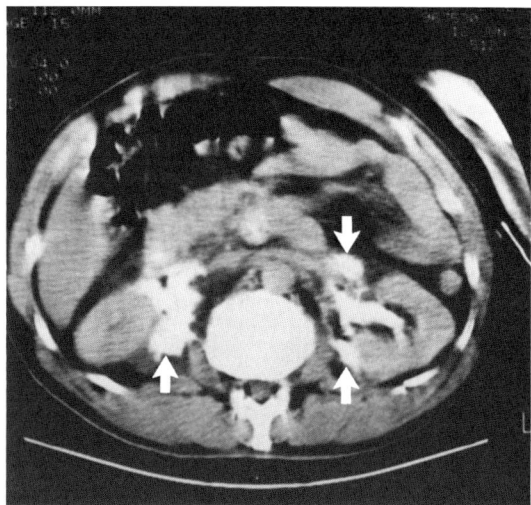

Figure 14–11. Abdominal CT scan of patient who suffered bilateral ureteral injury after a 40-foot fall. Extensive extravasation is noted in the region of the ureteropelvic junction bilaterally (*arrows*). (From Presti, et al.[44] Reprinted with permission.)

Exploration and Exposure

Owing to the high probability of concomitant associated organ injury, ureteral injury should be approached through a midline, transabdominal incision as previously described. Timing is important in the evaluation of ureteral injuries. Immediate recognition provides the best opportunity for successful repair. Treatment of those injuries that were recognized late should be individualized. If the injury is recognized within 10 to 14 days and no infection, abscess, or urinoma exists, immediate reexploration with subsequent repair is indicated. However, many such injuries are associated with urinary extravasation, abscess formation, and hydronephrosis. In these patients, proximal urinary drainage with a percutaneous nephrostomy is indicated initially. Reconstruction should be delayed for 6 to 8 weeks. Injuries that were recognized late are most often explored through an extraperitoneal approach to minimize peritoneal infection.

The left ureter is best approached by incising the retroperitoneum lateral to the left colon and mobilizing the colon medially. The ureter is most easily identified in its midportion as it crosses the common iliac vessels. Once identified, superior and inferior dissection can be performed. In most instances, it is safer to identify the normal ureter above or below the area of injury rather than to dissect into the area of damage. Hematoma and heavy bleeding may complicate exposure and identification of the ureter. An attempt should be made to minimize extensive mobilization of the ureter in order to preserve its blood supply maximally.

The right ureter is approached by incising the retroperitoneum over the common iliac vessels. Mobilization of the cecum and the right colon medially will provide for additional exposure of the abdominal ureter.

Reconstructive Techniques

Repair of ureteral injuries depends on many factors including the time of diagnosis, the type and position of injury, and the presence of any associated medical or surgical illnesses.

General principles of ureteral repair include debridement of nonviable tissue, a tension-free spatulated anastomosis, watertight closure, precise mucosal approximation, ureteral stenting in most cases, coverage of the repair with fat or omentum, and retroperitoneal drainage.[52,56]

Partial transections can often be managed by primary closure with interrupted 4-0 or 5-0 absorbable sutures. Complete transections or ischemic injuries of the abdominal ureter can usually be repaired by resection of the injured segment followed by ureteroureterostomy with interrupted sutures (Fig. 14–12). Complete debridement should be performed until bleeding ureteral tissue is identified. Spatulation of the distal and proximal ends of the ureter will enlarge the lumen size and minimize contracture during healing. Precise mucosal approximation should be performed using interrupted or running 4-0 or 5-0 absorbable suture material. All ureteral repairs should be drained extraperitoneally.

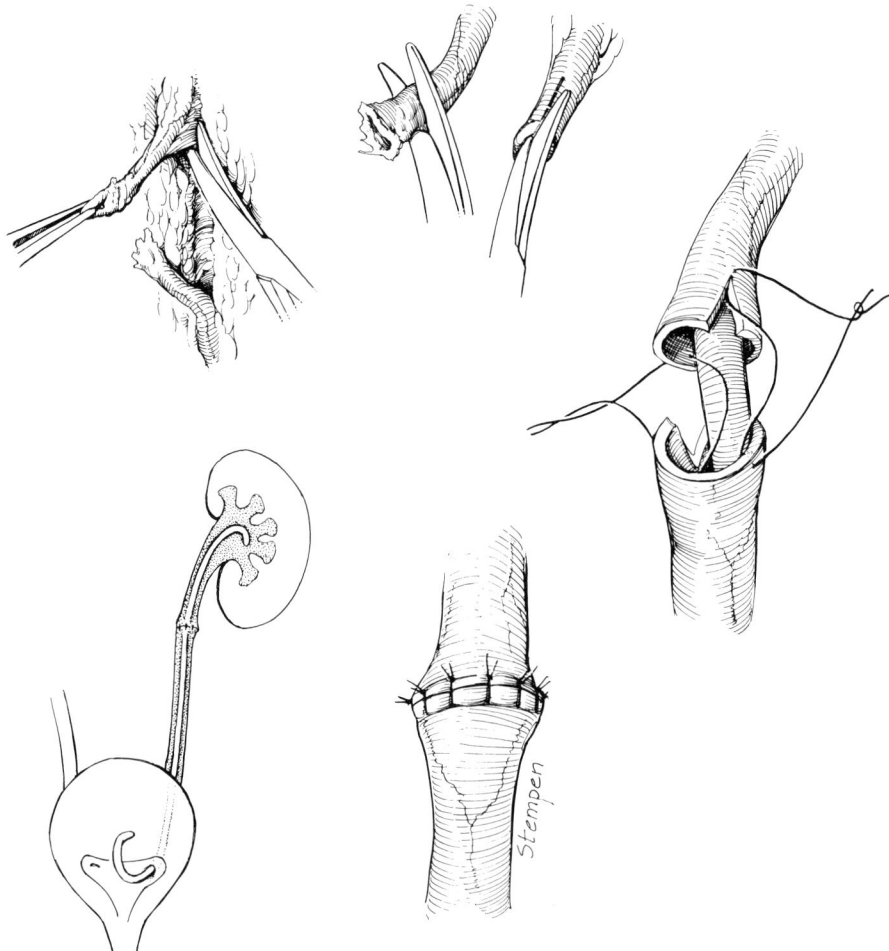

Figure 14–12. Spatulation of ureteral ends before uretero-ureterostomy over an internal ureteral stent. Precise mucosal approximation in the watertight closure is performed. (From Presti and Carroll.[56] Reprinted with permission.)

In patients with concomitant infection, the repair may be further isolated with fat or omentum. All complete and most partial transections should be stented, if possible. This can be achieved using a variety of catheters including standard ureteral catheters, pediatric feeding tubes, or "double-J" stents. Double-J ureteral stents are composed of inert polymers that minimize precipitation of urinary crystals and mucoproteins. These stents are available in a variety of diameters and lengths. Generally, 7 or 8 F stents should be used. These stents are passed over an angiographic guide wire. The stent is directed to the renal pelvis and bladder using the guide wire. Once a wire is removed, the tips of the stent will coil to prevent migration (Fig. 14–12).

Transuretero-ureterostomy can be used in cases of loss of long segments of the mid- and lower ureter. The opposite ureter is identified and exposed with as little manipulation as possible. A 1.5-cm ureterotomy is made in the contralateral ureter, while an equidistant spatulation is done on the anastomotic end of the injured ureter (Fig. 14–13). The anastomosis is completed using running or interrupted 5-0 absorbable sutures. Renal autotransplantation offers a solution for renal salvage when long ureteral segments are lost and no other technique is acceptable. Replacement of the ureter with ileum is possible, but rarely indicated because of the extent of associated injury, the possibility of metabolic abnormalities, and the fact that better reconstructive techniques exist. Complete transection or extensive ischemic injury of the pelvic ureter is often managed by direct ureteral reimplantation (Fig. 14–14). The ureter is brought to the posterior bladder wall in a position medial to the original ureteral hiatus. A submucosal tunnel, sufficiently long to avoid reflux (a ratio of length to diameter of 3 to 1) should be developed carefully. The ureter is brought through the submucosal tunnel and is then spatulated and sutured to the bladder with interrupted 4-0 or 5-0 polyglycolic suture material. The mucosal defect at the site

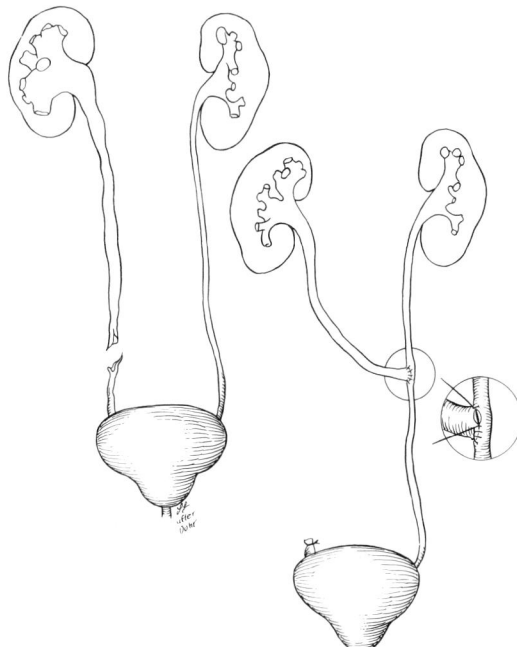

Figure 14–13. Technique of transuretero-ureterostomy.

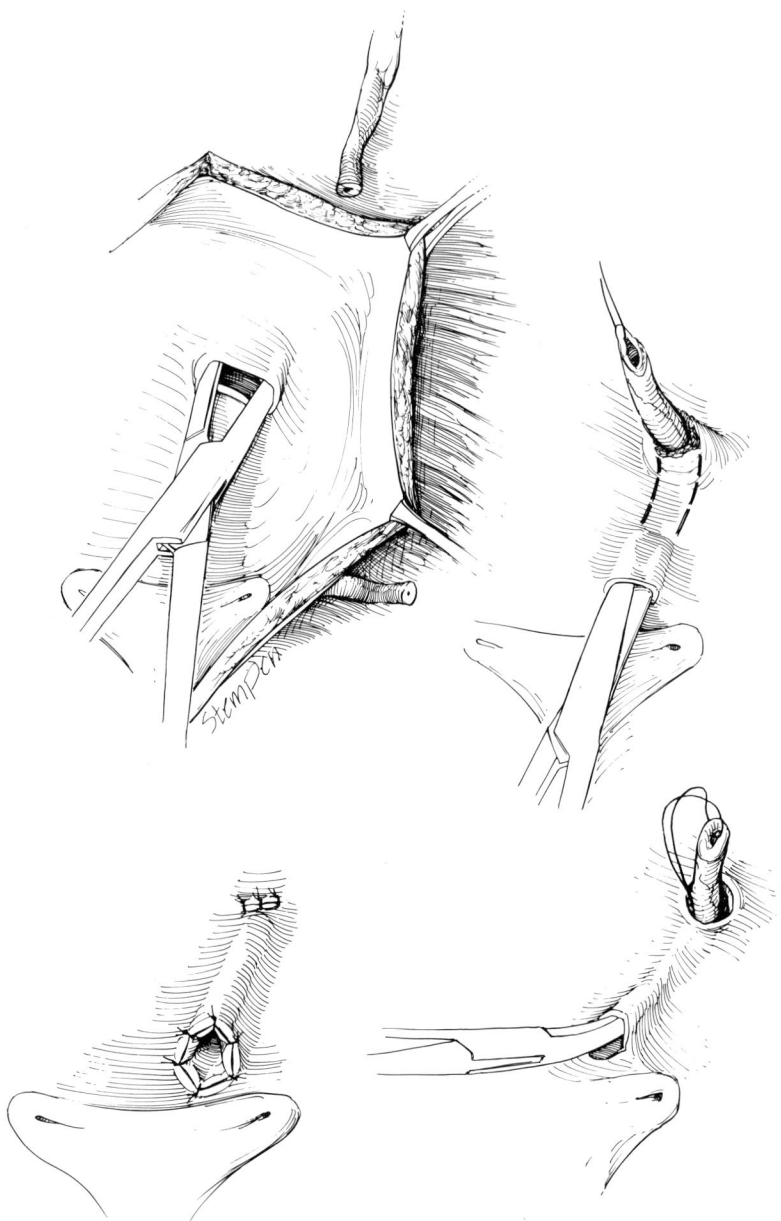

Figure 14–14. Technique of ureteral implantation after ureteral injury. (From Presti and Carroll.[56] Reprinted with permission.)

of entry of the ureter into the bladder should be closed with interrupted 4-0 polyglycolic sutures. The ureter should be stented with a double-J catheter or pediatric feeding tube. The cystotomy may be closed in two layers: the mucosa with running suture and the muscularis with interrupted sutures. Drains should be placed posteriorly at the site of the ureteral hiatus and anteriorly by the cystotomy. Catheter drainage of the bladder should be maintained

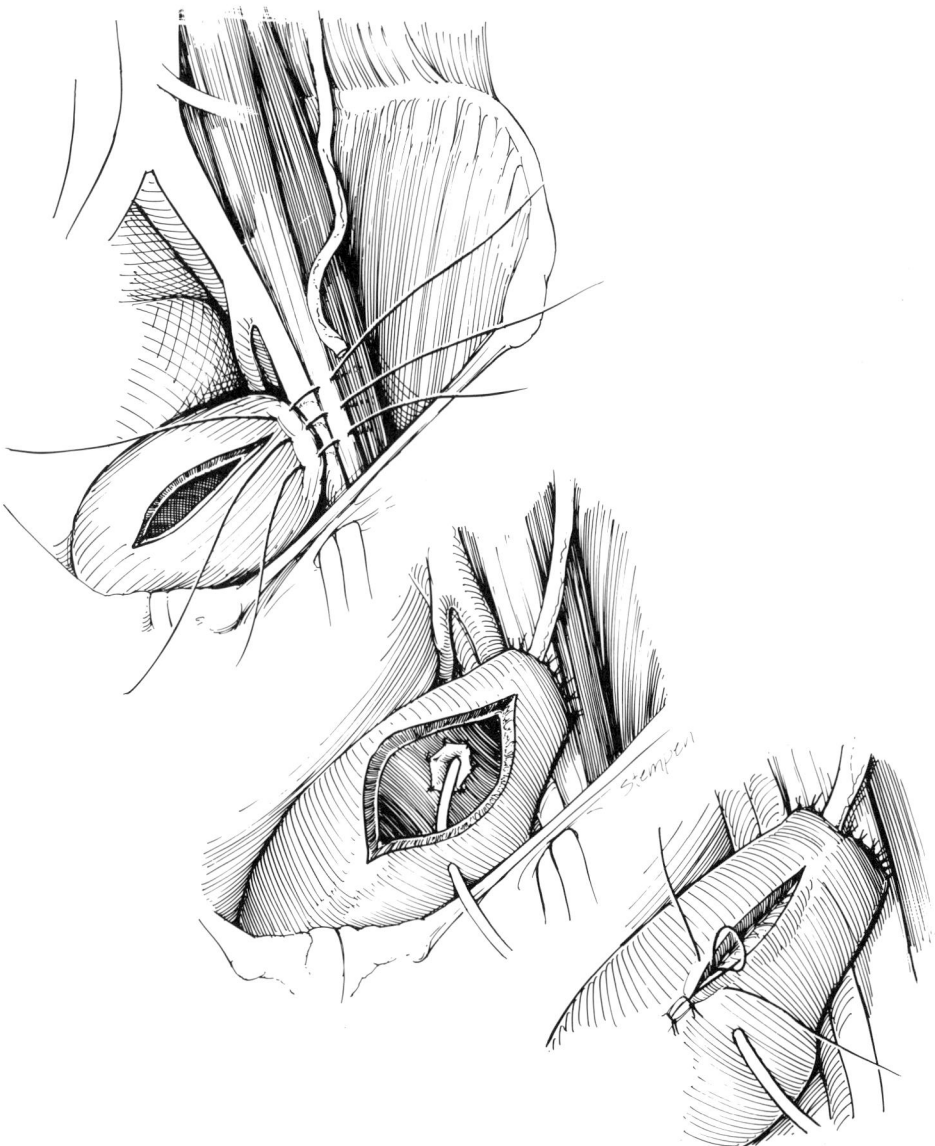

Figure 14–15. Psoas hitch maneuver to allow for tension-free ureteral reimplantation. (From Presti and Carroll.[56] Reprinted with permission.)

for approximately 7 days. If a pediatric feeding tube is employed for stenting, it may be removed at approximately 7 days. If a double-J catheter is employed for stenting, it is usually removed at 4 weeks. Cystography and intravenous urography should be performed at approximately 1 month to exclude vesicoureteral reflux and ureteral obstruction, respectively. In some cases, injury to the lower ureter is so extensive that the proximal ureter cannot be brought to the bladder without tension. Under such circumstances, a psoas hitch or bladder flap (Boari) can be performed (Fig. 14–15).[56] These procedures allow the bladder to be mobilized to provide the necessary length for a tension-free anastomosis. In the case of a psoas hitch, the peritoneum is stripped from the dome of the bladder and the bladder is separated from the cervix and proximal vagina in women and from the rectum in men. Division and ligation of the ipsilateral, obliterated umbilical vessels and, in more difficult cases, the contralateral superior vesicle vessel may allow additional mobilization. The bladder is brought to the psoas minor tendon by placement of the index finger in the cystotomy. The bladder is secured to the tendon with 2-0 absorbable suture material. These anchoring sutures should not be secured until the submucosal tunnel has been created. The ureter should enter the bladder medial to these fixation sutures and travel in a straight course along the posterior bladder wall to avoid kinking of the ureter.

Complications

Complications of ureteral injuries may be severe and complex.[57] Stricture formation and resulting hydronephrosis may occur at the site of repair. Urinary extravasation of the repair area may induce retroperitoneal fibrosis sufficient to cause ureteral obstruction. This type of fibrosis is generally more severe when the area has not been drained. A urinoma may develop in the retroperitoneum from slow extravasation and eventually may develop into a large abdominal mass. Such urinomas may cause minimal symptoms when the urine is uninfected. However, if the urine is infected, sepsis may set in rapidly. Pyelonephritis is a potential complication when any degree of ureteral obstruction exists. It is important in the follow-up period that urine cultures be monitored carefully and appropriate antibiotics administered to control bacteruria. Ureteral obstruction after repair may be silent and, therefore, follow-up studies are mandatory. Excretory urography should be performed within 4 to 8 weeks of repair. A repeat IVU should be performed 1 year after injury.

REFERENCES

1. Carroll PR, McAninch JW, Klosterman P, Greenblatt M. Renovascular trauma: risk assessment, surgical management and outcome. *J Trauma*. 1990; 30:547–554.
2. Mee SL, McAninch JW, Robinson AL, Auerbach PS, Carroll PR. Radiographic assessment of renal trauma: a ten year prospective study of patient selection. *J Urol*. 1989; 141:1095–1098.
3. Scott R, Carlton CE Jr, Goldman CE. Penetrating injuries: an analysis of 181 patients. *J Urol*. 1969; 101: 247–253.
4. Carroll PR, McAninch JW. Operative indications in penetrating renal trauma. *J Trauma*. 1985; 25:587–593.
5. Brodel M. The intrinsic blood vessels of the kidney and their significance in nephrectomy. *Bull Johns Hopkins Hosp*. 1901; 12:10–13.
6. Sclafani SJA, Becker JA. Interventional radiology in the treatment of retroperitoneal trauma. *Urol Radiol*. 1985; 7:219.
7. Carroll PR, McAninch JW. Staging of renal trauma. *Urol Clin North Am*. 1989; 16:193–201.
8. Bright TC, White K, Peters PC. Significance of hematuria after trauma. *J Urol*. 1978; 120:455.
9. Stables DP, Foch RF, van Neikerk JP de V, Cremin BJ, Holt SA, Peterson NE. Traumatic renal artery occlusion: 21 cases. *J Urol*. 1976; 115:229–233.
10. Chandhoke P, McAnich JW. Detection and significance of microscopic hematuria in patients with blunt renal trauma. *J Urol*. 1988; 140:16–17.
11. Hardeman S, Husmann DA, Chinn HKW, Peters PC. Blunt urinary tract trauma: identifying the patients who require radiological studies. *J Urol*. 1987; 138:99.

12. Tynberg PLH, Hoch WH, Persky L, Zollinger RM Jr. The management of renal injuries coincident with penetration wounds of the abdomen. *J Trauma.* 1973; 13:502.
13. Whitney RF, Peterson NE. Penetrating renal injuries. *Urology.* 1976; 7:7.
14. Jackson GL, Thai ER. Management of stab wounds of the flank and back. *J Trauma.* 1979; 19:660–664.
15. Bernath AS, Schutte H, Fernandez RRD, Addonizio JC. Stab wounds of the kidney: conservative management in flank penetration. *J Urol.* 1983; 129:468–470.
16. Mahoney SA, Perskey L. Intravenous drip nephrotomography in the evaluation of renal injury. *J Urol.* 1968; 90:513.
17. Elken M, Meng CH, de Paredes RG. Correlation of intravenous urography and renal angiography in kidney injury. *Radiology.* 1966; 86:496–498.
18. Glenn JF, Harvard BM. The injured kidney. *JAMA.* 1960; 173:1189–1195.
19. Lange EK, Trichel BE, Turner RW, Fontenot RA, Johnson B, St. Martin EC. Arteriographic assessment of injury resulting from renal trauma: an analysis of 74 patients. *J Urol.* 1971; 106:1–8.
20. Orkin LA. Evaluation of the merits of cystoscopy in retrograde pyelography in the management of renal trauma. *J Urol.* 1950; 63:9–29.
21. Nicolaisen G, McAninch JW, Marshall GA, Bluth RF Jr, Carroll PR. Renal trauma: reevaluation of indications for radiographic assessment. *J Urol.* 1985; 133:183.
22. Bretan PN, McAninch JW, Federle MP, Jeffrey RB Jr. Computerized tomographic staging of renal trauma: 85 consecutive cases. *J Urol.* 1986; 136:561–565.
23. Phillips T, Sclafani SJA, Goldstein A, Scalea T, Panetta T, Shaftan G. Use of contrast enhanced CT enema in the management of penetrating trauma to the flank and back. *J Trauma.* 1986; 26:593.
24. Sclafani SJA, Goldstein AS, Panetta T et al. CT diagnosis of renal pedicle injury. *Urol Radiol.* 1985; 7:63.
25. Steinberg DL, Jeffery RB, Federle MP, McAninch JW. The computerized tomographic appearance of renal pedicle injury. *J Urol.* 1984; 132:1163.
26. Kantor A, Sclafani SJA, Scalea T, Duncan AO, Atweh N, Glanz S. The role of interventional radiology in the management of genitourinary trauma. *Urol Clin North Am.* 1989; 16:255–265.
27. Uflacker R, Paolini RM, Lima S. Management of traumatic hematuria by selective renal artery embolization. *J Urol.* 1984; 132:662–667.
28. Holcroft JW, Trunkey DD, Minagi H, Korobkin MT, Lim RC. Renal trauma and retroperitoneal hematomas: indications for exploration. *J Trauma.* 1975; 15:1045–1052.
29. Cass AS, Bubrick M, Luxenberg M, Gleich P, Smith C. Renal trauma found during laparotomy for intraabdominal injury. *J Trauma.* 1985; 25:997.
30. McAninch JW, Carroll PR, Klosterman PW, Dixon CM, Greenblatt MN. Renal reconstruction after injury. *J Urol.* 1991; 145:932–937.
31. Carroll PR, Klosterman PW, McAninch JW. Early vascular control for renal trauma: a critical review. *J Urol.* 1989; 141:826–829.
32. Carroll PR, Klosterman PW, McAninch JW. Surgical management of renal trauma: analysis of risk factors, technique and outcome. *J Trauma.* 1988; 28:1071–1077.
33. McGonigal MD, Lucas CE, Ledgerwood AM. The effects of treatment of renal trauma on renal function. *J Trauma.* 1987; 27:471–476.
34. Narrod JA, Moore EE, Posner M, Peterson NE. Nephrectomy following trauma—impact on patient outcome. *J Trauma.* 1985; 25:842–844.
35. Mounzer AM, McAninch JW, Schmidt RA. Polyglycolic acid mesh in repair of renal injury. *Urology.* 1986; 28:127–130.
36. Maggio AJ, Brosman S. Renal artery trauma. *Urology.* 1978; 11:125–130.
37. Barry JM, Hodges CV. Revascularization of totally occluded renal arteries. *J Urol.* 1978; 119:412–415.
38. Clark DE, Georgitis JW, Ray FS. Renal arterial injuries caused by blunt trauma. *Surgery.* 1981; 90:87–96.
39. Brown M, Graham JM, Mattox KL, Feliciano DV, DeBakey ME. Renovascular trauma. *Am J Surg.* 1980; 140:802–805.
40. Fay R, Brosnan J, Lindstrom, Cohen A. Renal artery thrombosis: a successful revascularization by autotransplantation. *J Urol.* 1974; 111:572.
41. Peterson NE. Complications of renal trauma. *Urol Clin North Am.* 1989; 16:221–236.
42. Holden S, Hicks CC, O'Brien DP III, Stone HH, Walker JA, Walton KN. Gunshot wounds to the ureter: a 15-year review of 63 consecutive cases. *J Urol.* 1976; 116:562–564.
43. Walker JA. Injuries of the ureter due to external violence. *J Urol.* 1969; 102:410–413.
44. Presti JC, Carroll PR, McAninch JW. Ureteral and renal pelvic injuries from external trauma: diagnosis and management. *J Trauma.* 1989; 29:370–374.
45. Rao CR. Ureteral avulsion secondary to blunt abdominal trauma. *J Urol.* 1973; 110:188–190.
46. Reznichek RC, Brosman SA, Rhodes DV. Ureteral avulsion from blunt trauma. *J Urol.* 1973; 109:812–816.
47. Dowling RA, Corriere JN, Sandler CM. Iatrogenic ureteral injury. *J Urol.* 1986; 135:912.
48. Higgins CC. Ureteral injuries during surgery. *JAMA.* 1967; 199:82.
49. McGinty DM, Mendez R. Traumatic ureteral injuries with delayed recognition. *Urology.* 1977; 10:115–117.

50. Peterson NE, Pitts JC III. Penetrating injuries of the ureter. *J Urol*. 1981; 126:587–590.
51. Lirof SA, Pontes JES, Pierce JM Jr. Gunshot wounds of the ureter: five years of experience. *J Urol*. 1977; 118:551–553.
52. Carlton CE Jr, Scott R, Guthrie AG. The initial management of ureteral injuries: a report of 78 cases. *J Urol*. 1971; 105:335–340.
53. Eickenberg H-U, Amin M. Gunshot wounds to the ureter. *J Trauma*. 1976; 16:562–565.
54. Lankford R, Block NL, Politano VA. Gunshot wounds of the ureter: a review of ten cases. *J Trauma*. 1974; 14:848–852.
55. Cass AS. Ureteral contusion with gunshot wounds. *J Trauma*. 1984; 24:59–60.
56. Presti JC Jr, Carroll PR. Intraoperative management of the injured ureter. In: Schrock TR, ed. *Perspectives in Colon and Rectal Surgery*. St. Louis: Quality Medical Publishers; 1988: 98–106.
57. Marshall FF, Ureteral injuries. In: Marshall F, ed. *Urologic Complications*. Chicago: Year Book Medical Publishers; 1986: 208–209.
58. Carroll PR, McAninch JW. Renal trauma. In: Droller M, ed. *The Anatomical Basis of Genitourinary Surgery*. St. Louis: CV Mosby; 1992.
59. McAninch JW. Surgery of renal trauma. In: Novick AC, Pontes ES, Stroem SB, eds. *Stewart's Operative Urology*. 2nd ed. Baltimore: Williams & Wilkins; 1989.

15
Urethral and Bladder Injuries

CHRISTOPHER M. DIXON, M.D.
JACK W. McANINCH, M.D.
PETER R. CARROLL, M.D.

HISTORY: While the initial operations on the bladder (lithotomy) are lost in history, those on the urethra are easier to document. Heliodorus, sometime prior to Celsus (14 A.D.) was the first to operate on the urethra, treating urethral stricture with internal urethrotomy.[33] Richard Wiseman, in his treatise on gonorrhea, mentions the first case of external urethrotomy for stricture.[34]

As regards operations on the bladder, Pierre Franco, circa 1500, was the first to perform suprapubic cystotomy.[35] Daniel Ayre is credited by Garrison for the first successful repair of exstrophy of the female bladder (1859), and Joseph Pancoast (1872) the first successful repair of exstrophy of the male bladder.[36]

As regards bladder injury, there was no greater unsolved problem in gynecology than vesico-vaginal fistula. Many surgeons from the time of Ambroise Paré had operated unsuccessfully for this condition, only adding to the misery of the patients. In 1852, James Marion Sims revolutionized treatment.[37] He invented a special curved speculum that permitted excellent visualization of the injury. He utilized a suture of silver, to avoid sepsis, and a catheter for emptying the bladder while the fistula was healing.

URETHRAL INJURIES

Urethral injuries are uncommon. Most are caused by blunt trauma, but penetrating injuries occur rarely. They can be anatomically classified into anterior or posterior injuries, but almost all result from pelvic fractures or straddle injuries.[1,2] They are infrequent in women.[3,4] In men, rupture of the prostatomembranous urethra is potentially the most debilitating of all urologic injuries because of the possibility of incontinence, stricture formation, and impotence.

A management protocol for suspected lower tract injury is presented in Figure 15–1.

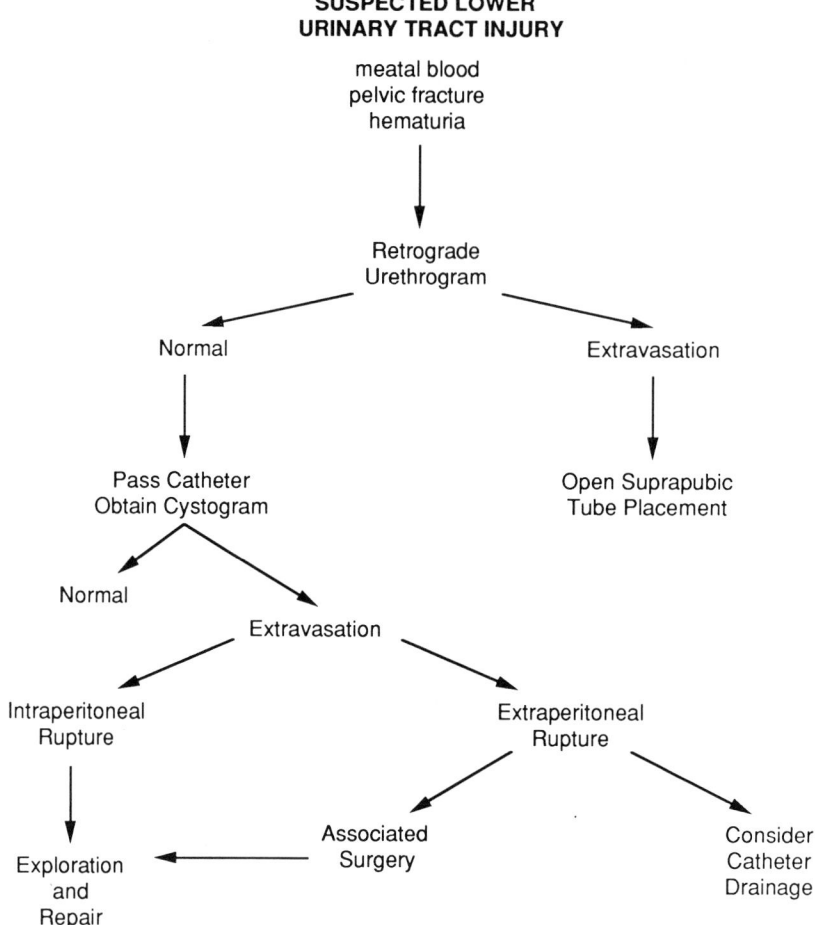

Figure 15–1. Management protocol for suspected lower urinary tract injury.

Even though a lower tract injury (urethra or bladder) may be diagnosed, the upper urinary tract (kidney and ureter) should also be assessed.

Anatomy

The male urethra is separated into two broad anatomic divisions: the posterior urethra, consisting of the prostatic and membranous portions, and the anterior urethra, consisting of the bulbous and pendulous portions. The proximal urethra, approximately 5 cm long, begins at the bladder neck and passes through the prostate; it then becomes the short membranous urethra (2 cm) as it passes through the urogenital diaphragm. The bulbous urethra then begins and is entirely in the perineum. The bulbous and pendulous portions are surrounded by the corpus spongiosum, which is held firmly to the ventral surface of the erectile bodies by Buck's fascia. The corpus spongiosum is a vascular structure and when ruptured can cause significant bleeding into the perineum. Buck's fascia is an adherent fascial layer completely surrounding the erectile bodies and corpus spongiosum. It attaches to the deep perineum over the bulbocavernous and ischiocavernous muscles and prevents urinary extravasation beyond its limits. In anterior urethral disruptions in which Buck's fascia is transected, extravasation of urine can occur with voiding, the only limit being Colles' fascia[5] (Fig. 15–2). Urine can extravasate to the level of the clavicles. If Buck's fascia remains intact, extravasation will be confined to the penile shaft, resulting in fusiform swelling.

The posterior urethra receives its blood supply from branches of the hypogastric artery by way of prostatic vessels; the anterior urethra, which is surrounded by the corpus spongiosum, receives arterial branches from the paired bulbar arteries by way of the internal pudendal artery. Venous drainage flows off the anterior urethra by way of the deep dorsal vein and empties into Santorini's plexus deep in the pelvis lateral to the apex of the prostate. The dorsal vein is located between the paired puboprostatic ligaments and, when lacerated, tends to retract, making hemostasis difficult. Trauma to this vein or the large venous plexus surrounding the prostate and urogenital diaphragm causes massive bleeding and large hematomas; in acute injuries, this makes attempts at visual reconstruction hazardous. Knowledge of this anatomy is useful for rapid vascular control. The urethra is endowed with an abundant blood supply and devascularization is rare.

In the male, two areas are responsible for maintaining urinary continence. The first, the internal sphincter, is at the bladder neck. When injured, this area must be meticulously

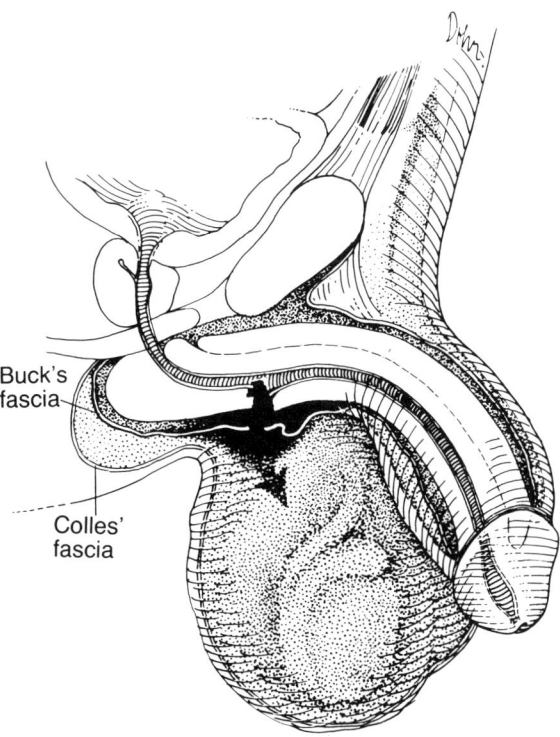

Figure 15–2. Illustration demonstrating urinary extravasation with rupture of Buck's fascia.

reconstructed. The second area is the external sphincter, which is located just distal to the apex of the prostate where the urethra passes through the urogenital diaphragm. In prostatomembranous disruption this sphincteric mechanism is destroyed and urinary continence is maintained by the internal sphincter alone.

Assessment of Urethral Injuries

A history of perineal trauma such as a kick or straddle injury is suggestive of an injury to the bulbous urethra. Straddle injuries to the perineum may present with minimal physical findings or large perineal hematomas and bloody urethral discharge. Classically, a "butterfly perineal hematoma" is present. Often this is an isolated injury, but associated injuries may be present. Pendulous urethral injuries are uncommon, but are associated with penile fractures in 20% of cases.[6]

Patients with rupture of the prostatomembranous urethra almost always have severe associated injuries. Pelvic fractures occur in 90% of cases[7,8] and may result in life-threatening hemorrhage from pelvic bleeding. Patients with this injury are unable to void and have a palpably distended bladder. On rectal examination, the prostate may not be palpable if it has been lifted from the pelvic floor by a developing hematoma. Rectal examination can be misleading because tense hematomas may sometimes mimic prostatic tissue. The prostate may not be displaced superiorly if the puboprostatic ligaments remain intact attached to the pubis, or if prostatomembranous disruption is only partial. It is important to note whether rectal bleeding is present so that a rectal laceration is not missed.

Careful examination of the urethral meatus is essential for patients with pelvic fractures or trauma to the perineum and genitalia. Blood at the urethral meatus is the single most reliable sign of urethral disruption,[4,9] but this may not always be present.[10] Therefore, the threshold for performing a retrograde urethrogram should be low. The study is quick, accurate, and carries almost no risk or complication. If blood is observed, a urethrogram is mandatory before catheter passage. If a pelvic fracture is identified (in particular, rami fractures) but meatal blood is not present, a urethrogram is strongly recommended. Attempts to pass a catheter before studying the urethra may cause infection of the retroperitoneal hematoma and convert incomplete tears to complete lacerations.

Once signs and symptoms suggest urethral injury, the diagnosis is confirmed with the help of retrograde urethrography (Table 15–1).[11–13] This is best accomplished with an irrigating syringe filled with contrast material injected in a retrograde fashion, the patient being placed in a slightly oblique position. The meatus is sterilely catheterized, the penis placed on gentle stretch, and angled about 45° from midline toward the side of the patient nearest the table. The x-ray is centered at the base of the penis and exposed during

Table 15–1 Technique for Cystography and Urethrography

	CYSTOGRAM	URETHROGRAM
Volume	300 ml	35–40 ml
Type of contrast	Cystographic or undiluted contrast	Undiluted contrast medium
X-ray films	Bladder filled and postevacuation	During injection
Position	Supine	Oblique

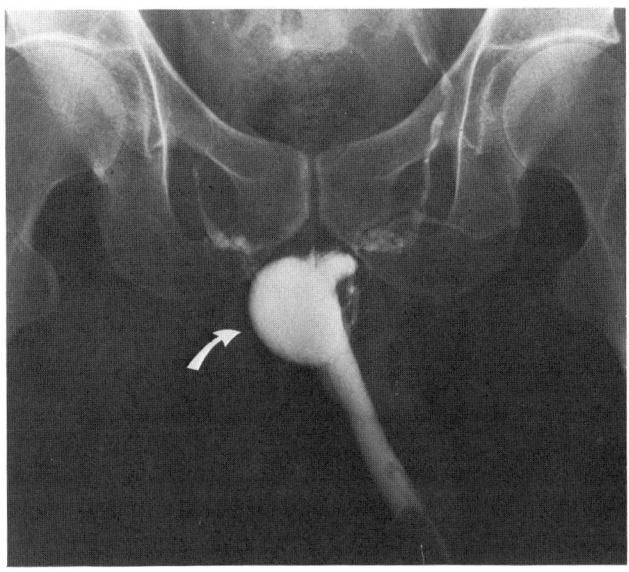

Figure 15–3. Retrograde urethrogram demonstrating an acute straddle injury.

injection of 35 to 40 ml of undiluted contrast. Usually only a single injection is required in the trauma patient.

The normal urethrogram often does not distend the prostatic urethra, but a thin line of contrast should be seen. In straddle injuries, extravasation will be seen in the bulbous urethra inferior to the urogenital diaphragm (Fig. 15–3); in prostatomembranous disruption, it will be visualized in the retropubic space superior to the urogenital diaphragm (Fig. 15–4). When the disruption is partial, small amounts of contrast enter the prostatic urethra and bladder, although significant amounts extravasate at the site of disruption.[12]

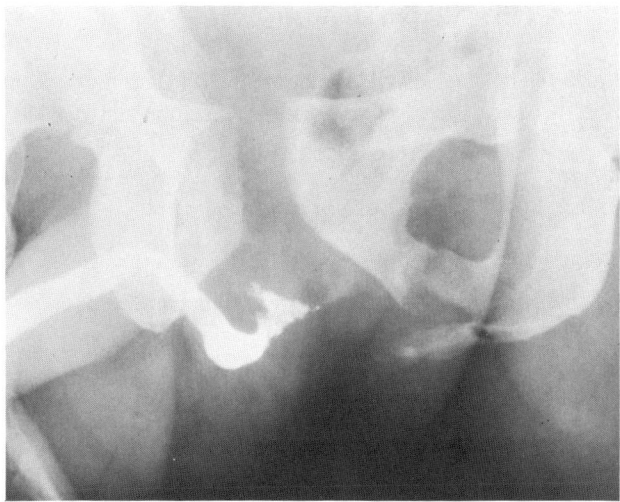

Figure 15–4. Retrograde urethrogram demonstrating a complete prostatomembranous disruption.

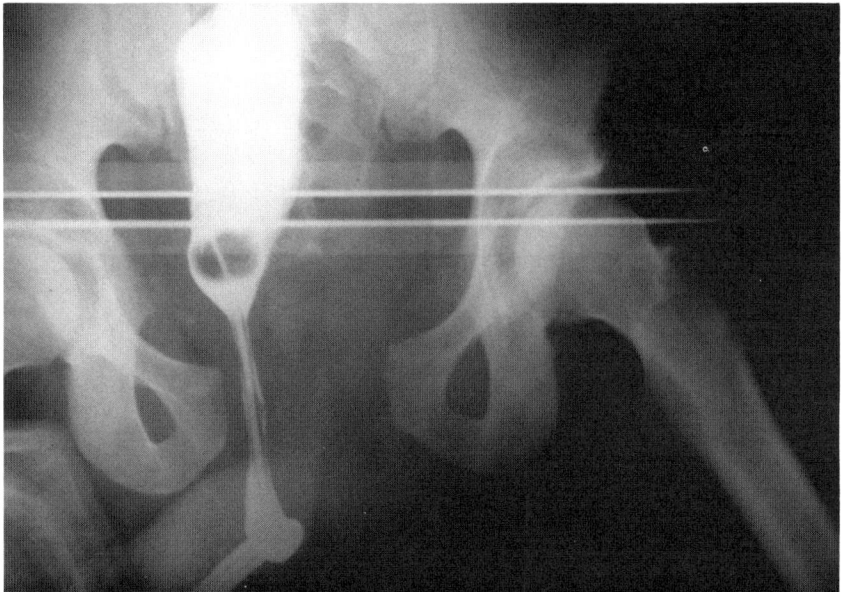

Figure 15–5. Combined retrograde urethrogram and cystogram demonstrating marked stretching of the prostatomembranous urethra but no extravasation. Note the wide separation of the pubic symphysis.

Occasionally, the urethra is stretched but not disrupted by a large pelvic hematoma (Fig. 15–5). These patients may have difficulty voiding and require catheter drainage until the hematoma begins to resolve. Penetrating injuries to the prostatic urethra are rare (Fig. 15–6). Blunt pendulous urethral injuries are also uncommon because of its mobility. In this injury, extravasation is seen along the shaft.

Preoperative Preparation

Prophylactic antibiotics are administered for all urethral injuries. For penetrating injuries or soft-tissue disruption, tetanus immunization may need to be updated. Patients sustaining straddle injuries usually do not require transfusions, but those with prostatomembranous disruption require adequate resuscitation because large amounts of blood can be concealed in the pelvis. An additional 4 to 6 units of blood should be available at operation.

Initial Management and Operative Exploration

Successful management of patients with urethral injuries requires suprapubic urinary diversion.[4,14] More than half of straddle injuries will heal with diversion alone.[15] This is best accomplished through a lower midline incision, which can be extended if necessary for intraperitoneal exploration. Only the anterior aspect of the bladder near the dome should be exposed. The space of Retzius and lateral perivesical area should be avoided so as not

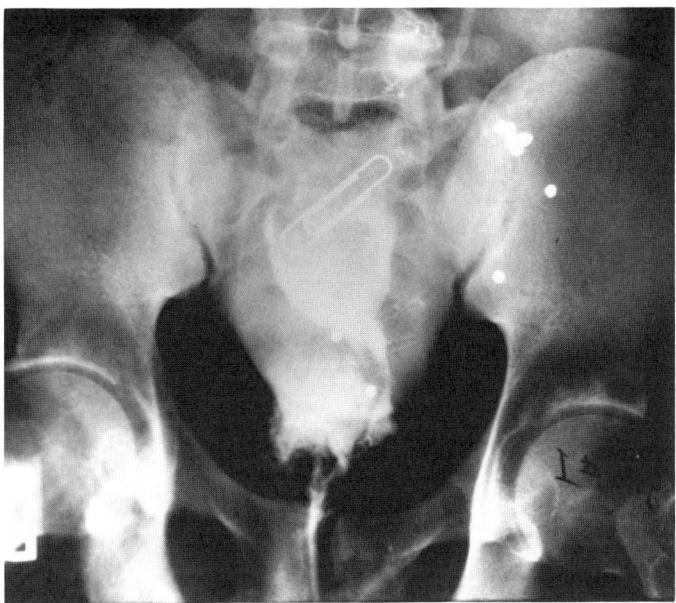

Figure 15–6. Gunshot injury to the prostatic urethra. A concomitant rectal injury was present. The paper clip marks the entrance wound and the bullet lodged in the perineum. The buckshot is from a previous gunshot injury.

to enter the pelvic hematoma. Once the bladder is identified, a vertical incision is made and a 28 F Malecot catheter is inserted. The urine is usually clear, unless bladder rupture is also present. In this case, the rupture must be repaired as discussed in the following section. In general, drains are not used to avoid infection of the hematoma. A two-layer, watertight closure of the bladder is performed with a running 4-0 chromic suture for the urothelium and a running 2-0 polyglycolic acid suture in Lembert fashion for the bladder wall. The suprapubic tube should exit the skin close to the midline. This facilitates antegrade passage of a sound into the prostatic urethra during definitive reconstruction. No attempt should be made to stent the urethra.

Percutaneous placement of a suprapubic catheter is generally not recommended because large pelvic hematomas or intraperitoneal blood may displace the bladder from its normal position, resulting in extravesical or intraperitoneal tube placement.

Penetrating injuries of the anterior urethra should be explored because of the high incidence of corporal injury. Debridement may be required and primary repair over a urethral catheter is usually possible.

Evaluation and Initial Management of Female Urethral Injuries

Although this injury is rare because the female urethra is short, severely displaced pelvic fractures may transect or lacerate it. The injury is usually obvious or discovered when catheterization is attempted. Palpation of the urethra may disclose bony fragments and vaginal lacerations. Life-threatening associated injuries are usually present. Urethrography is not practical but cystography should be done if possible. This injury should be managed by immediate repair with reconstruction of the bladder neck and repair of urethral, bladder, and vaginal lacerations. The goal of early repair is to prevent urinary incontinence and fistula formation.

Evaluation and Management of Anterior Urethral Injuries

Suprapubic urinary diversion is maintained for 2 weeks, and then voiding cystourethrography is performed by filling the bladder through the tube. If the injury has healed, the tube is clamped and the patient allowed to void. The tube is then removed 24 to 48 hr later if there are no complications. If extravasation is still present, the tube is left open until healing is complete. When the tube is removed, oral antibiotics are administered for 2 weeks. If a clinically significant stricture develops (as evidenced by voiding symptoms and decreased urinary flow), surgical intervention is required. Retrograde urethrography and sonourethrography will define the length of the stricture (Fig. 15–7, 15–8). If it is short, visual urethrotomy can be attempted, but most often open urethroplasty is required.

Evaluation and Management of Posterior Urethral Injuries

Suprapubic diversion is maintained for at least 3 months after prostatomembranous disruption or until patients have recovered from all other injuries. This allows resolution of the pelvic hematoma. Patients with this injury usually have a much longer convalescence owing to associated injuries. The patient with massive injuries that prevent ambulation

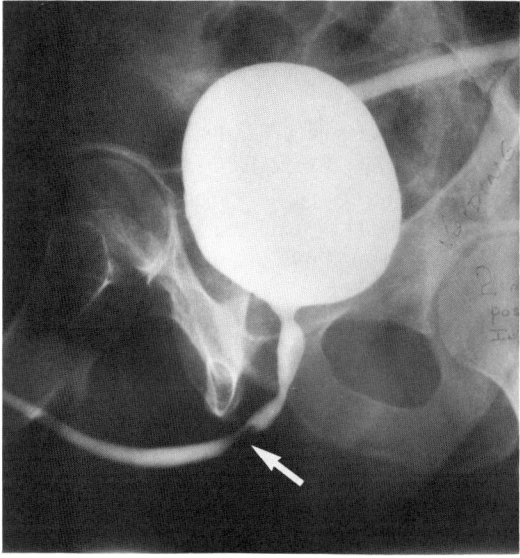

Figure 15–7. Retrograde urethrogram demonstrating a short stricture from a straddle injury.

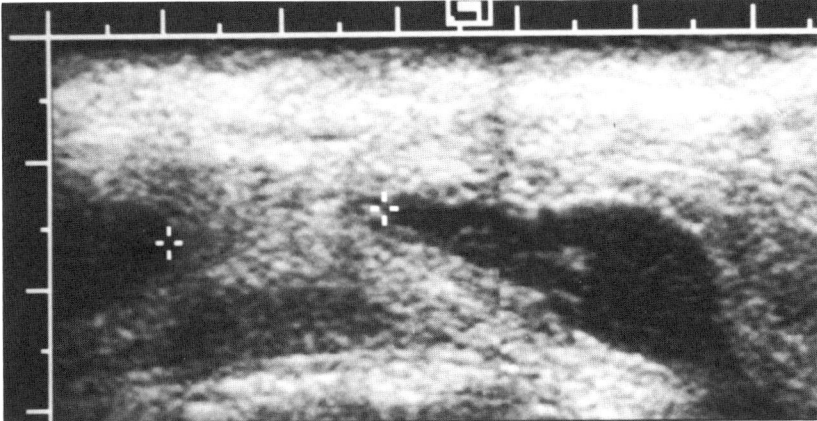

Figure 15–8. Sonourethrogram of a bulbar stricture from a straddle injury. Note the occluded lumen.

should undergo urethral repair later, after walking has resumed. Invariably, the urethra will be completely occluded from scar formation.

The status of the bladder and urethra must be assessed radiographically to determine the length and position of the resulting stricture, which will require repair. Simultaneous cystography and retrograde urethrography will provide such information (Fig. 15–9).[16] As the bladder is filled with contrast medium, the patient is asked to strain, thereby filling the prostatic urethra. The anterior urethra is simultaneously filled in a retrograde fashion, thereby delineating the length and location of the urethral defect. Definitive reconstruction can then be planned.

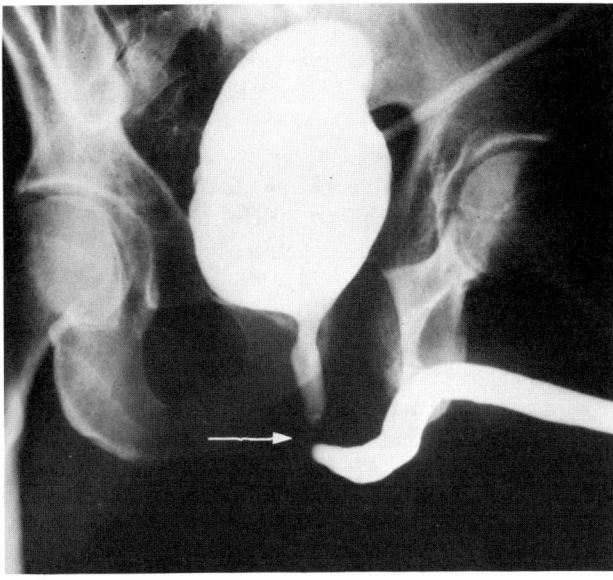

Figure 15–9. Combined cystogram and retrograde urethrogram several months after prostatomembranous disruption.

Patients with partial prostatomembranous urethral disruption can often safely void in 3 to 4 weeks after injury and cystostomy. A voiding cystogram will assure that no extravasation or stricture is present, so that the suprapubic catheter can be removed. If an obstructive stricture develops, reconstruction is usually required.

Operative Treatment

Definitive repair of the resulting urethral stricture from a straddle injury or prostatomembranous disruption is similar. In most instances, a 1- to 2-cm stricture will be present after injury, and the repair is best done through a perineal approach. Usually, the stricture can be excised and an end-to-end anastomosis performed. Strictures in the bulbous urethra, as occur from straddle injuries, are easier to approach because they are not located as deep in the perineum as membranous disruptions.

The patient is placed in an exaggerated lithotomy position to expose the perineum. Careful padding is necessary to prevent compression nerve injuries. A midline incision is made and a urethral catheter gently passed to the level of the stricture. The catheter can be palpated in the perineum, which helps to localize the stricture and guide the dissection. The bulbospongiosus muscle is exposed and then divided vertically in the midline. This exposes the corpus spongiosum and urethra. The bulbous urethra is then completely mobilized and stay sutures are placed at the level of the stricture. The urethra is then sharply transected and the strictured segment completely excised. The distal urethra is then mobilized to allow a tension-free anastomosis. The urethral ends are spatulated and calibrated to at least 26 F. The anastomosis is performed over an 18 F Silastic catheter with multiple interrupted 6-0 Maxon (Davis and Geck) sutures. In the bulbous urethra, the spongiosum is quite thick on the ventral side, allowing a two-layer anastomosis to be performed. The first layer approximates the urothelium and the second repairs the fascia of the spongiosum.

For prostatomembranous defects, the approach is similar, except that the dissection must continue deep into the perineum to the apex of the prostate. The tip of the urethral catheter is palpated at the obliterated urethra and then the urethra is divided. By transecting the urethra right at the level of the stricture, normal urethra is not inadvertently discarded, allowing an end-to-end repair. After dividing the urethra, the proximal lumen is often not visible. A urethral sound can be gently guided through the suprapubic tract into the prostatic urethra and palpated in the perineum. By cutting on the sound, the proximal lumen is identified. The distal urethra is mobilized and all surrounding scar tissue must be excised before proceeding with the anastomosis. Both ends are spatulated and an end-to-end anastomosis performed as above.

Occasionally, severe prostatomembranous disruptions require a partial inferior pubectomy or a combined perineal and transpubic approach to complete the anastomosis.[17] After determining that the perineal approach alone does not provide adequate exposure, a second vertical incision is made in the lower abdomen and carried around the base of the penis. The bladder is opened and the previous suprapubic tract excised. Attention is directed to the area of the pubis where the entire ventral surface of the symphysis is exposed. The suspensory penile ligament is transected inferiorly. The space of Retzius will be obliterated by fibrous reaction from injury and will be densely adherent to the posterior pubis. The posterior periosteum is sharply dissected inferiorly until the entire posterior symphysis is freed. Gigli saws are passed around the bone so that a wedge of symphysis can be removed. The anterior surface of the prostate is now exposed, and a urethral sound passed through the bladder into the prostatic urethra will demonstrate the prostatic apex and the stricture. All fibrous tissue at the apex must be excised. To avoid heavy bleeding and iatrogenic damage to the erectile nerves, no attempt should be made to mobilize the prostate. The anastomosis is then completed as described above. A suprapubic cystostomy is placed and the bladder is closed. Dead space where the pubis was removed is not filled. A closed system drain can be placed, but care must be taken to avoid infection in this space. It should be removed in 24 to 48 hr.

Postoperative Care

Patients undergoing a perineal repair have minimal pain and are usually ready for discharge in 3 or 4 days. In patients undergoing transpubic repair, the pelvis remains stable and pain from pubectomy is minimal. Ambulation is allowed on the third postoperative day, and most patients are discharged by the seventh day. Antibiotic coverage is maintained up to the time of hospital discharge, then discontinued.

Four weeks after the procedure, the urethral catheter is removed and a voiding cystourethrogram is obtained through the suprapubic catheter. A patent, open anastomosis is usually noted (Fig. 15–10). The cystotomy tube is clamped, permitting the patient to void for 48 hr, and then removed. Oral antibiotics are started and continued for 2 weeks. Flow rates and a repeat urethrogram should be obtained at 3, 6, and 12 months after catheter removal. Strictures seldom occur with this repair. If they do, they are usually short and amenable to visual urethrotomy.

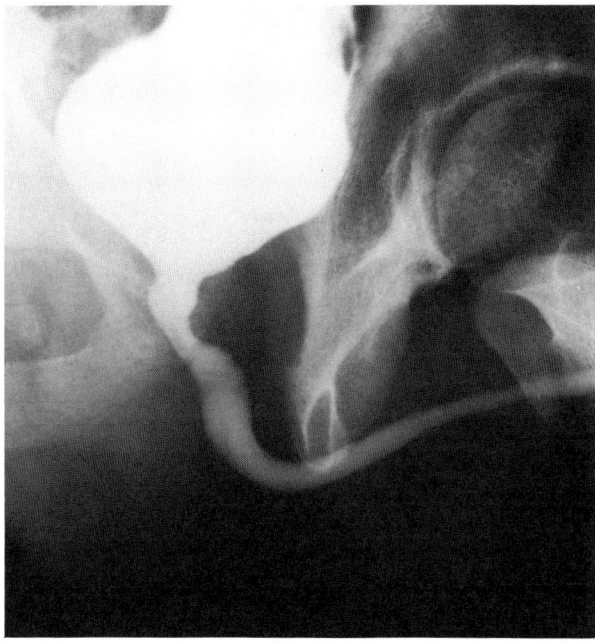

Figure 15–10. Follow-up voiding study after repair of prostatomembranous disruption.

Complications

Posterior urethral injuries create some of the most severe and debilitating complications seen in trauma to the urinary system. Impotence, particularly, can be a devastating complication. With management by suprapubic urinary diversion and delayed repair, impotence occurs in about 10% of cases. Although the literature suggests that primary repair has a higher incidence (50%),[18,19] such conclusions are based on retrospective clinical reviews. In more recent reports, it compares favorably with delayed repair.[20] Impotence is probably most often caused by the initial injury.[21]

Stricture may develop. In perineal or transpubic repair, incidence is less than 10%.[4,16,22–24] Direct vision urethrotomy has proved to be successful in managing these short fibrous strictures. Dilatation represents a temporary measure until more definitive repair can be done.

Incontinence, previously noted in 33% of patients having had initial primary repair, is less than 5% with the delayed combined perineal transpubic approach.[4,8,14,25]

BLADDER INJURIES

Bladder ruptures are most often seen in association with pelvic fractures from blunt trauma.[26] Approximately 15% of pelvic fractures (usually from automobile/pedestrian accidents) have concomitant bladder or urethral disruption. Gunshot and stab wounds rarely transect the bladder. Surgical injury to the bladder, if unrecognized, may lead to development of vesicovaginal fistula or pelvic urinomas.

Anatomy

The urinary bladder, with a capacity of 400 to 500 ml, lies well protected in the lower anterior bony pelvis. However, in young children and in adults with a full bladder, the position is more intraabdominal. This makes injury more likely when a blow strikes the lower abdomen or pelvis. The bladder receives its major blood supply from branches of the hypogastric artery—the superior, middle, and inferior vesical branches. Venous drainage corresponds to the arterial supply.

On the lateral trigone is the entrance of each ureter, which firmly attaches to the underlying trigonal musculature. Bladder function depends on nerve supply from the sacral parasympathetic nerves S2, S3, and S4, which course through a plexus along the posterior aspects of the bladder. Extensive dissection in this area can cause nerve interruption and functional problems.

Assessment of Injury

The diagnosis is easily made, assuming the examining physician suspects bladder rupture. The patient often has lower abdominal pain and is unable to void. There may be obvious signs of lower abdominal contusion and fracture of the pubic rami or symphysis. Gross hematuria is frequent and microhematuria almost always present. Definite diagnosis is made by cystography (Table 15–1). If urethral trauma is suspected, a urethrogram should be obtained before catheterization is attempted. If normal, a Foley catheter may be inserted and cystography performed. The bladder should be filled with at least 300 ml of contrast by gravity. This volume allows for complete expansion and helps to establish all areas of extravasation (Figs. 15–11, 15–12). If the initial x-ray does not demonstrate extravasation or the bladder does not appear full, additional contrast may be gently instilled via a syringe. Intraperitoneal rupture commonly occurs at the dome where, occasionally, bowel or omentum adheres. Installation of additional contrast will push the bowel away, identifying the injury. To minimize false negative studies, adequate bladder distention must be achieved and a drainage or washout film obtained. At least two films are required— one when the bladder is full and the other after it has been completely drained. Multiple films are not usually necessary in the trauma patient.

The increasing use of computed tomography (CT) scanning to evaluate traumatized patients does not eliminate the need for the cystogram. Routine abdominal pelvic CT cannot be relied on to exclude bladder rupture.[27] Cystography will most accurately diagnose an intra- or extraperitoneal rupture, but the degree of extravasation will not indicate the size of the laceration.

Evaluation and Repair

A review of several large series indicates that extraperitoneal ruptures are seen in 58% of cases and typically result from penetration of the bladder by bony fragments.[28–30] They rarely occur without a concomitant pelvic fracture. Extraperitoneal bladder ruptures from

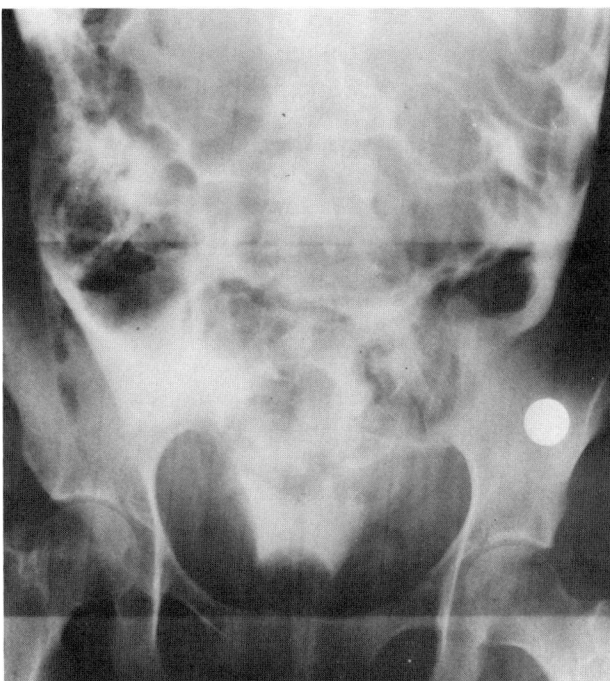

Figure 15–11. Cystogram demonstrating intraperitoneal rupture of the bladder. Note contrast surrounding the loops of bowel.

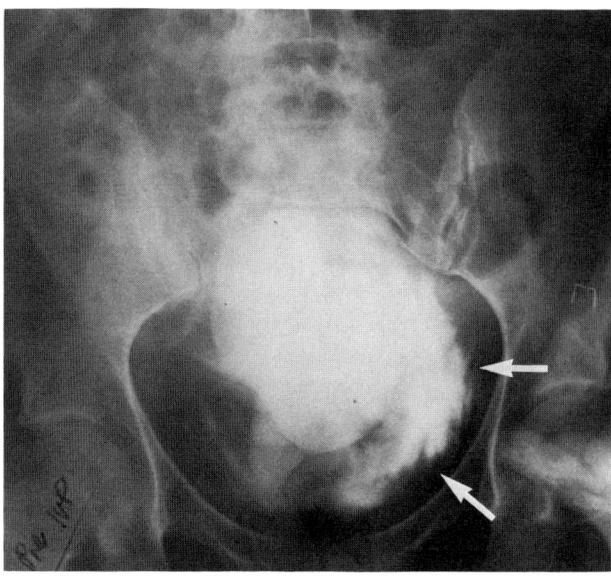

Figure 15–12. Cystogram demonstrating extraperitoneal rupture from blunt trauma.

blunt trauma have been treated successfully by catheter drainage alone,[30] but should be repaired surgically if abdominal exploration is planned for other injuries. Heavy blood loss and shock may occur from pelvic crush injuries. Resuscitation must be prompt and abundant blood available at operation. Thirty-four percent of cases show intraperitoneal rupture, and 8% have both an intra- and extraperitoneal injury. Intraperitoneal ruptures should be repaired surgically, as this will prevent continued spillage of urine into the peritoneal cavity or herniation of the abdominal contents into the bladder. Regardless of the perforation site, penetrating injuries require exploration because of the high incidence of associated injuries.

A lower abdominal midline incision allows opening of the peritoneum and, if indicated, exploration for possible visceral injury. A peritonotomy can be done; if no free blood is noted, it would seem safe to assume that no major intraperitoneal organ has been injured. Attention is then directed to the bladder. The surgeon should keep the exploration in the midline and not move laterally or into the space of Retzius, where heavy bleeding from the pelvic hematoma may ensue.

After the bladder wall is exposed, a vertical incision is made well above the bladder neck to expose the lumen. Once the bladder is open, the location and extent of damage can be identified from inside. Extraperitoneal perforations are closed from within the bladder with running 2-0 polyglycolic acid sutures for the muscle wall and a running 4-0 chromic suture for the urothelium. Intraperitoneal perforation should have a three-layer closure in which the bladder mucosa and musculature are closed separately from the peritoneum.

Occasionally, lacerations extend into the bladder neck. Repair in this area should be done with great care to avoid the danger of incontinence or bladder neck contracture. Precise interrupted suturing prevents secondary damage to other structures.

Suprapubic drainage with a 28 F Malecot catheter should be done.[31,32] Bladder ruptures occasionally have significant gross bleeding for several days after repair, and a large suprapubic catheter offers easy drainage without risk of obstruction by blood clots. The bladder incision is closed in two layers, with 4-0 chromic for the urothelium and a running 2-0 polyglycolic acid suture in Lembert fashion.

Heavy bleeding from rupture of pelvic vessels may be uncontrollable even though one does not violate the hematoma. Packing the pelvis with laparotomy tapes may control the problem. Persistent bleeding may necessitate leaving the tapes in place for 24 hr and removing them at reoperation. Placement of an external pelvic fixture may also help to control hemorrhage. Another alternative is embolization of pelvic vessels under angiographic control.

Penetrating bladder injuries require special consideration. As gunshot wounds to the bladder may cause extensive tissue loss, thorough debridement must be done before closure.[33] Distal ureteral and rectal injuries should be considered with gunshot wounds to the bladder. The ureteral orifices should be observed carefully for efflux of clear urine. Indigo carmine can be administered intravenously and the ureteral orifice observed for efflux; blue-stained urine suggests an intact ureter. Should there be a question of ureteral injury, catheterization and ureteral exploration are indicated. Bullets pass below the peritoneal reflection and penetrate the rectum and lower sigmoid without creating signs of obvious bowel injury. If rectal injury is suspected, sigmoidoscopy should be done at the time of operation. Missed rectal injuries result in serious morbidity and mortality.

Postoperative Care

Drainage should be maintained for 7 to 14 days, depending on the extent of injury. The catheter should not be irrigated unless it is obstructed by a clot. A low pressure cystogram can be performed before tube removal to be certain that the repair has healed. After suprapubic tube removal, the tract usually closes in 24 to 48 hr. If drainage persists, a urethral catheter can be placed for several days to allow the tract to close. Oral antibiotics are administered for 5 to 7 days after tube removal.

Complications

Once repaired, bladder injuries have a remarkable ability to heal. The incidence of dysfunctional voiding, incontinence, and fistulae is extremely low. Vesicovaginal fistulae are perhaps the most common and result from unrecognized injury at operation. Infected pelvic hematomas may require long-term care, but one can expect an eventual good result.

REFERENCES

1. Coffield KS, Weems WL. Experience with management of posterior urethral injury associated with pelvic fracture. *J Urol*. 1977; 117:722.
2. Peltier LF. Complications associated with fractures of the pelvis. *J Bone Joint Surg*. 1965; 47:1060.
3. Bredael JJ, et al. Traumatic rupture of the female urethra. *J Urol*. 1979; 122:560.
4. McAninch JW. Traumatic urethral injuries. *J Trauma*. 1981; 21:291.
5. Pontes JE, Pierce JM Jr. Anterior urethral injury: four year experience at Detroit General Hospital. *J Urol*. 1978; 120:563.

6. Orvis BR, McAninch JU. Penile rupture. *Urol Clin North Am.* 1989; 16:69.
7. Colapinto V, McCollum RW. Injury to the posterior urethra in fractured pelvis: a new classification. *J Urol.* 1977; 188:575.
8. Morehouse DD, MacKinnon KJ. Urological injuries associated with pelvic fractures. *J Trauma.* 1969; 9:479.
9. Cass AS, Godec CJ. Urethral injury due to external trauma. *Urology.* 1978; 11:607.
10. Lowe MA, Tate Mason J, Luna GK, Maier RV, Copass MK, Berger RE. Risk factors for urethral injuries in men with traumatic pelvis fractures. *J Urol.* 1988; 140:506–507.
11. Glassberg KI, et al. The radiographic approach to injuries of the prostatomembranous urethra in children. *J Urol.* 1979; 122:678.
12. Glassberg KI, et al. Partial tears of the prostatomembranous urethra in children. *Urology.* 1979; 13:500.
13. Moulonguet A. Ruptures traumatiques de l'urethra posteriur. *J Urol Nephrol.* 1965; 71:96.
14. Morehouse DD, MacKinnon KJ. Management of prostatomembranous urethral disruption: 13 year experience. *J Urol.* 1980; 123:173.
15. Pierce JM Jr. Disruptions of the anterior urethra. *Urol Clin North Am.* 1989; 2:329.
16. Waterhouse K, Laugani G, Patil U. The surgical repair of membranous urethral strictures: experience with 105 consecutive cases. *J Urol.* 1980; 123:500.
17. McAninch JW. Pubectomy in repair of membranous urethral stricture. *Urol Clin North Am.* 1989; 16:297.
18. Gibson GR. Impotence following fractured pelvis and ruptured urethra. *Br J Urol.* 1970; 42:86.
19. Gibson GR. Urologic management and complications of fractured pelvis and ruptured urethra. *J Urol.* 1974; 111:353.
20. Patterson DE, Barrett DM, Myers RP, et al. Primary realignment of posterior urethral injuries. *J Urol.* 1983; 129:513–516.
21. Dhabuwala CB, Hamid S, Katsikas DM, Pierce J Jr. Impotence following delayed repair of prostatomembranous urethral disruption. *J Urol.* 1990; 144:677.
22. Allen TD. Transpubic approach for strictures of the posterior urethra superior to the urogenital diaphragm. *Urol Clin North Am.* 1977; 4:95.
23. Malloy TR, Wein AJ, Carpiniello L. Transpubic urethro. 1980; 124:359.
24. Webster GD. Perineal repair of membranous urethral stricture. *Urol Clin North Am.* 1989; 16:303.
25. DeWeerd JH. Immediate realignment of posterior urethral injury. *Urol Clin North Am.* 1977; 4:75.
26. Montie J. Bladder injuries. *Urol Clin North Am.* 1977; 4:59.
27. Mee SL, McAninch JW, Federle MP. Computerized tomography in bladder rupture: diagnostic limitations. *J Urol.* 1987; 137:207–209.
28. Carroll PR, McAninch JW. Major bladder trauma: mechanisms of injury and a unified method of diagnosis and repair. *J Urol.* 1984; 132:254–257.
29. Cass AS. The multiple injured patient with bladder trauma. *J Trauma.* 1984; 24:731–734.
30. Corriere JN Jr, Sandler CH. Management of the ruptured bladder: seven years' experience with 111 cases. *J Trauma.* 1986; 16:830–833.
31. Ochsner TC, Busch FH, Clark BG. Urogenital wounds in Vietnam. *J Urol.* 1969; 101:224.
32. Salvatierra O Jr. Vietnam experience in 252 urological war injuries. *J Urol.* 1969; 101:615.
33. Garrison JF. *History of Medicine.* Philadelphia: WB Saunders Co. Publ. 1929:109.
34. Garrison JF. *History of Medicine.* Philadelphia: WB Saunders Co. Publ. 1929:276.
35. Garrison JF. *History of Medicine.* Philadelphia: WB Saunders Co. Publ. 1929:508.
36. Garrison JF. *History of Medicine.* Philadelphia: WB Saunders Co. Publ. 1929:504.
37. Sims JM. Treatment of vesico-vaginal fistula. *Am J Med Sci.* 1852; xxiii:59–82.

16
Genital Injuries

JACK W. McANINCH, M.D.
CHRISTOPHER M. DIXON, M.D.
PETER R. CARROLL, M.D.

HISTORY: Very little is written on the history of genital injuries. Regner de Graaf in 1668 described the histology of the testicle. He noted that it was made up of small tubules folded into lobules.[20] The interstitial cells of the testis were first investigated by Franz Leydig (1850) and their secretions were held by Ancel and Bouin (1923) to maintain male sexual characteristics.[21]

There were 147 wounds described in the Iliad with an overall mortality of 77.6%. The first attention the wounded received was a seat, lots of storytelling and a cup of Pramnian wine sprinkled with grated goat cheese and barley meal, served by a beautiful woman. Plato found this treatment was too much—not the woman, but the cheese and the barley which he said were surely inflammatory.[22]

Genital injuries are most often associated with other major injuries and can have a devastating effect on the skin, penis, and testes. Management is directed at preserving function and providing an acceptable cosmetic appearance. Of primary importance is the maintenance of erectile capability, which depends to a large extent on hormonal function. Spermatogenesis is of particular concern for younger patients. When undertaking surgical reconstruction of these severe injuries, age, associated injuries, and disabilities must be taken into account.

PENILE RUPTURE

Traumatic rupture of the corpus cavernosum, or fracture of the penis, is uncommon. Indeed, in 1936 Fetter and Gartman reported that blunt trauma of the penis was responsible for 1 of 175,000 hospital admissions.[1]

Approximately 200 cases have now been reported in the world literature and many more probably go unreported, as evidenced by a recent survey of Arkansas urologists that revealed 25 additional unreported cases in that state alone.[2] Owing to the limited number of cases and consequent lack of a prospective trial, no universally accepted method of diagnosis and treatment exists.

Mechanisms of Injury

All reported injuries have occurred to the erect penis as a result of direct blunt trauma that bends the organ abnormally. The resultant injury is a tear in the tunica albuginea, usually in a transverse orientation. During erection, the tunica albuginea of the corpora cavernosa is susceptible to injury owing to its relative inelasticity when distended and the pronounced thinning that occurs with sinusoidal engorgement. Its usual thickness of 2 mm is reduced to 0.25 to 0.50 mm.

Rupture occurs most commonly during coitus, with reports ranging from 33% to 58% of all injuries.[3] Usually the penis slips out of the vagina and is thrust against the perineum or symphysis pubis. The remainder of the cases are caused by abnormal bending of the penis during masturbation, by trying to place the erect penis into the pants, or by other trauma such as rolling over in bed, bumping into furniture in the dark, a kick from a horse, etc.

The site of injury is variable. Some report that the distal third of the penile shaft is most common, but injury may occur anywhere along the shaft, including the base where the corpora are somewhat fixed by the penile suspensory ligament.

Generally, only one corporal body is injured, but both corpora can be affected depending on the nature and severity of the trauma. Injury to the corpus spongiosum and urethra can also occur.

Clinical Findings

The events that follow the injury are characteristic. Typically, the patient reports a cracking or popping sound accompanied by immediate pain and rapid detumescence.[4] In cases without urethral injury, most patients are able to urinate normally, but occasionally hematoma and edema may cause external urethral compression, leading to obstructive symptoms or urinary retention.

Urethral injury occurs in approximately 20% of cases. In a 1983 literature review, Nicolaisen et al.[3] found that of 50 patients with penile rupture, 11 (22%) had urethral injuries, all but one of which were partial disruptions. Ten of the 11 patients presented with either gross hematuria or blood at the meatus. The 11th patient was unable to void and the injury was identified at surgical exploration. Of 18 patients with normal results on urinalysis, none had sustained urethral injury.

Physical findings include swelling and ecchymosis, sometimes of massive proportions. Typically, the penis is deviated toward the side opposite the injury owing to the mass effect of the hematoma. Usually the hematoma is confined to the penile shaft; however, if Buck's fascia is torn, blood or urinary extravasation may occur along fascial planes into the scrotum or perineum. The site of fracture is frequently apparent from the overlying hematoma, focal tenderness, or a palpable defect in the tunica albuginea.

Diagnosis

In the great majority of cases, the diagnosis is easily made on the basis of the typical history and physical findings, and no further studies are required. Not all patients present in typical fashion, however, and not all patients with the typical signs and symptoms have penile rupture. In these instances, an accurate diagnostic test would be useful.

For this purpose, many investigators have proposed cavernosography, as extravasation from the corpora is diagnostic.[4] A small butterfly needle (21–25 gauge) is inserted into the dorsolateral uninvolved corpus cavernosum. The patient is placed in an oblique position and, after a scout film, 30 to 50 ml of half-strength contrast medium (Renograffin 60) is instilled, preferably under fluoroscopic control. During infusion, an early filling defect may be present at the fracture site owing to hematoma, but this is not diagnostic in the absence of extravasation. Static films are then taken in the opposite oblique position after an additional 10 to 20 ml of contrast is instilled. Finally, a delayed film is taken at 10 min to identify delayed extravasation that may occur as contrast saturates the hematoma overlying the injury.

Therapy

Overall, the data from the recent reports of penile rupture strongly suggest that early surgical intervention should be the preferred form of management. The risks of unacceptable penile angulation, progressive hematoma, and abscess are significantly lower than with nonoperative management. In addition, the hospital stay is shorter and a faster return to normal function can be expected.

Surgical treatment consists of evacuation of hematoma, control of hemorrhage, and debridement and closure of the defect in the tunica albuginea, preferably with interrupted absorbable sutures. The preferred incision is a distal circumferential incision with "degloving" of the penile skin down to the area of injury. The advantage of this approach is that it allows not only excellent exposure of the ruptured corpus (Fig. 16–1) but adequate assessment of the contralateral corpus and corpus spongiosum.

Others advocate a direct incision over the suspected site of rupture,[1] since in most cases the site is apparent from the overlying hematoma, palpable defect with point tenderness, and deviation of the penis to the side opposite the injury. In cases in which the site of rupture is identified, especially if it is in the proximal shaft, and urethral injury is ruled out (negative results on urinalysis or retrograde urethrography), this approach may be useful, thereby avoiding unnecessary dissection. If any doubt exists, however, or if the site is on the distal shaft, a distal circumferential incision should be used.

Urethral lacerations should be repaired primarily over a urethral stenting catheter. In the case of complete transection, debridement, spatulation, and approximation of the margins with 4-0 interrupted absorbable sutures will provide an excellent result. Partial transections are often very small. These may heal over the stenting catheter in a few days; otherwise, closure of the injury with interrupted absorbable sutures provides rapid healing.

Although urethral catheterization in the presence of suspected urethral injury is advocated by some, we feel that it risks converting a partial tear to a complete transection.

Postoperative care in patients without urethral injury consists of urethral catheterization and a gentle pressure dressing. The routine use of systemic antibiotics is not necessary. Fibrinolytic agents and antiinflammatory agents are not required, since the evacuation of the hematoma and closure of the tunica should prevent excessive fibrosis. If pain with erection persists, diazepam, diethylstilbestrol, or amyl nitrite have been used with some success.

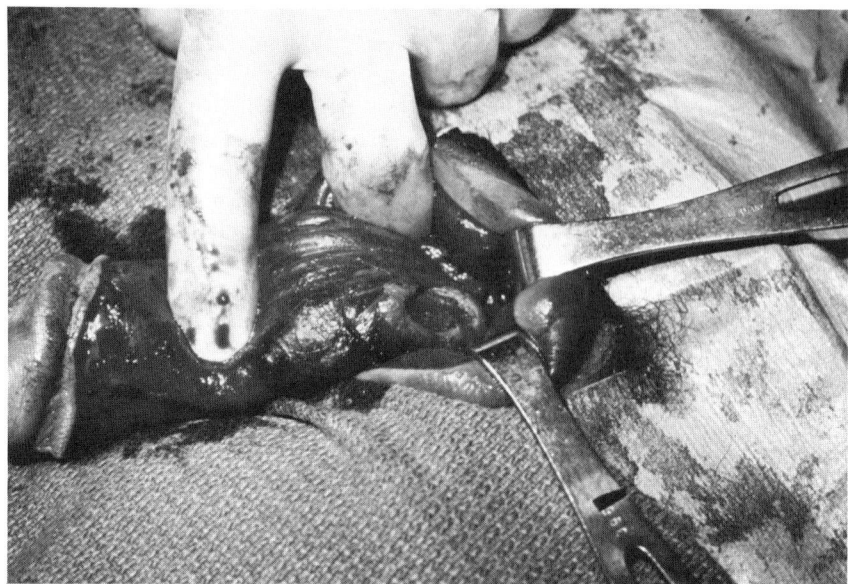

Figure 16–1. Intraoperative photograph demonstrating a tear of the corpus cavernosum. (From Orvis and McAninch.[4] Reprinted with permission.)

Certainly not all ruptures of the corpus cavernosum require surgical treatment. Most patients managed nonoperatively do well, and it is likely that many patients with minor ruptures never seek medical attention. One can assume that their risk of long-term complications is less than in those who obtain medical evaluation. When the history is suggestive, but the physical findings do not reveal an obvious injury, cavernosography may be useful. If extravasation is present, the tunical defect should be repaired. If no extravasation is identified and the hematoma is minimal, conservative treatment is reasonable. If the hematoma expands, delayed exploration should be undertaken.

TESTICULAR RUPTURE

Signs and Symptoms

Rupture of a testis from blunt trauma is a violent and immediately painful event. Wasko and Goldstein[5] have estimated that a force of 50 kg of pressure is needed to rupture the tunica albuginea in blunt scrotal trauma. Nausea and vomiting are frequently associated and occasionally syncope. The amount of scrotal swelling and ecchymosis can vary. Rupture of the tunica albuginea behind the tunica vaginalis can be associated with no ecchymosis and minimal to moderate testicular enlargement because bleeding and the extruded seminiferous tubules will be contained by the tunica vaginalis. On the other hand, if subalbugineal arterioles are involved, the hematocele can be quite large and may compress the parenchyma, eventually leading to parenchymal atrophy. If the rupture involves the junction of the tunica albuginea and tunica vaginalis in the area of the epididymis, the bleeding will extend into the scrotal sac proper and lead to a scrotal hematoma, which can vary in size.

Findings on physical examination may vary. Occasionally, the testis may be displaced to the inguinal canal and not be palpable in the scrotum. The most consistent sign is exquisite pain with palpation. Scrotal ecchymosis and swelling are also frequent, although their absence does not rule out a rupture. The differential diagnosis includes simple hematocele without rupture, torsion of the testis or one of the appendices, testis tumor, epididymitis, reactive hydrocele, or hematoma of the epididymis and spermatic cord. An accurate history should be taken, if possible, to ascertain the magnitude of the force causing the injury. Cassie[6] has reported that an associated neoplasm may predispose to rupture after apparently minor injuries. In this case, testicular rupture was manifested by swelling and pain some 16 hours after a fall down a flight of stairs. Patients with normal testes will report scrotal trauma that is much more violent and directly localized and they usually experience pain and swelling immediately, or they may have been in an accident resulting in multiple injuries.

Diagnosis

The definitive diagnosis of testicular rupture rests with surgical confirmation. Most urologists would probably explore the scrotum if there were any question of a rupture. Scrotal ultrasonography, which has improved the preoperative diagnosis, serves two useful functions: it can demonstrate whether or not acute disruption has occurred (extremely useful information when deciding which patients require emergency surgery), and it can evaluate the testicular parenchyma in a patient who presents with epididymitis several days after what might be deemed by history to be significant scrotal trauma. In this instance, if findings on physical examination are equivocal, a normal parenchymal echo pattern and an enlarged epididymis on ultrasonography would lead one to treat the patient medically. A recent review of the experience at San Francisco General Hospital demonstrated that preoperative scrotal ultrasonography correctly predicted the presence of a ruptured testis in 94% of patients with scrotal injuries.[7] No false negative results occurred, although an occasional false positive result was encountered when a large scrotal hematoma precluded adequate identification of the testis. The key findings for testicular rupture are an abnormal parenchymal echo pattern, resulting from extrusion of the tubules, and intraparenchymal contusion and hemorrhage.[7] In the trauma setting, the latter is quite specific for rupture; however, an abnormal parenchymal echo pattern is also seen in testicular neoplasms and infarction and its significance will be dictated by the clinical situation.

Approach to Management

Exploration with repair of the acutely ruptured testis has been advocated for some time.[7–9] The objectives of surgical exploration are testicular salvage, prevention of infection, control of bleeding, and reduction of convalescence.

In a review of 20 years' experience, which spanned an era when nonoperative management was common, del Villar et al.[8] reported a 45% failure rate (i.e., exploration was eventually required because of complications such as persistent pain and infection).

Additionally, 45% of those patients in whom exploration was delayed required an orchiectomy, as opposed to 5% of patients who underwent exploration within 3 days of injury. Furthermore, the hospital convalescence after surgery was 63% longer in those patients undergoing delayed exploration. At our institution patients without any associated injuries can be discharged 1 to 2 days after early exploration.

In addition to suspected rupture of the testis, the presence of a large hematocele is also an indication for exploration. Distinctions in size are somewhat subjective, but if the hematocele enlarges the palpable size of the affected gonad by a factor of 3 or more, we consider it large. Infection can result and is associated with a high risk of orchiectomy. In our experience smaller hematoceles do not require surgery, although other authors are more aggressive.[8] A major deficiency in the literature of testicular trauma is the lack of adequate long-term follow-up of patients undergoing early exploration. Unfortunately, the nature of the patient population is such that compliance with careful follow-up is not the norm. At our institution, follow-up is sporadic at best, but as yet no testis successfully repaired has atrophied.

Surgical Reconstruction

The testis is usually accessed through a scrotal incision, either midline longitudinal or transverse. In the rare case of an unreducible inguinal translocation, an inguinal incision is used. If a testicular tumor is suspected, an inguinal incision should be used; the spermatic cord should be occluded with a ¼-inch penrose drain or umbilical tape; the testis should be delivered through the incision and examined; if need be, an orchiectomy should be performed after high ligation of the cord. Hematoceles are drained by incising the tunica vaginalis. The tunica albuginea is repaired by debriding any necrotic tubules, controlling arterial bleeding with suture ligatures of 4-0 or 5-0 chromic catgut or electrocoagulation, and closing the tunica albuginea with a 3-0 or 4-0 running absorbable suture. Inguinal testes that cannot be replaced in the scrotum manually are fixed by orchiopexy. The intrascrotal portion of the spermatic cord should be thoroughly examined, although its contents should not be dissected unless there is a large hematoma, which suggests arterial injury that would require ligation or fulguration. Large scrotal hematomas are evacuated as much as possible by evacuating the major clot collections, but an exhaustive attempt at evacuating all the blood is futile, because at some point one begins to cause more bleeding by dissection. A ¼- or ½-inch Penrose drain is left in place and removed with the first dressing change within 24 hr. The scrotum is closed with interrupted 4-0 chromic vertical mattress sutures and dressed with a sterile, fluffy gauze dressing supported by either a large scrotal support or a burn net panty dressing.

Prophylactic antibiotics are not usually used for blunt injuries, unless infection is evident on urinalysis. For penetrating injuries, antibiotics with good gram-positive coverage, such as cephalosporins, are used. In gunshot wounds especially, the contralateral testis should be explored if the path of the projectile traversed its hemiscrotum or if a large scrotal hematoma precludes adequate ultrasound examination of it. If hematuria is present, injury to the urethra or bladder should be ruled out with preoperative retrograde urethrography and cystography.

In summary, the early surgical repair of testicular injuries has led to reduced morbidity and increased testicular salvage. Orchiectomy can be avoided in about 90% of cases.

Ultrasound has increased our ability to diagnose parenchymal injury preoperatively and thus to advise the frightened patient more authoritatively and assure ourselves of the necessity of surgical exploration. In most cases, the patient can expect a short convalescence and preservation of his injured gonad.

GENITAL SKIN LOSS

Etiology and Initial Management

Avulsion Injuries

Accidents with power farm machinery were at one time the common cause of avulsion injuries, but improved safety measures have greatly reduced the incidence.[10] Avulsion is more likely to occur from deceleration injuries, with the genitalia being caught on some stationary object. Motorcycles, bicycles, and other vehicles are the more frequent source of such injuries in current times.

Avulsed skin that is still attached to the body by a pedicle can often be salvaged and used to cover the defect. It should be gently cleaned and then reapplied. If it does not survive, debridement and skin grafting can be done. Avulsed skin without an attached pedicle often is totally nonviable and can be reapplied only in selected cases.

Infection

Synergistic necrotizing infections of the genitalia represent the most common cause of skin loss.[11,12] Colorectal or urologic disease accompanies the process in a high percentage of patients.[12,13] Fournier's original description in 1882 has been more completely delineated by recent authors.[12,13]

Commonly a perirectal abscess will penetrate Colles' fascia and quickly spread in the subdartos space to involve the skin. It is this same tissue plane that is involved on the penis. If not promptly treated by aggressive debridement and antibiotics, the infection can progress up to the abdominal wall. If the source is a periurethral abscess, it can penetrate through Buck's fascia, allowing the infection to spread below the penile and scrotal skin. Skin death is caused by thrombosis and destruction of the fine vasculature supplying the skin. The process can be rapidly progressive and destroy large areas of skin within hours.

The bacteria causing such massive destruction have been shown to be a combination of anaerobes and aerobes. Carroll et al.[12] found that *Bacteroides* species, facultative enterobacteria, and aerobic streptococci are commonly involved. *Escherichia coli* was the most common negative aerobe in their report, but a mean of 3.4 organisms were identified in the tissue cultures.

Patients present with pain and swelling of the genitalia. Crepitus is often palpable. Fever and skin necrosis are usually present and leukocytosis is expected. Many patients have evidence of systemic sepsis.

Initial management should consist of triple antibiotics providing broad spectrum coverage.[11] Commonly, aminoglycosides, high dose penicillin, and metronidazole are given systemically. Patients should have the inciting cause treated (i.e., the abscess should be drained). With extensive perirectal abscess, diverting colostomy is best done early. Urine can be diverted by cystostomy.

Aggressive and immediate surgical debridement is mandatory to control the rapidly spreading infection. All nonviable skin should be removed. The underlying penis and testicles usually are uninvolved and should be protected in the postdebridement period with moist saline-soaked dressings. Repeated debridement may be required.

Burns

Flame burns to the genital area are uncommon and rarely cause major skin loss. Most first- and second-degree burns will heal with local topical care; debridement is seldom required. Third-degree burns indicate complete full thickness destruction: the skin is charred, dry, and without sensation. When autograft skin is available, excision and grafting within the first week of injury is advantageous.

Electrical burns often cause severe damage to the skin as well as to the underlying soft tissues of the penis and testicles. Conservative debridement is recommended until the full extent of the injury can be determined. Then only nonviable tissue should be removed and local care given until reconstruction can be done.

Chemical burns to the genitalia are rare. Initial therapy should be irrigation of the wound with copious amounts of water to neutralize the chemicals. In some cases, radical skin debridement may be necessary to prevent progression of caustic agents into the underlying soft tissues. Once controlled, local wound care can be given in preparation for reconstruction.

Constrictive Bands

A variety of constrictive bands ("cock-rings," rubber bands, etc.) have been used to increase sexual gratification and prolong erections. When these are left in place too long, the penile skin and shaft become edematous and compromise blood flow. The skin can then be lost. Most commonly a portion of the proximal skin becomes ischemic and is lost. The remaining distal skin will become edematous and deformed because of interrupted lymphatic drainage. This severe edema does not ordinarily occur if any significant skin bridges the proximal and distal defect. Proximal circumferential skin loss with distal skin edema requires that the distal skin be removed and replaced by grafting or other measures.

PENILE SKIN LOSS

When penetrating injuries cause extensive skin loss, the penile soft tissue and urethra should be repaired and reconstructed before skin coverage, which usually can be done immediately.

When infection is the cause, the nonviable skin should be removed; moist dressings should be applied locally and changed twice daily. This process actively debrides and removes any infected tissue and develops a healthy tissue base for reconstruction. Once all surgical debridement is complete and infection controlled, reconstructive procedures can usually begin within 5 to 7 days.

Free Skin Grafts

Free skin taken from the host provides an excellent method of covering the penile shaft. This technique becomes necessary when skin loss is complete or when circumferential proximal skin loss has caused severe distal skin edema. In such cases, the residual edematous skin should be excised and new skin replaced over the entire penile shaft (Fig. 16–2).

Preparation of the penis for grafting is important. Any granulation tissue should be removed. This chronically infected tissue is high in fibroblasts. Removal down to the normal structures by sharp scraping will provide a well vascularized bed for skin grafts. After granulation tissue removal, hemostasis on the penile shaft must be excellent to prevent hematoma formation under the graft and ultimate graft loss.

Donor Site and Graft Procurement

The donor site for free grafts must be carefully selected. Ordinarily the anterior lateral aspect of the thigh will provide the thickness, texture, and color that will work well for penile skin. The area should be shaved free of existing hair and draped into the operative field. The graft site should be lubricated with mineral oil to help the dermatome glide smoothly over the surface.

The air dermatome is the preferred instrument. It can be used on the thigh or torso to harvest grafts and has the advantage of providing uniform graft thickness and a straight graft margin. The width of the usual dermatome is 10 to 12 cm and yields a graft that is nearly ideal to cover the penile shaft. After grafting, fine mesh gauze should be applied to the donor site and left in place.

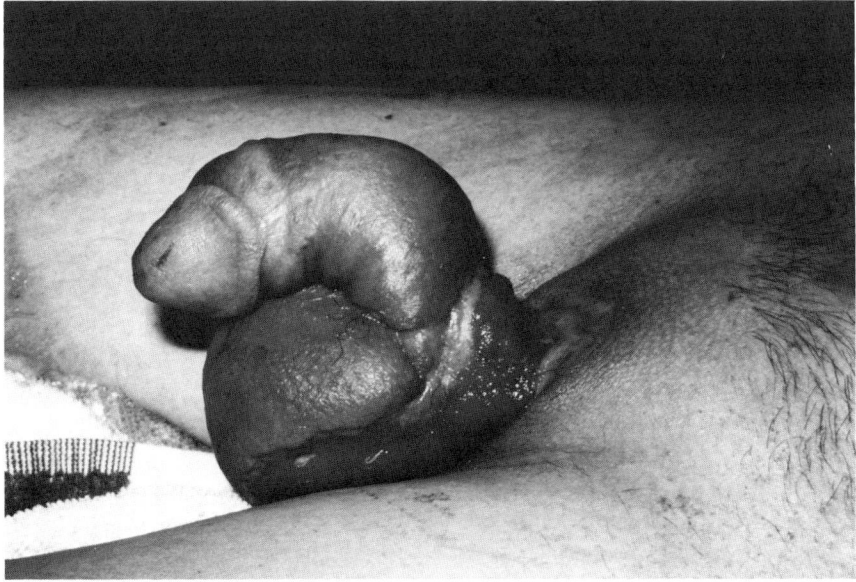

Figure 16–2. In this patient with circumferential skin loss at the base of the penis and scrotum, severe distal skin edema developed. (From McAninch.[14] Reprinted with permission.)

Selection of Graft Thickness

Full thickness grafts have epidermis and a full thickness of dermis. They produce minimal contracture after healing and thus provide an excellent functional result. Their major disadvantages are hair growth, a more difficult take, and the requirement of split thickness grafting to the donor site. Although the full thickness graft works well on the penis because the resultant minimal contracture allows unrestricted erections, the thick split thickness graft has similar characteristics and is ideal for penile reconstruction.

Split thickness grafts include the epidermis and varying degrees of dermis. The donor site will contain epidermal cells that can reepithelialize the donor area. Hair growth seldom occurs. Thick split thickness grafts (0.018 inch) taken from the thigh will cause only small degrees of contracture and thus are most appropriate for potent patients in whom retention of unrestricted erectile function is a consideration.

Thin split thickness grafts (0.008–0.014 inch) take rapidly in a high percentage of patients. No hair growth occurs and rapid reepithelialization of the donor site can be expected. More contracture develops than with the thicker split thickness grafts and will cause restricted erections in some patients.

Meshed split thickness grafts give excellent expanded skin coverage and have an excellent take.[14] Any fluid collection can drain freely, reducing the risk of graft loss. However, this type of graft has a higher rate of contracture than other split thickness grafts and thus is appropriate only for impotent patients.

Graft Technique

The existing proximal and distal skin margins should be debrided and any remaining skin should be excised up to the coronal margin (Fig. 16–3). The graft is applied to the penile shaft with the seam on the ventral surface. Ventral placement of the seam prevents the development of chordee and improves the cosmetic appearance by the formation of a medial raphe.

The seam margins are approximated with interrupted 5-0 chromic sutures. A urethral catheter should be in place to maintain easy control of the penis. The proximal and distal graft margins are approximated to the skin. A portion of these sutures should be long enough to tie over a large bolster dressing.

Fine-mesh impregnated gauze is applied directly to the graft, which must be in complete contact with the underlying tissue with all folds removed. Thin cotton padding soaked in mineral oil is applied to the gauze and then fluff dressing. The long suture ends are tied over the dressing to maintain constant graft position.

The penis should be maintained in the vertical position postoperatively. This is aided by the bolster dressing. However, to ensure immobilization in the proper position, a plastic housing is placed around the penis as a splint.

Postoperative Care

The penis should be maintained in the vertical position and a urethral catheter left in place unless cystostomy diversion has been done. Perioperative antibiotics should be given. The donor site should be kept dry and the fine mesh gauze covering should be open to the air. Exposure to a heat lamp for 15 min twice daily aids rapid eschar formation and encourages reepithelialization. In 14 to 20 days the donor site has usually healed.

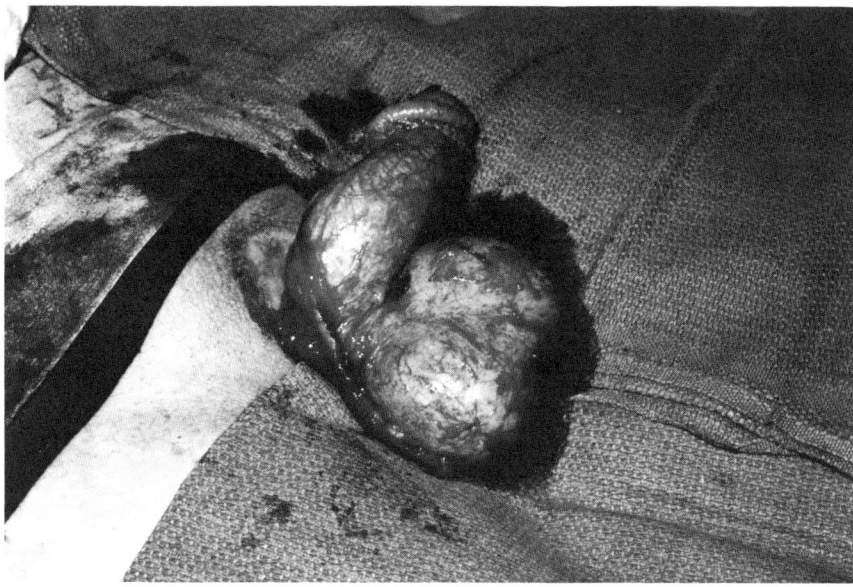

Figure 16–3. With total removal of edematous skin, the underlying testes and penis were found to be normal and grafting could be immediately undertaken. (From McAninch.[14] Reprinted with permission.)

The penile dressing should be taken down by the fifth postoperative day unless infection is present. The graft has capillary ingrowth from the vascular bed by the third day and is relatively fixed by the fifth day. Graft take in most cases exceeds 90% (Fig. 16–4).

Graft failure can be caused by infection, sheering, movement of the graft in the early postoperative period, or hematoma under the graft. Many of the efforts in grafting technique, wound preparation, and care are directed at preventing these major causes of graft loss. A high success rate can be expected with the given guidelines.[14]

Penile Flaps

Flaps maintain a vascular supply and are attached to the surrounding tissue by a pedicle. In many instances, partial skin loss of the distal shaft can be corrected by using the remaining skin as a pedicle flap. Total skin loss of the penis can be covered by pedicle flaps based on the lower abdomen or thigh, but these have a less acceptable cosmetic result than free grafts.[15] When erections are not expected and the scrotum is uninvolved, a scrotal flap can be raised. The penis is then placed in the scrotum and the glans is left exposed.

SCROTAL INJURIES

Partial Scrotal Loss

Partial loss of scrotal skin can be managed by debridement and closure. The scrotum has great compliance and elasticity, which allow even small remnants to be enlarged to cover large areas. Blood supply is excellent and scrotal flaps can be created with a high margin of

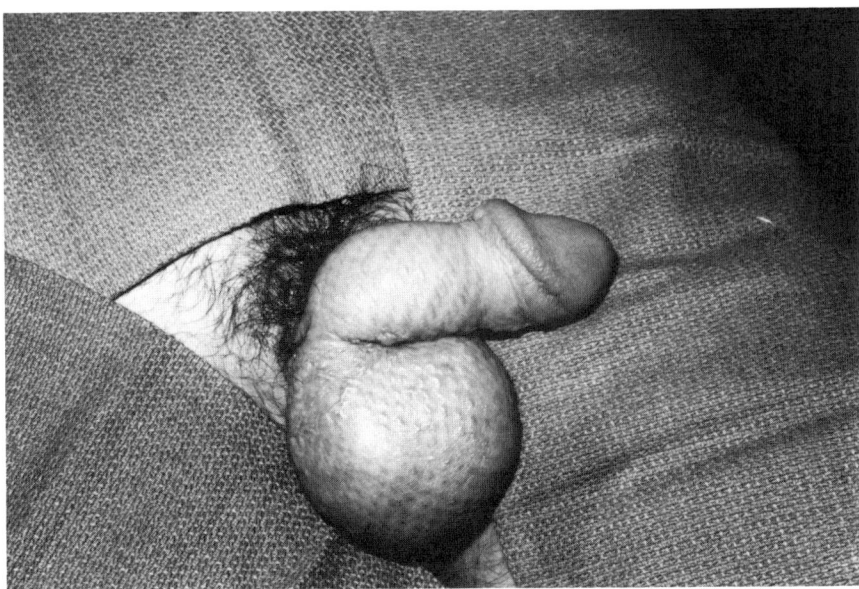

Figure 16–4. Three months after grafting, the cosmetic appearance of both scrotum and penis was excellent. (From McAninch.[14] Reprinted with permission.)

safety. It has also been suggested that the scrotum can regenerate, but detailed study in this area is lacking.

Total Scrotal Loss

Total loss of the scrotum presents a challenge for management and reconstruction. When severe contamination or infection is present, the initial care of the testicles is the use of moist dressing to the area with the testicles remaining exposed. Extensive perirectal infections require diverting colostomy. In some instances, medical colostomy can be achieved by parenteral hyperalimentation and cessation of oral food intake.[11,12] When infection originates in the urethra or prostate, a cystostomy is necessary for urinary diversion.[12,13]

Use of Thigh Pouches

Once infection is controlled, the testicles and spermatic cords can be protected by placement in two subcutaneous thigh pouches. This usually can be done 5 to 7 days after initial presentation and is a temporary measure until scrotal reconstruction can be initiated. The testicles should be placed on the medial aspect of each thigh. The skin and subcutaneous tissue are dissected from the thigh fascia to create a pocket for the testicle (Fig. 16–5). These subcutaneously constructed pockets are known to increase testicular temperature,

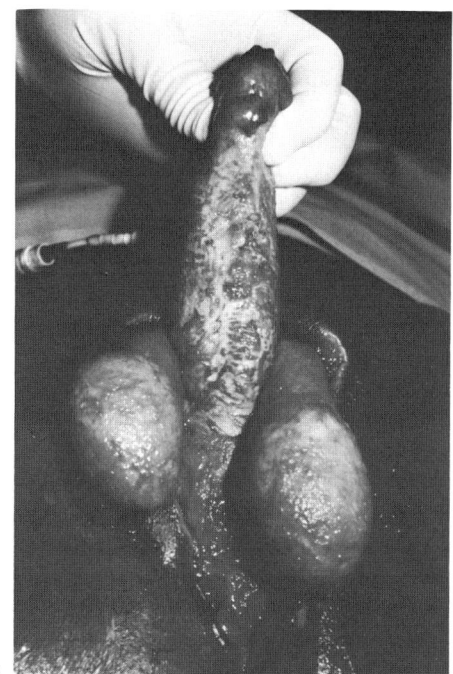 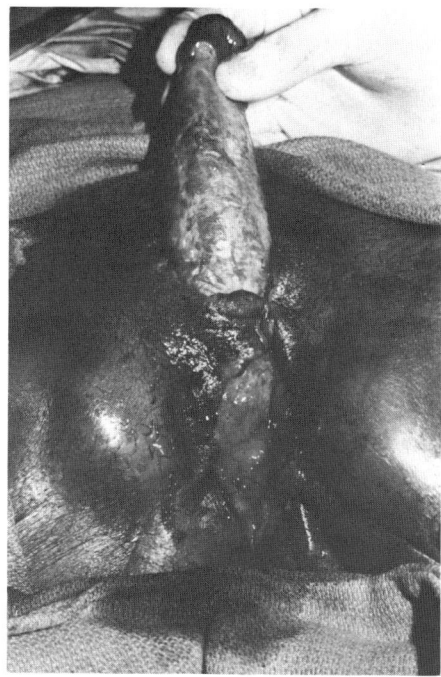

Figure 16–5. **A:** Testes before pouch placement are free of surrounding infection. **B:** After placement in the medial thigh pouch, the large perineal defect is greatly reduced and the testicles are protected from the environment. (From McAninch.[14] Reprinted with permission.)

which would impede spermatogenesis over the long term.[16] However, scrotal reconstruction can usually begin within 4 weeks.

In some instances the testicles may be placed in permanent thigh pouches. Elderly bedridden patients not concerned about reproduction would be best suited for permanent pouches. However, in younger patients testicular placement superficial to the subcutaneous tissue will permit maintenance of spermatogenesis.

Grafts in Scrotal Replacement

Total loss of scrotal skin requires complete replacement with new tissue. Split thickness skin grafts provide one method of scrotal reconstruction.[14] The testicles should be removed from thigh pouches and brought into the wound (Fig. 16-6A). A split thickness graft (0.014–0.018 inch) should be taken and meshed. All granulation tissue should be removed from the testes and they should be sutured together in the midline before the graft is applied. The meshed graft is applied such that the entire surface of the spermatic cords and testes is covered (Fig. 16–6B). The testicles must have a very dependent position. Fine-mesh impregnated gauze is used to cover the graft and will help maintain graft position in the early postoperative period. Fluff gauze constitutes the outside dressing, which is left

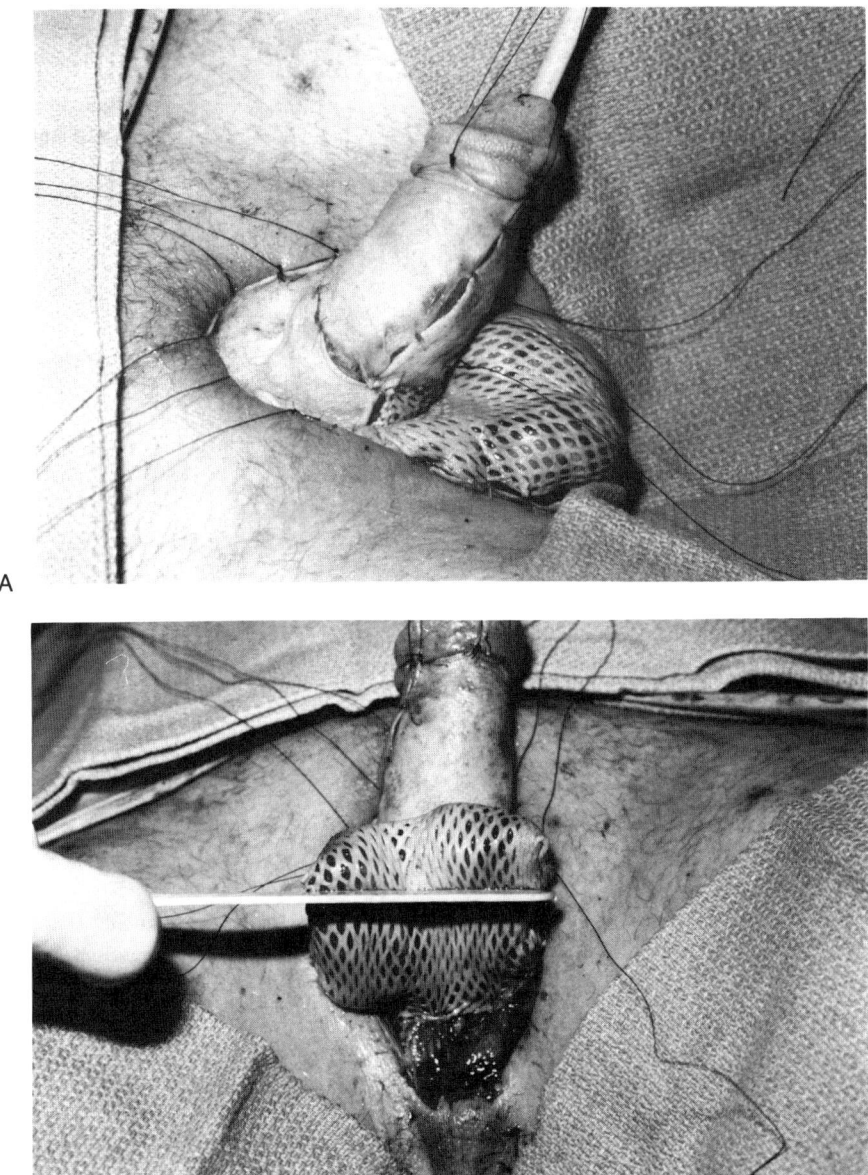

Figure 16–6. **A:** Mesh grafts are used to make the new scrotum. Nonmeshed split thickness grafts were needed for penile reconstruction in this patient. **B:** The testicles and cords should be covered entirely, anteriorly and posteriorly.

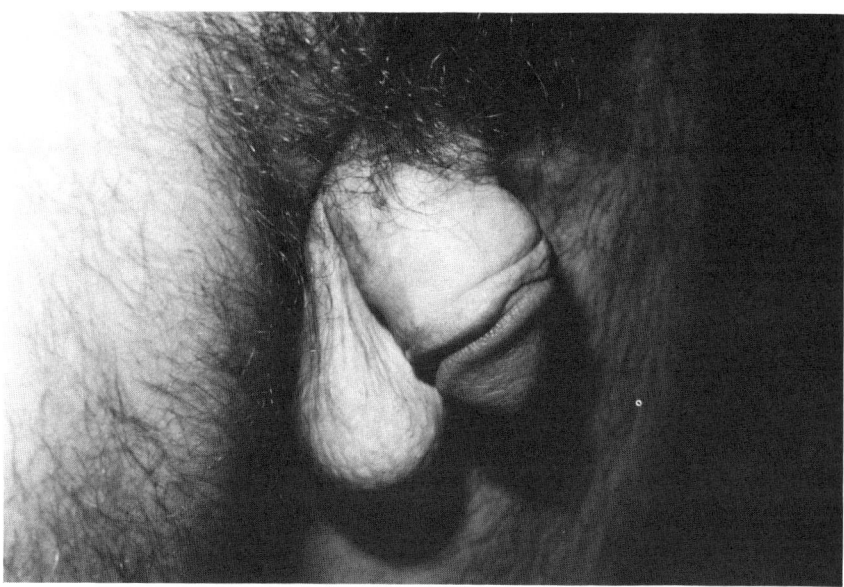

Figure 16–6, cont. C: One year after reconstruction, the cosmetic appearance of this patient's completely grafted genitalia is excellent and erectile function is normal. (From McAninch.[14] Reprinted with permission.)

in place for 3 to 5 days. In most cases graft take is greater than 90%. Infection and graft motion (sheering) are major causes for graft loss.

The dependent position of the testicles in the neoscrotum is especially important in the early postoperative period. This allows constant tissue expansion as reepithelialization occurs in meshed segments of the graft. This continuous expansion decreases graft contracture and produces a more normal-appearing scrotum. In addition, the cosmetic result is enhanced by the rugate appearance of the healed meshed graft (Fig. 16–6C). The testicular temperature in this type of scrotal reconstruction should be satisfactory for spermatogenesis.

Flaps in Scrotal Replacement

Numerous techniques for scrotal reconstruction with thigh flaps have been described.[10,17–19] Most use pedicle flaps and achieve acceptable results. These flaps have the advantages of being well vascularized and possessing a neural innervation similar to that of the normal scrotum (Fig. 16–7). Only patients with a small amount of soft subcutaneous tissue and relatively loose thigh skin can be considered for this procedure.

The testes are removed from the thigh pouch and sutured together in the midline. The thigh flaps are then raised. To maintain an excellent vascular and neural supply, we have the thin subcutaneous tissue with the flaps. The presence of loose thigh skin will allow primary skin closure on the thigh, and skin grafts can be avoided. The area under the neoscrotum should be well drained to control transudate accumulation and infection.

Postoperatively these patients should not ambulate too soon in order to minimize tension on the flaps.

Testicular Function After Scrotal Reconstruction

Limited information is available on patients with complete scrotal replacement. We have managed 10 such patients, but follow-up has not been uniform. At the time of the initial injury and debridement, testosterone dropped to near castrate levels in most patients, but rebounded to within the normal range after a few months. In only one patient was a sperm count obtained. One year after reconstruction with a meshed split thickness graft, he had severe oligospermia, but configuration, motility, and semen volume were normal.

In summary, it appears that Leydig cell function is depressed but returns after reconstruction with either the flap or graft technique. It is unclear when or if spermatogenesis returns.

Figure 16–8 is an algorithm outlining the methods of management. In most patients, partial skin loss can be managed by closure with local remaining skin. Tensive partial loss of penile skin may require grafting. Potent patients should have thick split thickness grafts or full thickness grafts. Impotent patients should have coverage with meshed split thickness grafts or scrotal flaps when available.

Partial scrotal loss is seldom a problem. Local flaps and closure of the defect with the remaining scrotal skin can usually be accomplished. After total scrotal loss the testicles should be placed temporarily in thigh pouches. Later, a new scrotum can be created with

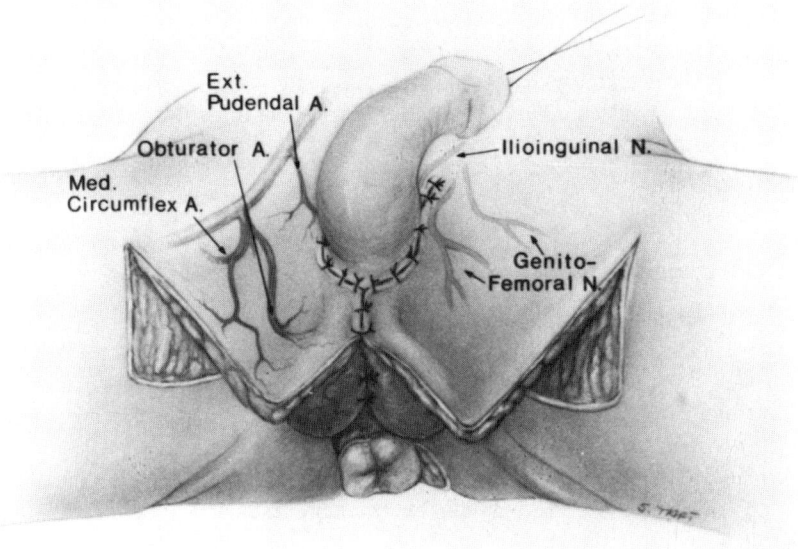

Figure 16–7. The arterial and neural supply of the cutaneous flaps used in scrotal reconstruction. (From McAninch.[14] Reprinted with permission.)

GENITAL SKIN LOSS

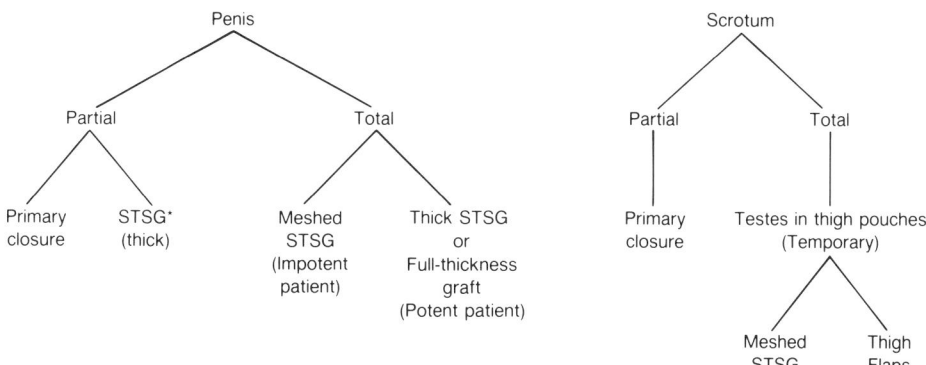

*STSG = Split-thickness skin graft

Figure 16–8. An algorithm for the suggested management of major genital skin loss. (From McAninch.[14] Reprinted with permission.)

meshed split thickness grafts or thigh-based cutaneous flaps. Aggressive wound care, appropriate timing of reconstruction, and adherence to basic principles of reconstructive surgery will result in functional recovery and a cosmetically acceptable appearance.

REFERENCES

1. Fetter TR, Gartman E. Traumatic rupture of the penis. *Am J Surg.* 1936; 32:371.
2. Redman JF, Miedmerma EB. Traumatic rupture of the corpus cavernosum: a case report and survey of the incidence in Arkansas. *J Urol.* 1981; 126:830.
3. Nicolaisen G, Melamud A, Williams RD, et al. Rupture of the corpus cavernosum: surgical management. *J Urol.* 1983; 130:917.
4. Orvis BR, McAninch JW. Penile rupture. *Urol Clin North Am.* 1989; 16:369.
5. Wasko R, Goldstein AG. Traumatic rupture of the testicle. *J Urol.* 1966; 95:721.
6. Cassie GF. Rupture of the testis: seminoma. *Br J Urol.* 1956; 28:283.
7. Fournier GR Jr, Laing FC, McAninch JW. Scrotal ultrasonography and the management of testicular trauma. *Urol Clin North Am.* 1989; 16:377.
8. Del Villar RG, Ireland GW, Cass AS. Early exploration following trauma to the testicle. *J Trauma.* 1973; 13:600.
9. McAninch JW, Kahn RI, Jeffrey RB, et al. Major traumatic and septic genital injuries. *J Trauma.* 1984; 24:291.
10. Culp DA. Genital injuries: etiology and initial management. *Urol Clin North Am.* 1977; 4:143.
11. Baskin LS, Carroll PR, Cattolica EV, McAninch JW. Necrotizing soft tissue infections of the perineum and genitalia. *Br J Urol.* 1990; 65:524.
12. Carroll PR, Cattolica EV, Turzan CT et al. Necrotizing soft-tissue infections of the perineum and genitalia, etiology and early reconstruction. *West J Med.* 1986; 144:174.
13. Spirnak JP, Renick MI, Hampel N et al. Fournier's gangrene: report of 20 patients. *J Urol.* 1984; 131:289.
14. McAninch JW. Management of major genital skin loss. *Urol Clin North Am.* 1989; 16:387.

15. Iturregui-Pagan JR. Scrotal flaps for penile denudation. *J Urol*. 1982; 127:989.
16. Culp DA, Huffman WC. Temperature determination in the thigh with regard to burying the traumatically exposed testis. *J Urol*. 1956; 76:436.
17. McDougal WS. Scrotal reconstruction using thigh pedicle flaps. *J Urol*. 1983; 129:757.
18. Reid CF, Wright JH Jr. Scrotal reconstruction following an avulsion injury. *J Urol*. 1985; 133:681.
19. Tiwari IN, Seth IIP, Mehdiratta KS. Reconstruction of the scrotum by thigh flaps. *Plast Reconst Surg*. 1980; 66:605.
20. Garrison FS. *History of Medicine*. Philadelphia: WB Saunders, 1929: 264.
21. Garrison FS. *History of Medicine*. Philadelphia: WB Saunders, 1929: 684.
22. Majno G. *The Healing Hand: Man and the Wound in the Ancient World. Commonwealth Fund Publ*. London: Harvard Univ Press. 1975: 142.

17
Female Genital Trauma and Sexual Assault

M. MARGARET KNUDSON, M.D.
WILLIAM R. CROMBLEHOLME, M.D.

". . . a cedar pencil, five inches long, and cut to a point, had been forced up through the posterior wall of the vagina into the abdominal cavity. Here it transfixed two coils of the small intestines, and after a sojourn of eight months was extracted by an incision through the anterior abdominal wall, midway between the umbilicus and Poupart's ligament, where the point was engaged in the fascia transversalis. It has occasioned repeated attacks of peritonitis, and after its extraction death resulted from the cause."

J. Erichsen, 1858
The Science and Art of Surgery

Sexual crimes against women and children continue to be the most common etiology of injury to the female genital tract. Iatrogenic injuries occurring during induced abortions or with other types of gynecologic surgery have also been well recognized. In more recent years, severe blunt trauma has resulted in an increasing number of genital tract injuries in both pregnant and nonpregnant women. Penetrating trauma may also result in injury to the intraabdominal reproductive organs. The promotion of women in both professional and amateur sports has led to an increased incidence of genital injuries in female athletes. Early recognition and definitive treatment of female genital trauma is essential to avoid the potential complications of hemorrhage, sepsis, and loss of endocrine and reproductive function.

ANATOMY

The perineum is the region at the inferior end of the trunk, situated between the thighs and the lower part of the buttocks.[27] The perineal region can be divided into two regions, anterior and posterior, by a line drawn between the two ischial tuberosities, passing anterior to the anus (Fig. 17–1). The anterior triangular area created by this line is referred to as the urogenital triangle and the posterior area as the anal triangle. The external genitalia located within the urogenital triangle are collectively termed the vulva, and include the labia majora, labia minora, the body and the glans of the clitoris, and the vaginal orifice.[27] The urethral orifice is adjacent to and superior to the vaginal orifice. The posterior or anal triangle contains the anal canal, which is surrounded by the fatty area and termed the ischiorectal fossa. The principal blood supply to the perineum arises from the internal pudendal artery, which transverses the ischiorectal fossa in the pudendal canal along with the pudendal nerve and veins, and enters the urogenital triangle.

The pelvic viscera, which include the urinary bladder, urethra, vagina, uterus, ovaries, fallopian tubes, and rectum, are supported inferiorly by the pelvic and urogenital diaphragms.[5] The pelvic diaphragm, comprising the levator ani and the coccygeus muscles and their investing fascia, arises from both sides of the pelvic wall and passes downward toward the midline to surround the terminal portions of the anus, vagina, and urethra.[5,27] The urogenital diaphragm extends across the anterior part of the pelvic outlet and contains the deep transverse perineal muscle and the sphincter muscle of the membranous urethra. The

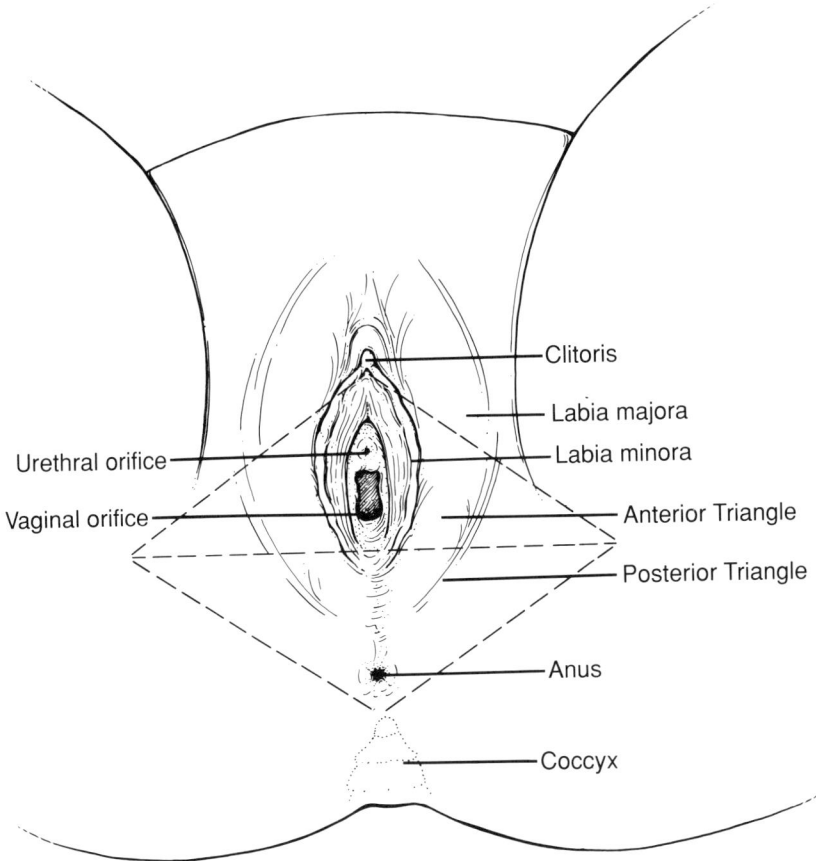

Figure 17–1. Anterior and posterior triangles of the female perineum.

anatomy of this area is complex and there exist distinct anatomical compartments that define how hematomas and sepsis are confined or the extent to which they spread.[5]

In the nongravid state, the organs of the upper female reproductive tract are well protected within the bony pelvis (Fig. 17–2). The uterus is a muscular organ located in the pelvis between the rectum and the bladder. In the nulliparous state, the uterus is 8 cm long and 5 cm at its widest part.[27] The uterus is surrounded on both sides by the broad ligaments, which contain the fallopian tubes, the round ligaments of the uterus, as well as the ovarian and uterine vessels arising from the internal iliac arteries. The fallopian tubes course through the upper portion of the broad ligaments, and can be divided into four parts moving medial to lateral: the interstitial part beginning at the angle of the uterus, a short isthmus, the long ampulla, and the infundibulum, which ends in the fimbriae. The ovaries lie deep in the pelvic side wall in front of the broad ligament. Their blood supply is derived directly from a branch of the aorta.[27]

The cervix is the narrow, distal portion of the uterus that ends in the vagina. The vagina passes through the urogenital diaphragm and opens into the perineum. Anteriorly, the vagina lies in close proximity to the bladder and ureters, and posteriorly it relates to the rectum.[27] The major blood supply to the vagina, the vaginal artery, arises from the internal iliac artery and enters laterally on each side.

MECHANISM OF INJURY

Blunt Trauma

Injuries to the nongravid female pelvic viscera after blunt trauma are rare. Dyer and Barclay reported that up until 1962, there were no recorded nonpenetrating injuries to the nonpreg-

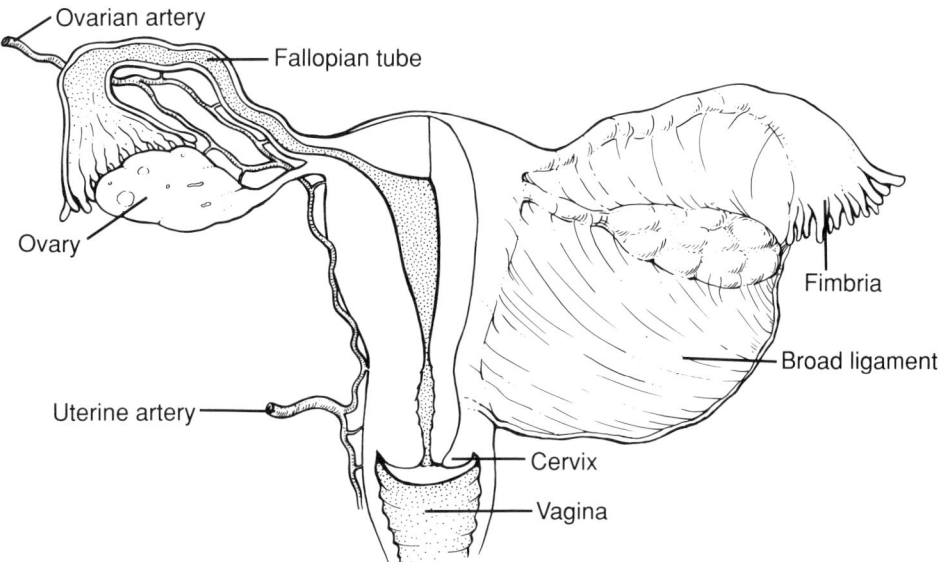

Figure 17–2. Female pelvic organs—uterus, ovaries, and fallopian tubes.

nant uterus.[3] Although there have been a few reports since that time, injuries to these relatively well protected organs are uncommon unless they are enlarged or diseased.[5,14]

In 1982, Grossberg and Druitt reported a case of traumatic rupture of the nonpregnant uterus that resulted from a crush injury.[7] This was only the second published case in the world literature on this entity, and both were associated with pelvic fractures. Kuntz described a patient with a partial avulsion of the uterine cervix that occurred after a fall while water skiing.[10] An isolated case of ovarian vein rupture sustained in a motor vehicle accident was published in 1982.[1] This patient presented with hemoperitoneum and was found to be bleeding from an ovarian cyst and adjacent vein.

Stone et al. reported the Maryland Institute of Emergency Medical Services Systems' experience with gynecologic injury in the nongravid female during blunt trauma occurring between 1975 and 1980.[26] During that time, 220 patients underwent exploratory laparotomy and 15 were found to have gynecologic injuries. All of the patients had a positive diagnostic peritoneal lavage before surgery. Thirteen of these patients were found to be bleeding from ovarian cysts (corpus luteum or lutein), one had sustained an ovarian laceration, and one patient who was postpartum suffered lacerations of the uterus and vagina. All of the patients had associated multiple trauma, with 40% having pelvic fractures.

The incidence of nonobstetric female genital tract trauma occurring in New Guinea was described by Sill in 1987.[25] During a 3-year period, there were 25 admissions to the Port Moresby General Hospital because of nonobstetric female genital injuries. Fifty-two percent of the injuries resulted from voluntary coitus, 20% from rape, 16% from assault, and 12% were related to falls. The most frequent injury was a laceration to the posterior fornix of the vagina. All of the falls occurred in children who sustained labial and perineal tears by falling on a hard object during play.

The most common injury to the female genital tract after blunt trauma is a vaginal laceration occurring with pelvic fractures. These injuries are discussed below.

Sports Injuries

The most common mechanism of injury to the female genitalia associated with athletic endeavors is the straddle injury.[11] Such injuries are caused by falling on an object with the legs spread, allowing the perineum to absorb most of the impact. These injuries typically result from landing forcefully on the crossbar of a bicycle or on gymnastic equipment. Such injuries have also followed falls while snow- or waterskiing.[6,10] The spectrum of injuries includes labial hematomas or tears, vaginal lacerations, clitoral tears, and urethral injuries.[11]

Penetrating Trauma

Gunshot wounds are the most common cause of injury to the genital organs in nonpregnant women.[14] An early report from Houston described 27 cases involving traumatic wounds of the female reproductive organs.[20] Gunshot wounds were responsible for 16 injuries and stab wounds for 7. (Four patients in this report had sustained blunt trauma). Although only 10 patients were pregnant at the time of injury, 71% were felt to have enlargement of the involved reproductive organs, due to either a recent pregnancy or ovarian pathology.

Penetrating trauma is most likely to injure the uterus, followed by the tube, ovary, and then the cervix.[14] Associated injuries to bowel and vascular structures are common. In the series from Houston, two-thirds of the patients had other abdominal injuries, with most involving the small bowel.[20]

INITIAL ASSESSMENT AND MANAGEMENT

Perineal Injuries

The two major areas of clinicopathological concern in regard to perineal trauma are hemorrhage and infection.[5] The perineum is one of the most highly vascularized areas of the body, and blunt trauma can result in hematomas that reach 4 to 5 cm in diameter. The source of such subcutaneous bleeding can be the anastomoses between the external and internal pudendal vessels contained within the fatty tissue of the labia majora or the vessels in the bulbs of the vestibule. With sufficient force, either of these vessel clusters can burst and lead to hematoma formation, which can dissect to the skin surface and rupture. Urinary retention may accompany these injuries, and in younger patients, may actually be the presenting complaint.[4,11]

The management of perineal injuries begins with a careful examination. This may be extremely difficult in young children and in patients who are anxious, bleeding extensively, or in pain. There should be no hesitation to administer sedation or an anesthetic in these situations to avoid underestimation of the injuries. The examination should include a complete inspection of the area, including vaginal and anal inspection for associated injuries. The possibility of urethral or bladder lacerations must be entertained and radiological evaluation with cystourethrograms obtained when indicated.

The treatment of perineal hematomas depends on the size and whether or not the hematoma is expanding. Small, nonexpanding hematomas can be managed with initial cold compresses, followed later by local heat, anticipating resolution within 3 to 5 days. Large hematomas (>4–5 cm in diameter) or those continuing to enlarge are best managed by incision and evacuation. At the time of evacuation, any obvious bleeding vessels should be ligated. However, since the source of bleeding is usually small venous anastomoses, searching for vessels to ligate may create more bleeding. The cavity created by the hematoma can be large and may require packing if oozing persists. Alternatively, the skin incisions can be closed with interrupted or continuous absorbable sutures with a drain left in place for 24 hr. Secondary infection is a potential risk after evacuation but is usually avoided with adequate drainage. "Prophylactic" antibiotics are not indicated. If urinary retention accompanies the injury, temporary drainage may be required.[11]

Lacerations of the vulva or periuretheral area require careful inspection for foreign material and debridement of all necrotic tissue. Hemostasis should be secured and the lacerations closed with fine absorbable sutures attempting to reestablish normal anatomic relationships. Irrigation and drainage may be indicated, and consideration given to antibiotics and the tetanus status of the patient. In evaluating penetrating injuries to the vulva that result from falling on sharp objects, the adjacent vagina, bladder, and rectum must be thoroughly inspected for associated injury. These injuries have occasionally penetrated the abdominal cavity, thus requiring exploration.

Vaginal and Cervical Injuries

The evaluation and management of vaginal lacerations depend on the circumstances of the injury and the likely site of the laceration. Lacerations sustained at the fourchette or just inside the introitus in adult women can usually be managed with sedation and local anesthesia. Children or young girls with lacerations resulting from sexual assault or blunt trauma will require a general anesthesia for both inspection and repair. Adults with forniceal lacerations will also generally require either a general or regional anesthetic as cul-de-sac perforation with entrance into the peritoneum is not an infrequent finding. In this latter instance laparotomy is usually appropriate to rule out intestinal injury.

The presenting complaint of vaginal injury is bleeding, which may range from minor to life-threatening hemorrhage with shock.[5] Both the anterior and posterior walls of the vagina must be inspected as well as the fornices. Retroperitoneal hematomas may be associated with these injuries and can be detected on bimanual examination.[5]

The vascular supply of the vagina is such that the bleeding points are usually along the cut edges of the vaginal mucosa. Hemostasis is secured as the tissue is reapproximated with running stitches of absorbable suture material. Vaginal packing alone is usually ineffective, but can be attempted when the injury is too great to repair primarily, or as a temporizing maneuver.[5] Penetrating injuries to the inferior lateral vaginal wall may involve the pudendal artery or vein, which run inferior and lateral to the ischial spine. These injuries result in large hematomas that bulge into the vagina along its lateral and inferior wall and may compress the lumen of the rectum. A substantial amount of blood can also dissect into the ischiorectal fossa with little external evidence of hematoma formation. Such hematomas need to be evacuated through the vagina with hemostasis secured by deep ligatures around the pudendal vessels. Drains brought out through the vagina may be necessary after closure.

Vaginal mucosal lacerations tend to heal rapidly without secondary infections unless contaminated with foreign material. Deeper lacerations or wounds into the supporting tissues of the vagina or hematoma cavities with excess dead space pose a greater potential risk for secondary infection. Patients with the latter injuries should receive broad spectrum antibiotics appropriate for the contaminating aerobic and anaerobic vaginal flora. Examples include an aminoglycoside in combination with either clindamycin or metronidazole, or a single agent such as cefoxitin.

The repair of cervical lacerations is also performed with absorbable suture material.[5] Postoperative edema of the cervix and vagina may be severe, and sutures tied too tightly may promote ischemia. Both the cervical mucosa and the fibromuscular stroma must be closed together, and a careful search made for any extension of the laceration into the uterine isthmus or bladder.[5]

Injuries to the Uterus, Fallopian Tubes, and Ovaries

Trauma to the intraabdominal reproductive organs is rarely isolated and is usually detected at laparotomy for associated blunt or penetrating injuries. If the patient is stable and other life-threatening injuries have been addressed, consideration can be given to preservation of reproductive and hormonal function. Lacerations of the uterus can often be repaired in layers with interrupted absorbable sutures. Hysterectomy is reserved for substantial destruction of the uterine tissue or in cases where the uterine arteries have been lacerated or avulsed at the level of the uterocervical junction. Omental or peritoneal grafts have been advocated to promote a clean and smooth closure when there is extensive serosal damage.[5] Ovarian lacerations are closed with simple suturing.[26] Occasionally, extensive damage or profuse bleeding may require removal of one tube or ovary, but in most cases the opposite adnexae can be spared.

Open Pelvic Fractures

Vaginal lacerations that result from pelvic bone fracture are considered open fractures and are associated with an increased morbidity and mortality. Although these injuries are not common, in a recently published series of 114 women with pelvic fractures, there were four patients with vaginal lacerations (3.5%).[16] The overall mortality associated with closed pelvic fractures is in the range of 9% to 30%, whereas patients with open pelvic fractures have mortality rates of 25% to 60%.[4,13,15,16,18,21,22] Deaths from open pelvic fractures are usually the result of hemorrhage or sepsis.[13,15]

The laceration of the vagina may be caused by direct penetration of a bone fragment through the vaginal wall (Fig. 17–3). Diastasis of the symphysis pubis, as occurs with straddle injuries, causes a lateral tearing force on the perineum, which may also result in vaginal lacerations.[16] Shearing lacerations of the vagina have been associated with bilateral ischiopubic rami fractures when the anterior pelvic ring is severed from the weight-bearing portion of the pelvis.[14,16] Foreign bodies present in the vagina at the time of impact, such as tampons or contraceptive devices, increase the risk of vaginal tears.[16]

Vaginal bleeding is the most common finding in most women with open pelvic fractures. However, the diagnosis may be missed in patients who are menstruating or

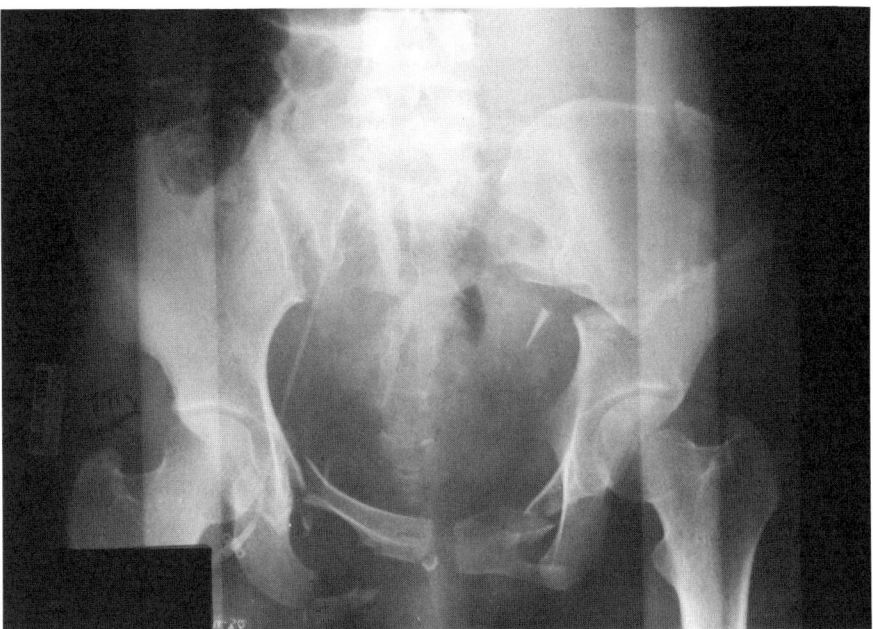

Figure 17–3. X-ray demonstrates severe open pelvic fractures with associated vaginal lacerations.

when spasm of the walls of the vagina traps blood in the vault.[14,16] Therefore, all female patients with pelvic fractures must undergo vaginal examination. The presence of hematuria, vaginal urine or stool, or difficulty in urinating or in passing a Foley catheter are other signs of severe perineal trauma that may accompany vaginal injury.[16]

The initial management of open pelvic fractures is directed at controlling hemorrhage. Rothenberger et al. have described two types of hemorrhage occurring with these fractures: a diffuse bleeding in the retroperitoneal space and an accompanying disruption of a major vessel to the lower extremities.[22] Major vascular trauma to the common iliac, external iliac, common femoral arteries, or veins that were directly related to the open pelvic fracture has been described, and will obviate initial operative management.[22] Excessive bleeding from the retroperitoneal space is best managed with angiographic localization and embolization techniques. Most patients with these severe fractures will have a number of other injuries that will also influence their initial management. In the series of patients reviewed by Rothenberger et al., there was an average of 2.8 additional major injuries per patient.[22] In another report of 16 patients who sustained open pelvic fractures after blunt trauma, 9 required laparotomy for associated abdominal injuries, and in 6 these injuries were multiple.

With the patient under anesthesia, a thorough perineal examination is conducted. This includes a complete examination of the vagina with a speculum, as well as an inspection of the rectum with a sigmoidoscope. The urethra should be examined and a cystogram obtained in search of an associated bladder disruption. The vaginal laceration is then irrigated, debrided, and closed with absorbable sutures. Systemic antibiotics are initiated and continued postoperatively as in other open fractures. However, the antibiotics used must be active against vaginal flora, as outlined above. Patients with rectal injuries will require diverting colostomy and distal rectal washout. Deep perineal tears also require diverting colostomy to prevent recurrent soiling and allow healing without sepsis.[14,16] Patients with widely separated fractures may be candidates for external fixation during their initial operation. In addition to increasing stability, these fixators may decrease bleeding from fracture sites. The initial treatment of open pelvic fractures is outlined in Table 17–1.

In addition to hemorrhage, other complications associated with open pelvic fractures include sepsis, pelvic abcess formation, vaginal stricture, dysparunia, vaginismus, urethrovaginal, vesicovaginal, and rectovaginal fistula formation, anal sphincter dis-

Table 17–1 The Initial Management of Open Pelvic Fractures

1. Suspect an open pelvic fracture in all females
2. Begin aggressive and early fluid resuscitation; transfuse as needed
3. Identify and treat the associated, life-threatening injuries of the head, chest, and abdomen
4. Surgically control concomitant major vessel injuries
5. Control pelvic hemorrhage with application of MAST suit, external fixation device, or angiographic embolization
6. Thoroughly examine the vagina, rectum, urethra, bladder
7. Debride, irrigate, and close vaginal lacerations
8. Perform a diverting colostomy and distal rectal irrigation in the presence of rectal injury or deep perineal wound
9. Administer broad spectrum antibiotics aimed at vaginal flora
10. Inspect, debride, and dress perineal wounds frequently

ruption, and osteomyelitis.[14,17,21,22,24] The prevention of abscess formation and sepsis begins with prompt recognition of the vaginal injury and attention to the perineal wound. In addition to the initial diverting colostomy and rectal irrigation, frequent inspection of complex perineal wounds in the operating room is indicated, especially if packing is required. Aggressive treatment of these complex fractures and their associated injuries will offer the best chance of survival with the least morbidity.

SEXUAL ASSAULT

Sexual assault can be considered under two headings: rape or molestation. Rape is defined as forced vaginal penetration by a penis without the female's consent. Molestation is defined as noncoital sexual contact without consent. In either circumstance, significant physical injury can occur during sexual assault, necessitating a careful and detailed assessment by the examining physician. Further, since sexual assault is uniformly accompanied by varying degrees of psychological trauma, the victim's physical needs will best be identified and treated by the physician's maintaining an awareness of the patient's emotional needs as well.

Because of the medical importance as well as the sensitive legal implications of the assessment of a victim of sexual assault, it is essential that the evaluation be performed in a systematic and thorough fashion. A suggested approach has been outlined in a Technical Bulletin from the American College of Obstetricians and Gynecologists[23] and forms the basis of the present discussion. The order of this approach assumes a clinically stable patient without life-threatening trauma or hemorrhage.

Support Services

Sexual assault is a violation of the victim's autonomy and self-determination. Once freed of immediate physical threat by the departure of the assailant, the most common response is one of withdrawal and distrust of unfamiliar faces and surroundings. Yet for reasons of her own physical health and for the purpose of legal documentation, the victim is confronted with an array of hospital personnel unknown to her, including clerks, nurses, and physicians and possibly also law enforcement officers. For this reason, support services tailored exclusively for victims of sexual assault exist in most communities. Such a service should be activated as soon as possible after the patient's arrival. In some areas the service will have specially trained nurses experienced in counseling assault victims and in assisting in evidence collection. Others may use psychiatric social workers focused on crisis intervention. Still other communities avail themselves of volunteer women's support groups whose members serve as patient advocates to assist victims in the initial phase of their ordeal and to provide ongoing support in the days and weeks after the incident.

Consent

A careful, detailed consent should be obtained from the patient at the outset, even before a history is taken. Obtaining consent should cover the need to elicit past medical history, the details of the assault, a complete physical examination, and anticipated treatment to be offered. In addition, the patient needs to be consented for evidence collection, which includes obtaining laboratory specimens, the taking of photographs if appropriate, the retention of articles of clothing for evidence, and the release of information to the authorities. The patient is entitled to consent to some, all, or none of these aspects of the evaluation and coming to a decision about the extent of the examination can be difficult for some patients. Nonetheless, as the ACOG bulletin points out, it is important for the victim of sexual assault to regain control of what will or will not happen to her, including an assessment of her injuries.

History

With the patient's consent, the examination begins with a detailed history of the assault. As much as possible the description of events should be recorded in the patient's own words. The sequential details of the circumstances of the assault are relevant for two reasons. First, in the case where legal proceedings eventuate from the assault, the patient's description of the assault will form the basis for her later testimony. Second, and of more immediate importance, the patient's description of what was physically done to her, or what she was required to do to her assailant, will indicate the likely site(s) and extent of possibly injury. In this regard, one should remember that patients can vary markedly in their sensibilities and degree of embarrassment when discussing sexual acts. A patient may be willing to describe forced vaginal intercourse without too much difficulty. However, eliciting that oral or anal penetration also occurred may be accomplished only by gentle but directed questioning.

Physical Exam

The physical examination begins with a thorough inspection of the skin surfaces of the patient's body. Any scrapes, cuts, or ecchymoses should be described in detail with respect to size and location and whenever possible, with the patient's permission, photographs should be taken. The previously obtained description of the assault will pinpoint those areas where signs of injury are most likely to be found, such as lacerations or fractures, and that will certainly require careful inspection and treatment. However, in the course of a struggle or fight with an assailant other injuries may be sustained of which the victim may be unaware but needs to have identified.

Ecchymoses or even hematomas of the perineum and vulva can be seen when these areas are pummelled or kicked in the course of an assault. Similarly, vaginal lacerations can be extensive and involve the fourchette, the hymenal ring, the vaginal walls, or even the posterior fornix. The degree of damage can be striking even when due only to an erect penis without the insertion of other implements such as a dildo. During consensual sexual arousal and intercourse, a normal lengthening and accommodation of the vagina has been demonstrated by Masters and Johnson.[12] This natural preparation is unlikely to occur in the perpetration of a sexual assault. As a result, shearing forces may develop with forced penetration that cause the severe lacerations that can be seen. When foreign objects are known or suspected to have been used, the possibility of penetration into the peritoneal cavity through the vagina must be considered and ruled out. Depending on the specifics of the assault, the oral cavity and anal canal may similarly require a detailed inspection for signs of injury that will require treatment.

Laboratory Specimens

A number of laboratory specimens need to be collected as evidence in the course of the physical examination of the patient. There is a fairly standard series of specimens to be obtained from the victim. Table 17–2 lists those specimens recommended by the American College of Obstetricians and Gynecologists[12] as appropriate to the evaluation of a female victim of sexual assault. As these specimens may become evidence in a future legal action, meticulous identification and labeling of samples must be assured. In addition, careful transfer of the specimens to police authorities must be accomplished so as to maintain an unbroken "chain" of evidence collection.

Treatment

Treatment of physical injuries should follow standard guidelines as described earlier in this chapter. Although the frequency of the victim's acquiring a sexually transmitted disease as a result of sexual assault is low, prophylaxis should be offered. Current Centers for

Table 17–2 Laboratory Specimens*

Pubic hair
  Combed (assailant)
  Plucked (patient control)
Vaginal fluid
  Wet mount
    Motile sperm
  Fixed smear
    Sperm
  Swab or saline wash
    Acid phosphatase
    ABO (H) antigen
    Sperm precipitins
Culture for *N. gonorrhea*
  Endocervix
  Rectum
  Mouth
Debris under fingernails
Dried secretions from hair, scraped from skin, or from clothing stains
  Acid phosphatase
  ABO (H) antigen
Blood
  VDRL serology
  B-HCG
  Alcohol and/or drug level
Urinalysis

*Adapted with permission from Haggard.[23]

Disease Control recommendations[29] suggest an initial dose of ceftriaxone 250 mg intramuscularly. This should be followed by a 7-day course of doxycycline, 100 mg orally twice a day. This regimen will cover virtually all gonococci including beta-lactamase producing strains, chlamydia, and most likely incubating syphilis. For patients allergic to penicillin, spectinomycin, 2 g intramuscularly, may be substituted. However, this will not provide coverage for incubating syphilis. A repeat serology 4 to 6 weeks after the assault should be performed regardless of which regimen the patient receives to rule out acquisition of syphilis.

The blood sample for beta–human chorionic gonadotropin for pregnancy testing at the time of the assault will rule out a preexisting pregnancy. The risk of rape-related pregnancy is quoted as 1% to 2%[23] and "prophylaxis" should be discussed with the patient. Estrogen administered within 72 hr of an assault has been shown to be quite effective in preventing pregnancy. In the past, diethylstilbestrol, 25 mg orally twice a day for 5 days, or ethinyl estradiol, 5 mg orally once a day for 5 days, has been used. These high dose estrogen regimens have been associated with significant nausea, requiring antiemetics. More recently, birth control pills containing ethinyl estradiol, 50 μg, combined with norgestrel, 0.5 mg, have been used with roughly equivalent efficacy in a regimen of two pills orally, twice, 12 hr apart.

Follow-up

Follow-up of treatment of physical injuries and of prophylaxis for sexually transmitted diseases and pregnancy should be arranged at appropriate intervals after the assault. Of equal importance is the psychological support and counseling that is likely to be needed by the victim in the days and weeks after the incident. Feelings of shame and guilt are not uncommon among victims and difficulties with family members at home or associates in the workplace are not infrequent. An additional benefit of the support services activated at the initial assessment of a victim of sexual assault is the ongoing counseling and follow-up such groups provide to these patients. Unfortunately for some victims of sexual assault, the assessment and treatment of their injuries is in some ways only the beginning, and not the end, of their postrape ordeal.

REFERENCES

1. Blumenthal NJ, Burgin S. Ovarian vein rupture sustained in a motor vehicle accident: a case report. *S Afr Med J*. 1982; 62:907.
2. Claytor RN, Barth KL, Shubin CI. Evaluating child sexual abuse: observations regarding ano-genital injury. *Clin Pediatr*. 1989; 28:419–422.
3. Dyer I, Barclay DL. Accidental trauma complicating pregnancy and delivery. *Am J Obstet Gynecol*. 1962; 83:907–929.
4. Gilliland MD, Ward RE, Barton RM, et al. Factors affecting mortality in pelvic fractures. *J Trauma*. 1982; 22:691–693.
5. Gould SF, Delaney JJ. Obstetrical and gynecological injuries. In: Zuidema GE, Rutheford RB, Ballinger WF, eds. *Management of Trauma*. 4th ed. Philadelphia: WB Saunders; 1985.
6. Gray HH. A risk of waterskiing for women. *West J Med*. 1982; 136:169.
7. Grossberg P, Druitt D. Traumatic rupture of the non-pregnant uterus. *Med J Aust*. 1982; 1:310–311.
8. Ikpeme JO, Morison CR. Vaginal avulsion complicating pelvic fracture. *Br J Surg*. 1970; 57:317–318.
9. Jackson FC. Accidental injury: the problems and the initiatives. In: Buchsbaum H, ed. *Trauma in Pregnancy*. Philadelphia: WB Saunders; 1979.

10. Kuntz WD. Water-ski spill and partial avulsion of the uterine cervix. (Letter) *N Engl J Med*. 1983; 309:990.
11. Mandell J, Cromie WJ, Caldamone AA, et al. Sports-related genitourinary injuries in children. *Clin Sports Med*. 1982; 1:483–493.
12. Masters W, Johnson V. *Human Sexual Response*. Boston: Little, Brown. 1966; 68–100.
13. Maull KI, Sachatello CR, Ernst CB. The deep perineal laceration: an injury frequently associated with open pelvic fractures: a need for aggressive surgical management. *J Trauma*. 1977; 17:685–696.
14. Maull KI, Rozycki GS, Pedigo RE, et al. Injury to the female reproductive system. In: Mattox KL, Moore EE, Feliciano DV, eds. *Trauma*. San Mateo: Appleton-Lange; 1988.
15. Naam NH, Brown WH, Hurd R, et al. Major pelvic fractures. *Arch Surg*. 1983; 118:610–616.
16. Niemi TA, Norton LW. Vaginal injuries in patients with pelvic fractures. *J Trauma*. 1985; 25:547–551.
17. Patil U, Nesbitt R, Meyer R. Genitourinary tract injuries due to fracture of the pelvis in females: sequelae and their management. *Br J Urol*. 1982; 54:32–38.
18. Patterson FR, Morton KS. The cause of death in fractures of the pelvis. *J Trauma*. 1973; 13:849–856.
19. Peltier LF. Complications associated with fractures of the pelvis. *J Bone Joint Surg*. 1965; 47:1060–1069.
20. Quast DC, Jordan GL. Traumatic wounds of the female reproductive organs. *J Trauma*. 1964; 4:839–844.
21. Raffa J, Christensen N. Compound fractures of the pelvis. *Am J Surg*. 1976; 132:282–286.
22. Rothenberger D, Velasco R, Strate R, et al. Open pelvic fractures: a lethal injury. *J Trauma*. 1978; 18: 184–187.
23. Sexual Assault. ACOG Technical Bulletin, no. 101, February, 1987.
24. Siegel RS. Vesico-vaginal fistula and osteomyelitis. *J Bone Joint Surg*. 1971; 53:583–586.
25. Sill PR. Non-obstetric female genital tract trauma in Port Moresby, Papua, New Guinea. *Aust NZ J Obstet-Gynaecol*. 1987; 27:164–165.
26. Stone NN, Ances IG, Brotman S. Gynecologic injury in the nongravid female during blunt abdominal trauma. *J Trauma*. 1984; 24:626–627.
27. Thorak P. *Anatomy in Surgery* 2nd ed. Philadelphia: JB Lippincott; 1962; 554–629.
28. Trunkey DD, Chapman MW, Lim RC Jr, et al. Management of pelvic fractures in blunt trauma injury. *J Trauma*. 1974; 14:912–923.
29. 1989 Sexually Transmitted Diseases Treatment Guidelines. CDC, MMWR, vol. 38, no. S-8, September 1989.

18
Trauma in Pregnancy

M. MARGARET KNUDSON, M.D.

"I dressed his wounds; God healed him."

Ambroise Paré, 1536 [23]

HISTORY: Penetrating injuries to the gravid uterus date back to antiquity, when wounding instruments included such objects as spears, sticks, and animal horns. Wounds resulting from more modern warfare were well described by the military surgeon Ambroise Paré in the 16th century. Paré wrote of his experience with gunshot wounds to multiple sites, including the uterus. He rejected the then customary hot oil treatments of these wounds in favor of clean dressings, and is credited with popularizing ligature control of disrupted vessels. Paré, who was also an obstetrician, wrote of trauma during pregnancy: *"when the womb is wounded, the blood cometh out at the privites, and all other accidents appeare . . ."*[32]

INTRODUCTION

In contrast to penetrating trauma, severe blunt abdominal trauma occurring during pregnancy is truly a disease of modern women. According to Savage, in the period between 1950 and 1960 in Baltimore, there were no maternal deaths attributed to injury during pregnancy, and only 11 stillbirths that could be related to trauma.[19] The leading causes of maternal death during that time period were infection, cardiac disease, and hemorrhage. A recently published study from Massachusetts, however, now lists trauma as the major cause of maternal death.[46] It is estimated that 6% to 7% of pregnancies are currently complicated by some form of trauma.[40]

ANATOMY IN PREGNANCY

The uterus increases in size during pregnancy from a 7-cm length and 70-g weight to a 36-cm length and an 800- to 1200-g weight.[7] Although it remains an intrapelvic organ during the first 12 weeks of pregnancy, during the second trimester the uterus leaves the protected intrapelvic location, displacing some of the abdominal viscera. The normally thick muscular wall of the uterus thins during late pregnancy, making it more susceptible to

Table 18-1 Physiologic and Anatomic Changes of Pregnancy

Cardiovascular system	Increased heart rate (15–20 bpm)
	New systolic murmur
	ECG: left axis deviation, flat T waves
	Increased blood volume—50%
	Increased cardiac output—40% (1–1.5 L/min)
	Decreased blood pressure (5–15 mm Hg)
Gastrointestinal system	Decreased lower esophageal sphincter pressure
	Delayed gastric emptying
	Decreased intestinal motility
	Increased alkaline phosphatase (placenta)
	Decreased abdominal sensitivity
	Displaced intraabdominal contents
Genitourinary system	Dilated collecting system
	Increased GFR, increased plasma flow
	Decreased BUN, creatinine
	Decreased bladder tone
	Enlarged, thin uterus
	Increased uterine blood flow
Hematologic system	"Physiologic anemia" (Hct 32–37%)
	Increased WBC (18,000/mm^3)
	Increased serum fibrinogen
	Decreased plasminogen activator
	Increased Factors VII, VIII, IX, X
Respiratory system	Increased minute ventilation (50%)
	Increased tidal volume (40%)
	Decreased pCO$_2$
	Decreased serum bicarbonate (4 mEq/ml)
	Increased oxygen consumption

trauma.[35] Uterine blood flow increases to 500 to 700 cc/min and at term, the entire blood volume of the mother circulates through the uterus approximately every 8 to 11 min.[7]

The placenta reaches its maximum size at 36 to 38 weeks of pregnancy. The placenta is usually in a state of relaxation, although it remains sensitive to catecholamine stimulation.[35] The lack of elasticity in placental tissue as compared to uterine tissue may explain the tendency of the placenta to tear away from the more pliable uterus during blunt trauma.

Despite the fact that the fetus has risen out of the pelvis by the second trimester, it usually remains cushioned by the amniotic fluid envelope. In late pregnancy, the fetal head engages in the pelvis and can be injured by compression against the pelvic bones during blunt trauma. As the uterus grows, the fetus becomes the most likely target for penetrating abdominal trauma (Fig. 18–1).

PHYSIOLOGY OF PREGNANCY

A thorough understanding of the complex physiological changes that occur during pregnancy is necessary to care properly for the injured pregnant patient. These changes affect almost all systems during a normal pregnancy, and may profoundly alter the responses to trauma.

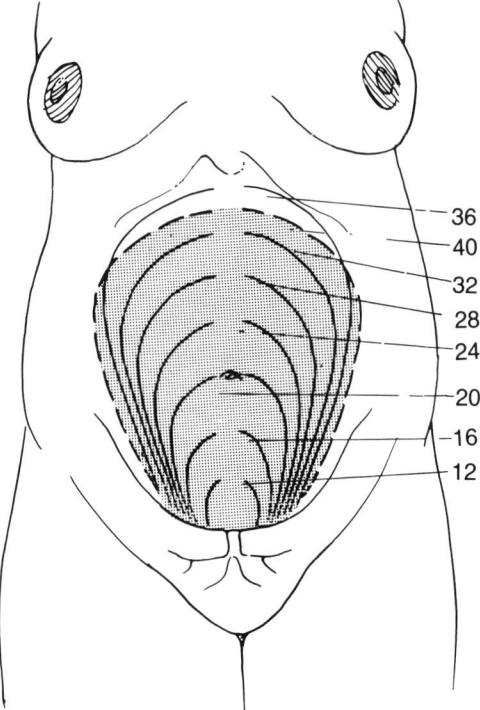

Figure 18–1. Abdominal heights of uterine fundus over gestation.

Cardiovascular System

The cardiac output increases throughout pregnancy, starting during the 10th week and reaching a maximum level of 6.0 to 7.0 L/min by 30 weeks.[7] Heart rate also increases by 15 to 20 beats/min by the third trimester. Both systolic and diastolic blood pressure fall 5 to 15 mm Hg below normal at midterm. Electrocardiogram changes include a left axis deviation as the diaphragm is pushed upward by the enlarging uterus.[25] The T waves may be flattened or inverted in the AVF or III positions. Ectopic beats, usually supraventricular, are more frequent during pregnancy, and a new soft systolic murmur may become audible. Although the venous pressure in the lower extremities is increased, changes in central venous pressure still reflect the patient's response to volume resuscitation.

During late pregnancy, the patient is extremely sensitive to position, as the enlarged uterus may impair flow back to the heart from the vena cava. This so-called supine hypotension syndrome can be particularly deleterious to the patient in hypovolemic shock.[7] Elevation of the right hip, manual displacement of the uterus off the cava, or positioning the patient on her left side will result in increased cardiac output.

Hematologic System

The plasma volume also starts to increase during the 10th week of pregnancy, and is expanded by 50% at term.[25,33] The erythrocyte volume increases as well, but by only

18% to 25%. This dilutional change results in a lowered measured hematocrit, which averages 37% at term, but may be as low as 32% in patients not receiving iron supplementation.[7] Pregnancy induces a leukocytosis, which may reach 18,000 white blood cells (WBC)/mm³ at term and 25,000 during labor. Clotting factors VII, VIII, IX, and X are elevated during pregnancy, although there are decreased levels of plasminogen activator.[33] Measured clotting studies are usually normal, but fibrin split products are often present.[25] Although these changes are protective for the mother during labor and delivery, they are accompanied by a tendency toward venous thrombosis throughout pregnancy, especially if prolonged bedrest is required.

Respiratory System

Changes in the respiratory system during pregnancy allow for the increased oxygen consumption necessary to meet the needs of the growing fetus and placenta.[25] Due to the elevation of the diaphragm by the uterus, the functional residual capacity of the lungs is diminished, although minute ventilation is increased by 50%. The pO_2 changes little, but pCO_2 decreases. This hyperventilation may be the direct result of the action of progesterone on the medullary respiratory center and results in a mild respiratory alkalosis. There is a compensatory decrease in the serum bicarbonate and thus a decrease in blood buffering capacity.[40] Pregnant women exhibit a more rapid induction during anesthesia as a result of these changes.[33] In addition, hypoxemia can develop rapidly if inspired oxygen is decreased. Chest x-rays obtained during late pregnancy may be erroneously interpreted as characteristic of pulmonary edema, as lung markings are increased from diaphragmatic elevation and the pulmonary vessels appear prominent.[12]

Gastrointestinal System

The motility of the gastrointestinal tract is decreased during pregnancy. The lower esophageal sphincter tone is also diminished, and the combination of these factors places the pregnant patient at higher risk for aspiration during induction of anesthesia or after a severe closed head injury. It is felt that the stretching of the abdominal wall results in diminished sensitivity to peritoneal irritation, thus making physical examination misleading on occasion.[7] In the third trimester, the intraabdominal organs are displaced, changing the perceptions of pain. Although the liver remains basically unchanged during pregnancy, the measured serum alkaline phosphatase may be 2 to 3 times normal, as this enzyme is released from the placenta. The incidence of cholestasis and cholelithiasis is increased with pregnancy.[25]

Urinary System

Beginning early in pregnancy, the renal collecting system is dilated, especially on the right side. Renal blood flow increases and the creatinine clearance may exceed 150 ml/min.[2] There is a corresponding decrease in both blood urea nitrogen and serum creatinine. Glucosuria is common in pregnancy because of both the increased glomerular filtration rate and a reduced tubular threshold for glucose.[25] The bladder is displaced anteriorly and superiorly, and suffers from lack of tone, making it more susceptible to injury.[7,40] These normal anatomical changes in the urinary tract must be kept in mind when interpreting radiographs. In addition, dosage changes may be required for those medications cleared by the kidney.

Musculoskeletal System

The increased venous pressure in the lower extremities during pregnancy can result in excessive bleeding around femur and tibial fractures. Fractures of the pelvis occurring in late pregnancy can cause massive retroperitoneal hemorrhage and profound shock. Pelvic films obtained during the last trimester may demonstrate a normal widening of the symphysis pubis (up to 8 mm at term)[7] (Fig. 18–2).

Central Nervous System

Changes in the central nervous system that occur with eclampsia of pregnancy can be confused with head injury. Both may present as seizures and be associated with hyperreflexia. If there are no obvious signs of head trauma, a history of hypertension during pregnancy should be sought, and the urine checked for the presence of protein. Seizures due to eclampsia are best treated with magnesium sulfate and emergency delivery; post-traumatic seizures may require anticonvulsants and emergency head scanning in search of mass lesions.[2]

MECHANISM OF INJURY

Blunt Trauma

Although sporting accidents and falls result in some serious injuries during pregnancy, the major cause of nonobstetrical maternal and infant mortality is motor vehicle trauma.[2,25,35] Motor vehicle accidents are 10 times more likely to result in death of women during their reproductive years than any other mechanism of injury.[7] The exact number of pregnant patients injured nationally in traffic accidents is currently unknown, but the number is certainly on the rise, with more women continuing to work into the last trimester.

The mother commonly suffers severe multisystem injuries as the result of motor vehicle accidents. In addition, blunt trauma to the abdomen during pregnancy can cause injury to the uterus and its contents. Rupture of the uterus after motor vehicle trauma occurs in approximately 1% of pregnant patients, and is usually associated with ejection from the vehicle.[15,48] Separation of the placenta is a more frequent consequence of blunt abdominal trauma, and is the most common cause of fetal death after trauma if the mother survives.[40] The lack of elastic tissue in the placenta may contribute to its tendency to shear rather than flatten with the uterus during compression injury.[14] Disruption of 25% of the placenta is still consistent with fetal survival, although premature labor may be induced. Disruption of 50% or more of the placenta is fatal to the fetus.[14]

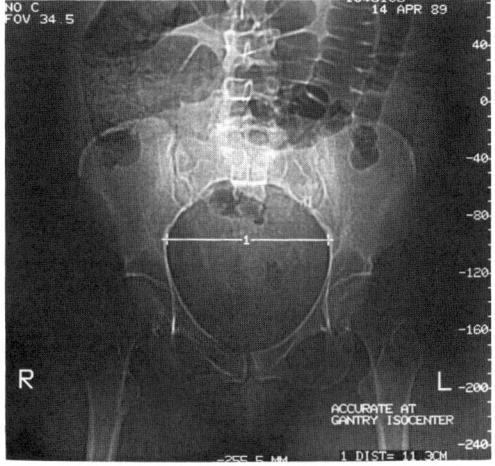
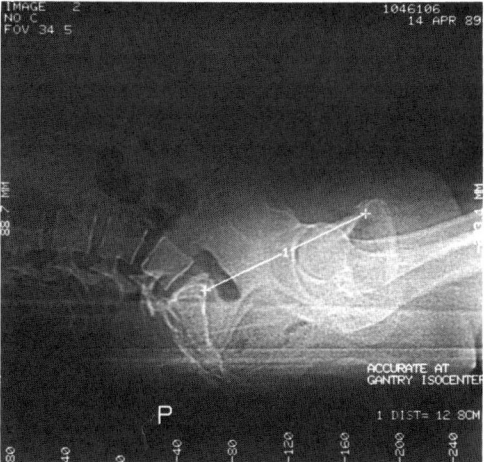

Figure 18–2. A, B: Pelvic radiologic assessment in the latter stages of pregnancy. The pelvic outlet appears adequate. The symphysis is beginning to widen.

Pelvic fractures are common as a result of motor vehicle accidents and are particularly hazardous during pregnancy. Hemorrhage from massively dilated retroperitoneal vessels can readily result in hemorrhagic shock.[19,33,49] Pelvic fractures are the most common injury to the mother that results in intrauterine death. Speer and Peltier reported a series of pregnant patients with pelvic fractures with a 25% incidence of fetal death.[49] Fetal death may result from direct injury to the fetus (usually to the head) or by indirect injury from maternal shock or placental separation.[35]

The initial experimental work by Crosby,[14] which demonstrated high intrauterine pressure generated by flexion over a lap belt, caused a concern that the use of seat belts would lead to increasing rates of uterine rupture during pregnancy.[3,9,14] Subsequently, however, Crosby and Costiloe reported a 33% death rate among unbelted pregnant women involved in severe collisions as opposed to 5% in those not ejected.[16] There was no associated increase in fetal loss with the use of the belt. Modern three-point restraints, when worn properly, prevent forward flexion, making them safer for both the mother and the fetus.[25]

Penetrating Trauma

Gunshot wounds are the most common form of penetrating trauma to the pregnant uterus. The true incidence of these injuries is unknown, but a number of factors are contributing to the increasing number of cases, including the availability of handguns, the prevalence of drug-related crime and gang violence, and maternal suicide attempts.[29] As the uterus grows, it becomes the most likely target for penetrating abdominal trauma, especially if the entrance wound is in the lower abdomen. On the other hand, if the entrance is in the upper abdomen, extensive gastrointestinal and vascular injuries can be anticipated, as the viscera are compressed into a small space.[35] Death of the mother after abdominal gunshot wounds is rare, and only 20% to 30% have injuries outside of the uterus.[7,35,40] However, 70% of the fetuses will sustain injuries from abdominal gunshot wounds and 40% to 65% will die, depending on the injury and the degree of prematurity.[40] In contrast, lower velocity stab wounds are less likely to cause injury to either the mother or fetus.[33]

Burns

The incidence of severe burns complicating pregnancy is fortunately rare, occurring in less than 0.1% of pregnant patients.[45] If the mother suffers burns during pregnancy, fetal wastage may result, although fetal death cannot be directly related to the extent of the burn.[17]

Extensive burns (exceeding 33% of the body surface area) occurring during the second trimester are associated with a high percentage of fetal deaths.[35] Maternal deaths as a result of burn injuries are usually the result of renal, respiratory, or liver failure, or overwhelming sepsis.[3] Infant mortality is related to sepsis, hypoxia, and the degree of prematurity. In general, however, maternal survival is accompanied by fetal survival.[3,54]

INITIAL ASSESSMENT AND TREATMENT

There are few situations in the trauma resuscitation room that provoke more anxiety for the trauma team than in the initial care of the seriously injured pregnant woman. During the preoccupation with the outcome of both the mother and fetus, the basic trauma resuscitation guidelines are sometimes overlooked. It is most important to keep in mind that if the fetus arrives alive, its best chance for continued survival rests with maternal survival. Thus, certain areas of the initial management deserve special mention.

Resuscitation

Whenever possible, the trauma patient in late pregnancy should be transported while in the left lateral position to avoid supine hypotension, which may aggravate hypovolemic shock.[15,48] When a spinal injury is suspected, the patient can be secured to a backboard and the entire board then tilted to the left.[27] Alternatively, the right hip can be elevated slightly. The positioning should be kept in mind throughout all phases of the initial evaluation and diagnostic procedure, and during induction of anesthesia.

The physiologic hypervolemia of pregnancy allows the mother to maintain her blood pressure at near normal levels, despite the loss of 20% to 30% of her blood volume.[35,40]

Although maternal blood pressure may be normal, the fetus may be in shock, as the release of maternal catecholamines causes vasoconstriction of the uterine artery. A 30% to 35% reduction in maternal blood volume reduces uterine blood flow by 10% to 20%.[40] Rothenberger et al., in a review of 103 cases of blunt maternal trauma, reported a fetal mortality of 80% when the mother arrived in hemorrhagic shock.[44] Thus, aggressive fluid administration with crystalloid and/or blood when appropriate should be initiated promptly. As with all trauma patients, vasopressor agents are rarely indicated. In the unusual situation of spinal shock unresponsive to fluid therapy, the vasopressor of choice would be dopamine, which, at least in low doses, has little effect on uterine blood flow.[40]

In addition to hypovolemia, hypoxemia must be avoided. Supplemental oxygen is applied during transport and oxygen saturation and arterial blood gases monitored continually after arrival at the hospital. Fetal hemoglobin functions in the lower portion of the oxygen hemoglobin dissociation curve.[37,45] Supplemental oxygen has little effect on the mother whose hemoglobin is normally saturated on room air. However, increasing oxygen tension will increase fetal saturation and oxygen reserve. There should be no hesitation to intubate the mother if her oxygen saturation deteriorates. Uncorrected fetal hypoxia can result in permanent central nervous system disorders in those infants who survive the insult.[7]

Primary Assessment of the Mother

After the initiation of resuscitative measures and the treatment of any potentially life-threatening injuries identified during the primary survey, a thorough history should be obtained from the stable patient. The history of the pregnancy should include the date of the last menses and any known complications of the current or previous pregnancies. Also pertinent is the immunization history, known drug allergies, and current medications. The events surrounding the accident are reviewed. The patient's obstetrician should be contacted if possible. Ideally, an obstetrician would be a member of the trauma team during the initial evaluation.

Monitoring during the initial assessment should include at least continuous pulse oximetry (oxygen saturation), electrocardiogram, blood pressures, and urinary output. The initial laboratory evaluation should include the studies listed in Table 18–2. A thorough physical examination is then conducted with special attention directed toward the abdomen and pelvis.

Primary Assessment of the Fetus

Evaluation of the fetus after trauma should include several modalities as outlined below.

Palpation of the Uterus

Examination of the height of the uterus will give an estimate of the gestational age (see Fig. 18–1). In general, the fundus can be palpated at 12 weeks of pregnancy, and reaches the umbilicus at 20 weeks.[2] A fundal height that is inconsistent with the reported duration of the pregnancy suggests uterine rupture, whereas an enlarging uterus that is tetanic can indicate abruption of the placenta.[35] Fetal parts easily palpated through the abdominal

Table 18–2 The Initial Management of Trauma in Pregnancy

1. Maintain left lateral position
2. Apply supplemental oxygen
3. Intubate promptly for hypoxia or airway compromise
4. Place IV catheters, Foley catheters, and nasogastric tube
5. Begin vigorous fluid resuscitation with crystalloid
6. If shock is present, transfuse O, Rh⁻ blood
7. Treat life-threatening injuries identified on primary survey
8. Monitor:
   —EKG
   —Oxygen saturation (pulse oximetry)
   —Urinary output
   —CVP in patients in shock
   —Uterine contractions and fetal heart rate
9. Laboratory studies to include:
   —CBC
   —Electrolytes, BUN, creatinine
   —Platelet count, fibrinogen level
   —Partial thromboplastin time, prothrombin time
   —Blood for type and crossmatch
   —Kleihauer-Betke smear
10. Conduct a secondary survey: history and physical exam
11. Contact the obstetrician
12. Initiate diagnostic procedures, including x-rays

---

wall also signifies uterine rupture. Tenderness elicited during palpation of the uterus may accompany uterine injury. Contractions, if present, suggest premature labor. The mother should be questioned regarding perceived fetal movement.

Vaginal Examination

If the patient is stable, a vaginal exam with a sterile speculum is performed. The uterine os is inspected for signs of dilation or effacement.[33,45] Cervical bleeding suggests abruptio placenta. The presence of amniotic fluid should be recognized and confirmed by testing with nitrazine paper (amniotic fluid has a pH of 7). However, this test may be erroneous in the presence of blood or urine in the vagina. A more specific test for the presence of amniotic fluid is to allow a sample of the fluid to dry on a microscope slide. A "ferning" pattern is observed under the microscope because of the crystallized sodium chloride.[6]

Fetal Heart Tones

Fetal heart tones can usually be detected by Doppler ultrasound at 12 weeks, and by fetoscope by 20 weeks.[2] The normal heart rate ranges from 120 to 160 beats/min. Fetal bradycardia is associated with hypoxia and is an ominous sign.

Real Time Ultrasound

Real time ultrasound is excellent for detecting fetal cardiac movement, and the B mode estimates fetal size and the location of the placenta.[45] The sonogram can also detect uterine rupture, but is of limited use in confirming the diagnosis of abruptio placenta.[4,22]

Continuous Electronic Fetal Monitoring

Electronic monitoring can provide early warnings of fetal distress. Marginal placental reserve (fetal hypoxia) is detected by the response of the fetal heart rate to fetal movement (nonstress test) or to uterine contractions (stress test).[3] Late decelerations of heart rate occurring with uterine contractions signify fetal compromise and demand immediate investigation.

Fetal monitoring is useful in detecting fetal distress resulting from abruptio placenta, a leading cause of fetal death after abdominal trauma. Whereas most cases of placental disruption are recognized by vaginal bleeding and abdominal pain, lesser degrees of placental separation may be clinically silent.[14] Placental abruption usually occurs within hours of injury. However, Higgins and Garite reported a case where abruptio placenta was not evident until 5 days after the accident.[28] Other case reports have documented placental disruption after relatively minor maternal trauma.[20,51]

Based on a review of the literature, it would seem that all symptomatic patients with potentially viable infants should they require delivery (generally 25 weeks gestation) be monitored continuously. The recommendations for continuous monitoring should also be extended to asymptomatic patients with significant mechanisms of injury.[11] These patients require 24 to 48 hr of monitoring, during which the majority of significant abruptio placenta will become evident.[28,45]

Amniocentesis

Sampling of amniotic fluid can also detect fetal distress in some cases. The presence of meconium staining indicates a period of acute anoxia, and bloody fluid suggests intrauterine bleeding.[3,14,35] The amniotic fluid can also be analyzed for the ratio of lecithin: sphingomyelin (LS). A ratio of greater than 2 correlates with fetal pulmonary maturation.[3,14,35] The detection of phosphatidyl glycerol (PG) on a sample of amniotic fluid also predicts fetal maturity and correlates with survival outside of the womb.[35]

Diagnostic Procedures

After the initial survey of both the mother and the fetus, the diagnostic studies required to evaluate fully the extent of maternal injuries should proceed promptly. There should be no hesitation to perform x-ray studies that are considered essential (Fig. 18–3). Whenever possible, the fetus is shielded, and duplication of studies is avoided. However, most emergency x-rays can be accomplished at well below the accumulative maximum dose recommended for the fetus (less than 10 rads).[25,37]

The hazards of radiation during pregnancy depend on both the dose and the stage of organogenesis. Three distinct phases of radiation damage have been described.[25] During the preimplantation stage (less than 3 weeks of gestational age) radiation damage causes death of the embryo. As little as 5 to 15 rads can cause death in mice at this stage, but the corresponding dose in humans is not known.

During organogenesis (23 days to 16 weeks) radiation damage results in fewer deaths but more anomalies, especially to the skeletal and genital systems.

After completion of organogenesis, fetal damage from radiation is more likely to be functional than structural, resulting from central nervous system damage. Neuroblasts are extremely radiosensitive throughout gestation and may be destroyed by 25 rads.

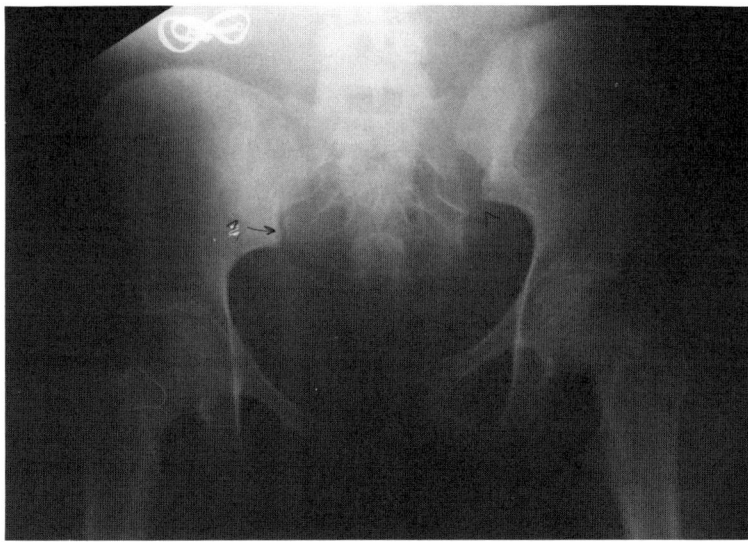

Figure 18–3. Malgaigne fracture of the pelvis with marked diastasis of the left sacroiliac joint in a 19-year-old woman who was 7 months pregnant. Note the fetal skull marked by the arrow.

Prenatal irradiation may also increase the risk of later development of childhood cancer.[24] It must be remembered, however, that the relative risk to the fetus from needed emergency films is much less than the risk to both the mother and fetus resulting from the complications of a missed injury.

Abdominal computed tomography (CT) scanning is also safe to perform during pregnancy. The dose is about 3 rads per slice to the tissue directly irradiated. Thus, if duplication and overlap are avoided, and a small gap allowed between slices, the accumulated dose is small.[25]

As mentioned above, the stretched abdominal musculature and peritoneum may decrease the sensitivity to irritation. Abdominal examination, which is always difficult in the multiple-injury patient, becomes even more unreliable. Peritoneal lavage, which is highly sensitive to detecting intraabdominal hemorrhage, was initially felt to be contraindicated during pregnancy. Buchsbaum wrote that abdominal paracentesis was not warranted in pregnant women because the gravid uterus compartmentalized the abdominal cavity and prevented the spread of intraperitoneal blood.[7] The displaced small intestine in the upper abdomen was felt to be at increased risk of injury from the lavage catheter. However, Rothenberger et al. found peritoneal lavage to be both safe and accurate in detecting abdominal injuries during pregnancy.[43] When lavage is conducted, it should be carried out with an open technique in the supraumbilical location. A return of excess fluid (amniotic fluid) may occur if the uterus has been ruptured.[2]

Experience with abdominal CT scanning during pregnancy is limited but, as mentioned above, it can be performed without undue risk and would be expected to detect injuries with the same accuracy as in the nongravid patient. Some authors have suggested that fetal injuries could be detected *in utero* by CT scanning.[10]

MANAGEMENT OF MATERNAL INJURIES

Central Nervous System Injuries

Neurologic injury during pregnancy is no longer a rare event. Initially, conditions associated with secondary brain injury must be avoided, such as hypoxia and hypotension. Prompt identification and treatment of intracranial hemorrhage will afford the best outcome for the mother and ultimately the fetus. There are reports of delivery of a normal child months after the onset of posttraumatic coma in the mother.[47] In these cases, the secondary complications of prolonged coma, such as infections, seizures, malnutrition, and deep venous thrombosis must be avoided to allow for normal fetal growth and development. Occasionally, maternal hypothalamic and pituitary dysfunction may accompany catastrophic brain injuries, and replacement of cortisone, thyroid, and vasopressin hormones is required.[25]

Injuries to the Chest

After maternal chest injury, fetal well-being and survival are threatened by both the direct damage from blunt or penetrating trauma and by the indirect effects of the resulting hypoxia or shock.[25] Therefore, potentially life-threatening injuries, including hemothorax, pneumothorax, vascular or cardiac disruptions, must be recognized early and promptly treated.[15] One thoracic injury that is particularly dangerous if missed during pregnancy is diaphragmatic laceration. The high intraabdominal pressures created during pregnancy and labor can increase the size of the rent, causing herniation and perforation into the chest.[26]

Abdominal Injuries and Operative Management

Patients who present in shock or with evidence of ongoing blood loss or peritonitis after abdominal trauma should be taken directly to surgery. There is some controversy as to the management of the stable patient who has sustained penetrating abdominal trauma during pregnancy. Iliya et al.[29] and Patterson[40] have argued that aggressive management of penetrating wounds to the lower abdomen does not seem to affect fetal outcome, and rarely injures the mother. These authors advocate expectant management of even gunshot wounds to the abdomen if the entrance wound is below the level of the uterine fundus, the mother is stable, and the bullet is radiographically located in the uterus.[29] However, as the complications of missed intraabdominal injury far outweigh the risks of anesthesia and laparotomy, and the path of the bullet is not always appreciated, operative exploration is still recommended by most trauma surgeons for gunshot wounds to the abdomen occurring during pregnancy. Lower velocity abdominal stab wounds may qualify for selective evaluation, such as with peritoneal lavage or close observation if the mother is stable.

If surgical treatment is indicated for abdominal injuries after either penetrating or blunt abdominal trauma, it should be accomplished without delay. A standard midline approach gives the best exposure. An autotransfusion device should be on hand for major trauma. The safety of autotransfusion in the presence of uterine rupture has not been established, however. A thorough abdominal exploration is conducted as with any other trauma patient. This may require retraction or packing of the uterus for adequate exposure. In general, the uterus can be gently maneuvered to examine the retroperitoneal area without inducing labor.[25] Aggressive retraction may injure the uterus or precipitate bleeding from the dilated uterine venous plexus and must be avoided.[54] Injuries to the mother resulting from blunt trauma that have been repaired during pregnancy include splenic, hepatic, pancreatic, intestinal, and mesenteric tears. These injuries are treated in the standard fashion.

Even though a laparotomy is being performed, concomitant cesarean section is only rarely indicated. Labor and vaginal delivery are usually well tolerated even in the immediate postoperative period.[25] If the fetus is dead at the time of surgery, spontaneous vaginal delivery can be anticipated within hours. If a uterine injury is encountered, it can be surgically repaired with the use of absorbable suture in a layered closure.[54] Even these patients can subsequently deliver vaginally. A cesarean section prolongs the operation and increases the blood loss by at least 1000 cc.[8] Occasionally, however, the uterus will be injured so severely that it cannot be repaired, or the resulting uterine hemorrhage cannot be controlled. In these cases, cesarean section may be required. Rarely, the uterus may prevent adequate repair of maternal injuries to the pelvis, necessitating uterine evacuation. Fetal distress during laparotomy or the precipitation of diffuse intravascular coagulopathy require emergency cesarean section. The indications for emergency cesarean section in the trauma patient have been summarized by numerous authors and are listed in Table 18–3 below.[2,27,35,45,54] Elective cesarean section should be anticipated for those patients who sustain unstable thoracolumbar spine fractures.

Post mortem cesarean section may be performed emergently after maternal death, or more electively after brain death has been established in the mother. Fetal survival correlates with both the duration of gestation and the interval of time between maternal death and delivery.[7,27] Cesarean section should be initiated within 10 min of maternal death. The birth of a healthy infant by post mortem section is more likely to follow head trauma than after an injury that results in hemorrhagic shock.

Injuries to the Uterus and Placenta

Placental Injury

As mentioned above, placental separation (abruptio placenta) is the most common cause of posttraumatic fetal death if the mother survives. Findings of placental disruption include

Table 18–3 Indications for Cesarean Section After Trauma

1. Uterine injury that is massive and cannot be repaired
2. Hemorrhage from the uterus that cannot be controlled
3. Fetal distress in a potentially viable fetus
4. Need for exposure for repair of maternal injuries
5. Imminent maternal death
6. Development of DIC

vaginal bleeding, uterine tenderness, increased uterine tone, and shock from blood lost into the uterus.[2,15] Disseminated intravascular coagulation may follow placental injury as thromboplastin is released from the placenta. When abruptio placenta does not result in symptoms or cause immediate fetal distress, it may go unrecognized. A Kleihauer-Betke smear is a sensitive test for detecting fetomaternal transfusion as the result of placental disruption. The Kleihauer-Betke test mixes a sample of maternal blood with alkali. Fetal cells are resistant to alkali, but the mother's are lysed. The ratio of lysed to unlysed cells predicts the volume of fetal blood cells in the maternal circulation.[37] In the case where the fetus has survived placental injury, the mother must be monitored closely for the development of disseminated intravascular coagulation (DIC) and the fetus for signs of distress.

Uterine Rupture

With major uterine rupture, the mother will present in shock. Fetal parts may be palpated separately from the uterus and a peritoneal lavage will return both blood and amniotic fluid. With more minor uterine injuries, ultrasound may be helpful in detecting blood outside of the uterus.[2] Although minor uterine ruptures may be repairable, in most cases the fetus has already died, and salvaging the mother will require uterine evacuation or hysterectomy.[2,15,33]

Premature Rupture of Amniotic Membranes

Rupture of membranes can follow either blunt or penetrating abdominal trauma. If the fetus is immature and the membranes are documented to be ruptured, prompt delivery is no longer recommended without fetal distress or amnionitis.[3] With careful monitoring, the fetus may be allowed to remain *in utero* while surfactant production and pulmonary maturity are induced with steroid therapy.

DIRECT FETAL INJURY

The fetus may suffer from fatal and nonfatal injuries after either blunt or penetrating trauma. Gunshot wounds have resulted in intrauterine injuries to almost every organ, including the heart, intestine, lung, liver, spleen, and diaphragm. Fetuses have survived penetrating wounds to the extremities, including gunshot wounds. In one reported case, a mother who was stabbed during her eighth month of pregnancy was successfully operated on for her injuries. Her child was delivered and also underwent surgery.[34] Blunt trauma suffered *in utero* results primarily in head injuries, especially during late pregnancy when the head is engaged in the pelvis.[33] Extremity fractures are also common.

If the neonate is delivered by cesarean section or vaginally after trauma, he or she should then be treated like any pediatric trauma victim. A thorough examination must be conducted for any signs of trauma. CT or ultrasound may be required to evaluate head injuries. Subcapsular hemorrhage of the liver and intestinal perforations that resulted from blunt maternal trauma have required treatment in the newborn.[25] After successful management of identified injuries, neonatal outcome will be determined by the degree of prematurity, as well as by pulmonary and central nervous system complications.

COMPLICATIONS AND POSTOPERATIVE CARE

Premature Labor

Premature labor may follow blunt abdominal trauma. The presence and frequency of uterine contractions can be monitored with a tocodynameter. Premature labor is defined as the onset of contractions before 36 weeks gestation that are forceful enough to cause cervical dilation and effacement.[2] Hypoxia and hypovolemia may also induce labor, and these conditions must first be corrected. If the mother is stable, however, tocolysis may be attempted. The agents used most frequently are beta-adrenergic agonists, in particular terbutaline and ritodrine.[54] These drugs are not without complications and should be used with caution in patients with hypertension, cardiac arrhythmias, and diabetes. Ritodrine causes tachycardia, hypokalemia, and hemodilution.[2] Contraindications to the use of these drugs include a heart rate greater than 120 beats/min, hypotension, fetal distress, hemorrhage, lung disease, cervical dilation greater than 4 cm, fetus less than the age of viability, and abruptio placenta.[2,37,54] Magnesium sulfate may be somewhat safer in the posttrauma setting, but it is also less effective. In the presence of severe maternal or uterine injury, it is doubtful that any tocolytic agent will be capable of suppressing labor.

Disseminated Intravascular Coagulation

DIC after trauma in pregnancy is caused by the release of thromboplastic substances from the placenta or decidua in the process of placental separation, resulting in massive uncontrollable hemorrhage.[2] If the fetus dies as the result of placental rupture, DIC will follow in approximately 30% of cases, but is rare when the infant survives. When this complication does develop, however, maternal shock and death can occur precipitously, and emergency evacuation of the uterus is required to salvage the mother.[35]

DIC may also result from amniotic fluid embolism. Disruption of the amniotic membrane causes a release of fluid and particulate matter into the circulation. The effect of the embolus on the pulmonary system includes mechanical obstruction and reflex bronchospasm, resulting in severe hypoxia.[2,45] Cardiovascular collapse, cyanosis, bleeding, and seizures may follow. Treatment, in addition to immediate evacuation of the uterus, includes the administration of fluid, blood, and blood products as needed to reverse the coagulopathy. Despite supportive care, amniotic fluid embolism carries a mortality of 75% to 80%.

Fetal Death

As tragic as fetal death is after trauma, a causal relationship between the traumatic event and subsequent abortion is not always easily established. It must be remembered that 10% to 20% of all pregnancies abort spontaneously, and that an abortion may have been in progress at the time of the accident.[3] Conversely, embryonic injury caused by trauma may not result in an abortion for several weeks or even months after the accident.[16] According to Crosby, a causative relationship between the traumatic event and subsequent fetal death requires that the pregnancy be known to be progressing normally before the traumatic event, and that the signs of impending fetal death be evident within 48 hr after trauma, with autopsy confirmation of placental separation or fetal injury.[14] It is hoped that with attention to the details of maternal resuscitation and prompt identification and treatment of her injuries, the best possible outcome for the fetus that does arrive at the hospital alive will be insured.

PREVENTION

No chapter on trauma can be complete without a word about prevention of injuries. Although it is doubtful that the pregnant woman will refrain from driving until delivery, the proper use of seat belts can be part of her prenatal instructions. The properly worn three-point restraint is both safe and effective. According to the American College of Obstetricians and Gynecologists, the pregnant woman is 25 times more likely to stay alive in the car, and the fetus has 4 times the chance of survival than if the mother is ejected.[48] No advancements in the care of the mother or her fetus are likely to approach these numbers in improving survival.

REFERENCES

1. Agran PF, Dunkle DE, Winn DG, et al. Fetal death in motor vehicle accidents. *Ann Emerg Med.* 1987; 16:1355–1358.
2. Augenstein JS. Trauma during pregnancy. In: Kreis DJ, Gomez GA, eds. *Trauma Management.* Boston: Little, Brown: 1989.
3. Baker DP. Trauma in the pregnant patient. *Surg Clin North Am.* 1982; 62(2):275–289.
4. Bedi DG, Salmon A, Winsett MZ, et al. Ruptured uterus: sonographic diagnosis. *J Clin Ultrasound.* 1986; 14(7):529–533.
5. Bickers RG, Wennberg RP. Fetomaternal transfusion following trauma. *Obstet Gynecol.* 1983; 61(2): 258–259.
6. Bocka J, Courtney J, Pearlman M, et al. Trauma in pregnancy. *Ann Emerg Med.* 1988; 17:829–834.
7. Buchsbaum HJ. *Trauma in Pregnancy.* Philadelphia: WB Saunders; 1979.
8. Buchsbaum HJ, Staples PP. Self-inflicted gunshot wound to the pregnant uterus: report of two cases. *Obstet Gynecol.* 1985; 65(3):325–335S.
9. Chetcuti P, Levene MI. Seatbelts: a potential hazard to the fetus. *J Perinat Med.* 1987; 15(2):207–209.
10. Civil ID, Talucci RC, Schwab CW. Placental laceration and fetal death as a result of blunt abdominal trauma. *J Trauma.* 1988; 28(5):708–710.
11. Combs TJ. Individualized monitoring after trauma in pregnancy. (Letter) *Ann Emerg Med.* 1988; 17(9):1000–1001.
12. Committee on Trauma, American College of Surgeons, Advanced Trauma Life Support Instructor Manual, 1988.
13. Connor E, Curran J. In utero traumatic intraabdominal deceleration injury to the fetus: a case report. *Am J Obstet Gynecol.* 1976; 125(4):567–569.
14. Crosby W. Trauma during pregnancy: maternal and fetal injury. *Obstet Gynecol Surg.* 1974; 29(10): 683–699.
15. Crosby W. Traumatic injuries during pregnancy. *Clin Obstet Gynecol.* 1983; 26(4):902–912.
16. Crosby W, Costiloe JP. Safety of lap-belt restraint for pregnant victims of automobile collisions. *N Engl J Med.* 1971; 284(12):632–635.
17. Deitch EA, Rightmire DA, Clothier JA, et al. Management of burns in pregnant women. 1985; 161(1):1–4.
18. Delaney JJ. Obstetrical and gynecological injuries. In: Zuidema GE, Rutherford RB, Ballinger WF, eds. *The Management of Trauma.* 4th ed. Philadelphia: WB Saunders: 1985.
19. Dyer I, Barclay DL. Accidental trauma complicating pregnancy and delivery. *Am J Obstet Gynecol.* 1962; 83:907.
20. Fries MH, Hankins GD. Motor vehicle accident associated with minimal maternal trauma but subsequent fetal demise. *Ann Emerg Med.* 1989; 18(3):301–304.
21. Greenspoon JS, Ault MJ. Trauma in pregnancy. (Letter) *Ann Emerg Med.* 1989; (3):332–333.

22. Grumbach K, Mechlin MB, Mintz MC. Computed tomography and ultrasound of the traumatized and acutely ill patient. *Emerg Clin North Am.* 1985; 3(3):607–624.
23. Haggard HW. *The Doctor in History.* London: Yale University Press; 1934.
24. Harvey EB, Boice JD, Honeyman M, et al. Prenatal x-ray exposure and childhood cancer in twins. *N Engl J Med.* 1985; 312(9):541–545.
25. Haycock CE, ed. *Trauma and Pregnancy.* PSG Publishing Co., 1985.
26. Henzler M, Martin ML, Young J. Delayed diagnosis of traumatic diaphragmatic hernia during pregnancy. *Ann Emerg Med.* 1988; 17(4):350–353.
27. Higgins SD. Trauma in pregnancy. *J Perinatol.* 1988; 8(3):288–292.
28. Higgins SD, Garite TJ. Late abruptio placenta in trauma patients: implications for monitoring. *Obstet Gynecol.* 1984; 63:10S–12S.
29. Iliya FA, Hajj SN, Buchsbaum HJ. Gunshot wounds of the pregnant uterus: report of two cases. *J Trauma.* 1980; 20(1):90–92.
30. Katz VL, Dotters DJ, Droegemueller W. Perimortem Cesarean delivery. *Obstet Gynecol Obstet.* 1986; 68:571–576.
31. Kettel LM, Branch DW, Scott JR. Occult placental abruption after maternal trauma. *Obstet Gynecol.* 1988; 71(3 pt 2):449–453.
32. Keynes G. *The Apology and Treatise of Ambroise Paré.* London: Falcon Educational Books; 1951.
33. Lavin JP, Polsky SS. Abdominal trauma during pregnancy. *Clin Perinatol.* 1983; 10(2):423–438.
34. McNabney WK, Smith EI. Penetrating wounds of the gravid uterus. *J Trauma.* 1973; 12(12):1024–1028.
35. Maull KI, Rozycki GS, Pedigo RE, et al. Injury to the female reproductive system. In: Mattox KL, Moore EE, Feliciano DV, eds. *Trauma.* Norwalk, Conn: Appleton and Lange; 1988.
36. Maull KI, Sachatello CR, Ernst CB. The deep perineal laceration: an injury frequently associated with open pelvic fractures: a need for aggressive surgical management. *J Trauma.* 1977; 17(9):685–696.
37. Neufeld JD, Moore EE, Marz JA, et al. Trauma in pregnancy. *Emerg Med Clin North Am.* 1987; 5(3):623–640.
38. Niemi TA, Norton LW. Vaginal injuries in patients with pelvic fractures. *J Trauma.* 1985; 25(6):547–551.
39. Obstetrics Advisory Committee of the Perinatal Advisory Council of Los Angeles Communities Prenatal and Intrapartum Protocols, 1987.
40. Patterson RM. Trauma in pregnancy. *Clin Obstet Gynecol.* 1984; 27(1):32–38.
41. Pierson R, Mihalovits H, Thomas L, et al. Penetrating abdominal wounds in pregnancy. *Ann Emerg Med.* 1986; 15:1232–1334.
42. Roberts JR. X-rays during pregnancy. *Emerg Med News.* 1989; 11(11):4–9.
43. Rothenberger DA, Quattlebaum FW, Zabel J, et al. Diagnostic peritoneal lavage for blunt trauma in pregnant women. *Am J Obstet Gynecol.* 1977; 129:479–481.
44. Rothenberger D, Quattlebaum FW, Perry JF, et al. Blunt maternal trauma: a review of 103 cases. *J Trauma.* 1978; 18(3):173–179.
45. Rozycki GS. Trauma in pregnancy. In: Moore EE, ed. *Early Care of the Injured Patient.* 4th ed. Toronto, Philadelphia: BC Decker; 1990.
46. Sachs BP, Brown DA, Driscoll SG, et al. Maternal mortality in Massachusetts. *N Engl J Med.* 1987; 316(11):667–672.
47. Sampson MB, Petersen LP. Post-traumatic coma during pregnancy. *Obstet Gynecol.* 1979; 53(suppl):2S–3S.
48. Schoenfeld A, Ziv E, Neri A, et al. Vehicular trauma in pregnancy: an algorithm for diagnosis and fetal therapy. *Fetal Ther.* 1987; 2(1):51–56.
49. Speer DP, Peltier LF. Pelvic fractures and pregnancy. *J Trauma.* 1972; 12(6):474–480.
50. Stone NN, Ances IG, Brotman S. Gynecologic injury in the nongravid female during blunt abdominal trauma. *J Trauma.* 1984; 24(7):626–627.
51. Stuart GCE, Harding PGR, Davis EM. Blunt abdominal trauma in pregnancy. *Can Med Ass J.* 1980; 122:901–905.
52. Taylor JW, Plunkett GD, McManus WF, et al. Thermal injury during pregnancy. *Obstet Gynecol.* 1976; (47):434–438.
53. Timberlake GA, McSwain NE. Trauma in pregnancy. A 10-year perspective. *Am Surg.* 1989; 55(3):151–153.
54. Zuidema GE, Rutherford RB, Ballinger WF. *Management of Trauma.* 4th ed. Philadelphia: 1985.

19
Abdominal Arterial Trauma

WILLIAM R. FRY, M.D.

HISTORY: Carrel and Guthrie, in 1906, published the foundations for current operative arterial repairs.[1] These technical advances lacked the support of anticoagulants, blood transfusions, adequate anesthesia, and prehospital transport. As a result, intraabdominal arterial injuries remained almost uniformly fatal.

From 1914 to 1921, Weglowski repaired 51 arterial injuries, including three iliac artery injuries.[2] These were repaired with venous interposition grafts. One year after Weglowski's publication in German, Wildegans reported a successful repair of a stab wound to the abdominal aorta.[3]

Despite increasing application of technical skills and the availability of anticoagulants and blood transfusions, abdominal aortic trauma continued to prove fatal during World War II. In DeBakey and Simcone's series of 2471 arterial injuries incurred by Allied Forces in the Mediterranean Theater, only three patients with major abdominal injuries survived to receive medical intervention.[4] During the Korean War, arterial injuries to the extremities were reconstructed, but almost all patients with injuries to major abdominal arteries died.[5]

During the Vietnam War, however, use of helicopter evacuation allowed some patients with injured abdominal arteries to survive long enough for attempted definitive treatment. Modern methods of reconstruction were available and consistently applied. As a result, Bill and colleagues[6] reported 14 survivors out of 33 patients with abdominal aortic trauma, and recent civilian experience with injuries to major abdominal arteries has been similarly encouraging.[7-11]

Despite application of field hospital techniques, abdominal arterial trauma continues to be a highly lethal injury. The results of management have improved very little in the two decades since Vietnam, possibly because as treatment has improved, parallel improvements in prehospital care result in cases that previously would not have survived to reach the hospital. Only with aggressive management and further investigations into the immunologic and cellular dysfunctions caused by hemorrhagic shock will patients survive the immediate and late complications of the postoperative period.

PATHOPHYSIOLOGY

Depending on the wounding agent, arteries can be transected, lacerated, or contused; they can sustain intimal injury or thrombose. Intrinsic hemostatic functions to contain bleeding rely primarily on the tamponade effect of the surrounding tissue layers. These tissues include not only the vessel's own adventitia, but also peritoneum, mesenteric leaves, or in certain instances, fascia. The high flow rates through the major abdominal vessels only rarely allow for the coagulation cascade to achieve hemostasis (see illustration, page 344).

Cleanly transected nondiseased arteries, even arteries as large as the aorta, may stop bleeding spontaneously. The transected intima curls inward to narrow the lumen. Contraction and shortening of the divided media further constrict the arterial lumen. With constriction of the media, the vessel wall thickens, reducing its wall tension and allowing the cut ends to collapse. The adventitia is pulled over the end of the constricted artery by the retracted media, creating additional resistance to the flow. Tamponade of the flow is achieved then through a combination of Poiselle's and Laplace's laws. In contrast, partially lacerated, diseased, and atherosclerotic arteries seldom stop bleeding spontaneously because these mechanisms cannot come into play.

With either transection or a partial laceration, blood will extravasate into the surrounding tissues. During a diagnostic work-up or at operation, this can present in several ways. If the artery is tamponaded by surrounding tissue, it can present as a hematoma, either stable in size or expanding. Since the adventitia as well as the retroperitoneum represent potential spaces, a hematoma may expand or a false aneurysm can develop as blood continues to extravasate.

If arterial and venous injuries occur in close proximity, blood flow may meet the least resistance going from the arterial injury to the venous injury. This results in the development of a traumatic arteriovenous fistula. A fistula may be obvious soon after the injury or may take months or years to manifest itself clinically. Some fistulae, such as some of those confined to vessels within the hepatic parenchyma, may be well tolerated or even thrombose spontaneously. Others, such as those involving somatic vessels, usually enlarge with time. Ultimately, the low resistance to blood flow directly into the venous system can result in a leak of the magnitude sufficient to precipitate high output cardiac failure.

Contusions vary from an insignificant disruption of the vasa vasora, resulting in minor periarterial hemorrhage, to disruption of all layers of the arterial wall. Contusion with disruption of the intima may result in partial obstruction of the artery—often misinterpreted as spasm. This can result in delayed thrombosis. The thrombus not only may occlude the artery, but may embolize to the distal arterial tree. In addition, a disrupted intima may progress to a subintimal dissection with the intima occluding the lumen of the artery.

False aneurysms result from disruption of all layers of the arterial wall with organization of the resulting periarterial hematoma. The outer layer of the aneurysm is organized fibrous tissue; the inner layer is organized thrombus. The wall of false aneurysms contains neither intima, media, nor adventitia. Rupture or thrombosis of a false aneurysm is unpredictable. Thrombus from inside the aneurysm may also embolize distally.

Blunt trauma to abdominal arteries most frequently produces avulsion-type injuries. A seat belt impingement or blow to the abdomen may displace the renal pedicle or the root of the mesentery. A forceful stretching of a renal or mesenteric artery results in fracture of the relatively nonelastic intima. With greater forces, medial and adventitial disruptions occur, causing renal or superior mesenteric artery avulsion from the aorta. Traction forces may produce a wide spectrum of arterial injuries including intimal tears, arterial laceration or rupture, branch artery avulsion, contusions, or thrombosis.

Spasm is mentioned only to be dismissed. Spasm is defined as severe constriction of the media in an otherwise undamaged larger artery. Constriction of large arteries, demonstrated by physical examination, arteriography, or operative exposure, suggests trauma to the artery and its intima. The surgeon must prove that the intima is intact in the presence of such severe constriction either by obtaining a definitive arteriogram, often with the help of intraarterial vasodilators, or by direct inspection of the intima at the presumed site of injury.

MECHANISM OF INJURY

The incidence of injuries to major abdominal arteries is unknown since most patients with such injuries die at the scene of the accident, and postmortem examinations are unlikely to list the precise injury beyond the general statement of exsanguination due to abdominal hemorrhage. In a recent series of arterial injuries in patients who survived to reach the hospital, 32.1% of the cases involved injuries to abdominal arteries; 67.9% involved injuries to vessels in the extremities, neck, or chest.[12] These injuries result most commonly from penetrating trauma but also occur as the result of blunt injury.

Arteries within the abdominal cavity are more often injured by penetrating trauma than blunt trauma. Penetrating injuries can be caused by shotgun, gunshot, and stab wounds. All types of arterial injuries previously discussed can occur with penetrating trauma. Dawidson reported that 18% of shotgun and gunshot wounds to the abdomen caused a major vascular injury.[13] With penetrating injuries of all types, approximately 60% of all clinically significant abdominal vascular injuries are arterial.[14] In addition, gunshot wounds to the lower chest have a 4% incidence of abdominal arterial trauma.[15]

Blunt injuries to the abdominal arteries occur with less frequency than with penetrating injuries. In a recent report, 4.1% of blunt trauma victims sustained abdominal vascular injury.[16] These injuries are usually the result of rapid deceleration such as with motor vehicle accidents, falls, or impact with other blunt objects or weapons.

Arterial wall injuries from both penetrating and blunt trauma have similar possible presentations, e.g., thrombosis, expanding hematoma, false aneurysm, or free intraperitoneal bleeding. Although contusion can be caused by the shock wave generated by a high velocity missile, it is usually caused by blunt trauma with the damaging force applied directly to the artery itself. Arteriovenous fistulae as a result of blunt trauma are exceedingly rare. Blunt vascular trauma presents with thrombotic manifestations far more commonly than hemorrhage. This is because blunt trauma is usually a stretch-type injury in which intima and media separate, leaving an intact hemostatic adventitia.

ANATOMY

Many excellent texts give detailed descriptions of abdominal arterial anatomy.[17-20] It is absolutely essential that the trauma surgeon be knowledgeable in all aspects of the anatomy

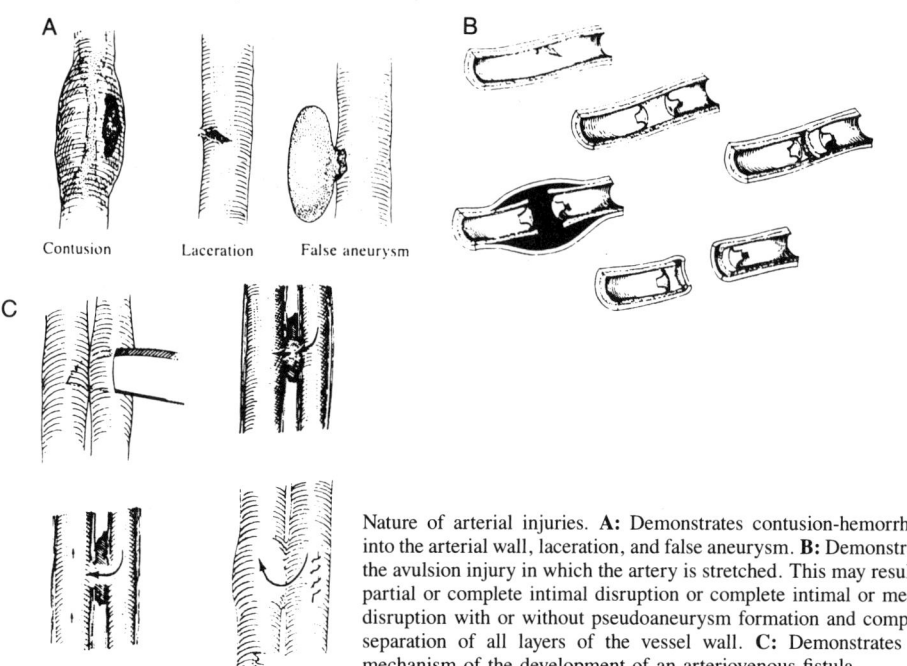

Nature of arterial injuries. **A:** Demonstrates contusion-hemorrhage into the arterial wall, laceration, and false aneurysm. **B:** Demonstrates the avulsion injury in which the artery is stretched. This may result in partial or complete intimal disruption or complete intimal or medial disruption with or without pseudoaneurysm formation and complete separation of all layers of the vessel wall. **C:** Demonstrates the mechanism of the development of an arteriovenous fistula.

of the region in which he is working. This knowledge facilitates the recognition of possible vascular injury and permits simultaneous determination of the best operative approach for repair.

The abdominal aorta begins at the aortic hiatus of the diaphragm, usually at the level of T-11 or T-12 vertebrae (Fig. 19–1). At this level, the aorta is covered by the left and right crus of the diaphragm as well as the median arcuate ligament. At the level of T-12, to L-1, the celiac axis originates from the anterior surface of the abdominal aorta. Immediately below this (at the level of L-1) the superior mesenteric artery originates. Due to the embryologic ascent of the kidneys, a bimodal distribution of the renal arteries exists. Although most renal arteries occur at the L1-2 level, accessory renal arteries usually occur at the L2-3 level. The gonadal vessels originate from the anterior lateral aorta just before the renal arteries and paired lumbar arteries arise opposite the mid–upper four lumbar vertebrae. The inferior mesenteric artery has its distribution centered at the level of L-3. The aorta bifurcates at the fourth lumbar vertebra into the right and left common iliac arteries, which have no major branches. The common iliac arteries bifurcate at the level of the sacroiliac synchondroses into the external and internal iliac arteries. The former gives off only two major branches, both in its distal portion near the inguinal ligament—the inferior epigastric and circumflex iliac arteries. The internal iliac artery divides into the anterior and posterior trunks, providing circulation to the pelvis and pelvic organs. Principal branches of the anterior trunk are the vesical, middle rectal, obturator, pudendal, and vesical arteries. Those of the posterior trunk are the gluteal, sacral, and iliolumbar branches (Fig. 19–1).

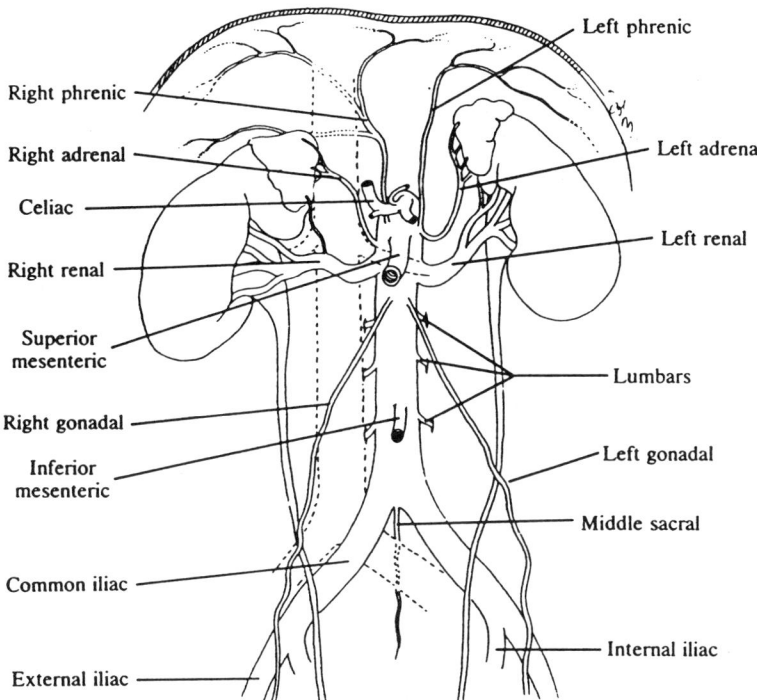

Figure 19–1. Anatomy of the abdominal aorta.

Collateral Circulation

Occasionally, the most prudent operative intervention may be ligation of a major arterial branch. To allow for end organ viability (liver, spleen, gastrointestinal tract, kidneys, and pelvic organs), knowledge of the collateral circulation in the abdomen is essential.

The celiac artery has anastomotic connections with the superior mesenteric artery through the pancreaticoduodenal arcade. This arcade includes the common hepatic artery and its second branch, the gastroduodenal artery, which in turn divides into the right gastroepiploic artery and the superior pancreaticoduodenal artery. The superior pancreaticoduodenal artery bifurcates into anterior and posterior branches, which anastomose with anterior and posterior branches of the inferior pancreaticoduodenal artery, the first branch of the superior mesenteric artery (Fig. 19–2).

On the basis of this important collateral circulation, either the celiac axis or superior mesenteric artery may be ligated proximally, provided the other artery is patent and collateral pathways are intact. Perfusion to the viscera supplied by the injured artery must be assessed before or immediately after definitive ligation.

The superior mesenteric artery has the main anastomotic connections with the inferior mesenteric artery through the meandering mesenteric artery, not the marginal artery of Drummond as is often taught. The second branch off the superior mesenteric artery is the middle colic artery. This artery divides into left and right branches. The left branch of

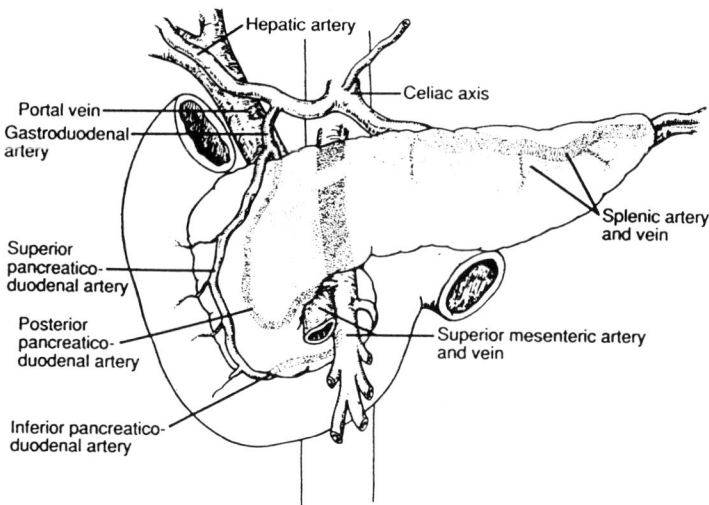

Figure 19–2. Collateral communications between the celiac axis and the superior mesenteric artery.

the middle colic artery anastomoses with the ascending branch of the left colic artery, a branch of the inferior mesenteric artery (Fig. 19–3).

The inferior mesenteric artery anastomoses with the internal iliac arteries via the rectal arteries. The superior rectal artery is the terminal branch of the inferior mesenteric artery. It has direct anastomoses with the middle and inferior rectal arteries. The middle rectal is usually a branch of the internal iliac artery or its branch, the internal pudendal artery. The inferior rectal artery is a branch of the internal pudendal artery.

The internal iliac artery communicates with the common femoral artery via the internal pudendal, obturator, and inferior gluteal arteries. These connect to the medial femoral circumflex and lateral femoral circumflex arteries, respectively.

ASSESSMENT

Any injury to the lower chest, abdomen, back, pelvis, buttocks, or perineum may cause an injury to an abdominal artery. Patients sustaining abdominal arterial injury present with hypovolemic shock in 55% to 58% of cases.[7,21] With aortic injuries, 60% to 100% of patients arrive in the emergency department in hypovolemic shock.[8–10,22]

Extraabdominal injuries should be investigated as a cause for hypovolemia and if present should be controlled. Maxillofacial, neck, thoracic, and extremity trauma can all cause significant blood loss. Pneumothorax, hemothorax, and cardiac tamponade should also be evaluated as a cause of hypotension. Use of physical examination to assess elevations in central venous pressure and chest x-ray facilitate evaluation of these factors. Continued unexplained blood loss is most likely due to intraabdominal injury, with a vascular injury often present.

Estimation of the level of arterial injury may provide useful information for planning operative intervention. Most patients should have entrance wounds, and, if present, exit

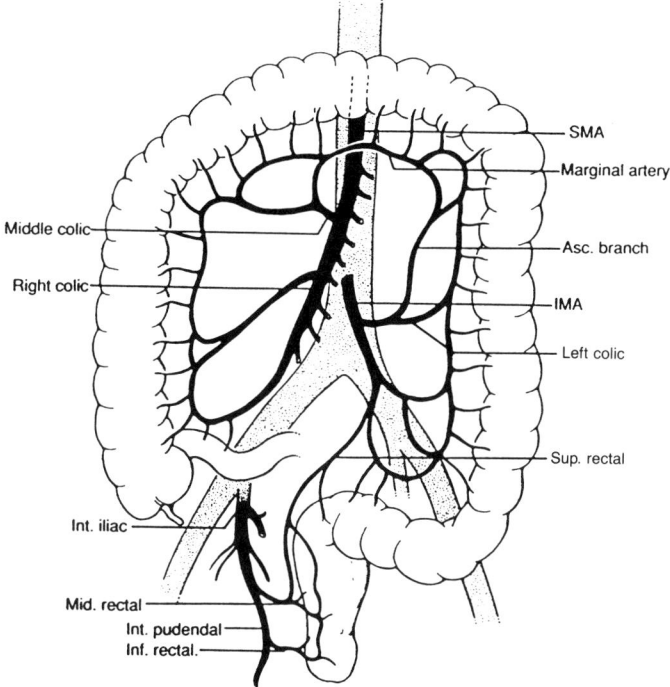

Figure 19–3. Collateral communications between the superior mesenteric and the inferior mesenteric artery and between the inferior mesenteric and the internal iliac arteries.

sites marked with paper clips or other radiopaque markers. With the help of chest and abdominal radiographs, the possible site(s) of arterial injury can be estimated by establishing the relationship of abdominal arterial anatomy to the vertebral column (Fig. 19–4). The identification of bullet fragments or bony injury in addition to lateral films can be valuable in assessing the course of a missile within the abdominal cavity.

If the missile(s) cannot be accounted for on chest or abdominal x-rays, missile embolism is a likely explanation and reexamination of peripheral pulses may help locate the foreign body. Otherwise, panradiographs are necessary to locate the missile(s). Bullet embolism, although rare, may occur in up to 1% of deaths by gunshot or shotgun wounds (Fig. 19–4B).[23,24] Bullet embolism is diagnostic of a major cardiovascular injury.

Arteriograms can be helpful in selected patients with suspected abdominal arterial injuries. They can pinpoint sites of occlusion, demonstrate extent of vascular injuries to organs that may not manifest ischemia acutely, and delineate unusual lesions such as arteriovenous fistulae or bullet embolism.

Blunt trauma more often presents with arterial occlusion rather than hemorrhage. This may be symptomatic, as with acute aortic occlusion and lower extremity ischemia, or relatively asymptomatic, as with renal artery thrombosis. Nonocclusive blunt vascular injuries may be initially asymptomatic, but may result in late thromboses or distal embolism.

Patients who have continued hypotension due to an intraabdominal cause should be taken expeditiously to the operating room for definitive care. Only those patients who

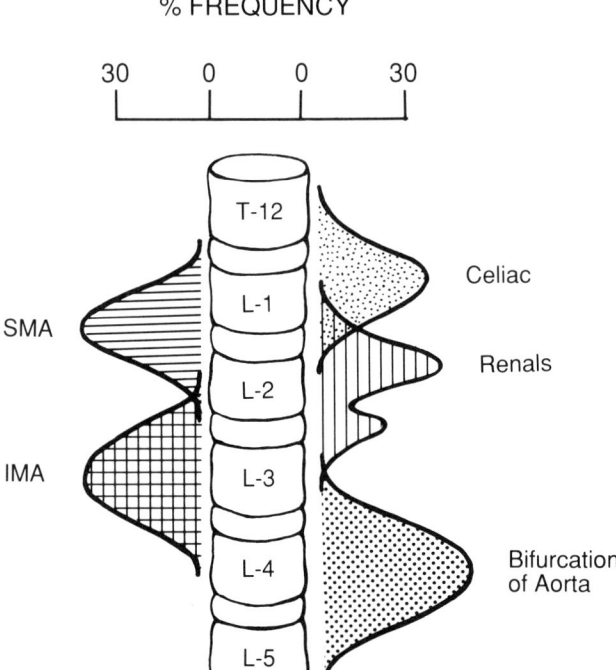

Figure 19–4. The relationship of the branches of the abdominal aorta to the vertebral column—with the relative frequency at each location.

are stable should be considered for preoperative diagnostic studies. Magnetic resonance imaging, angiography, and ultrasound are well outlined in Chapter 3.

Delays in operative repair are often associated with a poor outcome, be it loss of organ function, tissue viability, or patient morbidity/mortality. The trauma physician must consider whether a diagnostic study will alter treatment, or if a less sensitive or specific but shorter study may provide the needed information [e.g., intravenous pyelogram instead of computed tomography (CT) scan].

PREOPERATIVE MANAGEMENT

Most patients with injured abdominal arteries present with obvious signs of blood volume loss and the symptoms of hypovolemic shock. Once the airway and ventilation are secure, one should begin volume replacement rapidly by administering fluid through the largest cannula possible into the largest available vein.

Superficial veins in the upper extremity, collapsed secondary to hypovolemia, can be accessed for volume replacement by cutdown. A cutdown on the saphenous vein at the ankle or the medial antecubital vein permits the insertion of a large-bore catheter such as a 5-mm diameter infant feeding tube. Alternatively, one can cut down directly over the saphenous vein in the groin or the basilic vein itself on the medial aspect of the upper arm. By this route, the inferior or superior vena cava can be cannulated, allowing measurement of central venous pressure and providing a means of administering large volumes of fluid directly into the central vascular space. Percutaneous lines can be placed in the forearms with large plastic catheters. Resistance to flow increases proportionately to the length. Short catheters, then, permit the highest rates of fluid administration.

For initial resuscitation, a balanced salt solution such as Ringer's lactate is appropriate. If infusion of 2 liters of fluid resuscitates the adult to an awake, alert state with good vital signs, good peripheral perfusion, and a urine output of 0.5 ml/kg/hr, time is available for further diagnostic studies. On the other hand, if the infusion of 2 liters of fluid does not adequately resuscitate the patient, manifested by a strong pulse, good blood pressure and capillary filling, and establishment of urine output, it should be assumed that continuing bleeding is present. The patient may have sustained a major vascular injury, and requires immediate operation.

Once the patient is in the operating room, his entire chest, abdomen, and both groins should be prepped and draped. With the hemodynamically unstable patient, prepping and draping should be done before anesthetic induction. Vasodilation induced by anesthesia causes both arterial dilation and increased venous capacitance, both of which exacerbate hypovolemia. This, in combination with further decreases in venous return caused by the initiation of positive pressure ventilation and the negative inotropic effects of several general anesthetics, can precipitate cardiovascular collapse in the hypovolemic patient. If the patient suffers cardiovascular deterioration with induction of anesthesia, exposure and control of intraabdominal bleeding should be carried out rapidly.

Assuming the operating room is immediately available, blood should not be used in the initial resuscitation. Usually it should be possible to maintain the patient's hemodynamic status with balanced salt solution until the bleeding is controlled at surgery. If it is necessary to give blood before controlling bleeding, both the transfused blood and the patient's own blood will be lost. If transfusion can be delayed until bleeding is controlled, then vital resources will not be expended and availability of blood will be ensured for postresuscitation management.

Although the high incidence of associated intraabdominal injuries often leads to peritoneal contamination, the use of autologous blood recovery systems should be strongly considered in any case of abdominal vascular trauma. The risk of disease transmission and possible compromise of immunosuppression resulting from multiple transfusions of banked blood make autologous blood recovery appealing. Additionally, cost savings can be quite substantial when multiple units of blood are recovered.

If it is necessary to give blood on an emergency basis, type-specific uncrossmatched blood may be used. The typing of blood, as opposed to crossmatching of blood, should take but a few minutes. Type O$^-$ blood is reserved for patients with rare blood types.

Finally, broad spectrum antibiotics should be started as early in the hospital course as possible in any patient with a penetrating injury of the abdomen or lower chest. If no intraabdominal viscus has been compromised by the injury, the antibiotics can be stopped during the operation. If there is contamination of the peritoneal cavity with bowel contents, antibiotics should be continued during the perioperative period.

INITIAL OPERATIVE MANAGEMENT

A midline incision should be made from the xiphoid to below the umbilicus. If there is difficulty with exposure, the incision can be extended down to the pubis and/or up along the xiphoid. If bleeding appears to be from the vicinity of the proximal abdominal aorta, this can be converted to a thoracoabdominal incision. It cannot be overemphasized that adequate exposure is the key to successful salvage of patients with arterial injuries.

It can be difficult to locate the source of bleeding, especially in the presence of massive hemorrhage. Dry laparotomy tapes should be used to evacuate intraperitoneal blood and clots. Suction is often ineffective, as suction tubing becomes occluded by clotted blood. There should be a search for blood clots that adhere to any of the intraabdominal organs or to the parietal peritoneum. Blood clots tend to accumulate near the source of hemorrhage, thus helping locate the primary site of bleeding. Free nonclotted blood provides no information about the source of hemorrhage. As an example, free blood frequently accumulates in the pelvis because of its dependent position, even though there may be no primary bleeding in the pelvis itself.

The first encountered source of hemorrhage should not be mistaken necessarily for the sole source. As an example, the small bowel mesentery, an area that is easily observed upon opening the abdomen, frequently is a site of bleeding, but is infrequently a source of major hemorrhage. The spleen and the liver should also be inspected as another potential source of significant blood loss. Injuries of this sort, however, should not preclude the search for injuries to other less easily observed structures, such as retroperitoneal blood vessels.

Once a source of hemorrhage has been found it can usually be controlled by direct pressure while the remainder of the abdomen is quickly examined. This will allow the anesthesiologist to volume resuscitate and stabilize the patient. After stabilization, exposure and definitive control of the major bleeding site(s) can be obtained.

Palpation for pulses and thrills can help in the assessment of arterial injuries. The trauma surgeon should keep in mind that a weak pulse may be secondary to arterial injury or systemic hypotension. Thus, good communication between the trauma surgeon and anesthesiologist is essential throughout the operation. The celiac axis normally has a thrill palpable through the gastrohepatic ligament. When the gastrocolic ligament has been divided, it can be palpated through the lesser sac. The midportion of the superior mesenteric artery can be evaluated between the fingers and thumb of the right hand around the base of the small bowel mesentery. This artery normally has an easily palpable strong pulse. Pulses in nonexposed renal arteries may prove difficult to feel, even in thin patients. Occasionally in abdominal trauma it is possible to palpate a thrill in a damaged renal artery. The aorta and common iliac arteries are easy to palpate at the base of the small intestine mesentery with the small intestine eviscerated to the patient's right. The right external iliac artery can be felt as it nears the inguinal ligament just to the left of the cecum. The left external iliac artery is best felt by reflecting the sigmoid colon to the patient's right and palpating the artery just before it traverses the inguinal ligament.

Most major arterial injuries produce large retroperitoneal hematomas. These hematomas complicate the exposure of the damaged vessel since the exact location of injury may not be obvious. Generally, proximal and distal control of the potentially bleeding artery should be obtained before exposing the area of injury. The surgeon must decide how far away from the suspected injury to gain control. On the one hand, if the patient has a simple stab wound to the common iliac artery, it would be a mistake to expose the supraceliac abdominal aorta routinely to obtain proximal arterial control of bleeding. On the other hand, if the patient with a penetrating injury to the aorta at the level of the celiac axis has an extensive hematoma that extends from diaphragm to pelvis, it would be a mistake to limit the exposure to the abdomen and proximal control requires exposing the distal thoracic aorta.

When ongoing arterial hemorrhage or a large upper abdominal arterial hematoma is present, the chest can be rapidly opened by extending the abdominal incision upward in the sixth–seventh intercostal space and exposing the descending aorta where temporary cross occlusion can be done while the area of injury is exposed. When the presumed area of injury lies below the superior mesenteric artery, an aortic compressor can be used to compress the aorta at the level of the aortic hiatus (see Fig. 4–3). Pressure is exerted against the vertebral column and the instrument manipulated until the distal pulse disappears. At this point compression is maintained by an assistant until definitive proximal control is obtained.

Usually it is necessary to expose the damaged vessel at the time of the original exploration of the abdomen. On occasion, it may be wise to defer exposure of vascular injuries that appear stable and obtain arteriograms before operative exposure and definitive repair. Injuries to the suprarenal abdominal aorta are a case in point. If the hematoma around the suprarenal aorta is nonexpanding and nonpulsatile and if arteriography is most quickly obtained, it may be best to defer exposure. An operative arteriogram may be satisfactory in some instances, or the abdomen can be closed quickly with the patient taken to the arteriography suite. The patient can then be returned to the operating room for definitive repair. Arteriography should be used only when it is unlikely that the delay would decrease the patient's chances for survival. Thus, arteriography may be appropriate in certain proximal visceral arterial injuries and arteriovenous communications when the precise location and extent of the injury is uncertain. Although no published data exist, use of intraoperative ultrasound may also provide valuable information as to the precise location of the injury.

In the hypotensive patient, control of continued bleeding should take precedence over all other injuries. Once bleeding source(s) are identified, it (they) should be tamponaded by direct compression or occluded with vascular clamps. Because of the dramatic nature of abdominal vascular bleeding, surgeons often place vascular clamps much more tightly than necessary for hemostasis, exacerbating arterial injury. When placing vascular clamps, one must always be cognizant of the potential for arterial wall injury by the clamp itself. Vascular instruments should only approximate the vessel walls to arrest the intraluminal flow of blood. Compounding arterial trauma by crushing the arterial wall is always a potential hazard. A variety of vascular clamps should be included in the instrument packs available to the trauma surgeon. A straight or slightly curved aortic clamp allows for rapid clamping of the aorta without the need for circumferential mobilization. Satinsky partial occluding clamps and an assortment of angled vascular clamps should be available for simple lacerations that do not require cross-clamping to control branch vessels. Experience will guide the trauma surgeon to proper clamp selection in specific situations.

Most abdominal vascular injuries have associated visceral or solid organ injuries. After initial operative control of hemorrhage, bowel injuries can be rapidly controlled with suture or staples to minimize bacterial contamination. This will allow the anesthesiologist time to complete the fluid resuscitation.

EXPOSURE OF SPECIFIC INJURIES

Operative Exposure

The abdominal arteries can be functionally divided into four zones depending on their anatomic location and the exposure necessary for adequate evaluation and repair.[25] Operative exposure of the abdominal arteries for trauma has to be expedient and provide a wide operative field. Furthermore, because the best therapeutic intervention may not be known until the injury is exposed, the ability to preserve flexibility with respect to reconstructive options is essential. To clarify what is often perceived as complex operative exposure and anatomy, it is appropriate to divide the abdominal arterial tree into four anatomic zones based on their requirements for operative exposure. This classification allows for rapid and precise visualization of all major intraabdominal arteries.

Zone 1 includes the suprarenal aorta, the celiac axis, superior mesenteric artery, and the left renal artery. Surgical exposure of these vessels can be gained by dividing the peritoneal reflection over the descending colon, along with the splenorenal ligament (Fig. 19–5A). By reflection of the descending colon and spleen medially, the posterior surface of the pancreas and stomach are exposed. Division of the loose areolar tissue between the colonic mesentery and the posterior surface of the pancreas allows these organs to be reflected to the midline. The kidney should be left within Gerota's fascia at this point and not displaced to the midline. While rotating these viscera medially, the retroperitoneal portion of the stomach is mobilized by incising the peritoneal reflection over the cardia to the level of the esophageal hiatus (Fig. 19–5B). The supraceliac aorta, celiac axis, and superior mesenteric artery can now be exposed (Fig. 19–5C). The supraceliac aorta remains covered by the diaphragmatic crura, which can be divided to provide exposure of the aorta to the level of T-8. Care should be taken to avoid excessive traction or compression of the spleen, as it can be damaged easily by retractors.

To provide control of the thoracic aorta at a higher level, the laparotomy incision is extended to include a left thoracotomy. The diaphragm is then incised along its lateral attachments to the ribs. This allows entrance into the left chest with preservation of diaphragmatic blood supply and innervation. If access to the left posterolateral aorta is required, the kidney can be reflected medially with the rest of the viscera for exposure (Fig. 19–5D).

Zone 2 includes the right renal artery, the right side of the suprarenal aorta, the proximal right side of the superior mesenteric artery, and the common hepatic artery. Surgical exposure of the right renal artery can be accomplished by incising the peritoneal reflection of the right colon and releasing the hepatic flexure (Fig. 19–6A). With the ascending colon reflected medially, a Kocher maneuver is performed to reflect the duodenum and the head of the pancreas to the midline (Fig. 19–6B,C). These maneuvers expose the inferior vena cava, the right renal vein, and the origin of the left renal vein. The right renal artery can now be exposed with mobilization of the inferior vena cava (Fig. 19–6D). The origin of the left renal artery, common hepatic artery, and superior mesenteric artery can also be exposed through this technique.

Zone 3 includes the infrarenal aorta, the inferior mesenteric artery, and the proximal common iliac arteries. Access to this portion of the abdominal arteries can be gained by rotating the small intestine to the right upper quadrant (Fig. 19–7A). This exposes the third and fourth portions of the duodenum overlying the aorta. The peritoneal reflection is divided close to the duodenum where a relatively avascular plane exists. This approach also avoids injury to the inferior mesenteric vessels (Fig. 19–7B). The duodenum and pancreas can be mobilized cephalad to the level of, and often above, the left renal vein, if needed. The left renal vein can be divided, if necessary, to gain more proximal exposure, but should be divided as close to the vena cava as possible to avoid interrupting collateral venous drainage.[26,27] With this maneuver, the infrarenal aorta as well as the common iliac arteries can be controlled and dissected along their entire length (Fig. 19–7C). Alter-

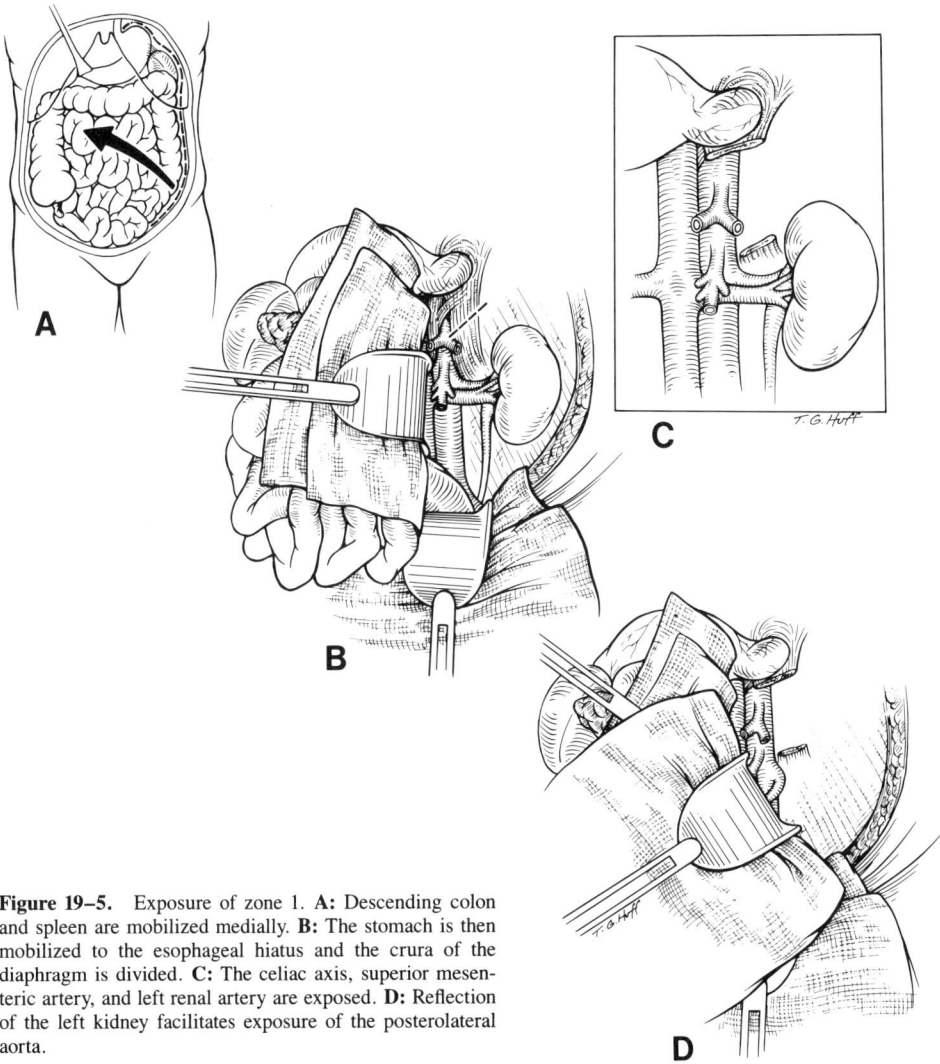

Figure 19–5. Exposure of zone 1. **A:** Descending colon and spleen are mobilized medially. **B:** The stomach is then mobilized to the esophageal hiatus and the crura of the diaphragm is divided. **C:** The celiac axis, superior mesenteric artery, and left renal artery are exposed. **D:** Reflection of the left kidney facilitates exposure of the posterolateral aorta.

natively, the exposure used for Zone 2 can be extended and will provide good exposure of the same area.

Zone 4 includes the distal common iliac arteries, the internal iliac and external iliac arteries. Access to these arteries may require no visceral mobilization. Typically, though, the ileocecal valve lies over the right iliac bifurcation. Thus, the cecum may need to be mobilized cephalad to gain adequate exposure of the right iliac system. The bifurcation of the left iliac artery is usually covered by the mesentery of the sigmoid colon. Rather than divide this mesentery, greater exposure can be gained by reflecting the sigmoid colon and distal descending colon superomedially to the right (Fig. 19–8). This will facilitate exposure of the left internal iliac artery as well as the left external iliac artery to the level of the inguinal ligament.

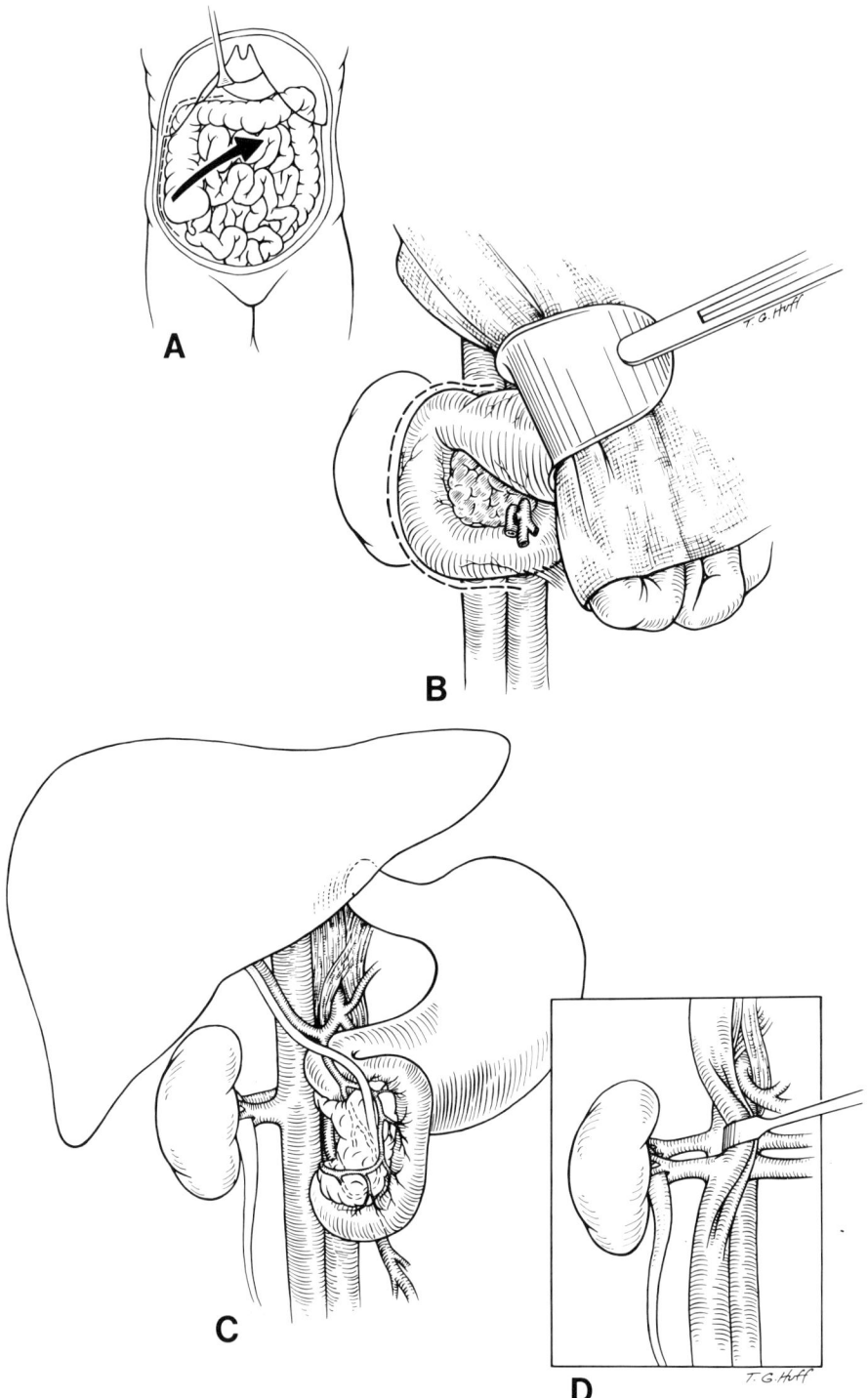

Figure 19–6. Exposure of zone 2. **A:** The right colon is mobilized to the left. **B:** An incision is made in the fascia lateral to the duodenum to initiate the Kocher maneuver. **C:** The duodenum and head of the pancreas are mobilized upward toward the midline. **D:** The inferior vena cava is mobilized as necessary to expose the proximal right renal artery.

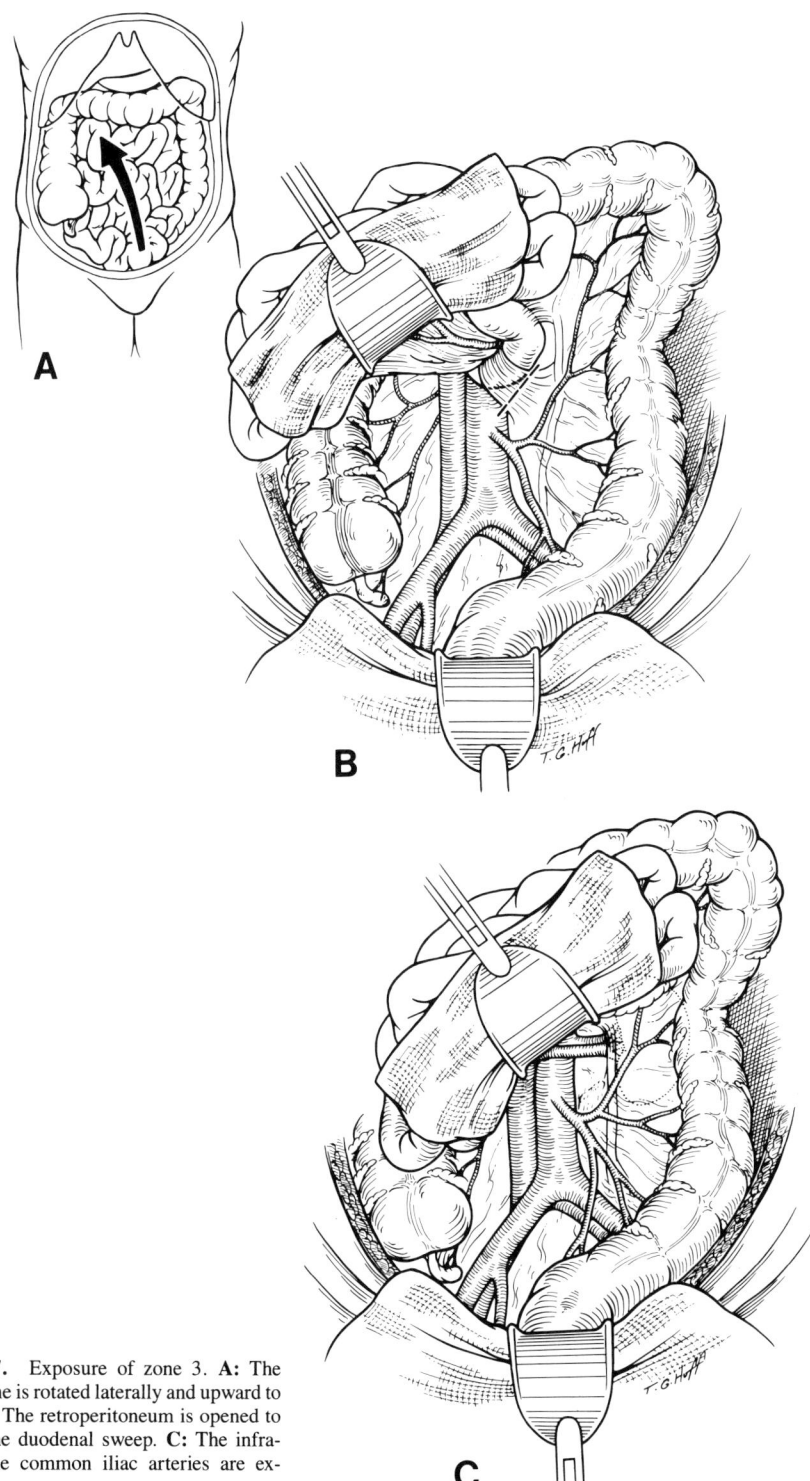

Figure 19–7. Exposure of zone 3. **A:** The small intestine is rotated laterally and upward to the right. **B:** The retroperitoneum is opened to the left of the duodenal sweep. **C:** The infrarenal and the common iliac arteries are exposed.

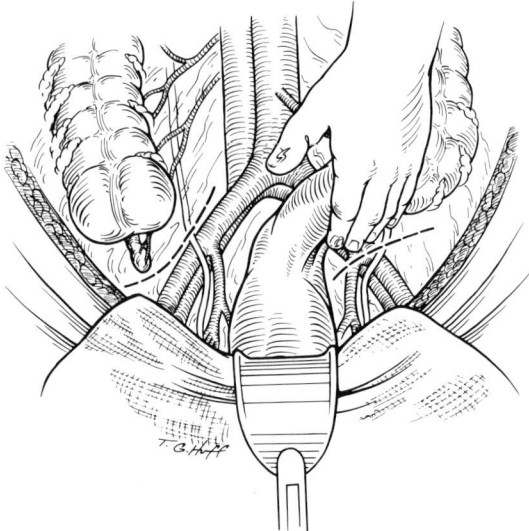

Figure 19-8. The sigmoid colon is mobilized to the right and its lateral attachment is divided and the retroperitoneum opened to expose the left external iliac artery.

MANAGEMENT OF SPECIFIC INJURIES

Supraceliac Aorta

The supraceliac aorta, because it is such a short segment, is rarely injured by either blunt or penetrating trauma. The optimal approach to this segment is through a thoracic or thoracoabdominal approach. Fortunately, lateral exposure and suture will accomplish repair in most supraceliac aortic injuries.[11] When more extensive repairs are needed, several methods are possible. Patch angioplasty can be accomplished using the autogenous saphenous vein or internal iliac artery. In the absence of bacterial contamination, a prosthetic patch may be employed. As an adjunctive measure, the diaphragmatic crura should be reapproximated to help protect the repair, and in the case of prosthetic repair, this viable muscle coverage may help prevent graft infection.[28] Circumferential loss of up to 1.5 cm of aortic wall may be closed with judicious mobilization of the thoracic aorta and primary anastomosis. If bacterial contamination is not present, a prosthetic tube graft can replace the injured segment.

In the stable patient with loss of a segment of supraceliac aorta and bacterial contamination, more complex repairs may be required. The aorta can be ligated proximally and distally to the injury. Reperfusion of the viscera can be accomplished by extraanatomic routes (axillofemoral or thoracic aorta to iliac artery bypass).

Another option may be to put a prosthetic graft into a contaminated field with irrigation catheters and coverage with a vascularized pedicle (muscle or omentum) and use long-term antibiotic suppression.

Owing to mortality rates of up to 70%,[11] complex autogenous repairs should probably not be attempted initially. The main goal is to restore continuity of the aorta and have an alive patient. If the patient survives the initial injury, then a work-up can be undertaken to assess the significance of any prosthetic graft infection that subsequently develops.

Celiac Axis and Its Branches

Injuries to the celiac axis can be managed with the same exposure as that used for the supraceliac aorta. Often a hematoma is present around the abdominal aorta as it comes through the diaphragm. The optimal method of control is to expose the descending thoracic aorta before entering the hematoma. The most difficult part in management of the injured celiac axis is obtaining exposure. This is due not only to its retroperitoneal location, but also to its covering of splanchnic nerves. Once the injury is exposed, reassessment of the patient's stability should take place.

In the unstable patient, the celiac axis can be ligated without sequelae so long as its collateral circulation to the superior mesenteric artery remains intact.[29,30] Primary reconstruction of the damaged celiac artery is difficult because the artery is thin-walled and branches early, so that mobilization for reconstruction is difficult. In the hemodynamically stable patient, the celiac axis should be repaired. Attempts at reconstruction of the celiac axis have failed in the past because of excessive mobilization. This mobilization may interrupt the collateral blood supply to the upper abdominal viscera. Additionally, excessive tension is unavoidable with primary reanastomosis of the celiac axis. Thus, it is best with most injuries causing segmental defects of the celiac axis to use interposition grafting.[31] On occasion, if there is a question of viability of the upper abdominal viscera after ligation, the splenic artery can be dissected from its bed, transected near its origin, and reimplanted in the supraceliac aorta so as to provide prograde flow. Splenic blood flow should be maintained through collaterals supplied by the left gastric and hepatic arteries.

Injuries to the left gastric artery and splenic artery can also be exposed as described for Zone 1. However, if the limited nature of injury is recognized, extensive exposure may not be necessary. The most direct approach to both left gastric artery and the splenic artery is through the lesser sac after dividing the gastrocolic ligament. The left gastric artery can be ligated without compromising the gastric blood supply. The splenic artery can be ligated and the spleen will remain viable so long as the short gastric arteries are intact. Before definitive ligation of the splenic artery, Doppler assessment of the splenic hilum should be done to assure adequate collateral blood flow through the short gastric arteries. If the short gastric arteries are taken and splenic artery ligation is necessary, splenectomy should be performed to avoid the sequelae of splenic infarction.

The common hepatic artery is best exposed through the gastrohepatic ligament. It too can be ligated if necessary. The proper hepatic artery should be repaired, if possible, but if necessary it can usually be ligated with minimal effects on liver function (see Chapter 10). The common hepatic artery is well demonstrated in utilizing Zone 2 exposure.

Superior Mesenteric Artery and Its Branches

The origin of superior mesenteric artery can be exposed as described for Zone 1 and Zone 2. The dissection of the proximal portion of the superior mesenteric artery is difficult, like the celiac axis, because of the dense plexus of nerves surrounding the vessel. Care must be taken not to damage the artery, particularly at its origin from the aorta during dissection. The superior mesenteric artery, if damaged in its proximal portion, should be repaired, as collateral flow may prove inadequate to maintain viability of the small intestine. Since the proximal 3 to 5 cm of the superior mesenteric artery has no branches, once the proper plane is entered and once the nerves around the proximal portion of the artery are cut, the first several centimeters of the artery can be dissected rapidly.[33,34]

Most injuries of the superior mesenteric artery will require patching with or an interposition graft of saphenous vein. Attempts to suture a longitudinally orientated laceration of the vessel without benefit of vein patch angioplasty will narrow the artery enough to jeopardize the small intestine's blood supply. If the origin of the superior mesenteric artery is avulsed from the aorta, one alternative is interposition grafting from the aorta to the superior mesenteric artery with vein. Another is to transect the splenic artery and create an end-to-end anastomosis with the distal mesenteric artery or use the internal iliac artery as vascular replacement. Injuries to the superior mesenteric artery in the mesentery of the small intestine can be patched with autogenous vein. Alternatively, the intestine supplied by the injured vessel can be resected if the injury is distal to the proximal intestinal branches.

Perirenal Aorta and the Renal Arteries

The left renal artery is exposed as described for injuries in Zone 1. The left renal artery can also be controlled at its origin through the base of the left colonic mesentery. Although this affords proximal control of the left renal artery, full exposure still requires mobilization of the left colon, pancreas, and spleen. Exposure of the left renal artery by reflecting the fourth portion of the duodenum off the aorta and extending the dissection underneath the inferior portion of the pancreas has limited utility for traumatic injuries.

If either renal artery is damaged near its origin and if it is necessary to cross-clamp the aorta, it may be most expeditious to apply the cross-clamp or a vascular compressor to the supraceliac aorta. The left renal artery may occasionally originate at the level of the superior mesenteric artery origin. Attempting to place a clamp between the superior mesenteric artery and the renal arteries or between the celiac axis and superior mesenteric artery when the interval is less than 1 to 2 cm can not only distort the aorta at the level of the renal arteries, making repair difficult, but it may also damage other major arterial branches as well. Thus, supraceliac control may be the safest and most expeditious. If the injury is to the ventral surface of the aorta near the origins of the renal arteries, the left renal vein may hinder exposure. The vein can be mobilized upward toward the midline. This requires dividing the adrenal, gonadal, and lumbar veins. This will allow movement of the vein cephalad and caudad and permit exposure of the ventral aorta at that level along with all of the left renal artery and some of the right renal artery. Transection of the left renal vein is also safe if done close to the inferior vena cava and the above described branches are retained.[26]

The right renal artery is best exposed as described for Zone 2. It can also be exposed through the base of the right colonic mesentery. Again, while this exposure allows proximal control, exposure for definitive repair is limited. Adequate exposure may require mobilization of the vena cava or the kidney from its bed.

Injuries to the renal arteries, unless repaired in a transverse manner or unless fairly minor, will require a vein patch to avoid anastomotic narrowing. In some cases, the splenic artery or gastroduodenal artery can be used to provide an end-to-end reconstruction. Prolonged attempts at renal artery repair are not warranted, assuming that the patient has a functioning kidney on the other side. If the repair requires an undue commitment of time, or multiple associated injuries exist, nephrectomy may be prudent. It is essential, before nephrectomy, to verify function of the opposite kidney by operative IVP if possible. In the rare instance in which there is a problem with function of the opposite kidney, *ex vivo* repair may be appropriate.[27]

Infrarenal Aorta

Initially, an infrarenal aortic injury may be controlled by direct pressure[32] or supraceliac aortic clamping or compression.[35] As with the suprarenal aorta, most injuries to the infrarenal aorta can be managed with lateral arteriorrhaphy or patch angioplasty. Transection can be managed with primary reanastomosis. Small segmental defects may be closed primarily with mobilization of the remaining aorta. Mobilization can be achieved by ligation of lumbar segmental branches. Defects up to 1.5 cm can be repaired by this method.

Large traumatic defects need interposition grafting. While synthetic interposition grafts may be useful in certain circumstances, an autogenous conduit can be constructed using internal iliac artery, saphenous vein, or a common iliac artery combined with femoral bypass[34] (Fig. 19–9). This method is of particular value in a grossly contaminated field. Extraanatomic bypass can also be used to restore infrarenal aortic perfusion should ligation be used.

Inferior Mesenteric Artery

The inferior mesenteric artery can be ligated at its origin provided it is less than 0.5 cm in diameter. The use of inferior mesenteric artery stump pressures to decide if ligation is safe[35] is often unreliable in the hypotensive trauma patient. If it is larger than 0.5 cm, the inferior mesenteric artery may be the dominant blood supply to the large intestine and should be repaired to avoid massive bowel infarction. When injury requires distal ligation so that the bifurcation into the left colic and superior rectal collateral is compromised, functional assessment by Doppler or fluorescein dye of the bowel should be done. If collateral circulation is inadequate, arterial repair or bowel resection should be carried out.

Iliac Arteries

As with other abdominal vascular injuries, lateral arteriorrhaphy can be used to repair most iliac arterial injuries. If a larger segmental defect does not lend itself to mobilization and primary reanastomosis, the common iliac artery can be reimplanted in the contralateral common iliac, as reported by Landreneau et al.[36] (Fig. 19–10).

The external iliac artery can be replaced with a segment of internal iliac artery or saphenous vein (Fig. 19–11). Because of the rich collateral blood supply, the internal iliac artery can be ligated proximally and distally if lateral arteriorrhaphy cannot be accomplished easily. Should both internal iliacs be injured, repair of one internal iliac should be attempted to assure adequate pelvic circulation. An interposition graft can be obtained from the internal iliac artery to be ligated or from the saphenous vein.

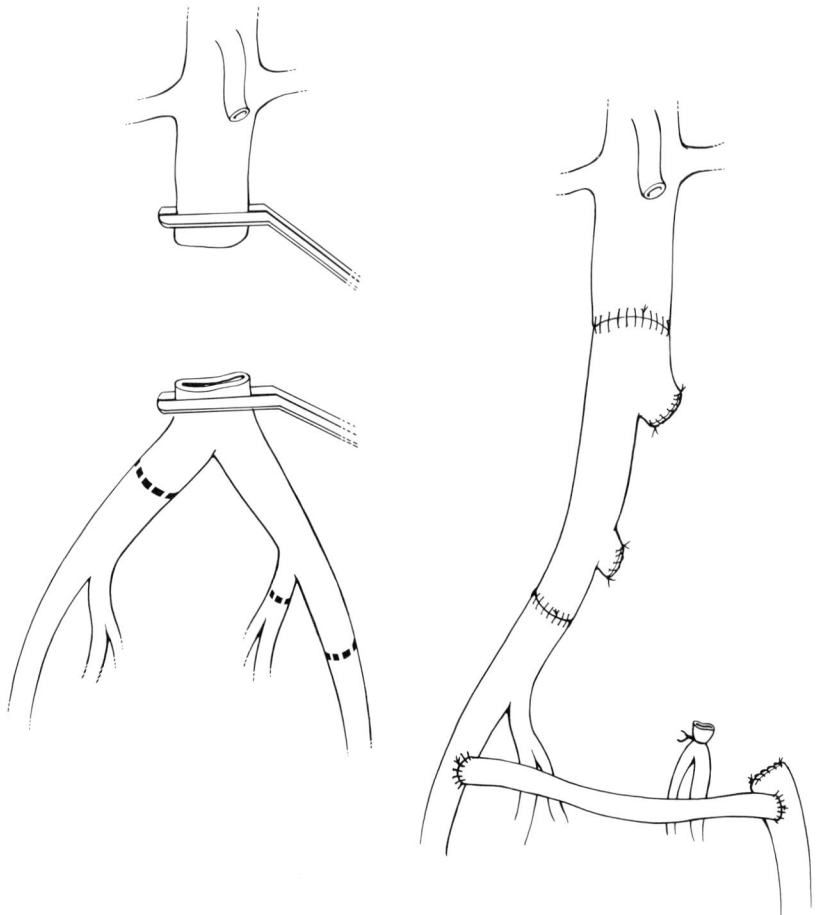

Figure 19–9. One iliac artery can be removed to provide an autogenous conduit to the opposite iliac artery and the ipsilateral leg revascularized utilizing a femoro–femoral bypass.

TECHNIQUES OF REPAIR

Most major abdominal vascular injuries should be repaired, when possible, by direct suture without using a graft. The best suture material is fine monofilament plastic. Generally, 1- to 2-cm defects of any of the abdominal arteries can be repaired by judicious mobilization of the proximal and distal segments of the artery and bringing the ends together for a primary anastomosis. Mobilization may require sacrifice of collateral branches. For vessels smaller than 4 mm, interrupted technique provides optimal results (Fig. 19–12). For 5- to 6-mm vessels, interrupted everting sutures at the ends with running sutures in between can be used (Fig. 19–13).

When a large vessel is encountered and narrowing of the anastomosis is not likely, a continuous running suture may be used (Fig. 19–14). The posterior wall can be sutured from within if branches prohibit rotation of the vessel.

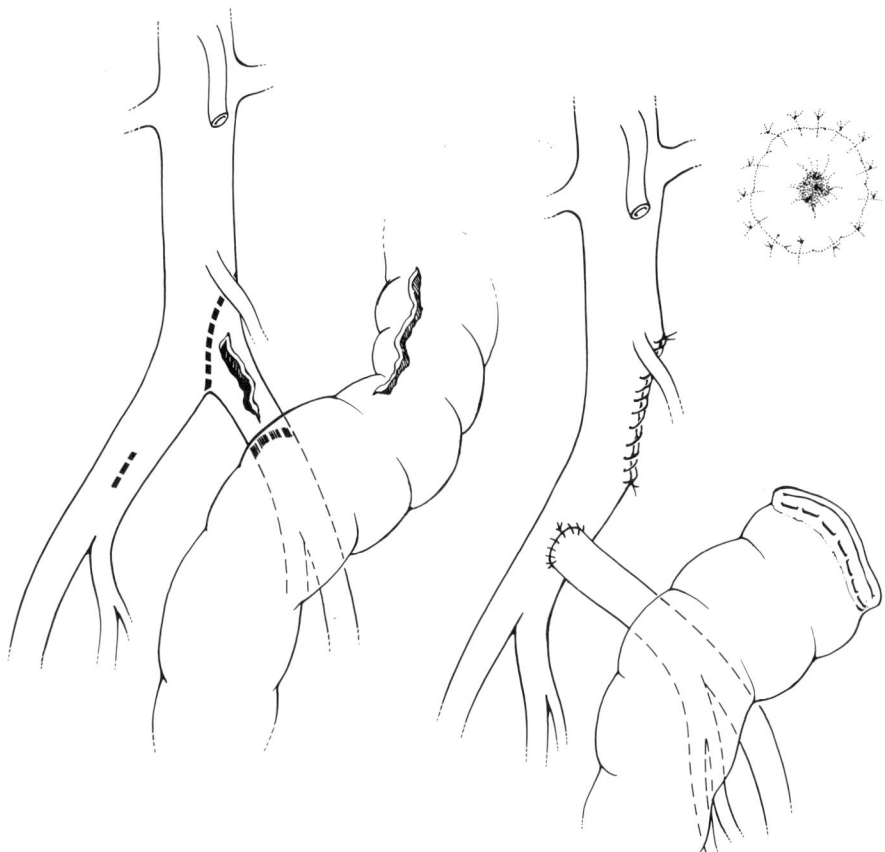

Figure 19-10. A damaged segment of a proximal common iliac artery can be excised and the vessel anastomosed to the opposite iliac.

When a primary repair would result in marked narrowing of an artery, a graft should be used either as a patch or as an interposition graft. Most major abdominal arterial injuries will be associated with contamination of the peritoneal cavity, since most of the major vascular injuries will be due to penetrating trauma. One should avoid putting prosthetic material into a contaminated field if there is a reasonable alternative. Every effort should be made to use autogenous tissue. The saphenous vein makes an excellent graft. The vein from the lower leg is thicker than the vein from the thigh and is easier to handle. However, the vein from the lower leg is smaller than the vein from the thigh, and its small size may make it an unsatisfactory replacement graft for many of the abdominal vessels. If the saphenous vein from the thigh is also too small, one can make a composite graft in which two segments of vein are sutured together to expand the cross-sectional area of the graft (see Chapter 20). Valve lysis may increase initial flow rates.[37]

Arteries taken from other areas can also be used as a graft. The first choice would be the internal iliac, since no replacement is necessary. The next choice would be the common femoral artery. If one of the groins is not contaminated, the femoral artery from

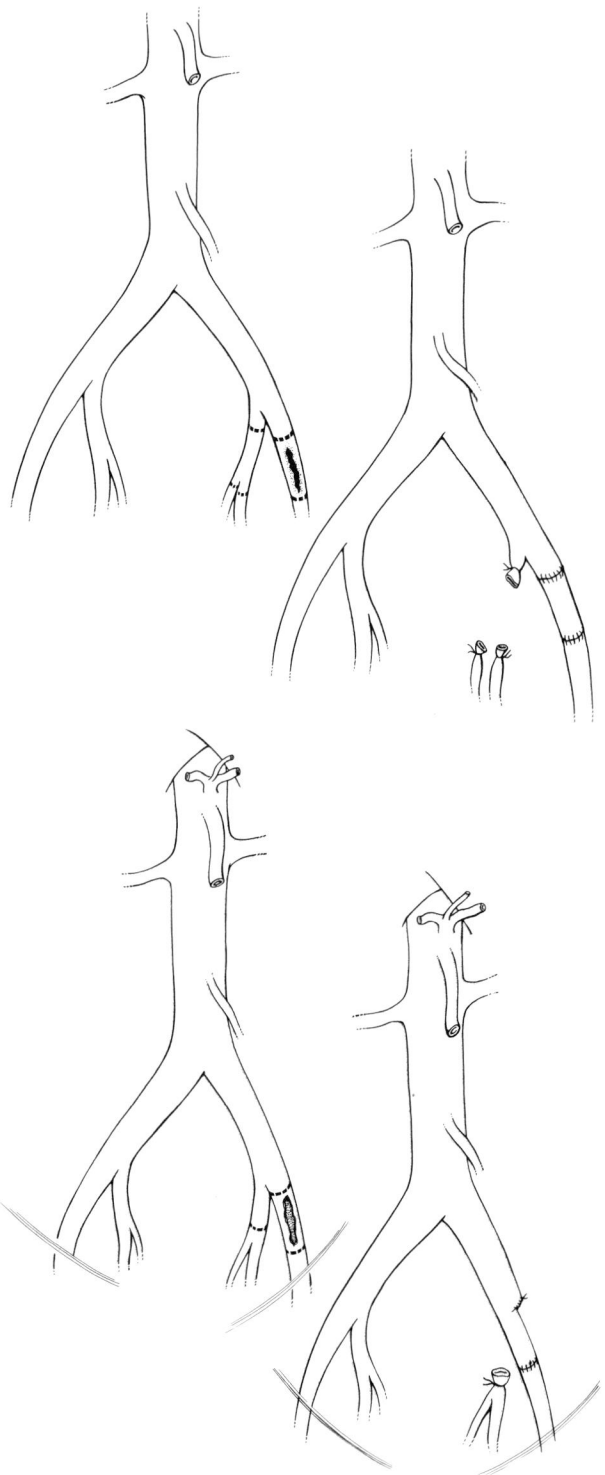

Figure 19–11. The internal iliac artery can be sacrificed to repair a common iliac or an external iliac injury.

Abdominal Arterial Trauma   363

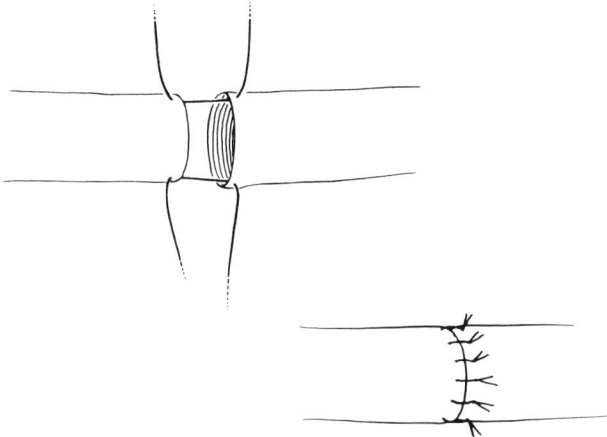

Figure 19–12. Simple interrupted vascular repair. This technique is most useful for small vessel anastomosis.

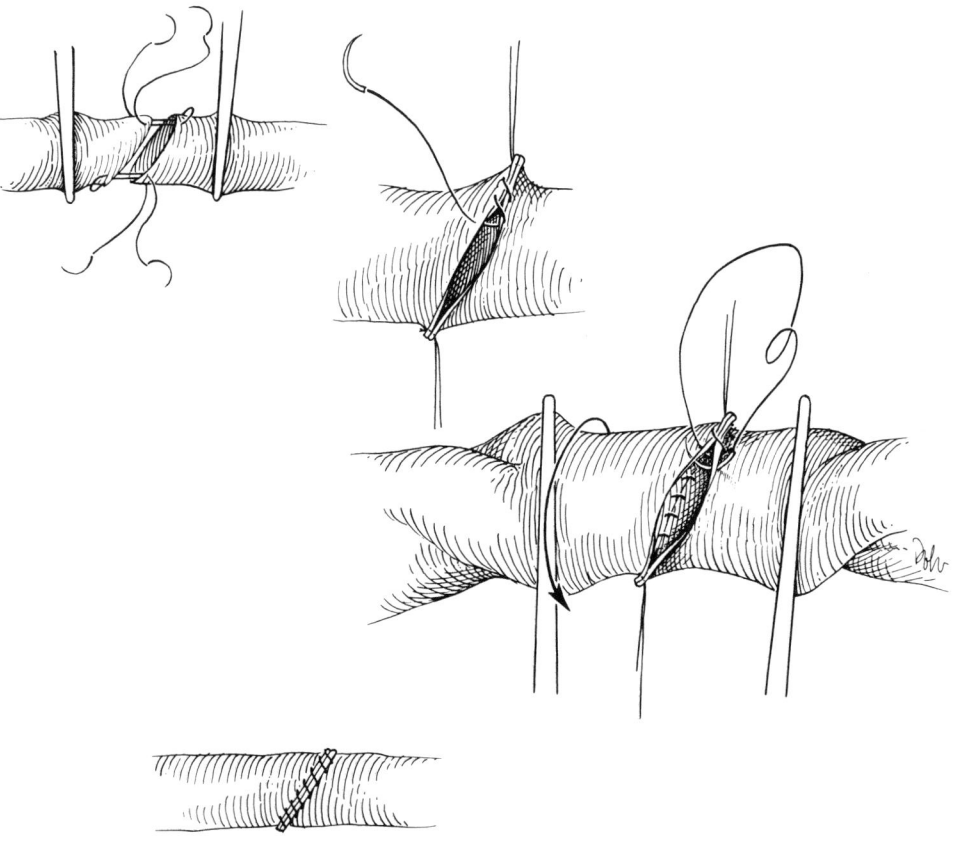

Figure 19–13. Standard technique for repair of medium size (4–6) vessels. Two everting mattress sutures are placed at opposite sides of the proposed repair to initiate arterial eversion. A running suture is placed between. The artery is then rotated to permit a running suture of the opposite side.

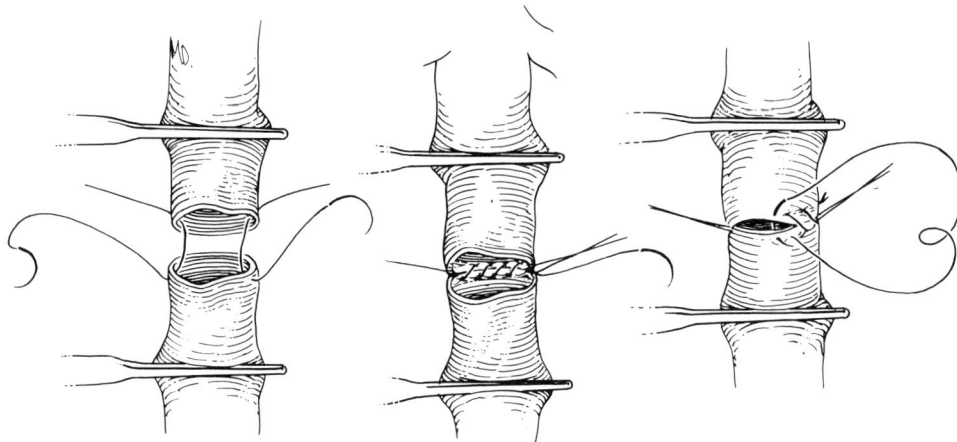

Figure 19–14. Large vessel anastomosis. A running suture can be used for the entire anastomosis or the anastomosis with two interrupted sutures at opposite sides of the vessel. The back row can be placed from within the vessel if it is technically easier.

that groin can be replaced with a prosthetic graft and the artery used in the contaminated abdominal field.

In elective cases, the external iliac artery can make the ideal arterial graft since it is large and long and has no large branches. Replacement of the artery is well tolerated with few complications such as infection, false aneurysm formation, or thrombosis, perhaps because the prosthesis lies in a protected, nonstressed location. Unfortunately, it is possible only rarely to use the external iliac artery in trauma cases because if the peritoneal cavity is contaminated, it is difficult to harvest the external iliac artery without contaminating its bed. If the external iliac artery is used, a femorofemoral crossover graft should be used to restore lower limb perfusion. This will avoid putting a graft in a contaminated field. In some cases, the splenic artery can be used to vascularize a critical organ. It can be divided distally and anastomosed to damaged arteries that lie near it, such as the superior mesenteric artery or either renal artery. It is not of sufficient caliber to revascularize the abdominal aorta, nor long enough to reach the iliac arteries.

If, by chance, an artery is injured and the peritoneum is not contaminated, then prosthetic material can be used for reconstruction. Even under this circumstance, however, it is best to use autogenous material if obtaining the autogenous material does not add excessive operative time.

As mentioned earlier, many of the major abdominal arteries can be ligated without ill effect. Ligation should be considered if the alternative requires repair with prosthetic material in a contaminated field. The celiac axis can be ligated, as long as its major branches are intact. Any of the branches of the celiac axis such as the splenic artery, the left gastric artery, or the proximal common hepatic artery can also be ligated, as long as the distal collateral circulation is intact. A renal artery can be ligated and the kidney removed if necessary. The inferior mesenteric artery can be ligated. The infrarenal abdominal aorta or either of the common iliac arteries can be ligated, but ligation will usually cause severe ischemia of the lower extremities. Nonetheless, in an emergency, ligation can be carried out and the patient systemically anticoagulated with heparin. After the abdomen is closed, the extremities can be examined. If limb-threatening ischemia is present, flow can be reestablished through bypass graft using the axillofemoral or femorofemoral route. Prosthetic material can be used in this reconstruction, assuming that the groins and the axilla and the graft tunnels are not contaminated.

ATHEROSCLEROTIC ARTERIAL TRAUMA

Although penetrating trauma is fortunately rare in patients with atherosclerotic arterial disease, several cases of acute aortic occlusion with blunt trauma have been reported.[38,42] These patients present with a wide range of complaints and physical findings. Patients with aneurysmal disease may present with symptoms of aneurysm rupture or thrombosis. Those patients with acute occlusion of the aorta often present with lower extremity rest pain. Lack of leg motion secondary to limb ischemia can be confused with a spinal cord lesion.

With a history and physical exam consistent with occlusion superimposed on chronic occlusive disease, liberal use of angiography and perioperative invasive monitoring should allow more successful operative strategies. In those patients with a history of aneurysm and signs of aortic rupture, diagnostic studies should not delay rapid abdominal exploration.

POSTOPERATIVE MANAGEMENT

Patients who suffer abdominal arterial trauma are at a high risk for developing complications in the postoperative period. Hypotension secondary to blood loss, associated injuries, and the possibility of problems related to the control and/or repair of vascular injuries all can provide challenging management problems. Visceral ischemia may occur secondary to thrombosis of repairs or deliberate ligation.

Patients suffering isolated injuries of major abdominal vessels may have an uncomplicated postoperative course if the injuries are expeditiously treated with minimal blood loss. The postoperative management of nonarterial injuries is discussed in other chapters.

Antibiotics given in the perioperative period should be continued postoperatively as dictated by the extent of peritoneal contamination. When autologous arterial reconstruction is done, antibiotic therapy is not necessary beyond that for associated injuries. When PTFE or Dacron grafts are used in the face of gross contamination, antibiotic therapy should be continued for at least 1 month. If prosthetic infection develops, life-long oral antibiotic suppression will be required or alternative options such as graft removal followed by extraanatomical reconstruction as necessary.[43] Choice of antibiotic should be based on intraoperative cultures. Although this will not sterilize a prosthetic graft, suppression of the infecting organism often allows a symbiotic relationship between the patient and a contaminated vascular conduit. Coverage of the prosthetic graft with a viable tissue pedicle should also be done at the initial operation when contamination of the graft occurs.

High flow rates in the abdominal aorta obviate the need for anticoagulation in the perioperative period. Any time a branch of the aorta is repaired with an interposition graft of autogenous or prosthetic materials, strong consideration should be given to the adjunctive use of antiplatelet agents. Dextran 40 has been demonstrated to increase 30-day and long-term patency rates in distal bypasses[44] and may be useful to prolong patency of abdominal arterial repairs. The role of postoperative heparinization is controversial.

If the patient develops a coagulopathy, the antiplatelet agent should be withheld until there is stabilization of coagulation parameters and no need for transfusions exists. Dextran probably has little use in this situation, but aspirin may improve long-term patency.

Cardiovascular monitoring can help in maximizing cardiac function. It may help minimize visceral sympathetic-mediated vasoconstriction, resulting in an increase in visceral vascular resistance. Concomitant higher graft blood flow may decrease the amount of thrombus lining the graft, which can be important for maintaining early graft patency.

COMPLICATIONS

Several aspects of the postoperative course need special attention. For all patients who have any major injury, postoperative bleeding is a potential hazard. Volume status should be monitored by following the patient's vital signs, abdominal girth, peripheral perfusion, urine output, and hematocrit. Vascular instability or signs of hemorrhage should prompt reexploration.

Bleeding can occur either as an early or late complication of any vascular reconstruction. Early bleeding can be secondary to technical inadequacies of the repair or it can be due to a bleeding diathesis resulting from shock or extensive soft tissue damage. Some of the bleeding diathesis may be due to dilution of the patient's own clotting factors with transfused blood. Most patients with a major bleeding diathesis, however, will have a consumption coagulopathy to explain their bleeding abnormalities. This bleeding may begin during the operation. Patients who spontaneously start to bleed from small vessels in the subcutaneous tissue, muscle, or from other areas that were dry usually have at least some degree of disseminated intravascular coagulation. In this circumstance, closing the abdomen may allow tamponade and slowing of the bleed. The hemodynamic status tends to improve when the abdomen is closed because the hypothermia and cardiac depression associated with an open abdomen and general anesthesia can be reversed. As the patient's hemodynamic status improves, tissue perfusion will improve and the stimulus for intravascular clotting and clot lysis will decrease.

If the abdomen is closed in the face of diffuse bleeding, the abdomen should be reexplored within 24 hr. Removal of clotted blood also forestalls further bleeding, and removes it as a culture medium for bacteria.

Late bleeding after a major revascularization is usually due to infection at the site of reconstruction. The threat of exsanguination from such a hemorrhage should prompt immediate operative exploration. It is usually necessary to ligate the bleeding reconstructed artery. Sometimes ligation will be well tolerated; sometimes it will not. In the latter case, reconstruction as described earlier will be necessary.

Thrombosis can occur after any arterial reconstruction. The thrombosis can be caused by inadequate inflow, inadequate outflow, or most commonly by technical errors in the reconstruction. Postoperative thrombosis in some reconstructed arteries will be obvious, as in the case of a thrombosed iliac artery. Thrombosis of other arteries may be difficult to detect early, such as thrombosis of reconstructed mesenteric artery. Patients with reconstructions of certain critical arteries that could become silently occluded in the immediate postoperative period should be routinely explored within 24 hr of the initial operation; the decision to reexplore should be made at the time of initial surgery. As an example, if a superior mesenteric artery is reconstructed and the surgeon decides at the time of surgery that reexploration should be carried out the following day, the patient should be reexplored even if doing well. The purpose of the reexploration is to find a correctable lesion before it progresses to a fatal issue. The best time to explore such a patient is when the patient is doing well. By the time the patient has begun to deteriorate clinically, serious complications have already begun and it may be too late to reverse the damage.

Thrombosis of a renal artery repair may be asymptomatic, or present with flank pain, oliguria, hematuria, or even hypertension. Duplex scanning, nuclear renograms, or arteriography will help in making appropriate therapeutic decisions. If rerevascularization is attempted, mannitol should be given. A calcium channel blocker, such as verapamil, can be injected directly into the distal renal artery and may also help preserve renal function.[45]

Ischemic changes are usually manifest in the early postoperative period. Bowel ischemia can be a difficult diagnostic problem. After thrombosis of a visceral artery reconstruction, acidosis may be the only significant finding before massive bowel necrosis. Thus, if unexplained acidosis develops, it should be quickly addressed. If other causes, such as poor ventilation or cardiac dysfunction, are corrected and acidosis remains, prompt consideration should be given to assessment of visceral blood flow. Arteriogram or abdominal duplex scan may be helpful in the evaluation of mesenteric blood flow.

Reperfusion injury with cellular damage and swelling can offset a technically adequate repair. Reperfusion of dead or severely ischemic muscle is associated with the release of procoagulants into the systemic circulation. This activates the coagulation cascade and with it inflammatory mediators. These tear up the vascular system and result in permeability alterations and third spacing. Increased vascular permeability results in respiratory distress syndrome. Therefore, assessment should involve monitoring arterial blood gases, cardiovascular function, and renal function. It should include peripheral pulses, neurologic and compartment pressure assessment. Pressures in all four lower leg compartments should be measured. Fasciotomy, if needed, is done through generous incisions.

Renal failure should be a rare complication of abdominal vascular injuries. Acute tubular necrosis can result from prolonged preoperative hypotension, prolonged clamping of the aorta, or direct renal artery or vein trauma. In the normovolemic patient, calcium antagonist may help improve renal function.[46] In the absence of these factors, renal failure is almost always due to either inadequate fluid resuscitation or to a delay in removing necrotic bowel or ischemic limbs. Renal failure is difficult to treat and carries a high mortality in the trauma setting. It may prove better to give too much fluid initially and risk pulmonary edema than to allow renal failure to develop. If doubt exists regarding the adequacy of fluid resuscitation, a pulmonary artery catheter should be used to guide fluid therapy and/or inotropic support.

Infection and intraabdominal abscess formation may provide a frustrating late complication after an initial therapeutic success. Because of extensive blood loss and associated visceral injuries, more than one-third of patients with abdominal vascular injury develop sepsis due to the immunosuppression that accompanies major injury and transfusion. Wilson et al.[47] have found a correlation between the number of transfusions and the development of serious infection or intraabdominal abscess (Table 19–1). A particularly high-risk group had an initial operating room systolic blood pressure of 70 mm Hg or less and received 10 or more units of blood. In this group 100% developed serious infections.

Table 19–1 Incidence of Infection in High-risk Patients Correlated with Initial Operating Room Blood Pressure and Units of Blood Transfused in the First 24 Hours

	TOTAL INFECTIONS
OR systolic BP <70 mm Hg or 10+ units blood given	77%
OR systolic BP >70 mm Hg or 9 units of blood or less	20%
OR systolic BP <70 mm Hg and 10+ units blood	100%

Adapted with permission from Wilson, et al.[47]
OR, operating room; BP, blood pressure.

When no obvious pulmonary or cutaneous soft tissue infection can explain a septic presentation, ultrasonography or CT should be used to evaluate the patient for an intraabdominal drainable source of serious infection.

If an intraabdominal abscess is present, drainage either by operative or percutaneous route is recommended. An abscess located near a vascular repair needs to be drained operatively. This allows for visual inspection of the area surrounding the vascular reconstruction. Hopefully, the vascular coverage provided at the time of initial repair may have precluded purulent material from having direct contact with the vascular suture line. This omentum or covering tissue should not be dissected off of the repair as vascular graft contamination could result. The peritoneal cavity should be washed copiously with antibiotic irrigation and appropriate systemic antibiotic therapy instituted.

A vascular repair contained within an abscess cavity has the potential for catastrophic consequences. If the area of repair appears viable, sump drains should be placed in proximity but not directly over the vascular repair. Dilute Betadine or antibiotic irrigation for 3 to 5 days may help prevent dehiscence of the repair or graft necrosis. If arterial or suture line necrosis is present, an alternative method of vascular reconstruction should be attempted, such as extraanatomic bypass. The arteries involved should be debrided to viable tissue in relatively noninfected areas. Closure of the arteries can be protected using anterior spinal ligament[48] or omentum.

Should the vascular repair in jeopardy not lend itself to alternate reconstruction, another alternative is to cover the graft with a muscular pedicle flap. An anterior rectus muscle flap to cover the aorta has been described.[26] Another source for muscular flap coverage may be the latissimus dorsi based on its thoracodorsal or lumbar blood supply. This can be brought through the lumbar triangle (preferably from the left) and cover a variety of arterial structures. Catheters placed between the artery and muscular flap allow dilute Betadine or antibiotic irrigation for a short length of time to help sterilize the area.

RESULTS

In DeBakey and Simcone's series of 2471 arterial injuries incurred by Allied Forces in the Mediterranean Theater during World War II, only three patients with injuries to major abdominal arteries survived to reach medical attention.[4] During the Korean War, arterial injuries to the extremities were reconstructed but almost all patients with injuries to major abdominal arteries died.[5]

During the Vietnam War, however, helicopter evacuation allowed some patients with injured abdominal arteries to survive long enough to be taken to the operating room in time to permit definitive treatment. Modern methods of reconstruction were available and consistently applied. As a result, Bill and colleagues were able to report 14 survivors out of 33 patients with abdominal aortic trauma, a survival rate of 42%.[6] Recent civilian experience with injuries to major abdominal arteries has been similarly encouraging.[49-53]

The survival rate after blunt aortic trauma is significantly more favorable than penetrating trauma.[54,55] Lock[55] reported a 73% survival rate and Neuman in a recent literature review summarized a total of 46 reported cases with an overall 83% survival rate. Burch et al. reviewed their experience with iliac vascular injury. The overall survival rate for all arterial and renal vascular injuries was 72%. For common iliac arterial injuries the survival rate was 58%, for the external iliac artery 59%, and for the internal iliac artery 70%. In isolated injuries of the same vessel survival was 69%, 71%, and 100% respectively.[54]

Prognosis in all injuries relates not only to the vessel injured but relates to whether shock or associated injuries are present. In Burch's series the mortality involved only 2 of 65 patients who had no shock at any time.[52] In contrast, 61 out of 93 patients died who had persistent shock in the preoperative period.

Georgi repeated an overall mortality rate of 36% in 42 patients with abdominal vascular injury secondary to penetrating vascular injury. However, 15 out of 18 patients died whose blood pressure was under 80 mm Hg (systolic) for more than 30 min.[53]

REFERENCES

1. Carrel A, Guthrie CC. Uniterminal and biterminal venous transplantations. *Surg Gynecol Obstet*. 1906; March.
2. Weglowski R. Ueber die Gefasstransplantation. *Zentral Chir*. 1925; 52:2241.
3. Wildegans HL. Vrlotzungen der aorta. *Dtsh Med Wochenschr*. 1926; 52:1810.
4. DeBakey MD, Simcone FA. Battle injuries in arteries in World War II: an analysis of 2471. *Ann Surg*. 1946; 123:534.
5. Hughes CW. Arterial repair during the Korean War. *Ann Surg*. 1958; 147:555.
6. Bill LF, Amato JJ, Rich NM. Aortic injuries in Viet Nam. *Surgery*. 1971; 70:385.
7. Sirinek KR, Gaskill HV, Root HD, Levine BA. Truncal vascular injury—factors influencing survival. *J Trauma*. 1979; 23:372–377.
8. Myles RA, Yellin AE. Traumatic injuries of the abdominal aorta. *Am J Surg*. 1979; 138:273–277.
9. Millikan JS, Moore EE. Critical factors in determining mortality from abdominal aortic trauma. *Surg Gynecol Obstet*. 1958; 160:383–386.
10. Brinton M, Miller SE, Lim RC, Trunkey DD. Acute abdominal aortic injuries. *J Trauma*. 1982; 22:481–485.
11. Accola KD, Feliciano DV, Mattox KL, et al. Management of injuries to the suprarenal aorta. *Am J Surg*. 1987; 154:613–618.
12. Feliciano DV, Bitando CG, Mattox KL, et al. Civilian trauma in the 1980's. A 1-year experience with 456 vascular and cardiac injuries. *Ann Surg*. 1984; 199:717–724.
13. Dawidson I, Miller E, Litwin MS. Gunshot wounds of the abdomen—a review of 277 cases. *Arch Surg*. 1976; 111:862–865.
14. Trunkey DD, Blaisdell FW. Abdominal vascular injuries. *West J Med*. 1975; 123:321–324.
15. Moore JB, Moore EE, Thompson JS. Abdominal injuries associated with penetrating trauma in the lower chest. *Am J Surg*. 1980; 140:724–730.
16. Omert L, Rodriquez A, Simon B, et al. Blunt vascular trauma: analysis of 484 cases. *J Trauma*. 1989; 29:1035.
17. McVay CB. *Anson and McVay's Surgical Anatomy*. 6th ed. Philadelphia: WB Saunders; 1984: 762–767.
18. Netter FH. *Atlas of Human Anatomy*. Summit: CIBA-Geigy; 1989.
19. Hollinshead WH. *Anatomy for Surgeons*. 3rd ed. Philadelphia: Harper and Row; 1982.

20. Henry AK. *Extensile Exposure*. 2nd ed. Baltimore: Williams and Wilkins; 1959: 160–171.
21. Wieneck RG, Wilson RF. Injuries to the abdominal vascular system: How much does aggressive resuscitation and prelaparotomy thoracotomy really help? *Surgery*. 1987; 102:731–736.
22. Reynolds RR, McDowell HA, Diethelm AG. The surgical treatment of arterial injuries in the civilian population. *Ann Surg*. 1979; 189:700–708.
23. Chapman AJ, McClain J. Wandering missiles: an autopsy study. *J Trauma*. 1984; 24:634–637.
24. Jones AM, Graham NJ, Looney JR. Arterial embolism of a high velocity rifle bullet after a hunting accident: case report and literature review. *Am J Forensic Med Pathol*. 1983; 4:259–264.
25. Fry WR, Fry WJ, Fry RE. Exposure of the abdominal arteries for repair of vascular injury. *Arch Surg*. 1991; 126:289–291.
26. Adar R, Rabbi I, Bass A, et al. Left renal vein division in abdominal aortic aneurysm operations. Effect on renal function. *Arch Surg*. 1985; 120:1033–1036.
27. Lim RC Jr, Eastman AB, Blaisdell FW. Renal autotransplantation: adjunct to repair of renal vascular lesions. *Arch Surg*. 1972; 105:847.
28. Mixter RC, Turnipseed WD, Smith DJ Jr, et al. Rotational muscle flaps; a new technique for covering infected vascular grafts. *J Vasc Surg*. 1989; 9:472–478.
29. Appleby LH. The coeliac axis in the expansion of the operation for gastric carcinoma. *Cancer*. 1953; 6:704–707.
30. Graham JM, Mattox KL, Beall AC, DeBakey ME. Injuries to the visceral arteries. *Surgery*. 1978; 84:835–839.
31. Rapp JH, Reilly LM, Ovarfordt PG, et al. Durability of endarterectomy and antegrade grafts in the treatment of chronic visceral ischemia. *J Vasc Surg*. 1986; 3:799–806.
32. Conn J Jr, Trippel OH, Bergan JJ. A new atraumatic aortic occluder. *Surgery*. 1968; 64:2258–2260.
33. Veith FJ, Gupta S, Daly V. Technique for occluding the supraceliac aorta through the abdomen. *Surg Gynecol Obstet*. 1980; 151:426–428.
34. Fry RE, Fry WJ. Aortoiliac, femoral, and popliteal artery occlusive disease. In: Hardy JD, ed. *Hardy's Textbook of Surgery*. Philadelphia: JB Lippincott; 1983; 894–911.
35. Ernst CB, Hagihara PF, Daugherty ME, Griffen WO. Inferior mesenteric artery stump pressure: a reliable index for safe IMA ligation during abdominal aorta aneurysmectomy. *Ann Surg*. 1978; 187:641–646.
36. Landreneau RJ, Mitchum P, Fry WJ. Iliac artery transposition. *Arch Surg*. 1989; 124:978–981.
37. Ku DN, Klafta JM, Giewertz BL, Savins CK. The continuation of valves to saphenous vein graft resistance. *J Vasc Surg*. 1987; 6:274–279.
38. Bergqvist D, Takolander R. Aortic occlusion following blunt trauma of the abdomen. *J Trauma*. 1981; 21:319–322.
39. Clyne CAC, Ashbrooke EA. Seat belt aorta: isolated abdominal aortic injury following blunt trauma. *Br J Surg*. 1985; 72:239.
40. MacBeth A, Malone JM, Norton LW, Peltier LF. Paralysis and aortic thrombosis following blunt abdominal trauma. *J Trauma*. 1982; 22:591–594.
41. Roehm EF, Twiest MW, Williams RC. Abdominal aortic thrombosis in association with an attempted Heimlich maneuver. *JAMA*. 1983; 249:1186–1187.
42. Lassonde J, Laurendeau F. Blunt injury of the abdominal aorta. *Ann Surg*. 1981; 194:745–748.
43. Crawford ES. Personal communication.
44. Rutherford RB, Jones DN, Bergentz SE, et al. The efficacy of dextran 40 in preventing early postoperative thrombosis following difficult lower extremity bypass. *J Vasc Surg*. 1984; 1:765–773.
45. Puschett JB. Calcium channel antagonists and renal ischemia. In: Epstein M, Loutzenhiser RD, eds. *Calcium Antagonists and the Kidney*. Philadelphia: Hanley and Belfus; 1989.
46. Wait RB, White G, Davis JH. Beneficial effects of erapamil on postischemic renal failure. *Surgery*. 1983; 94:276–282.
47. Wilson RF, Wiencek RG, Balog M. Predicting and preventing infection after abdominal vascular injuries. *J Trauma*. 1989; 29:1371–1375.
48. Fry WJ, Lindenauer SM. Infection complicating the use of plastic arterial implants. *Arch Surg*. 1967; 94:600–609.
49. Buscaglia LC, Blaisdell FW, Lim RC Jr. Penetrating abdominal vascular injuries. *Arch Surg*. 1969; 99:764.
50. Lim RC Jr, Trunkey DD, Blaisdell FW. Acute abdominal aortic injury. *Arch Surg*. 1974; 109:706.
51. Feliciano DV. Approach to major abdominal vascular injury. *J Vasc Surg*. 1988; 7:730.
52. Burch JM, Richardson RJ, Martin RR, Mattox KL. Penetrating iliac vascular injuries: recent experience with 233 consecutive patients. *J Trauma*. 1990; 30:1450.
53. Georgi BA, Massad M, Obeid M. Ballistic trauma to the abdomen: shell fragments versus bullets. *J Trauma*. 1991; 31:711.
54. Reisman JD, Morgan AS. Analysis of 46 intra-abdominal aortic injuries from blunt trauma. *J Trauma*. 1990; 30:1294.
55. Lock JS, Hasfman AD, Johnson RC. Blunt trauma to the abdominal aorta. *J Trauma*. 1987; 27:674.

20
Abdominal Venous Trauma

F. WILLIAM BLAISDELL, M.D.

HISTORY: In 1894, an Italian anarchist shot and mortally wounded the President of the French Republic. The inability of surgeons to repair his portal vein injury prompted Alexis Carrel, then a medical student, to study blood vessel suture techniques. His accomplishments in this area earned him the Nobel Prize for Medicine in 1912 and laid the groundwork for the emergence and development of modern vascular surgery.[1]

Other important milestones in the development of venous surgery are summarized by Rich and Spencer.[2] The first anastomosis between two blood vessels, the portal vein and the inferior vena cava, was performed in a dog by Eck in 1877. In 1882 Schede reported the first clinical application of a lateral suture in repairing a femoral vein laceration. Seven years later, Kummel performed the first clinical end-to-end anastomosis of a femoral vein. Clermont, in 1901, successfully sutured a transected canine inferior vena cava. Goodman, in 1918, advocated lateral suture repair of venous injuries resulting from war wounds despite Makins' assertion that venous injuries were best treated by ligation, especially if concomitant arterial ligation was necessary. The practice of ligation treatment for injured veins persisted throughout World War II. The considerable morbidity resulting from routine ligation treatment of venous injuries during the Korean War prompted Hughes and Spencer independently to begin repairing veins again. However, it was during the Vietnam conflict that a concerted effort was made by vascular surgeons to repair venous injuries routinely when possible.

Historical accounts of the management of portal and mesenteric vein injuries stressed the importance of repair rather than ligation because ligation was considered to be incompatible with life, owing to massive visceral congestion and portal hypertension. This dogma was based primarily on the results of canine and other lower animal experiments in which death invariably occurred after portal and superior mesenteric vein ligation.[3,4] However, Robson, as early as 1897, and others, subsequently reported cases in which the portal vein or superior mesenteric vein was ligated without adverse sequelae.[5-7] Child observed that acute portal vein ligation was possible in humans because of adequate portal collateral flow.[8] Fish reviewed the literature and summarized the techniques available for portal and mesenteric vein reconstruction including lateral repair, end-to-

end anastomosis, portacaval shunting, splenic to mesenteric vein anastomosis, and graft interposition.[9]

MECHANISM OF INJURY AND PATHOPHYSIOLOGY

The mechanism of venous injury is similar to that of arterial injury as described in an earlier chapter. Penetrating trauma is more apt to injure major veins than blunt trauma. However, major venous injury can occur in association with pelvic fractures, particularly unstable types associated with sacroiliac disarticulation or in association with massive liver injuries when major hepatic veins or intrahepatic portions of the vena cava may be lacerated. The vena cava is subject to injury during abdominal operations such as lumbar sympathectomy, nephrectomy, adrenalectomy, and aortic surgery. It can also be injured by trocars introduced for peritoneal dialysis or for the diagnosis of hemoperitoneum. The portal vein may be injured during hepatic, biliary, or pancreatic surgery.

Since the veins constitute a low pressure system, overlying tissues are capable of tamponading major lacerations, and the intact abdominal wall with increasing intraabdominal pressure following bleeding may result in a relative tamponade of bleeding from major injuries. For major ongoing hemorrhage to occur, venous injuries must decompress externally, into a body cavity or into a cavity produced by injury such as that which occurs in association with pelvic fractures. Since soft tissues effectively tamponade venous bleeding, missed venous injuries rarely result in secondary hemorrhage.

Trauma to the great intraabdominal veins when associated with hemorrhage presents a far more difficult problem than that of corresponding arterial trauma, for the following reasons:

1. Proximal control of arterial injuries usually stops hemorrhage, since with shock, distal collateral flow is relatively modest and back-bleeding is not a major problem. Venous injuries conversely require both proximal and distal control since distal pressure is raised, causing veins to bleed vigorously in both directions.
2. While cross-clamping of the artery during shock results in little change in collateral flow, cross-clamping of veins results in a marked increase in pressure and collateral bleeding is augmented dramatically in all branches entering the injured segment. Proximal and distal control therefore does not necessarily result in control of hemorrhage.
3. Arteries have integrity and hold sutures well. Veins often have the consistency of wet tissue paper and tear with the application of clamps or when sutured under tension.
4. Suture lines in large arteries rarely produce thrombotic problems, whereas suture lines in veins that expose raw surface produce a high risk of local thrombosis and embolism. Moreover, suture lines in veins tend to contract and obstruct flow with the passage of time, whereas this is unusual in arteries.
5. Prosthetic substitutes work relatively well in the arterial system and poorly, or not at all, in the venous system.

In partial compensation for these problems the veins can be ligated with relative impunity as compared to arteries, since collateral flow is much better. The exceptions are perhaps major segments of the mesenteric or portal vein or the suprarenal vena cava where serious consequences may occur if ligation is carried out.

ANATOMY

The external iliac veins originate at the inguinal ligament, pass just medial to the corresponding arteries, and course upward along the rim of the true pelvis at the medial margin of the psoas muscle. The internal iliac veins join the external iliac veins halfway between the inguinal ligament and the sacral promontory to form the common iliac veins (Fig. 20–1). The latter course upward to unite and form the vena cava. Branches of the external and common iliac veins are few and small. The internal iliac veins comprise multiple anastomosing branches originating from deep within the true pelvis. The left common and external iliac veins are covered by the mesosigmoid, the right common iliac veins by the retroperitoneum, and near the junction of the vena cava by the small bowel mesentery. Both are crossed by the ureters in the vicinity of the external iliac origin. The left common iliac vein passes under the aortic bifurcation and/or the common iliac artery, pursuing a longer course than the right iliac vein, which it joins to form the cava along the right anterior portion of the vertebral column. The right common iliac vein passes under the right common iliac artery, joining the common iliac vein to form the inferior vena cava.

The inferior vena cava passes upward from the sacral promontory to the L-2 level, where it is joined by the left and right renal veins. The lower portion of the cava lies in intimate contact with the aorta and progressively diverges so at the level of the renal veins, it lies approximately 1 cm to the right of the aorta. It is joined sequentially by paired lumbar veins, corresponding to the underlying vertebrae, and a number of smaller retroperitoneal collateral veins. Just below the renal veins, the vena cava is joined in most instances by the right gonadal vein. The base of the small bowel mesentery overlies the infrarenal vena cava. Just below the renal veins, the fourth portion of the duodenum passes over the cava.

The right renal vein is relatively short compared to the left and usually joins the vena cava 1 cm below that of the left and approximately at the level of L2-3 vertebral junction. The left renal vein in most instances passes over the aorta as it proceeds from the renal hilum to the cava. The left gonadal vein joins the left renal vein just lateral to the aorta. The left adrenal vein enters the left renal vein just above the gonadal vein.

The suprarenal vena cava courses upwards anterior to the L1-2 vertebral body, passes under the liver in the cava fossa, and in some instances is surrounded almost entirely by liver substance as it reaches the caval hiatus in the diaphragm. The cava at or just above the renal veins passes under the second portion of the duodenum, below the portal triad, and is covered by the retroperitoneum lining the foramen of Winslow. It is joined by a relatively large right adrenal vein just above the right renal vein, but usually no lumbar veins enter this segment of the vena cava.

The only tributaries of the suprarenal cava, in addition to the adrenal vein, consist of the hepatic veins, the largest of which, the main right and the left, enter the cava at the superior margin of the liver. Several small veins pass directly from the caudate lobe into the cava. These are of special significance when the liver is elevated to expose the suprarenal vena cava, as they may tear off the cava, adding to the local hemorrhage. Several small

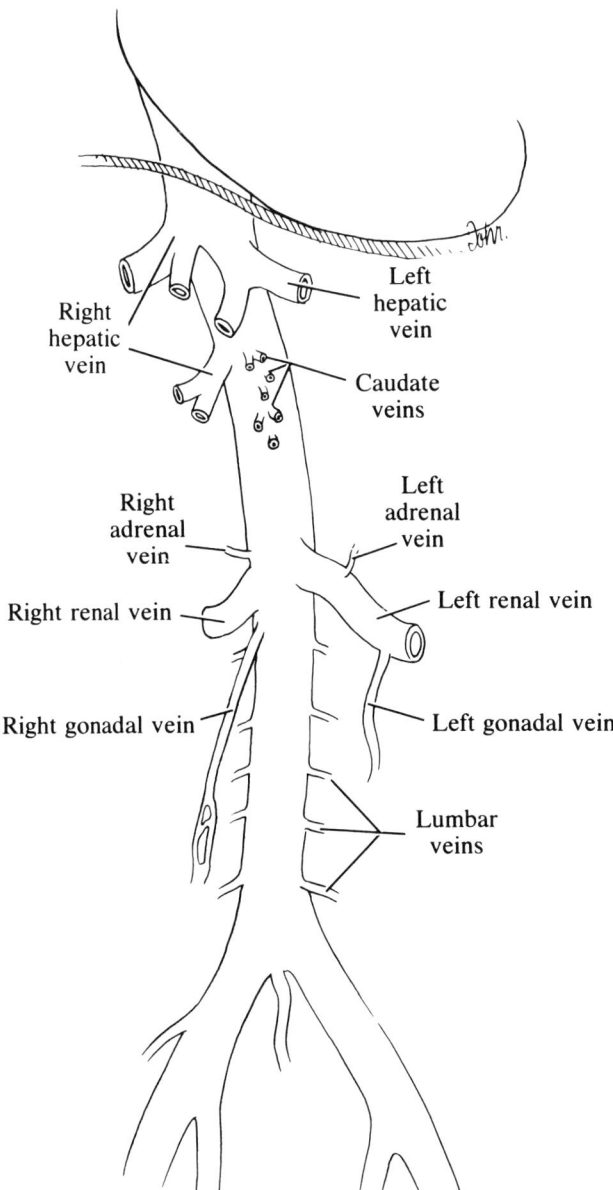

Figure 20–1. Anatomy of the vena cava and its tributaries.

phrenic veins constitute the only other veins entering this caval segment. Approximately 2 to 3 cm of cava lie above the diaphragm before the cava enters the right atrium. The supradiaphragmatic vena cava is surrounded over three-fourths of its surface by pericardium, and it lies almost entirely within the pericardial sac. It is therefore easily encircled by appropriate dissection.

The portal venous system comprises the splenic vein, the inferior and superior mesenteric veins, and their tributaries, which join to form the portal vein (Fig. 20–2). The inferior mesenteric vein passes upward in the root of the mesocolon just lateral to the aorta and joins the splenic vein just proximal to its junction with the superior mesenteric vein. The splenic vein takes origin at the splenic hilum, passes along the posterior midportion of the pancreas to join the superior mesenteric vein forming the portal vein. The superior mesenteric vein receives tributaries from the small bowel and colon and passes upward in the root of the mesentery posterior and to the right of the mesenteric artery, over the uncinate process of the pancreas and under the junction of the body and tail over the second vertebral body to join the splenic vein, forming the portal vein at approximately the inferior margin of the posterior surface of the pancreas. The portal vein passes upward under the junction of the body and head of the pancreas, under the second portion of the duodenum. Here it is joined by the hepatic artery and the bile duct to form the portal triad, which courses anterior to the foramen of Winslow. The portal vein lies posterior and between the common bile duct and the hepatic artery where it enters the liver (see Chapter 10). The only other large vein of consequence in the upper abdomen is the coronary vein, which courses in the gastrohepatic ligament to join the portal vein as it enters the portal triad just above the second portion of the duodenum.

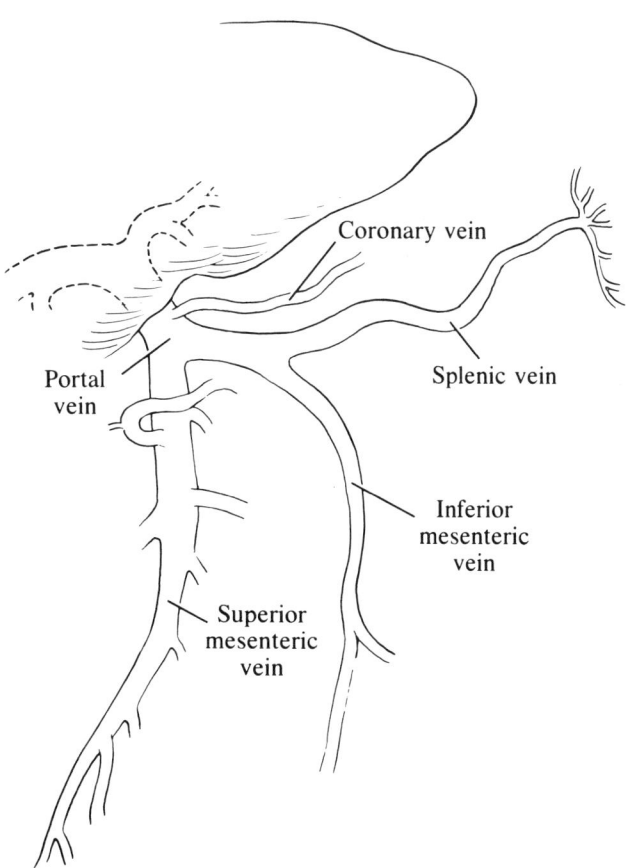

Figure 20–2. Portal venous anatomy.

ASSESSMENT

The assessment of the patient for possible major abdominal venous injury is similar to that for a patient with major arterial injury. The exception is that venography is used only rarely to assess for possible injury. The reason relates to the fact that the patients are rarely stable when there is a significant venous injury. Moreover, if the injury is not bleeding, the tamponade effect of soft tissue may result in a negative venogram even when a large laceration is present.

The possibility of major venous injury exists when any penetrating injury is located near the great veins. The patient who presents in shock a short period after injury should be assumed to have a major vascular injury. If the site of penetration corresponds to that of a major vein, there should be presumption of major venous injury. Injuries to the great veins are more deceiving than those of the arteries; being a low pressure system there is minimal resistance to blood flow in major channels and tissue resistance and hematoma formation adjacent to the injury may, for the most part, maintain blood flow in the major venous channel as previously noted. In addition, abdominal pressure serves to prevent exsanguinating hemorrhage, which occurs with arterial injuries of equivalent size. However, once positive pressure ventilation is instituted, central venous pressure in the abdomen is raised and major hemorrhage may ensue.

Several forms of blunt trauma are associated with major venous injury. These include major unstable pelvic fractures, particularly those associated with sacroiliac disarticulation, in which tearing of pelvic veins frequently occurs. As long as the retroperitoneum is intact, major exsanguinating hemorrhage is unlikely. In some instances, however, the peritoneum is disrupted at the time of pelvic fracture, and massive hemorrhage can occur. Liver injuries, particularly those occurring in falls from heights where victims land on their feet, may result in lacerations of the intrahepatic portion of the vena cava or major hepatic veins, as the liver is literally avulsed from the vena cava. The greater mass of the liver renders the right hepatic veins more vulnerable to these types of tears. Seat belt injuries may result in mesenteric lacerations, with corresponding venous hemorrhage.

PREOPERATIVE PREPARATION

As indicated in the previous sections, the intact abdomen and retroperitoneum tissues can tamponade venous bleeding much more readily than arterial bleeding. Typically, a patient with a major venous injury will respond to resuscitation but will crash on the institution of endotracheal intubation and the institution of positive pressure ventilation. This is because when the patient is breathing spontaneously, intrathoracic pressure is negative and abdominal venous pressure correspondingly low. Thoracic and abdominal venous pressure is abruptly raised to positive with institution of ventilatory support. In addition, a surgeon expecting to deal with a trivial abdominal injury may, on opening the abdomen, be confronted instead with massive venous hemorrhage, particularly if the retroperitoneum is exposed. It is for this reason that patients with major trauma, who present with evidence of major blood loss, routinely have at least one cutdown placed during resuscitation. This initial cutdown in reasonably stable patients is best performed in the antecubital fossa. An infant feeding tube approximately 5 mm in diameter threaded upward in the basilic vein to an intrathoracic position insures rapid fluid therapy and allows monitoring of central venous pressure. This can be supplemented by whatever percutaneous lines seem appropriate for the administration of drugs or for withdrawal of blood specimens. When the patient presents in severe shock, a second cutdown, usually the initial cutdown of choice, is placed in the saphenous vein at the ankle. This vein is readily accessible, accepts the entire cross-section of intravenous tubing in the average adult male, and permits resuscitation of any patient with reversible vascular injury. Despite the fact that the cava is injured, administration of fluid via the saphenous cutdown is just as effective in resuscitation as that administered through a jugular or subclavian catheter or cutdown, since the venous system constitutes one continuous pool, and raising the pressure in one portion raises the pressure in all portions of the thoracic and abdominal veins. Because of abundant collateral channels in the venous system, effective volume resuscitation can still be carried out with a saphenous cutdown, even with the vena cava clamped. Were this not the case, it would be impossible to cross-clamp the inferior vena cava, for, within a few minutes of caval occlusion in the absence of collaterals, the entire blood volume theoretically would be trapped below the occluding clamp.

Preoperative evaluation should include chest and abdominal films; if there is any possibility of renal or renal pedicle injury, intravenous pyelography should be performed. A urinary catheter is always indicated in the patient presenting in shock, and a nasogastric tube should be placed for gastric decompression. As is true with most trauma cases, blood should be reserved for administration in the operating room since badly needed reserves can be depleted attempting to resuscitate patients with vascular injury. Patients can temporarily tolerate a hematocrit of 10, provided volume is maintained, and it is better to use balanced salt solution rather than red blood cells during resuscitation before vascular control. Operative vascular control may on occasion be required as part of the resuscitation process.

OPERATIVE EXPLORATION AND EXPOSURE

Abdominal venous injuries, like arterial injuries, are best exposed through a generous midline incision running from xiphoid to pubis. The bowel should be eviscerated, blood evacuated from the abdominal cavity, and areas of major bleeding controlled temporarily with packs while a rapid gross assessment of the abdomen is carried out. Blood should be aspirated from all corners of the abdomen and these areas packed to isolate bleeding. By so doing there is less danger that the patient will exsanguinate from a second injury while the first is being treated. When a venous injury is identified, hemorrhage can be controlled in most cases by the judicious application of pack and pressure. This permits volume restoration before attempts are made to expose the site of injury. The reason for this relates to the fact that attempts to expose the injury result in further hemorrhage and, if the patient is hypovolemic, cardiac arrest may occur. Venous bleeding is also more subtle than arterial bleeding and the surgeon is often less aware of the magnitude of the hemorrhage in venous injury as opposed to that in arterial injury. For this reason, continuous application of suction to the area of injury should not be allowed, since the sucker may remove blood so rapidly that the extent of the hemorrhage may not be appreciated by the surgeon. It is better to have the assistant aspirate for a few seconds, remove the sucker from the field, and then reaspirate.

With the exception of the portal vein, exposure of the great veins is generally easier than that of the corresponding arteries. Local pressure can be used to control bleeding while proximal distal dissection is carried out. In some circumstances temporary intraluminal occlusion by balloon catheters can be used to control hemorrhage. The left external iliac vein is best exposed by severing the lateral attachments of the sigmoid colon and retracting it medially. This permits exposure of the entire left external and common iliac vein. With the exception of the ureter, all critical anatomy, including most importantly the mesenteric circulation of the large intestine, is retracted away.

The most difficult portion of the iliac system to isolate and control is the internal iliac vein or one of its major branches. This is particularly true with multiple injuries to the internal iliac vein that occur in association with major pelvic fractures. For this reason, venous hematomas in the vicinity of the pelvis are usually left alone unless there is an associated overlying peritoneal laceration that results in free intraabdominal bleeding. The problem with internal iliac vein injuries is that although proximal control is relatively easy, control of internal iliac vein tributaries can be exceedingly difficult, as dissection within the hematoma results in extensive hemorrhage from proximal smaller veins. Since both external iliac and common iliac veins have few, if any, branches, the area of injury can be compressed with sponge sticks and direct repair is relatively easily carried out.

The proximal common iliac veins also can be challenging to expose and control. This is because they are covered by the aortic bifurcation. Injuries to the veins often are associated with simultaneous arterial injuries. Arterial injuries should be controlled proximally while pressure is used to control venous hemorrhage. Once the distal aorta is encircled the dissection can proceed distally on the artery until an occluding vascular clamp can be placed on the aorta or proximal iliac artery.[10] Dissection with exposure of the external and internal iliac arteries will give distal control. At this point the artery can be retracted to expose the venous injury or the injured artery can be divided (Fig. 20–3) to provide direct venous exposure.[11,12] With the venous laceration controlled by sponge stick, proximal and distal venous exposure can be carried out. The laceration can then be isolated with vascular clamps or trapped proximal and distal to the injury with sponge sticks or fingers while the vein is ligated or repaired (Fig. 20–4).

The vena cava can be exposed from either the left or the right. The optimal method of exposure is to mobilize the ascending colon by severing its lateral attachment and retracting it along with the duodenum upward and to the left (Fig. 20–5). This permits exposure of the entire common iliac vein on the right and the entire length of the vena cava as far as the liver. This also mobilizes all the mesenteric vessels and moves them upward out of the field so that damage to the circulation of the intestinal tract is avoided. The right renal vein is readily exposed from this approach, as is 3 to 5 cm of the left renal vein.

Left renal venous injuries can be exposed in the area of the ligament of Treitz or by severing the lateral attachments of the descending colon and mobilizing it upward to the right (see Fig. 12–3). The latter is preferred because injuries near the left renal vein may involve the aorta and the left renal artery as well.

Injuries involving the extrahepatic suprarenal vena cava are readily exposed by a Kocher maneuver, mobilizing the duodenum upward to the left (Fig. 20–5). Proximal control can be obtained by temporarily trapping the vena cava with a pack or sponge stick at the level of the renal veins. Compression of the liver downward will usually tamponade the vena cava superiorly, thus permitting repair of a laceration, since the only vein entering the segment between the renal veins and the liver is the right adrenal vein, bleeding from which can usually be ignored temporarily.

The intrahepatic vena cava is the most inaccessible portion of the venous system. In

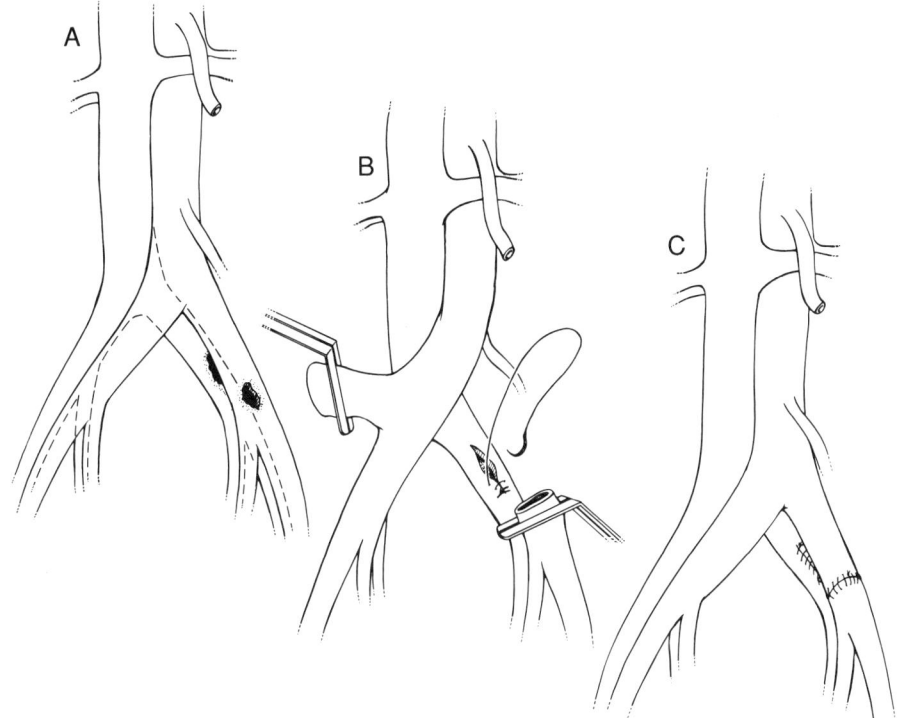

Figure 20–3. A: Location of simultaneous injury to the iliac artery and vein. **B:** Division of the iliac artery to permit exposure of the venous injury for repair. **C:** Resection of the arterial injury and primary anastomosis.

most instances the entire anterior surface of the vena cava is surrounded by liver. Multiple large right hepatic veins and the left hepatic vein enter this segment, and attempts to mobilize the liver upward may result in exsanguination before the area of injury can be exposed. For this reason, some method of isolating this segment before attempting repair is necessary. There are three ways to accomplish this. The first involves isolating and clamping the vena cava above and below the liver (Fig. 20–6).[13,14] This can be done in elective circumstances when the patient is normovolemic. This is rarely the case in trauma circumstances and the additional trapping of blood usually results in immediate cardiac arrest.

The second approach involves using a technique for isolation of this portion of the vena cava with the addition of an intracaval shunt. Although it is possible to place a shunt from below the liver, this is actually more difficult than placing a shunt from above through the atrium, since excessive bleeding may occur while manipulating the vena cava as the catheter is inserted from below.[15,16] A 1- to 2-cm diameter (34–40 F) catheter such as an endotracheal tube or chest tube passed through the right atrial appendage has proved to be more optimal (Fig. 20–7). The reason for this is that in the hypovolemic patient, left atrial pressure is low and blood loss is much less since the venous return is not interrupted during placement of the catheter. To accomplish this, the midline abdominal incision is extended up to the sternal notch as a midline sternotomy. The pericardium is opened and the right

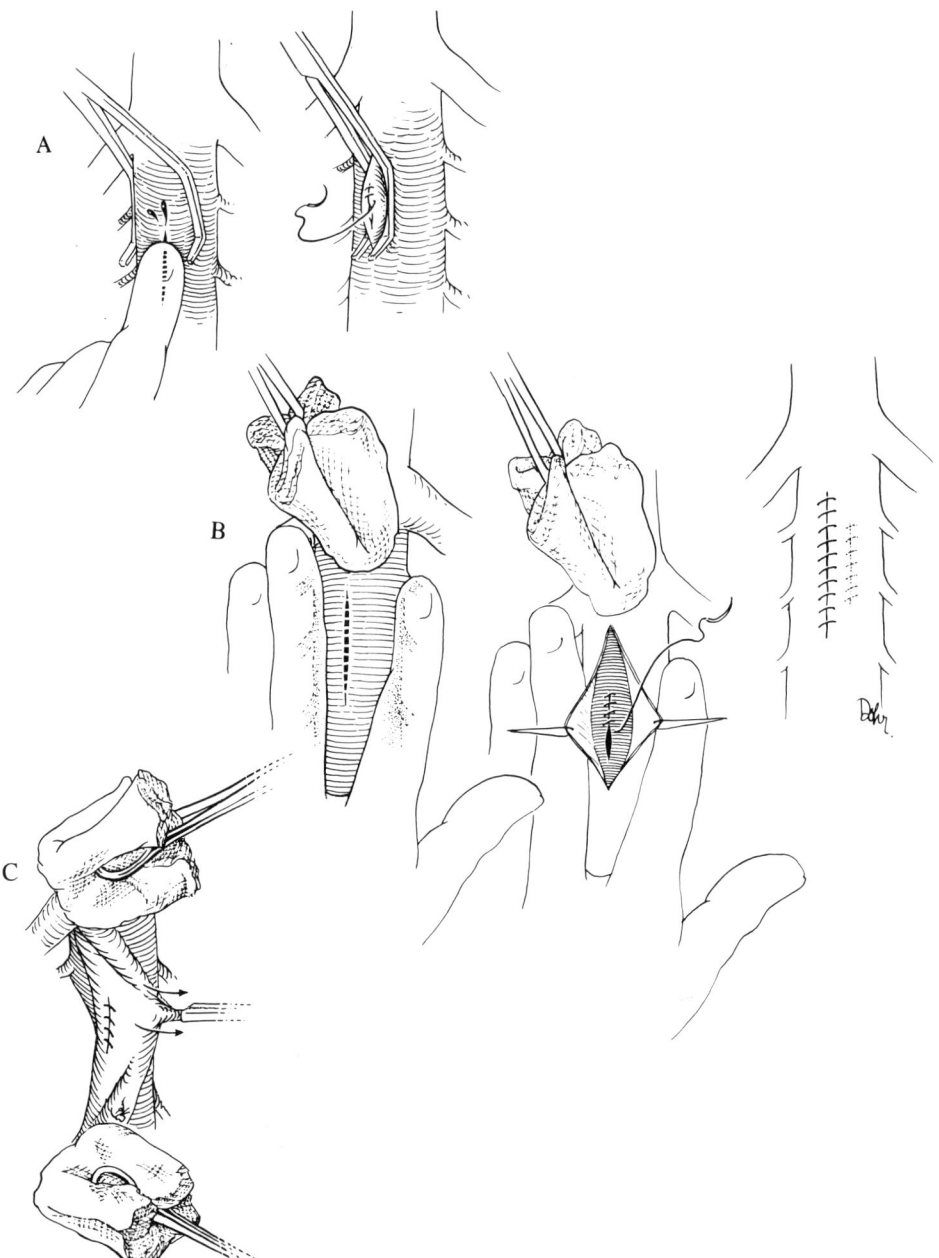

Figure 20–4. Vascular control of vena cava. **A:** Control of hemorrhage from vena cava would be by direct pressure, applying partial occluding clamp and suture repair. **B:** Management of through-and-through wound of vena cava. Hemorrhage controlled by direct pressure using sponge forceps proximally and distally and fingers on either side of the cava to compress lumbar veins. The anterior wound is enlarged, the posterior wound is repaired from within, and the anterior wound is then trimmed and closed. **C:** Vena cava rotated for repair of a posterior wound. Lumbar veins have been divided and ligated.

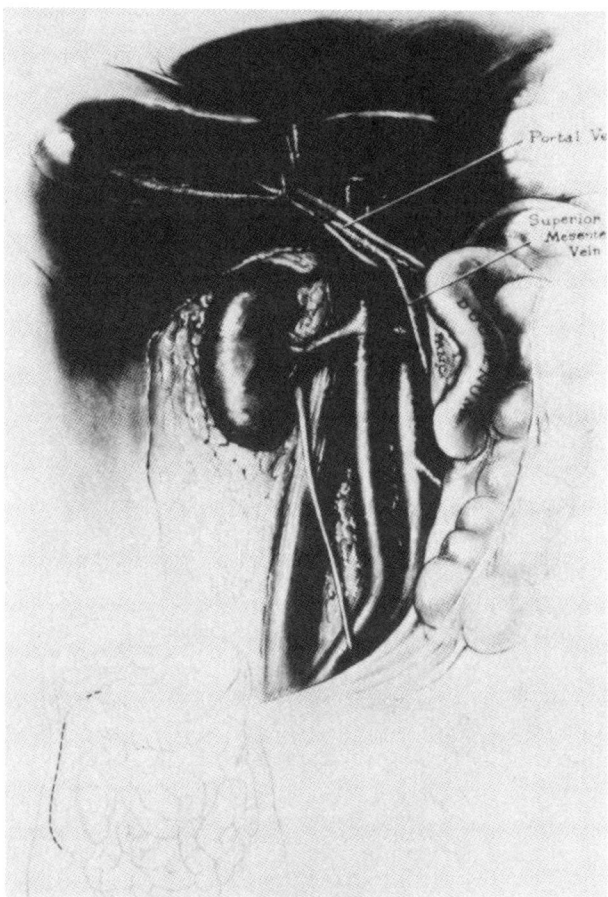

Figure 20–5. Right-sided approach to major vascular structures. Inset shows line of incision in posterior peritoneum. Right colon, duodenum, and head of pancreas are then mobilized upward to the left, exposing the intrahepatic vena cava and entire length of portal vein.

atrial appendage is identified. With a purse-string suture placed around the atrial appendage and an occluding clamp placed across the base of the appendage, the catheter is inserted into the atrium while the intracardiac portion of the vena cava is palpated to insure that the catheter passes into the inferior vena cava rather than the right ventricle. The catheter should be manipulated gently since it may pass through a large laceration or may enter the right hepatic vein, which can be 1½ to 2 cm in diameter. Gentle advancement and twisting of the catheter insures its appropriate passage, and palpation of the tip at the level of the renal veins verifies its proper location. As the tip of the catheter reaches the level of the renal veins, it is cross-clamped at the atrium, and a side hole is cut. The side hole is then advanced into the atrium as the purse-string suture is tightened. This hole provides for egress of blood from the shunt. It is preferable to leave the end of the catheter projecting from the atrium for use in rapidly infusing blood or crystalloid solutions (Fig. 20–8). In exsanguinating injuries the author has used the Bentley autotransfusion device, in the pump mode, to infuse

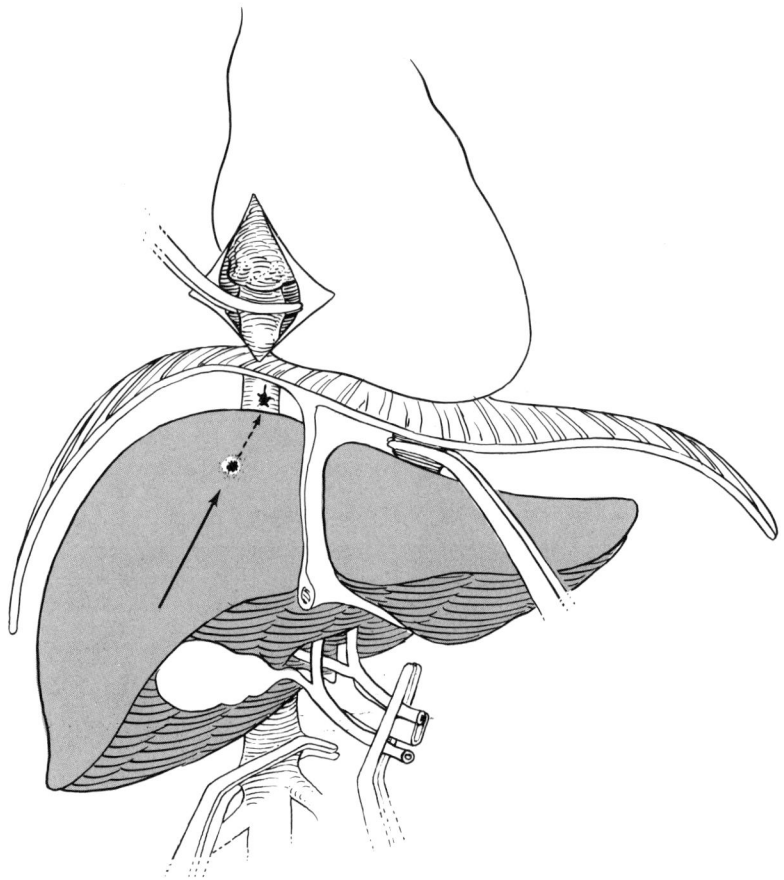

Figure 20-6. Vascular isolation of hepatic circulation for repair of vena cava laceration at diaphragm. This has been achieved by placing vascular clamps across the aorta, porta hepatis, and vena cava above and below the liver.

crystalloid. With this technique 500 ml/min can be infused. Crystalloid, balanced salt solution heated to 38°C is used to prevent hypothermia. Umbilical tapes can be placed rapidly around the intrapericardial and suprarenal portions of the vena cava with the catheter in place. When these are pulled up, the caval segment is isolated when simultaneous occlusion of the portal triad by a vascular clamp is carried out.

The third principle of liver isolation consists of using a bypass shunt of the type now popular in liver transplantation.[17] This involves the use of large caliber plastic tubing preferably containing bonded heparin, and a nonocclusive pump. The proximal end of the shunt should be inserted into the femoral or iliac vein. The distal end of the shunt can be inserted into a jugular or axillary vein or the right atrium if a midline sternotomy has been used for exposure of the liver injury (Fig. 20-9). The nonocclusive roller pump permits decompression of the inferior vena cava and maintains venous filling of the heart. Transplant surgeons have found that if flow rates through the tubing are maintained above 1000 cc per min, heparin is not necessary either in the shunt tubing or systemically.[17]

With the cava isolated, the liver can be rolled upward from the right by severing its attachments to the retroperitoneum and the length of the vein exposed. Should major

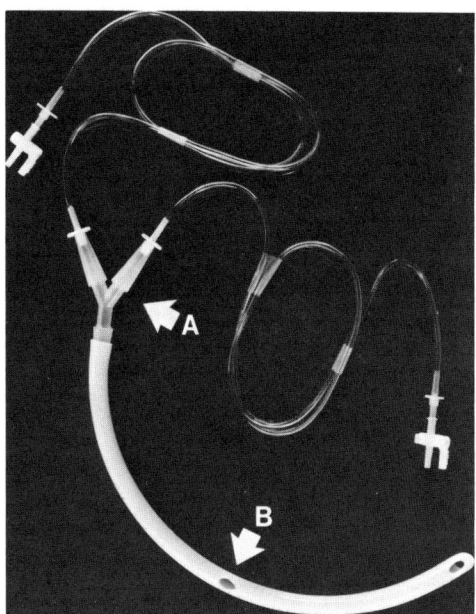

Figure 20–7. Endotracheal tube set-up used for intracaval shunting. **A:** "Y" connector with femoral ends of intravenous tubing attached to allow rapid infusion of crystalloid. Three-way stopcocks are connected to opposite ends of the tubing. **B:** Side hole cut at appropriate level to permit egress of blood into right atrium.

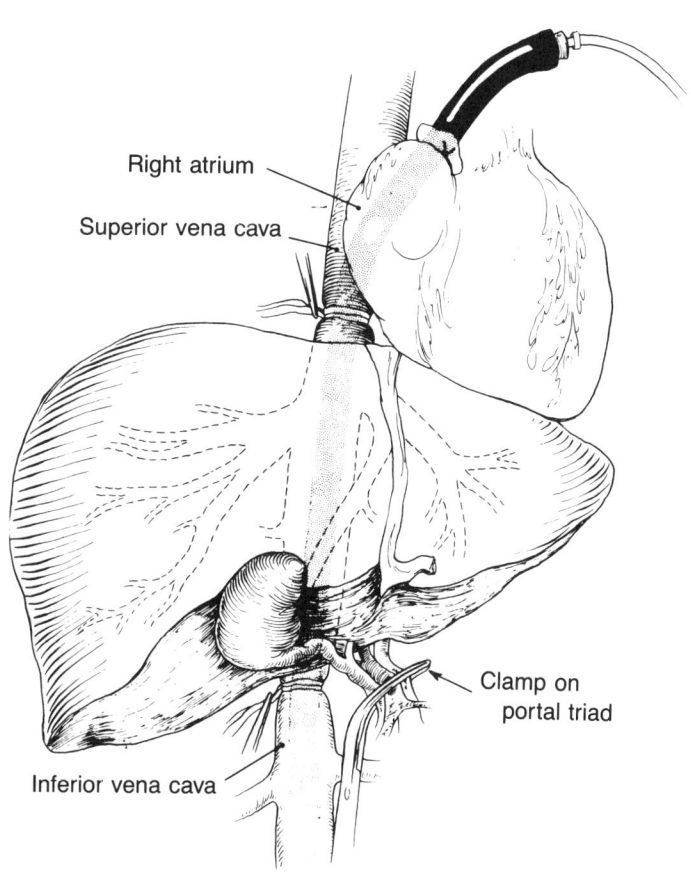

Figure 20–8. View shows a #36 F catheter inserted through the right atrial appendage into the inferior vena cava. The tip of the catheter lies just below the level of the renal veins. The side hole of the catheter, 20 cm from the tip, lies at the level of the right atrium. The proximal end of the catheter is connected to an infusion line as depicted. For more rapid infusion, a "Y" connector is provided.

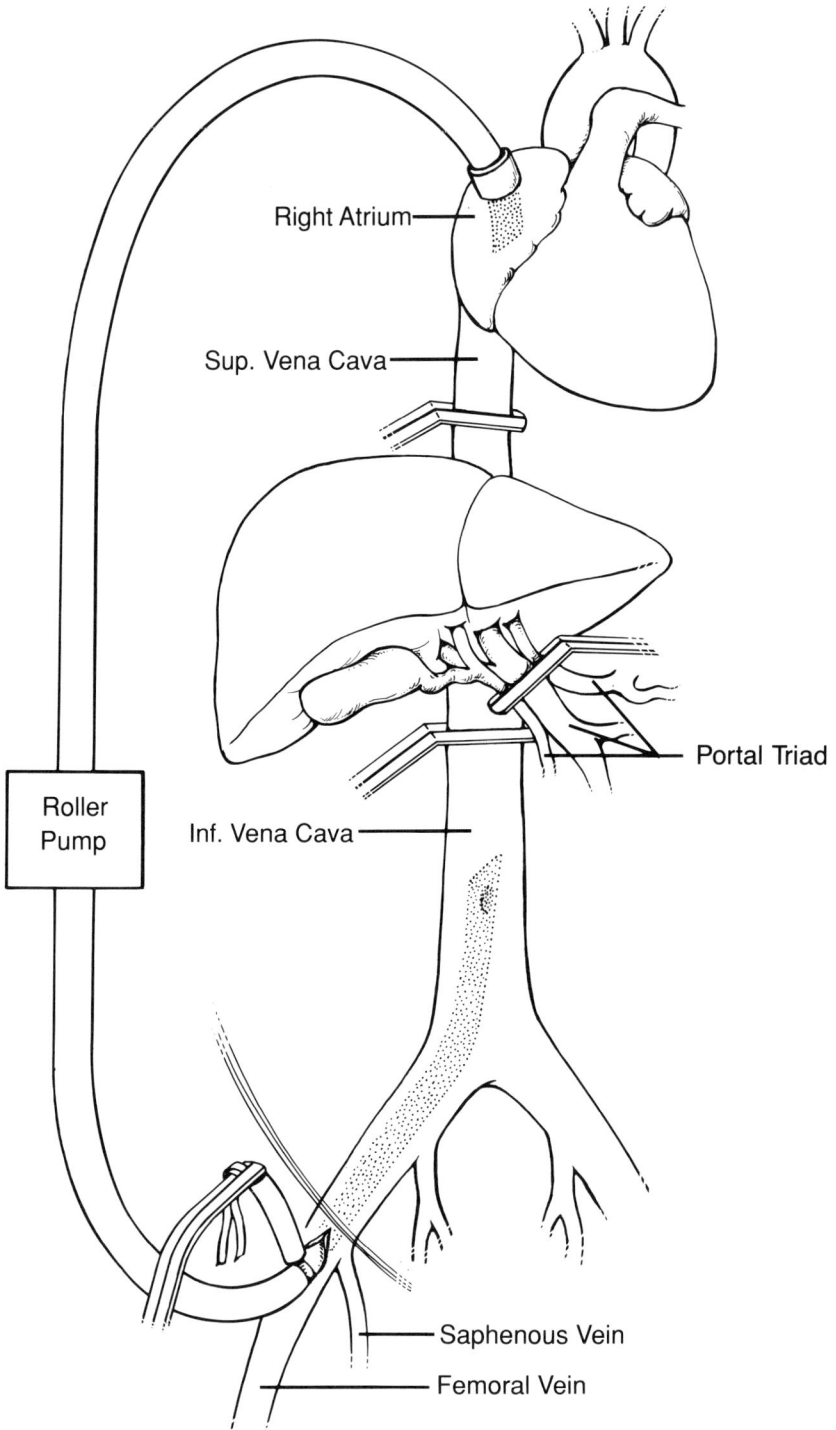

Figure 20–9. Using a nonocclusive pump, a bypass can be carried out by shunting blood around the liver. The proximal tubing can be placed in the inferior vena cava or the femoral or an iliac vein. The distal end can be placed in the right atrium or a jugular or axillary vein.

hepatic venous drainage of the right or left lobe be involved, lobar hepatectomy may be required. This can be accomplished rapidly in a relatively avascular field when the caval isolation technique is used.

Injuries to the intrapericardial portion of the vena cava usually result in intrapericardial hemorrhage with pericardial tamponade. Isolation of this portion of the cava is difficult because of its close proximity to the atrium, but isolation can be obtained as just described for the intrahepatic portion of the vena cava.

Recently, a fourth alternative has been used in what previously were nonrepairable caval and hepatic vein injuries. This consists of liver transplantation. The first two successful cases were reported from Pittsburgh by Esquivel et al.[18]

The splenic vein can be identified by mobilizing the base of the transverse mesocolon downward from under the inferior portion of the body and tail of the pancreas. This is accomplished by entering the lesser sac, separating the omentum from the transverse and descending colon, and mobilizing the spleen and the tail of the pancreas upward to permit exposure of the posterior surface of the pancreas. Injury to the splenic vein is often associated with injuries to the pancreas. Distal pancreatic resection for treatment of the pancreatic laceration simultaneously permits control of splenic vein bleeding. Distal pancreatic resection with or without splenectomy is often appropriate when exposure is difficult.

The superior mesenteric vein is controlled through the mesentery as it passes over the duodenum and uncinate process of the pancreas and down under the body of the pancreas. Exposure of the subpancreatic portion of the vein requires mobilization of the inferior surface of the pancreas, as previously described. Injuries to the junction of the splenic and mesenteric vein and the portal vein can be best exposed by carrying out a generous Kocher maneuver. This is facilitated by mobilizing the entire ascending colon along with the duodenum and head of pancreas and the entire base of the small bowel mesentery as necessary, as shown in Figure 20–10. Because the portal vein is a posterior structure in the portal triad, elevation of the head of the pancreas permits posterior exposure of the vein. Injuries to the anterior portion of the portal vein are best repaired through the posterior venotomy if necessary. The portal vein can be trapped by the first assistant's finger, dissected from the pancreas, and isolated for vascular repair. If the integrity of the pancreas has not been compromised, portal venous injuries are often best left untreated unless free intraperitoneal bleeding is present, since these complex injuries are difficult to expose, more difficult to repair, and can be associated with massive operative blood loss.

TECHNICAL CONSIDERATIONS

The results of anastomoses in the venous system do not parallel the excellent results that are seen almost routinely in the arterial system. Patency of venous anastomoses or grafts is more difficult to achieve for the following reasons:

1. The total diameter of the great veins is 1.5 or more times that of the corresponding arteries. Since venous return to the heart is identical to aortic outflow, there necessarily has to be a lower blood flow velocity in veins. Thus, platelet aggregates that form at the sites of anastomoses or in areas of local turbulence and stasis such as in valve pockets are less likely to be "washed away" by the bloodstream.

386 *Abdominal Trauma*

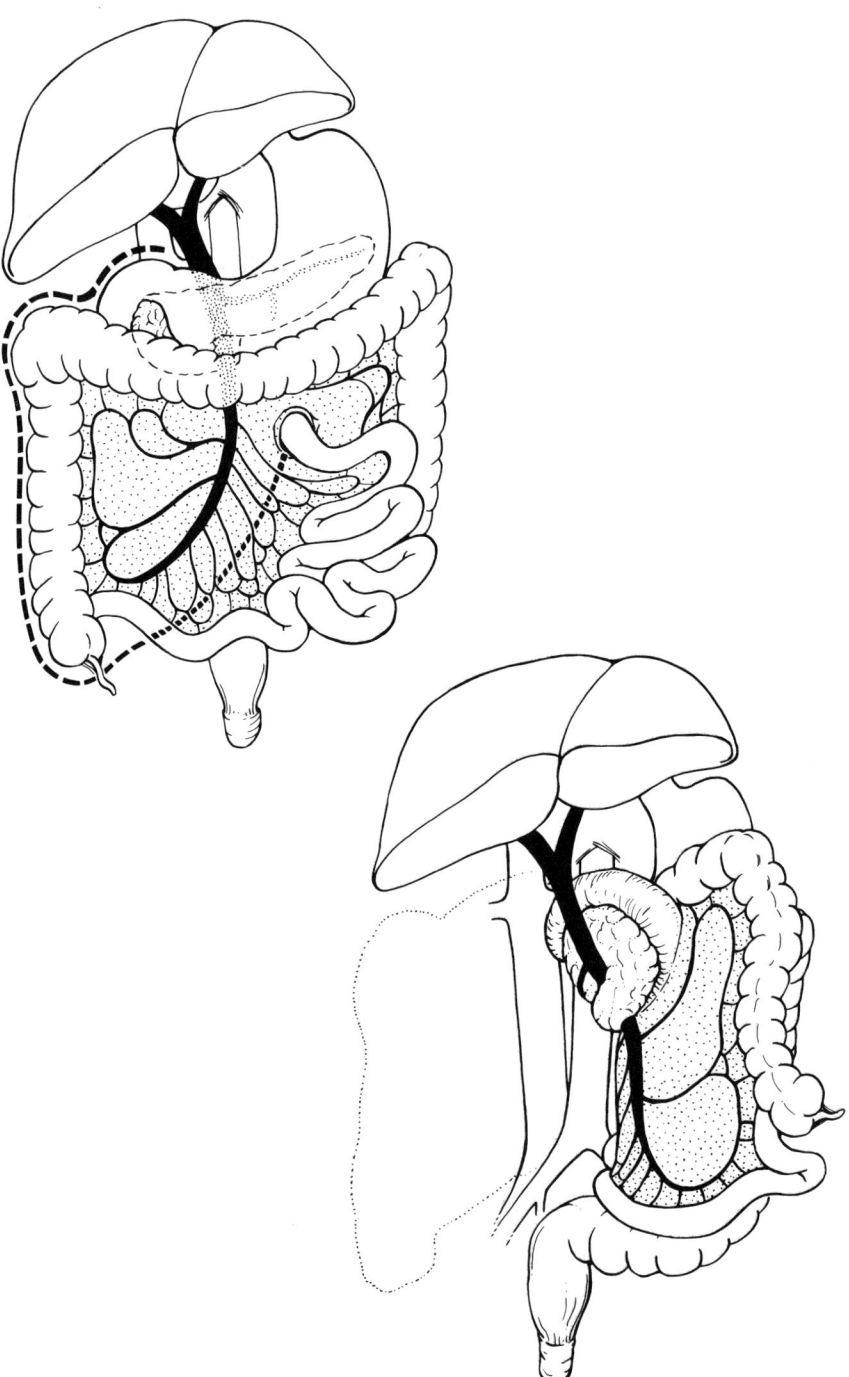

Figure 20–10. Exposure of the portal vein involves mobilizing the right colon, the duodenum, and the head of the pancreas upward and medially. This is facilitated by also mobilizing the root of the small bowel mesentery.

2. Veins are thin-walled and easily torn, and they collapse and retract when dissected away from supporting tissue. Twisting, buckling, and ridging all predispose to thrombosis.
3. The lower pressure in the veins results in the tendency for suture lines to shrink and anastomoses to stenose.

In performing venous surgery, a successful outcome depends on strict attention to technical details and to the use of adjuvant measures to improve patency. The principles formulated by Carrel in 1902 for the construction of a venous anastomosis are still relevant: strict asepsis, gentle handling of veins, use of fine suture materials, and simple continuous suture without tension to avoid narrowing.[19] Because of the lower pressure in veins, less tension on the stitches is required when using a continuous suture and purse-stringing is thereby avoided. Leaving the loops of a continuous suture somewhat loose may result in some leakage of blood, but this readily stops with gentle pressure. Care should be taken not to draw strands of adventitia into the lumen as these will serve as a nidus for thrombosis. For smaller veins the tripartite suture of Carrel (Fig. 20–11) permits greater precision in suture placement. Intimal apposition can be assured by using everting mattress sutures.

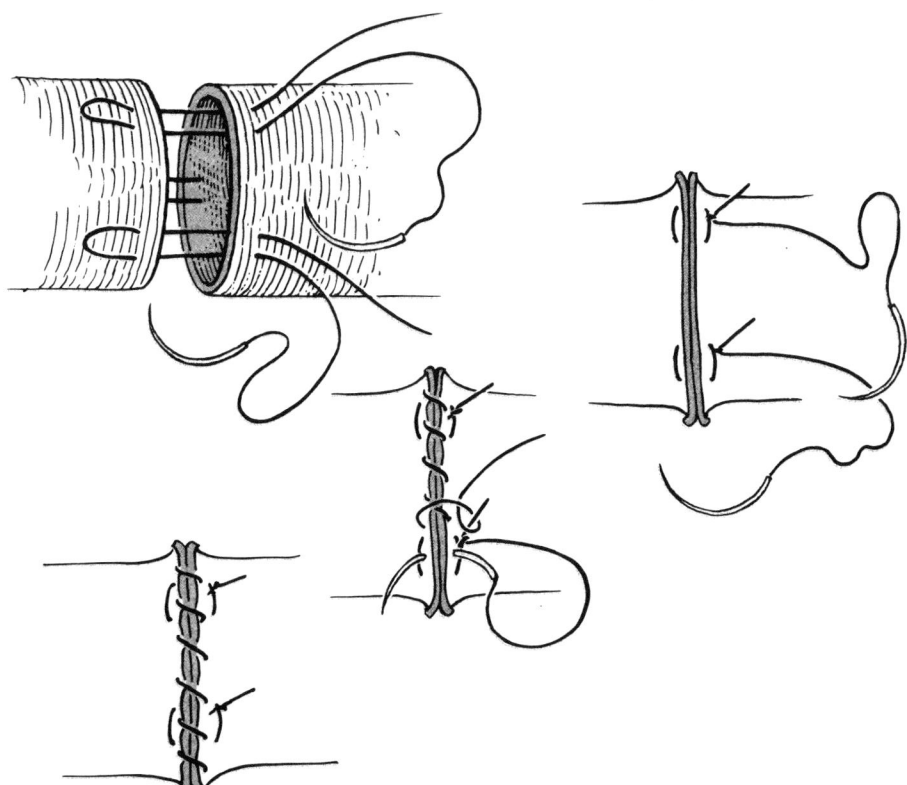

Figure 20–11. The tripartite suture of Carrel facilitates accurate placement of sutures. Mattress sutures ensure intima approximation. Less tension is required in venous anastomosis than in arterial anastomosis.

Magnification using operating loupes also permits more optimal suture placement. If grafts are required they should be somewhat longer than the defect to be repaired. Methods of enlarging the ends of veins should be used when possible to prevent anastomotic stenosis. These include diagonal cuts, "fish-mouthing," and the use of adjacent branches.[20]

The use of an oblique anastomosis may diminish the conscquences of vein collapse if it occurs. With a straight anastomosis, compression results in apposition of the entire suture line circumferentially. With an oblique anastomosis, however, apposition of edges occurs only if the suture line is compressed laterally (Fig. 20–12).

To prevent the collapse and cicatrization of a veno–venous anastomosis, suspension rings and nonsuture methods of anastomoses have been used. Mechanical suture techniques can shorten the time required for the anastomosis but the instruments are cumbersome and have not enjoyed widespread popularity. When replacement of a venous segment is needed there are a number of techniques possible, including use of the internal iliac vein to replace a segment of external iliac vein.

When autogenous material is needed for large vein replacement, composite tubular and bifurcation grafts can be constructed (Fig. 20–13). The longer suture lines, however, may predispose to thrombosis. In the absence of suitable autogenous tissue, prosthetic grafts may be used to replace large veins, provided adjunctive measures to improve patency are used. These consist of supporting rings built into the graft. Experimental and clinical studies cited by Scherck and colleagues indicate that without these adjunctive measures, patency of fabric grafts in the infrarenal vena cava is difficult to achieve.[21] Grafts in the superior vena cava are more likely to remain patent than those in the inferior vena cava. In the superior vena cava, negative thoracic pressure holds the grafts open, whereas positive abdominal pressure causes graft compression in the inferior vena cava. In addition, superior vena cava flow is isogravitational, whereas inferior vena cava flow is antigravitational.

Adjuvant therapy with antithrombotic agents has been shown to improve patency after experimental venous reconstruction and its clinical use is discussed in the section on postoperative management.

The use of temporary arteriovenous fistulae (AVF) to increase blood flow velocity has been shown to be a way of improving patency rates after venous reconstruction.[22-24] These have no place in the acute trauma setting but may be of value in delayed or elective reconstruction.[25] To maintain patency of grafts or anastomoses in the iliac veins, the saphenous vein or a major branch can be connected to the superficial femoral artery. For inferior vena cava grafts, a saphenous vein–superficial femoral artery anastomosis should be used (Fig. 20–14).[26] The fistula should be no larger than 5 mm in diameter. A larger

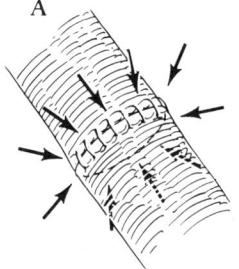
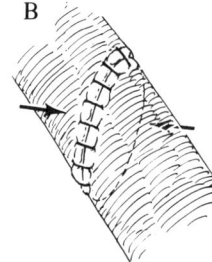

Figure 20–12. **A:** If a vein with a straight anastomosis is compressed, there will be circumferential suture contact. **B:** With an oblique anastomosis suture contact will occur in one plane only.

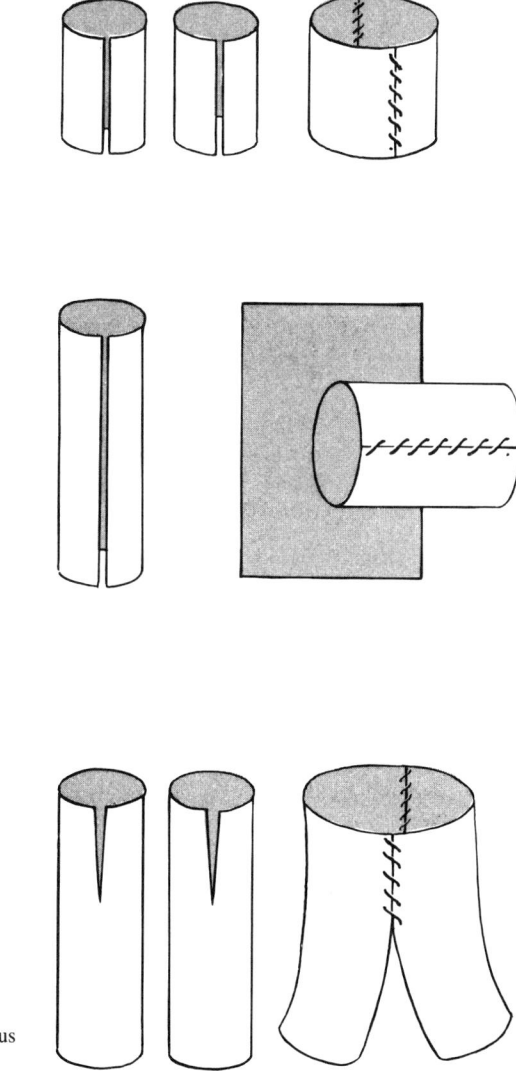

Figure 20–13. Methods of enlarging autogenous vein grafts to form tubular or bifurcation grafts.

fistula risks adverse hemodynamic effects. The arteriovenous anastomosis is marked by a loosely placed suture loop, the ends of which are left long and buried just underneath the skin. This facilitates later closure of the fistula. The recommended time that an AVF should be kept in place is 1 to 2 months.[25] Beyond this time venous grafts tend to stay open even with the AVF closed. Adverse effects from a temporary AVF include temporary limb edema and possible venous insufficiency if distal venous valves are rendered incompetent by the elevated venous pressure. There is, of course, the need for a second operation but, theoretically, a temporary AVF might be closed nonoperatively by angiographic catheterization and balloon tamponade.

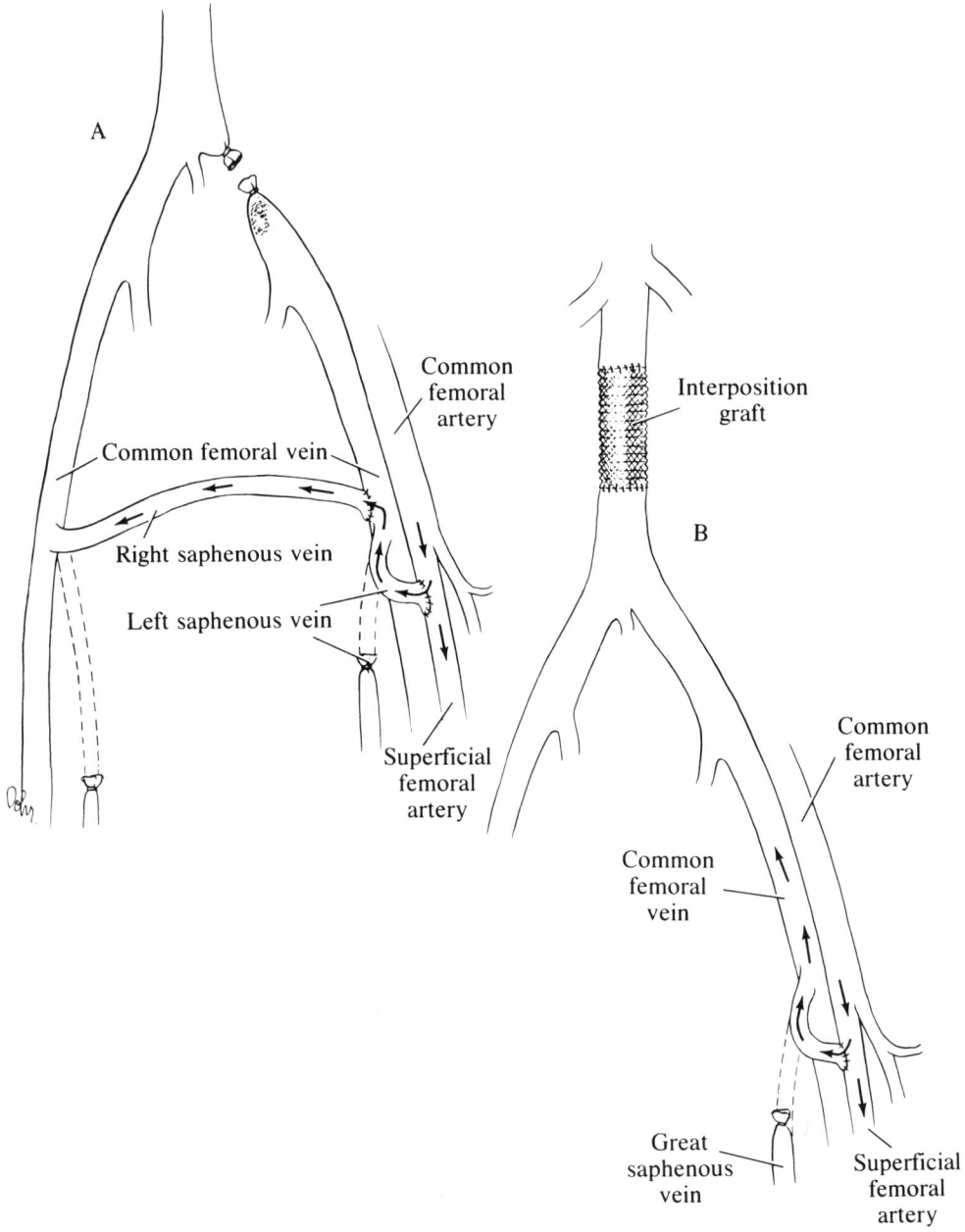

Figure 20–14. Temporary arteriovenous fistula to maintain patency in vein grafts. **A:** Branch of left saphenous vein sewn end-to-side to superficial femoral artery to increase flow velocity through cross-femoral saphenous venovenous bypass graft. **B:** Left saphenous vein sewn end-to-side to superficial femoral artery after inferior vena cava replacement.

OPERATIVE TREATMENT

The definitive treatment of injured veins involves lateral repair, ligation, and, on occasion, venous replacement. Venous injuries may be isolated by pressure or with a vascular clamp. Since the delicate nature of the veins is such that the application of clamps may result in further tearing, we prefer to trap the injured segment of the vein with fingers or a "sponge-stick" above and below and either side to control collaterals (Fig. 20–14).

Isolated injuries of the external, internal, or common iliac veins can be treated with ligation or repair. If the laceration is a simple one, meticulous repair with everting sutures (using fine monofilament sutures) is usually associated with a good result. However, complex injuries are difficult to repair without producing stenosis of the vein or leaving a raw intimal surface of the vein exposed. This is thrombogenic and may result in complications of thrombosis or, worse yet, embolism. Therefore, complex injuries to the iliac veins and the infrarenal vena cava are best treated by ligation of the injured segment. For complex vena cava injuries the distal ligature is best placed just below the renal veins and the intervening lumbar veins ligated if necessary, since stasis in a relatively blind segment above the ligature may be the source of thrombosis and subsequent embolism. If the injury is simple and can be repaired cleanly, this should be accomplished using atraumatic isolation techniques. Penetrating injuries involving both anterior and posterior walls of the vena cava are best managed by suturing the posterior laceration through a widened anterior hole or, alternatively, rotating the cava for exposure and repair.

Either renal vein can be ligated but the status of the opposite kidney should first be determined by IVP if possible. The distal 2 or 3 cm of the left renal vein can be ligated with impunity since collateral flow from the adrenal or gonadal veins provides sufficient drainage such that impaired function of the left kidney seldom occurs. Ligation of the right renal vein is not as likely to be associated with complete recovery of the kidney and a simple laceration should be repaired. Complex injuries may best be treated by nephrectomy, particularly if there is associated renal artery or renal parenchymal damage.

Ligation of the suprarenal vena cava is usually not compatible with survival, since two-thirds of cardiac venous return is compromised. Therefore, this segment should be repaired unless this is absolutely out of the question. Severe injuries to this segment are usually incompatible with survival long enough to reach a point of definitive treatment. The application of liver isolation techniques permitted isolation of this segment and repair. Occasionally, if vascular volume has been restored to normal, it may be possible to occlude this segment temporarily for repair, as previously described.

There is no technical challenge quite as great as a complex injury of the infrarenal vena cava. There may be massive bleeding from lumbar veins, and as the injury is exposed, collateral bleeding can be such as to result in exsanguination. The assistant should control the vein from above with a sponge stick and roll a pack from above downward, so as to expose a small segment of the laceration, initiate the suture, and then roll the pack further downward as suturing is carried out. As lumbar veins are identified they can be occluded temporarily with silver clips.

Mesenteric vein injuries also constitute a major challenge. When the injury is located well out in the mesentery, ligation can usually be safely carried out. Proximal injuries at the root of the mesentery can often be treated by closing the overlying peritoneum and ignoring the venous injury with planned reexploration within 12 or 24 hr to assess viability of bowel. Mesenteric vein injuries at the junction with the portal vein or splenic vein injuries at this level may be difficult to manage. The splenic vein can be ligated with impunity; therefore, repair of this vein is rarely indicated. Although the superior mesenteric vein can be ligated, thrombosis and loss of viability of bowel may result. Therefore, this vein and the portal vein should be repaired if at all possible using the techniques illustrated (Fig. 20–15).

Although severe injuries to the portal vein and the portal triad can be treated with a portacaval shunt, this is often difficult in unstable patients and furthermore is associated with severe morbidity due to protein intolerance. Ligation is an acceptable alternative if reconstruction is not possible. Injuries to the junction of the portal and mesenteric veins can be treated with a venous patch if the injury is complex or, alternatively, the splenic vein can be divided and used to reconstruct the superior mesenteric vein. The higher pressure portal system is associated with better results after suturing and repair, both on an immediate and long-term basis, than the lower pressure systemic veins. If an interposition graft is required, a segment of internal jugular vein, internal iliac vein, or external iliac vein is preferred, although there has been some limited success using prosthetic grafts in this position.[27]

POSTOPERATIVE CARE

Postoperative management problems presented by venous injuries are relatively mild compared to other types of vascular injury. Once control has been obtained, secondary

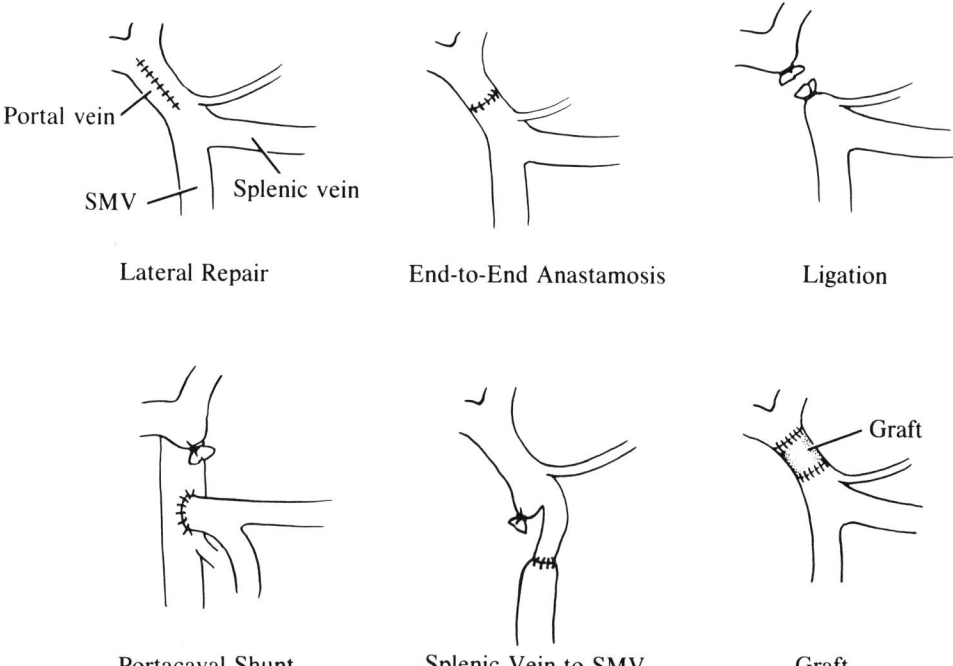

Figure 20–15. Methods used for reconstruction of the portal and superior mesenteric veins.

hemorrhage is unusual. However, because of massive associated blood loss and shock, coagulation defects may develop after multiple transfusions. This is initially a platelet defect that results in persistent oozing from wounds and suture lines. Catastrophic diffuse hemorrhage is usually a manifestation of disseminated intravascular clotting with consumption coagulopathy. This can result from a mismatched transfusion, from extensive soft tissue injury in shock, or from vital organ damage. Intravascular coagulation is aggravated by persistent hypovolemia, and treatment requires restoration of vascular volume, the adequacy of which can be monitored by urinary output and central venous pressure measurements. If the status of cardiovascular volume is uncertain, pulmonary artery wedge pressure monitoring with the Swan-Ganz catheter is used.

Although bleeding from venous suture lines is relatively rare, associated bleeding from other lacerations or associated organ injuries may result in unsatisfactory hemostasis at the time of closure. When this is the case, reintervention should be planned 12 to 24 hr later, after coagulation defects have been corrected. This permits removal of blood clots, assessment of the status of vital organ perfusion and the quality of venous repair.

After major venous injuries have been repaired, thrombotic complications are possible, and when major systemic veins such as iliac or cava have been repaired, extensive distal thrombosis is common. This can produce considerable morbidity, whereas clean ligation without thrombosis usually results in little immediate and late morbidity. Therefore, when the iliac vein or vena cava is ligated, or when venous reconstruction has been performed, postoperative management should include an antithrombotic regimen when possible. This can consist of the administration of low molecular weight dextran, 10 cc/kg for the first 24 hr and 5 cc/kg in subsequent days, until normal activity is resumed. Intermittent pneumatic compression, elastic wraps, and elevation of the extremities are essential to prevent morbidity, provided there has been no associated arterial injury. If prolonged immobility is anticipated, anticoagulation with warfarin sodium, keeping the prothrombin time elevated to twice normal, can be effective in preventing thromboembolic complications. With careful monitoring, bleeding complications from anticoagulants can be minimized.

COMPLICATIONS

Complications of venous injury consist of those related to bleeding, thrombosis, and ischemia. These include transfusion reactions and bleeding problems as previously mentioned. Coagulation factors should be monitored, particularly if circulation to the liver has been temporarily interrupted. These consist of prothrombin time and partial thromboplastin time. Coagulation defects noted should be treated with fresh frozen plasma. Disseminated intravascular coagulation with a consumption coagulopathy is best treated by restoration and maintenance of normal volume and by reoperation if there is a question of intestinal or liver ischemia, so that ischemic tissue can be removed.

Thrombosis of venous repairs is a major problem. This is usually manifested by swelling distal to the injury. If extensive thrombosis occurs, the swelling can be massive. If a visceral vein is involved, ischemia of the gastrointestinal tract or ascites may be the result. Renal infarction is a possibility following renal vein injury. The manifestation of caval or iliac vein thrombus[44] may be negligible if the clot is not firmly adherent to the vein wall, but this type of clot usually renders the patient vulnerable to pulmonary embolism 7 to 10 days postinjury, as he is being mobilized and/or venous pressure is raised by performance of a Valsalva maneuver. If there is no contraindication, major thrombosis or pulmonary embolism is most appropriately treated with heparin. The author uses 150 units/kg as an initial bolus in the average patient, followed by approximately 25 units/kg/hr by continuous infusion for thrombosis. Pulmonary embolism is best treated by high doses of heparin consisting of a 300-unit/kg initial bolus followed by 40 units/kg/hr by continuous intravenous infusion. If anticoagulation is contraindicated because of associated injuries, ligation of the vena cava or the placement of a caval filter just below the renal veins is the treatment of choice.

Since ligation of venous injury is frequently used, the anticipated complication might be incapacitating edema. We have found, however, that this is surprisingly rare and is less than that associated with repair of complex injuries. This is because clean ligation is less apt to be associated with extensive thrombosis. It is the latter that interferes with collateral flow. Mullins et al. tabulated the results of venous ligation after injury involving six vena cava, five external iliac, and three common iliac veins.[45] They found that three patients with caval ligation had no edema at discharge or follow-up. One had mild edema at discharge and none on follow-up and two with mild edema at discharge had moderate edema at follow-up. Of the five patients with external iliac ligation, three had no edema at discharge or follow-up. One with minimal edema at discharge had none at follow-up. The remaining patient was lost to follow-up.

Injuries to the portal venous system may result in bowel ischemia or in portal hypertension and ammonia intoxication if the portal vein is ligated or thrombosis of the repair occurs. If this is suspected in the immediate postoperative period, reoperation is indicated to evacuate clot from the portal or mesenteric vein and revise the repair. When this is accomplished, the risk of anticoagulation must be accepted to prevent recurrent thrombosis.

Renal function should be monitored whenever the renal veins or suprarenal vena cava have been injured and repaired. Renal infarction may be relatively silent or associated with prostrating symptoms. In the latter instance, nephrectomy may be indicated.

RESULTS

In the Vietnam Vascular Registry there were 194 venous injuries among 718 vascular injuries.[28] There were only 28 isolated injuries of major veins noted. (This relatively low incidence may not be accurate because documentation of venous injury is usually not as complete as for arterial injury.) Lower extremity venous injuries predominated, with popliteal and femoral vein injuries the most common. Venous repair was performed in 124 injuries and ligation was done in 253. Only 12 abdominal and pelvic venous injuries were included and of these, three were repaired. The lessons learned from this vast military experience are that venous repair could reduce the incidence of (1) acute venous hypertension resulting in a lowered amputation rate, and (2) the long-term stasis problems are frequently associated with chronic venous insufficiency.

Contrary to previous notions, thrombophlebitis and pulmonary embolism were not increased after venous repair. The value of attempting repair after venous trauma is that if the repair remains patent for 24 to 72 hr, this may allow for relaxation of the arterial spasm and the opening up of venous collaterals. Furthermore, veins that have thrombosed can recanalize, as can thrombosed autogenous vein grafts.

A civilian experience with venous trauma was reported by Gaspar and Treiman.[29] They concluded that the results after repair were superior to those achieved after ligation and that postoperative thrombophlebitis was not a major problem.

Early reports on the management of inferior vena cava (IVC) injuries stressed the rarity of survival, particularly after suprarenal IVC and associated hepatic vein injuries.

Abdominal venous trauma carries a high mortality. The victims often present in shock as there are frequently other associated vascular injuries. Inability to obtain vascular control rapidly results in death by exsanguination. Improved results can be expected if operative control of hemorrhage is carried out as part of the resuscitative process. The mortality rate for abdominal venous injury varies greatly, undoubtedly related to the number of associated injuries, degree of shock, and time interval before definitive repair.[30] The first large series treated surgically was that of Oschner and associates, who reported a 43% survival in 37 patients with inferior vena cava injury.[31] However, mortality rates for cava and iliac injuries have remained between 30% and 60%.[10,16,31–33] The advent of caval shunting permitted treatment of suprarenal and hepatic vein injuries that previously were uniformly lethal. However, mortality rates from this injury vary from 50% to 90%.[13,34–36]

Improved resuscitation techniques, better blood bank support, and more aggressive operative intervention all contributed to survival rates reported in a more recently published series.[37] An important advance was the clinical application of techniques to isolate the suprarenal vena cava and hepatic veins. Of interest is the report by Waltuck and colleagues, describing a case in which suprarenal vena cava ligation was successful in treating an avulsion injury at the level of the renal veins.[38] This was the fourth patient reported to survive suprarenal caval ligation for trauma.

Survival after abdominal venous injury depends on the nature of the wounding agent, the presence or absence of shock at the time of hospital admission, the level of injury, and the number and type of associated vascular injuries.[39,40] More destructive firearms and high-speed vehicular accidents are frequent wounding agents. With more efficient ambulance services, many patients who would otherwise die at the scene arrive at the hospital for treatment. It is this group of patients presenting in profound shock that accounts for most of the reported mortality.[16,30]

For portal and mesenteric vein injuries, the mortality rate averages 60% and ranges between 53% and 71%.[41,42] There are frequently multiple associated vascular injuries, and death, as in vena cava injuries, is usually caused by exsanguination or complications of hemorrhagic shock. In a collected review of portal vein injuries, Busuttil and colleagues found that the death rate with lateral repair was 30%, whereas that with ligation treatment was 78%.[40] Undoubtedly ligation was used in cases with more extensive trauma and this may account for the increased mortality. Stone reported the survival of 16 of 20 patients who required portal vein ligation for trauma.[41] Portal collateral channels appear to be sufficient in most cases to prevent portal hypertension and splanchnic venous infarction after portal or superior mesenteric vein ligation.[43] Portasystemic shunting has rarely been used as a primary procedure because of the frequent development of encephalopathy in patients with previously normal hepatic blood flow.

REFERENCES

1. Dale WA. In discussion of Mattox, et al., Traumatic injury to the portal vein. *Ann Surg*. 1975; 181:519–522.
2. Rich NM, Spencer RC. *Vascular Trauma*. Philadelphia: WB Saunders; 1979.
3. Boyce FF, Lampert R, McFetridge EM. Occlusion of the portal vein. *J Lab Clin Med*. 1935; 20:935.
4. Johnson CC, Baggenstross AH. Mesenteric vascular occlusion 1. Study of 99 cases of occlusion in veins. *Proc Staff Meet Mayo Clinic*. 1949; 24:618.
5. Colp R. Treatment of pylephlebitis of appendicular origin with report of three cases of ligation of portal vein. *Surg Gynecol Obstet*. 1926; 43:627.
6. Robson AWM. Case of perforating wound of abdomen. *Br Med J*. 1897; 2:77.
7. Wilms EF, cited by Harsha WN, Orr TG. Ligation of superior mesenteric vein. *Am Surg*. 1952; 18:148–155.
8. Child CG III. *The Hepatic Circulation and Portal Hypertension*. Philadelphia: WB Saunders; 1954.
9. Fish JC. Reconstruction of the portal vein: case reports and literature review. *Am Surg*. 1966; 32:472.
10. Burch JM, Richardson RJ, Martin RR, Mattox KL. Penetrating iliac vascular injuries: recent experience with 233 consecutive patients. *J Trauma*. 1990; 30:1450.
11. Salam AA, Stewart MT. New approach to wounds of the aortic bifurcation and the interior vena cava. *Surgery*. 1985; 98:105.
12. Vitelli CE, Scales TM, Phillips TF. A technique for controlling injuries of the iliac vein in patients with trauma. *Surg Gynecol Obstet*. 1988; 166:551.
13. Pachter H, Spencer FC, Hofstetter S, et al. The management of juxta hepatic venous injuries without an atriocaval shunt. *Surgery*. 1986; 99:569.
14. Williams CD, Brenowitz JB. Sequential aortic and inferior vena caval clamping for control of suprarenal vena caval injuries: case report. *J Trauma*. 1977; 17:164–167.
15. Schrock T, Blaisdell FW, Mathewson C. Management of blunt trauma to the liver and hepatic veins. *Arch Surg*. 1968; 96:698–704.
16. Allen RE, Blaisdell FW. Injuries to the inferior vena cava. *Surg Clin North Am*. 1972; 52:699.
17. Shaw BW, Martin DJ, Marquez JM, Starzl TE. Venous bypass in clinical liver transplantation. *Ann Surg*. 1984; 200:524–534.
18. Esquivel CO, Bernardos A, Makowa L, Starzl TE. Liver replacement after hepatic trauma. *J Trauma*. 1987; 27:800.
19. Carrel A. La technique operatoire des anastomoses vasculaires et la transplantation des visceres. *Lyon Med*. 1902; 98:859.
20. Rich NM, Hobson RW II, Wright CB, Swan KG. Techniques of venous repair. In: Swan KG, et al., eds. *Venous Surgery in the Lower Extremities*. St. Louis: Warren H. Green Publishers; 1975.
21. Scherck JP, Kerstein MD, Stansel HL. The current status of vena cava replacement. *Surgery*. 1974; 76:209–233.
22. Johnson V, Eiseman B. Evaluation of arteriovenous shunt to obtain patency of venous autograft. *Am J Surg*. 1969; 118:915.
23. Kunlin J, Kunlin A. Experimental venous surgery. *Major Prob Clin Surg*. 1979; 23:37–66.
24. Rabinowitz R, Golfarb D. Surgical treatment of axillo subclavian venous thrombosis: a case report. *Surgery*. 1971; 70:703.
25. Rich NM, Levin PM, Hutton JE. Effect of distal arteriovenous fistulas on venous graft patency. In: Swan KG, et al., eds. *Venous Surgery in the Lower Extremities*. St. Louis: Warren H. Green Publishers; 1975.
26. May R, De Weese JA. *Surgery of the Pelvic Veins*. Philadelphia: WB Saunders; 1979.
27. Norton L. Eiseman B. Replacement of portal vein during pancreaticoduodenectomy for carcinoma. *Surgery*. 1975; 77:280–284.
28. Rich NM, Hughes CW. Vietnam Vascular Registry, a preliminary report. *Surgery*. 1969; 65:218.
29. Gaspar MR, Treiman RL. The management of injuries to major veins. *Am J Surg*. 1960; 100:171.
30. Wilson RF, Wiencek RG, Balog M. Factors affecting mortality rate with iliac vein injuries. *J Trauma*. 1990; 30:320.
31. Oschner JL, Crawford ES, DeBakey ME. Injuries of the vena cava caused by external trauma. *Surgery*. 1961; 49:397–405.
32. Burch JM, Feliciano DV, Mattox KL. Injuries of the inferior vena cava. *Am J Surg*. 1988; 156:548.
33. Quast DC, Shirkey AL, Fitzgerald JB, et al. Surgical correction of injuries of the vena cava: an analysis of sixty-one cases. *J Trauma*. 1965; 5:1–10.
34. Beal SL, Ward RE. Successful atrial caval shunting in the management of retrohepatic venous injuries. *Am J Surg*. 1989; 158:409.
35. Buechter KJ, Gomez GA, Zeppa R. A new technique for exposure of injuries at the confluence of the retrohepatic veins and the retrohepatic vena cava. *J Trauma*. 1990; 30:329.
36. Kudsk KA, Sheldon GF, Lim RC Jr. Atrial–caval shunting after trauma. *J Trauma*. 1982; 22:81.
37. Rovito P. Atrial caval shunting in blunt hepatic venous injury. *Ann Surg*. 1987; 205:318.

38. Waltuck TL, Crow RW, Humphrey LJ, Kaufman HM. Avulsion injuries of the vena cava following blunt abdominal trauma. *Ann Surg*. 1970; 171:67–72.
39. Bricker BL, Morton JR, Okies JE, Beall AC. Surgical management of injury to the inferior vena cava: changing patterns of injury and newer techniques of repair. *J Trauma*. 1971; 11:725.
40. Busuttil RQ, Kitahanea A, Cerise E, et al. Management of blunt and penetrating injuries to the porta hepatic. *Ann Surg*. 1980; 191:641–648.
41. Stone HH. In discussion of Busuttil et al., ref. 40.
42. Peterson SR, Sheldon GF, Lim RC. Management of portal vein injuries. *J Trauma*. 1979; 19:616.
43. Schnug E. Ligation of the superior mesenteric vein. *Surgery*. 1973; 14:610–616.
44. Nagy KK, Duarte B. Post-traumatic interior vena caval thrombosis: case report. *J Trauma*. 1990; 30:218.
45. Mullins RJ, Lukas CE, Ledgerwood AM. The natural history following venous ligation for civilian injuries. *J Trauma*. 1980; 20:737.

21
Retroperitoneal Hematoma

ANTHONY A. MEYER, M.D.
KENNETH A. KUDSK, M.D.
GEORGE F. SHELDON, M.D.

HISTORY: *In 1941, Cushman and Kilgore provided the first description of retroperitoneal hematoma.[1] They described a series of signs and symptoms that they believed would lead to the diagnosis of "subperitoneal" hematoma. They reported 22 cases and indicated that the symptoms were dull constant abdominal pain usually accompanied by nausea and vomiting. Vomiting aggravated the discomfort instead of bringing relief. Examination disclosed local tenderness of the abdomen but no rigidity. A mass was often palpable in a central location. When intraperitoneal rupture occurred, the patients manifested shock, abdominal rigidity, and ileus.*

In the late 1950s and early 1960s, articles began to appear further identifying retroperitoneal hematoma as a clinical problem. At this point there were mixed views as to whether ligation of the internal iliac artery was appropriate to control the bleeding.[2-4] In 1962, Bayliss et al. believed that the morbidity of exploring the retroperitoneal hematoma outweighed the risk of nonoperative management and combined blood replacement,[2] whereas Seavers et al. advocated laparotomy for retroperitoneal hematoma and ligation of the internal iliac artery.[3] Ger et al. carried out experimental studies of retroperitoneal hemorrhage and noted that ligation of the internal iliac artery had no effect on the venous pressure in the pelvic veins.[5]

The problem related to ligation of the internal iliac artery was that, when the retroperitoneal hematoma was opened, venous bleeding was decompressed and was much more difficult to manage than the arterial bleeding.[4]

In a series reported by Allen et al., the overall mortality was 24% for 75 cases.[6] The mortality was 30% when the hematoma was explored versus a mortality of 10% when the hematoma was left intact. Allen also pointed out that in his series, ligation of the internal hypogastric artery was not effective in controlling the pelvic bleeding.

Because conservative management was still associated with high mortality from ongoing hemorrhage, alternative means of controlling bleeding were sought. Sheldon and Weinstock reoperated on a pelvic fracture with uncontrollable bleeding and after ligating the proximal iliac artery they were able to thread a small balloon catheter into the bleeding gluteal vessel that controlled the hemorrhage.[7] *Trunkey and colleagues advocated transfemoral catheterization of the femoral artery with muscle embolism of the internal iliac artery for bleeding control.*[8] *At the present time, conservative management of pelvic hematomas remains the standard treatment with selective embolization being indicated in those cases associated with major bleeding.*

Retroperitoneal hematoma is a serious problem encountered in the evaluation and treatment of patients with severe injury. Potential sources for retroperitoneal hemorrhage are the organs and major vascular structures in the retroperitoneum, the small vessels and soft tissue surrounding these organs and vessels, and the skeletal structures posterior to the retroperitoneum. Regardless of whether the hemorrhage is from any one or all of these sources, retroperitoneal hematoma can be a life-threatening problem, and its appropriate management requires understanding the anatomy, pathophysiology, and diagnostic tools available. Retroperitoneal hematomas that occur from nontraumatic causes or from iatrogenic vascular manipulation will not be included in this chapter.

Diagnosis and management of retroperitoneal hematoma has evolved considerably during the last 10 to 15 years. The development of sophisticated imaging techniques and interventional radiologic procedures has altered the way in which retroperitoneal hematoma is evaluated and treated. However, the fundamental pathophysiology and goals for optimal patient care remain the same.

Morbidity and mortality from retroperitoneal hematoma are associated with the magnitude of injury to retroperitoneal structures, the amount of blood loss, and associated injuries.[9] As in any injury, prompt resuscitation, diagnosis, and management of the injuries are essential to improve outcome for patients.

Retroperitoneal hematoma can be due to hemorrhage from any organs or major vessels of the retroperitoneum. In these circumstances management relates to the specific organ or structure injured and is described in the appropriate chapter in this volume. Retroperitoneal hematoma from the small vessels in the soft tissue surrounding these structures, however, is the clinical problem to be addressed in this chapter.

ANATOMY

The retroperitoneum is the area between the parietal peritoneum covering the back of the abdomen and pelvis and the musculoskeletal structures of the back. The retroperitoneum contains organs of the gastrointestinal, urinary, cardiovascular, and endocrine systems listed in Table 21–1. These organs and structures are shown in anatomic relationship in Figure 21–1. A thorough knowledge of the anatomy of the retroperitoneum is essential to understanding the mechanisms of injury, determining the need for surgery, and providing operative management for these injuries.

The volume of the retroperitoneum can increase with hemorrhage because of the limited resistance of the abdominal cavity. The retroperitoneum is also a potentially expandable space, which makes hemorrhage difficult to control. The retroperitoneal hematoma can expand cephalad into the chest, caudad into the thighs, anteriorly into the small bowel and transverse colon mesenteries, and laterally into the flanks. This huge

Table 21–1 Retroperitoneal Structures

GASTROINTESTINAL	GENITOURINARY	CARDIOVASCULAR	ENDOCRINE
Duodenum	Kidneys	Abdominal aorta	Adrenals
Pancreas	Ureters	Inferior vena cava	
Ascending colon	Bladder	Iliac arteries and veins	

potential space makes retroperitoneal hematomas a major concern because of the amount of blood loss that can occur without obvious external signs.

Location of retroperitoneal hematomas varies and in some patients may extend to the entire retroperitoneal area. The relative incidence of hematomas in the different areas of the retroperitoneum varies among studies. Table 21–2 shows the relative incidence of retroperitoneal hematoma in different areas of the retroperitoneum.[2,10,11] The nature of injury in the individual institution will determine whether there will be a greater number of pelvic retroperitoneal hematomas associated with blunt injury or central retroperitoneal hematomas seen more often with penetrating wounds.

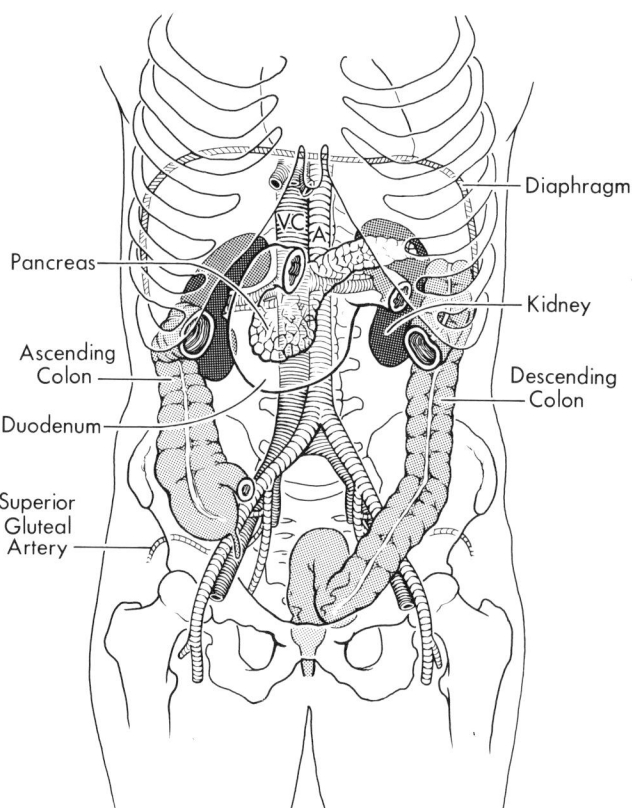

Figure 21–1. Retroperitoneal anatomy. Retroperitoneal hematomas originate from organs or vasculature of the retroperitoneum in which bleeding is contained by the retroperitoneum.

Table 21-2 Location of Retroperitoneal Hematomas

	PELVIC	PERIRENAL	OTHER*
Bayliss et al.[2]	33	9	8
Greico and Perry[10]	23	36	21
Nick et al.[11]	22	39	41
Total	78 (33.6%)	84 (36.2%)	70 (30.1%)

*Primarily central.

PATHOPHYSIOLOGY

When presented with a patient with possible retroperitoneal hematoma, it is essential to know the mechanism of injury. Depending on the severity and mechanism of injury, the management may be quite different. Generally, only injuries to organs or major vessels require urgent operative intervention.

With retroperitoneal hematomas, it is important to separate blunt from penetrating injuries when considering the pathophysiology of injury and in planning the evaluation and management of the patient. Blunt trauma is responsible for 70% to 80% of retroperitoneal hematomas. The single most common blunt injury causing retroperitoneal hematoma is pelvic fracture.[12] The causes of blunt trauma leading to retroperitoneal hematoma are listed in Table 21-3.[6,8,10,13-16]

Specific blunt injuries that should raise concern about possible retroperitoneal injury are steering wheel impact and isolated lap belt in motor vehicle accidents and any trauma associated with large amounts of force applied to a relatively small area of the torso. History of any of these types of injury should raise further the index of suspicion of retroperitoneal bleeding.

Penetrating trauma can be divided into stab wounds and gunshot wounds. Any patient with apparent retroperitoneal hematoma from penetrating injury where the weapon or projectile has traversed the peritoneal cavity has a high likelihood of abdominal visceral injury. Penetrating injuries that enter the flank or back and cause retroperitoneal hematoma may also have abdominal visceral injury, but the likelihood is much lower. This difference in pathophysiology determines management. In general, most patients with gunshot

Table 21-3 Etiology of Blunt Retroperitoneal Hematoma

	MVA	PEDESTRIAN	MOTORCYCLE	FALL
Retroperitoneal hematoma				
Allen et al.[6]	31	28	—	12
Greico and Perry[10]	35	12	14	10
Pelvic fracture				
Flint et al.[13] (severe injuries)	10	19	9	0
Hamilton[14]	31	—	—	9
Hawkins et al.[15]	16	16	2	1
Rothenberger et al.[16]	233	162	38	114
Trunkey et al.[8]	42	62	16	52

MVA, motor vehicle accident.

wounds are explored whereas many of those with stab wounds are managed expectantly if they are stable and have no signs of organ injury. It is incumbent upon the physician to rule out any likely organ injury rather than to expect it to be overly manifest.

When assessing a patient or communicating the facts to another physician, it is important to define the location of injury, structures involved, and magnitude of the retroperitoneal hematoma.

EVALUATION AND DIAGNOSIS

Many retroperitoneal hematomas that are currently identified would never have been noted without modern imaging techniques. Studies of the incidence of retroperitoneal hematoma before the availability of computed tomography (CT) scans would considerably underestimate the frequency with which this injury occurs. Little is found on physical exam in patients with isolated retroperitoneal hematoma, especially immediately after injury. The abdomen may be distended and the girth may be increased, but these findings can be due to distension of gut or accumulation of sequestered intravenous (IV) fluid given during resuscitation. Furthermore, abdominal girth is an extremely insensitive measurement of bleeding into a retroperitoneal hematoma. The volume and dimensions of the abdomen and retroperitoneum are such that a single unit of hemorrhage will produce no measurable change in abdominal girth.

Patients with retroperitoneal hematoma may also have pain, but they frequently have other injuries to account for the pain. Furthermore, evaluation of pain may be difficult because it may be masked by medications or altered mental status from head injury.

Late signs of retroperitoneal hematoma, such as the Grey-Turner's sign of ecchymosis in the flank, initially described in patients with hemorrhagic pancreatitis, is often not seen in the early evaluation of retroperitoneal hematoma. The treating physician should have the clinical suspicion that retroperitoneal hematoma may be present in any patient with a history of significant blunt or penetrating trauma to the torso. Retroperitoneal hematoma should be especially considered in patients who have evidence of significant blood loss without external evidence of bleeding.

Patients with retroperitoneal hematoma may be in shock at the time of their presentation.[17] The relative incidence of hypotension in any series will be partially determined by the relative ratio of penetrating versus blunt injury. The incidence of hypotension in those patients with retroperitoneal hematoma from pelvic fracture is listed separately. Excluding patients with major vascular injuries, the pelvic fracture patients have the greatest blood loss from retroperitoneal hematoma.

Evaluation of retroperitoneal hematomas is accomplished by serial exams and appropriate studies. The physical exam of the trauma patient should not be forgotten. Retroperitoneal injuries can be overlooked, especially when associated with penetrating wounds or soft tissue injuries of the flanks or back.[18] It is essential that the patient be carefully log-rolled to both sides to evaluate the flanks and back. The presence of soft tissue injuries should alert the physician to the possibility of major injury deep to that area. Point tenderness in the spine, ribs, or pelvis may indicate fractures. The presence of blood at the urethral meatus should raise a suspicion of urethral or bladder injury. Rectal exam should look for evidence of rectal injury or pelvic organ disruption such as prostatic separation.

Radiologic studies are important adjuncts to any patient with retroperitoneal hematoma. Patients with suspicion of retroperitoneal hematoma should have a chest x-ray, thoracic and lumbosacral spine films, and pelvic x-rays to evaluate possible bone injuries. Identification of specific fractures will indicate likelihood of possible associated injuries. Examples of this are pancreatic or duodenal injury associated with a lumbar spine fracture or pelvic arterial injury associated with pelvic fractures. The relationship of the arterial anatomy in the lower abdomen and pelvis with the bony structures of the pelvis is shown in Figure 21-2. Disruption of the pelvic ring can lead to laceration of one or more of these arteries resulting in massive pelvic retroperitoneal hematoma.[14,19,20] Complex pelvic fractures may indicate necessity for early arteriogram and possible arterial embolization. A more complete review of these pelvic fractures is found in Chapter 7.

Plain film x-rays are also used for gunshot wounds to evaluate bone injury and to locate missiles. Skin markers of entrance sites are often useful when reviewing these films. Chest x-rays should not be forgotten in evaluation of retroperitoneal injury because of the proximity of the diaphragm and association with pneumothorax or other chest injuries.

CT of the abdomen remains the most readily available and sensitive study for retroperitoneal hematoma and should be the diagnostic test of choice.[21] CT scans can estimate the severity of retroperitoneal hemorrhage and identify its location. Missed injuries associated with CT scans are more often due to errors in reading than insensitivity of the study.

Several series have documented the value of CT scans in injuries of specific retroperitoneal organs such as the pancreas, duodenum, and kidney.[22,23] Figure 21-3 shows an

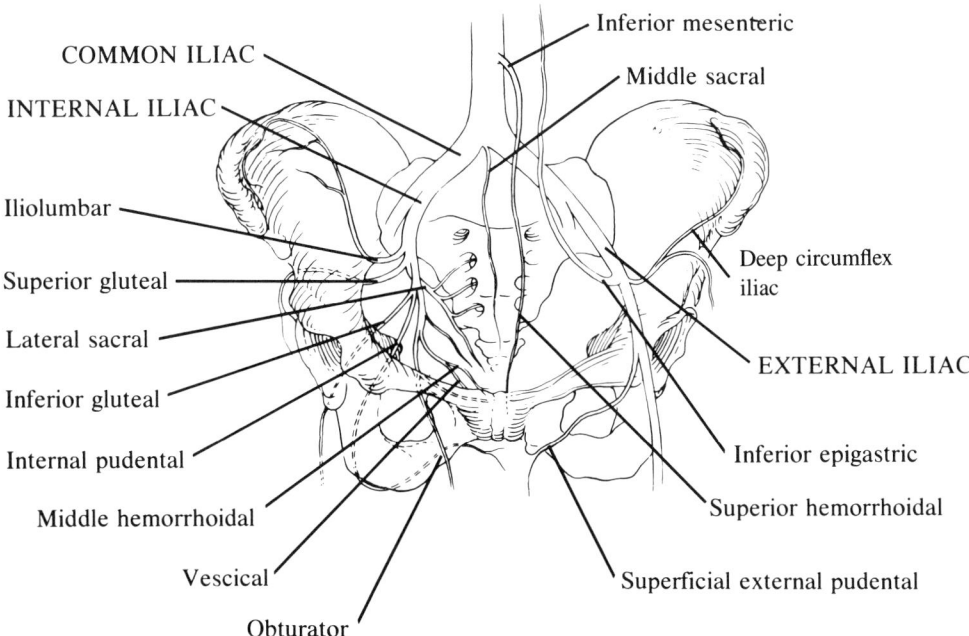

Figure 21-2. Arterial anatomy of the pelvis.

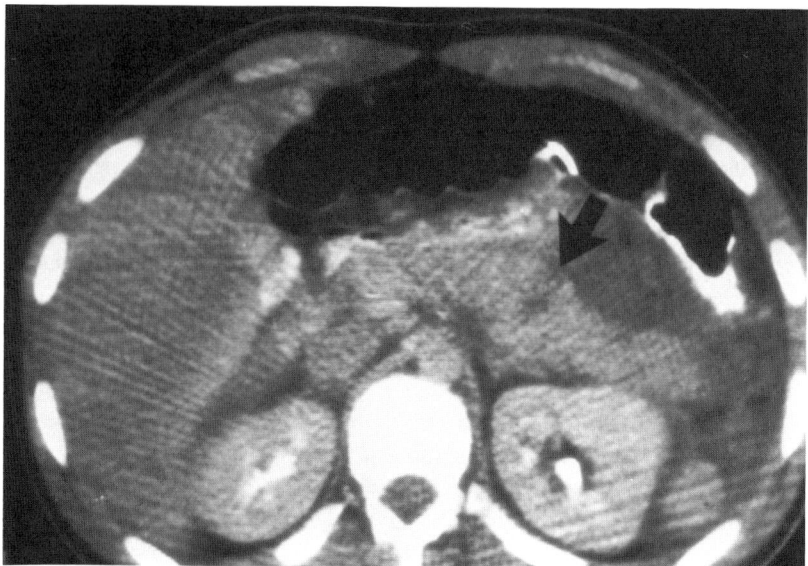

Figure 21–3. Pancreatic injury identified by CT scan (*arrow*).

example of a pancreatic injury identified by CT scan. Figure 21–4 demonstrates renal injury that is well delineated on CT scan. Figure 21–5 shows the CT of a patient who suffered blunt abdominal injury when he was crushed to the ground by a bull. The single cut on his CT scan identifies a pancreatic injury, an infarcted left kidney from a renal artery injury, and a liver injury with free intraperitoneal blood anterior to the kidneys. Abdominal CT scans for trauma should be done with intravenous and oral contrast. If specific concerns are present regarding the lower pelvis, rectal contrast can also be administered. The contrast is useful in outlining the stomach and duodenum, as well as vascular structures, kidneys, and ureters.

An IVP is an alternative test to study the kidneys and ureters. It is more sensitive for urinary extravasation but is inadequate for evaluating injury to the other retroperitoneal organs. It can be used in conjunction with an upper gastrointestinal test using water-soluble contrast to evaluate the duodenum and pancreatic head as an alternative when CT scans are not available. Ultrasound provides another option for imaging retroperitoneal hematomas, but is not widely used.

Cystograms are the best studies to evaluate bladder injury. A complete cystogram requires distention of the bladder and postevacuation films. Although the management of bladder injuries has changed and now includes percutaneous cystostomy or simple Foley catheter drainage for extraperitoneal rupture, the role of cystograms for the diagnosis of bladder injury has not changed.

Arteriography is specifically useful in identifying vascular injuries (Fig. 21–6).[24] These are more common in penetrating injuries but do occur in blunt trauma.[25] An arteriogram may identify a specific vascular lesion such as arteriovenous fistula, suspected on physical exam by a bruit, or acute onset congestive heart failure in an otherwise stable patient. Many times preoperative arteriography is not available to patients with penetrating

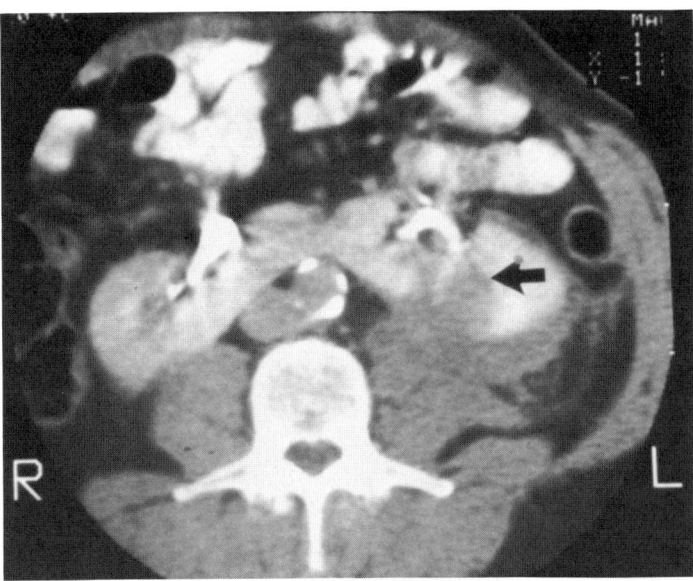

Figure 21–4. Renal injury identified by CT scan (*arrow*).

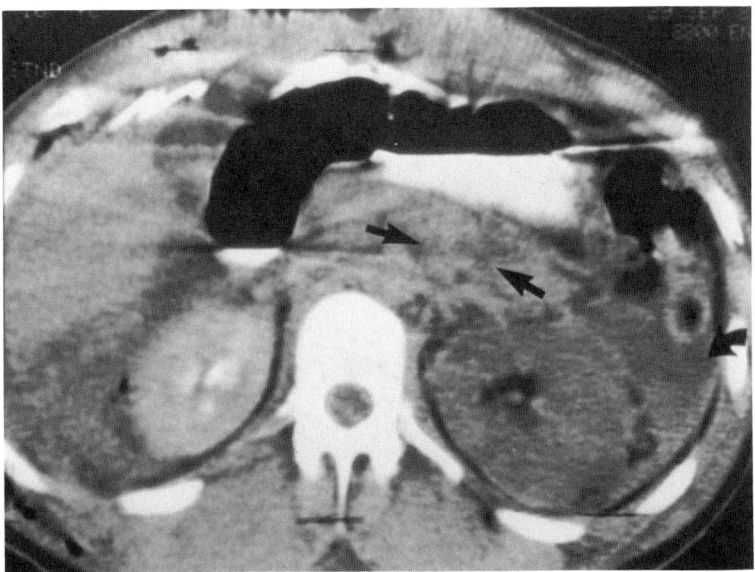

Figure 21–5. Pancreatic injury, left renal infarction, and renal injury demonstrated by the CT scan.

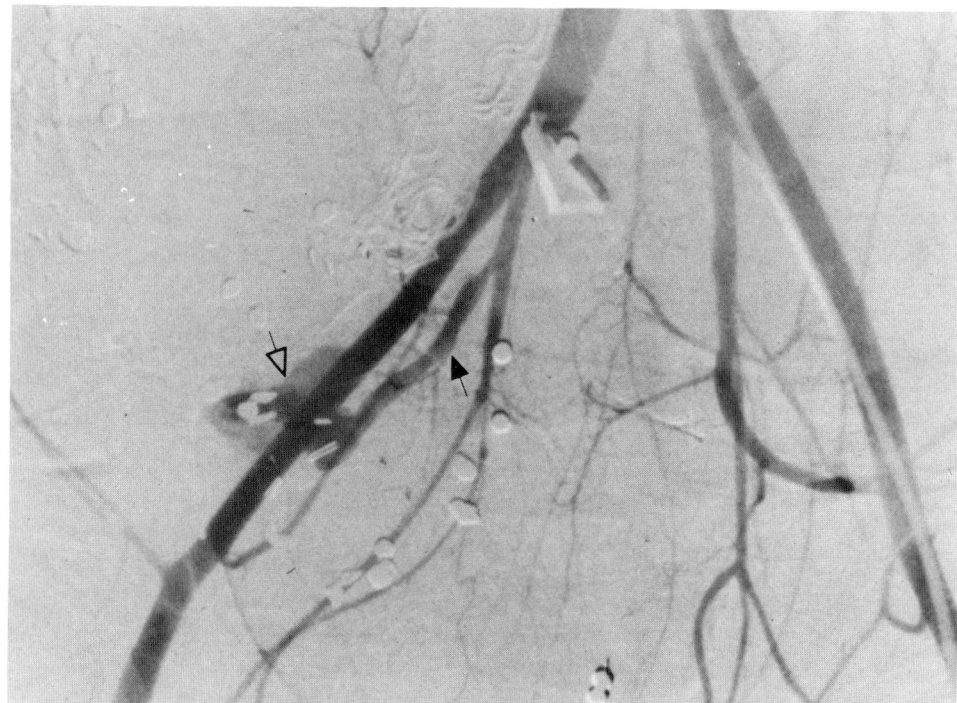

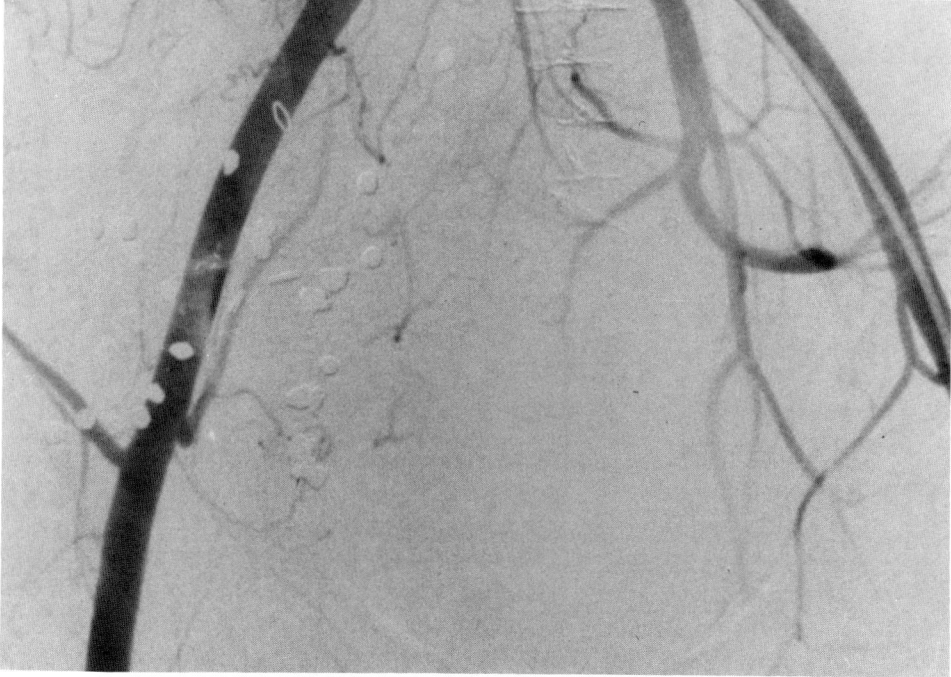

Figure 21–6. **A:** Distal aortogram (before balloon occlusion). Contrast has pooled (*open arrow*) after extravasation from the superior gluteal artery. **B:** Distal aortogram (after balloon occlusion). The internal iliac artery and its branches have been occluded and do not opacify. There is no longer extravasation of contrast. (From Sheldon.[7] Reprinted with permission.)

injuries because of hemodynamic instability and massive hemorrhage, but, when it is possible to obtain this examination, operative treatment is greatly facilitated.

Peritoneal lavage is not particularly helpful in evaluating retroperitoneal injuries. This study may be misleading because a positive peritoneal lavage is generally assumed to indicate abdominal visceral injury. False positive peritoneal lavages from retroperitoneal hematoma are well documented.[26-28] The retroperitoneal injuries responsible for these false positive studies frequently do not require surgery. Peritoneal lavage has also been used to screen for pancreatic, biliary, or duodenal injuries by examining the peritoneal lavage fluid for bile or amylase.[29] These remain relatively insensitive measures and are considered inferior to good imaging studies.

Sigmoidoscopy is useful in evaluation of the rectum and sigmoid colon. Penetrating injuries or lacerations from bone fragments can lead to early fatal sepsis in patients if the injury is not identified and treated appropriately. The presence of blood on rectal exam should raise suspicion about any major pelvic fracture, and any massive pelvic fracture should be evaluated for rectosigmoid injury. An alternative to sigmoidoscopy is a water-soluble contrast enema. It is more difficult to obtain such a study in some patients with pelvic fracture because of the pain resulting from moving and positioning the patient for x-rays.

MANAGEMENT

The principal considerations in the management of retroperitoneal hematoma are, first, whether operative intervention is required and, second, whether exploration of the retroperitoneal hematoma is indicated if the patient is undergoing laparotomy.[30] The presence of blood in the retroperitoneum itself does not indicate a need for surgery. Tests described in the last section on evaluation of retroperitoneal hematoma are designed to determine if there is specific organ injury and estimate the extent of bleeding. Knowledge of the mechanism of injury, the specific site of the hematoma, and any change in the patient's clinical status will determine whether or not exploration is indicated. Emergent surgery is often required in extremely unstable patients. However, operative intervention in stable patients without appropriate diagnostic tests may lead to unnecessary surgery. Furthermore, exploration of certain retroperitoneal hematomas may actually jeopardize the patient.

If a patient is stable and has no other clinical indications for emergency celiotomy, the following options for management can be followed:

Blunt Trauma

1. History of significant torso injury but no clinical symptoms: serial exam and hematocrits, plain film x-rays
2. Injury with pain and falling hematocrit and/or rising amylase: abdominal CT scan, alternately IVP with soluble contrast upper gastrointestinal test
3. Massive or rapidly expanding retroperitoneal hematoma noted on CT scan: arteriogram of abdominal and pelvic vessels.

Penetrating Trauma

1. Gunshot wound: celiotomy with preoperative IVP if concern for renal injury and patient stability tolerates this

2. Stab wound: if the patient is totally asymptomatic, simple observation may be appropriate. If suspicion of organ injury is significant, IVP and hypaque enema or abdominopelvic CT with rectal contrast. If the patient has peritoneal signs or shock, emergent celiotomy should be performed.

If the patient requires emergent abdominal exploration and diagnostic procedures are not done preoperatively, retroperitoneal hematoma may be encountered intraoperatively.[15,30] A management plan for the retroperitoneal hematoma must be made at that time. In considering operative management, the mechanism of injury and location of retroperitoneal hematoma are two important factors. The retroperitoneum can be divided into three zones for the purpose of considering exploration. These zones are shown in Figure 21–7. Zone I is the upper central area of the retroperitoneum. This corresponds to the area from the diaphragmatic hiatus of the aorta and esophagus and extends to the sacral promontory. Primary structures in this area are the aorta, vena cava, proximal renal vessels, portal vein, pancreas, and duodenum. Zone II consists of the right and the left flank. It contains the kidneys and suprapelvic ureters. Zone II on the right also includes the right colon and mesocolon, and Zone II on the left includes the left colon and mesocolon. Zone III consists of the pelvis and it contains the sigmoid colon and rectum, the bladder, and the distal pelvic segment of the ureters.

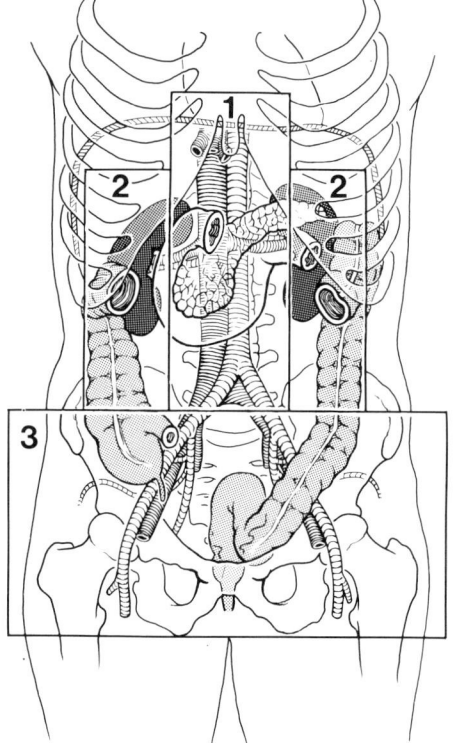

Figure 21–7. Relation of anatomic zones to indication for exploration of retroperitoneal hematomas, correlating the retroperitoneal anatomy with indications for operative management. *Zone 1*: Central–medial retroperitoneal hematomas. *Zone 2*: Flank retroperitoneal hematomas. *Zone 3*: Pelvic retroperitoneal hematomas.

Management of specific organ injuries is described elsewhere in this text. Pancreatic, duodenal, vascular, colonic, or renal injuries should be managed with established techniques. Consideration should always be given to the fact that other injuries may exist and thorough exploration may be necessary. The remainder of this chapter will concentrate on strategies for decision to explore the retroperitoneal hematoma and general principles of management. Management plans for retroperitoneal hematoma are separated by the nature of the injury. Decisions on operative exploration of retroperitoneal hematomas should be considered separately for blunt and penetrating trauma.

Blunt Injuries

Operative decisions for management of retroperitoneal hematomas for blunt injuries use the zones described in Figure 21–7 in the decision-making process.[12] Retroperitoneal hematomas in Zone I are usually not due to major vascular injury. There is considerable concern, however, for injuries to the pancreas and duodenum; therefore, Zone I retroperitoneal hematoma from blunt trauma should be explored. Generous exposure of the duodenum and posterior head of the pancreas by the Kocher maneuver and evaluation of the anterior surface of the pancreas by entrance into the lesser sac through the omentum near the stomach should be performed. Major vessels in Zone I can also be exposed and evaluated if appropriate. The tissue should be inspected for small bleeding vessels or evidence of bile or gas to suggest pancreatic or duodenal injury. If such injuries are identified, they should be managed as outlined in Chapter 9.

In general, simple retroperitoneal hematomas in Zone II are not explored unless they are rapidly expanding or there are signs of specific organ injury such as colon perforation.[31] If exploration is necessary, the colon is mobilized laterally to medially with care to not injure the mesocolon. Management of colon injuries is outlined in Chapter 12. If the hematoma relates to the kidney, it will most often resolve with time and require no operative intervention (see Chapter 14).[32] However, if the hematoma outside Gerota's fascia is enlarging rapidly, exploration may be necessary.[33] If the kidney is to be explored, it is important to gain control of the renal artery and vein at the aorta and vena cava before opening Gerota's fascia. It is also important to have some knowledge about the state of bilateral renal function before exploration of the kidney. If an IVP was not done preoperatively, one can be done before renal exploration in order to document presence of bilateral nephrograms. If the injured kidney is the only one with function, every effort should be made to preserve it.

Retroperitoneal hematoma in Zone III from blunt trauma usually should not be explored.[12] Nonexpanding retroperitoneal hematomas are treated with observation.[6] Patients with expanding Zone III retroperitoneal hematomas should be closed quickly and taken to arteriography. Not only will arteriography assist with the diagnosis, but it can be used to treat the hemorrhage itself.[13] Detachable balloons can be used to occlude major bleeding vessels and smaller bleeding arterial vessels can be embolized. Opening Zone III pelvic hematomas in an attempt to identify and oversew the bleeding source is relatively futile and is associated with further hemorrhage that may be impossible to control.

If pelvic fracture is the cause of Zone III retroperitoneal hematoma, immediate reduction and fixation usually stop the hemorrhaging and improve survival. This is usually accomplished with external pelvic fixation but can also be done with internal fixation in some cases.[34] This management is specifically described in Chapter 7. This is the optimal treatment and in almost all cases will result in prevention of further hemorrhage.

Pneumatic Anti-shock Trousers (or MAST suits) can be used to control lower retroperitoneal and pelvic hemorrhage in some patients.[19] This is usually used only in those patients in whom bleeding persists where there are not specific injuries or vessels to be ligated or occluded. Patients with pelvic fracture and continued nonarterial bleeding are those most likely to benefit from these devices. Inflation of the leg and abdominal compartments will provide some tamponade effect by increasing external pressure. It is important to monitor the patients closely when this device is used. These garments are associated with potential complications. Conversion of closed to open fractures as well as skin breakdown and necrosis have been described.

Penetrating Injuries

In general, all retroperitoneal hematomas from penetrating trauma should be explored if the abdomen is already open. If laparotomy is not otherwise planned, the specific nature of the penetrating weapon should be considered. Gunshot wounds to the trunk usually require laparotomy, and the evaluation of a retroperitoneal hematoma is part of that exploration.[35] Patients suffering stab wounds, however, are often not explored and are frequently managed by observation without further diagnostic tests.[31,36] If the patient with the stab wound is explored, however, the management is no different from that of a gunshot wound.

Stab wounds to the anterior chest or abdomen may cause retroperitoneal hematoma. Indications for abdominal exploration for stab wounds are outlined in Chapter 1. Stab wounds to the back and flank require surgical intervention less often than those to the abdomen. Chest x-rays, observation, and selected radiographic procedures are indicated.[31,36] If a vascular injury is suspected, proximal and distal control should be obtained before opening the hematoma at the point of penetrating injury.[37] The techniques for isolating vessels are described elsewhere in this text and in other texts.[9] The importance of these efforts cannot be emphasized enough.[38] If massive bleeding is present at the time of exploration, direct pressure at the point of bleeding may be necessary while proximal and distal control is obtained. It is important to coordinate these efforts with that of the anesthesiologist and the rest of the operating room team. This will ensure having blood, equipment, and instruments immediately available to accomplish repair once the task is undertaken. Repeated unsuccessful efforts with massive blood loss because of inadequate exposure, lack of blood for transfusion, or unavailability of appropriate instruments or supplies greatly increase the risk to the patient.

Retroperitoneal hematomas from stab wounds that are not associated with evidence of significant bleeding or specific organ injury can be observed. Observation includes repeated physical exams and serial determinations of blood count to assess perforation of hollow viscus or continued bleeding. Many retroperitoneal hematomas from stab wounds to the back will not require operative intervention, but it is essential that clinical deterioration be quickly evaluated and treated. Development of clinical signs of shock or peritonitis, even when diagnostic studies have been negative, indicates need for emergent exploration. All radiologic exams may have false negative findings, and the presence of clinical signs should themselves be adequate reason for exploration.

COMPLICATIONS

Retroperitoneal hematomas are associated with significant complications because of the magnitude of injury, the amount of blood loss, and problems due to occasional missed injuries. Most retroperitoneal hematomas from blunt trauma have other associated injuries. These additional injuries slow recovery and limit mobilization of the patient. This relative immobility increases risk for atelectasis, pneumonia, skin breakdown, and general debility. Efforts to prevent these problems by chest physical therapy, early ambulation when possible, and general protective care are important.[39] Attention to routine supportive measures including nutrition and physical therapy will limit complications.

Coagulopathy can occur in patients with retroperitoneal hematoma who require massive transfusions. This coagulopathy can lead to activation of humoral mediators that further impair other organ systems and may cause early adult respiratory distress syndrome or multiple organ failure.[40] Prompt attention to limit bleeding and resuscitate the patient rapidly is important to prevent coagulopathy. If it does occur, coagulopathy should be treated by replacement therapy and circulatory stabilization.[41]

Nutritional dysfunction from ileus and duodenal obstruction secondary to retroperitoneal hematoma can occur.[42,43] Parenteral nutrition is useful in many of these patients and provides caloric supplementation as well as correction of protein malnutrition. However, enteral feedings should be reinstituted as soon as possible. This can be done by placement of feeding jejunostomy at the time of exploration if celiotomy is undertaken. If this is not available, then placement of a feeding tube into the duodenum should be undertaken as a means to try to restore enteral feeding. Correction of nutritional deficiencies will permit a more normal healing rate and help to correct immune dysfunction associated with trauma and malnutrition.

Renal failure remains a concern in patients with retroperitoneal hematoma. Renal failure may develop as a consequence of diminished perfusion, injury to the kidney itself, myoglobulinuria, or even pressure from the retroperitoneal hematoma.[44] In evaluating patients with deteriorating renal function from retroperitoneal hematoma, it is essential to assess the adequacy of renal blood flow. If there is doubt about renal blood flow despite adequate cardiac output, a nuclear medicine renal scan or arteriogram can be obtained. Possible postrenal obstruction should be evaluated using ultrasound to evaluate any ureteral or bladder obstruction. Other uncommon complications include femoral neuropathy and pulmonary microembolism.[45–47]

RESULTS

Retroperitoneal hematoma is associated with considerable morbidity and mortality. However, there are no frequent long-term sequelae to the hematoma itself. If there are no organ injuries or major fractures, there will be little prolonged disability from retroperitoneal hematoma. Most morbidity in patients with retroperitoneal hematoma is from injuries to specific retroperitoneal organs or structures or from their associated injuries.

Mortality from retroperitoneal hematoma also is affected by concomitant injury, but the retroperitoneal hematoma itself can cause death.[16] The mortality of four series of patients with retroperitoneal hematoma is shown in Table 21–4.[2,10–12] The series de-

Table 21-4 Mortality Associated with Retroperitoneal Hematoma

	MORTALITY (%)	NO. OF PATIENTS
Bayliss et al.[2]	18	50
Allen et al.[6]	24	75
Nick et al.[11]	31	65
Selivanov et al.[12]	13	81

scribed by Selivanov had a higher mortality in pelvic fractures compared with all other causes of retroperitoneal hematomas.[12] Some of these patients had other injuries, but the considerable mortality indicates that the presence of retroperitoneal hematoma should demand close attention to its management.

REFERENCES

1. Cushman GF, Kilgore AR. Syndrome of mesenteric or subperitoneal hemorrhage. *Ann Surg*. 1941; 114:672.
2. Bayliss SM, Lansing EH, Glas WW. Traumatic retroperitoneal hematoma. *Am J Surg*. 1962; 103:477.
3. Seavers R, Lynch J, Ballard R. Hypogastric artery ligation for uncontrollable hemorrhage in acute pelvic trauma. *Surgery*. 1964; 55:516.
4. Ravitch MM. Hypogastric artery ligation in acute pelvic trauma. *Surgery*. 1964; 56:601.
5. Ger R, Condrea H, Steichen FM. Traumatic intrapelvic retroperitoneal hemorrhage. *J Surg Res*. 1969; 9:31.
6. Allen RE, Eastman BA, Haller BL, Conolly WB. Retroperitoneal hemorrhage secondary to blunt trauma. *Am J Surg*. 1969; 118:558.
7. Sheldon GF, Weinstock DP. Hemorrhage from an open pelvic fracture controlled intraoperatively with a balloon catheter. *J Trauma*. 1978; 18:68.
8. Trunkey DD, Chapman MW, Liss NC Jr, Dunphy JE. Management of pelvic fractures in blunt trauma injury. *J Trauma* 1974; 14:912.
9. Feliciano DV, Burch JM, Graham JM. Abdominal vascular injury. *J Trauma*. 1988; 31:519–536.
10. Greico JG, Perry JF. Retroperitoneal hematoma following trauma: its significance. *J Trauma*. 1980;16.
11. Nick WV, Zollinger RW, Pace WG. Retroperitoneal hemorrhage after blunt abdominal trauma. *J Trauma*. 1967; 7(5):653–659.
12. Selivanov V, Chi HS. Alverdy JA. Morris JA Jr. Sheldon GF. Mortality in retroperitoneal hematoma. *J Trauma*. 1984; 24:1022–1027.
13. Flint LM, Brown A, Richardson JD, Polk HC. Definitive control of bleeding from severe pelvic fractures. *Ann Surg*. 1979; 198(6):709–716.
14. Hamilton SG. Pelvic fractures and their complications. *Proc Roy Soc Med*. 1973; 66:629–631.
15. Hawkins L, Pomerantz M, Eisenman B. Laparotomy at the time of pelvic fracture. *J Trauma*. 1970; 10(8):619–623.
16. Rothenberger DA, Fischer RP, Strate RG, Velasco R, Perry JF. The mortality associated with pelvic fractures. *Surgery*. 1978; 84(3):356–361.
17. Manenti A, Malagoli M, Gibertini G, Miselli A, Rossi A. Shock and traumatic retroperitoneal hematoma: diagnostic and therapeutic problems. *Resuscitation*. 1989; 18(2–3):159.
18. Henao R, Aldrette JS. Retroperitoneal hematomas of traumatic origin. *Surg Gynecol Obstet*. 1985; 161: 106–116.
19. Moreno C, Moore EE, Rosenberger A, Cleveland HC. Hemorrhage associated with major pelvic fracture: a multi-specialty challenge. *J Trauma*. 1986; 26:987–993.
20. Trunkey DD, Chapman MW, Lim RC, Dunphy JE. Management of pelvic fractures in blunt trauma injury. *J Trauma*. 1974; 14(11):912–923.
21. Federle MP, Brant-Zawadzki M, eds. *Computed Tomography in the Evaluation of Trauma*. 2nd ed. Baltimore: Wilkins and Wilkins; 1986.
22. Jeffrey RB Jr, Federle MP, Crass RA. Computed tomography of pancreatic trauma. *Radiology*. 1983; 147:491–494.
23. McAninch JW, Federle MP. Evaluation of renal injuries with computerized tomography. *J Urol*. 1982; 128:456–460.

24. Levin DC, Watson RC, Baltaxe HA. Arteriography of retroperitoneal masses. *Radiology*. 1973; 108(3): 543–551.
25. Lois JF, Levin DC, Hooshmand I. Angiography of nonneoplastic retroperitoneal masses. *Cardiovasc Intervent Radiol*. 1982; 5(6):312–317.
26. de Vries JE, van der Slike W. False positive peritoneal lavage due to retroperitoneal hematoma. *Injury*. 1980; 12:191–193.
27. Hubbard SG, Bivins BA, Sachatello CR, Griffen WO. Diagnostic errors with peritoneal lavage in patients with pelvic fractures. *Arch Surg*. 1979; 114:844–846.
28. Parvin S, Smith DG, Asher M, et al. Effectiveness of diagnostic peritoneal lavage in blunt trauma. *Ann Surg*. 1975; 181:255–261.
29. Kearney PA Jr, Vahey T, Burney RE, Glazer G. Computed tomography and diagnostic peritoneal lavage in blunt abdominal trauma: their combined role. *Arch Surg*. 1989; 124:344–347.
30. Lambert CJ, Levin HJ, Bergman PA. Concomitant retroperitoneal exploration for abdomino-renal trauma: when and why? *Milit Med*. 1966; 131:277–280.
31. Weil PH. Management of retroperitoneal trauma. *Curr Probl Surg*. 1983; 20:539–620.
32. Lucey DT, Smith MJV, Koontz WW. A plea for the conservative treatment of renal injuries. *J Trauma*. 1971; 11(4):306–316.
33. Holcroft JW, Trunkey DD, Minagi H, Korobkin MT, Lim RC. Renal trauma and retroperitoneal hematomas: indications for exploration. *J Trauma*. 1975; 15(12):1045–1052.
34. Goldstein A, Phillips T, Schafuni SJA, et al. Early open reduction and internal fixation of the disrupted pelvic ring. *J Trauma*. 1986; 26:325–333.
35. Steichen FM, Dargan EL, Pearlman DM, Weil PH. The management of retroperitoneal hematoma secondary to penetrating injuries. *Surg Gynecol Obstet*. 1966; 123(1):581–591.
36. Shaftan GW. Retroperitoneal trauma. *Contemp Surg*. 1980; 16:25–35.
37. Costa M, Robbs JF. Management of retroperitoneal hematoma following penetrating trauma. *Br J Surg*. 1985; 72:662–664.
38. Feliciano DV. Management of traumatic retroperitoneal hematoma. *Ann Surg*. 1990; 211:109–123.
39. Meyer AA, Trunkey DD. Critical care as an integral part of trauma care. *Crit Care Med*. 1986;2: 673–682.
40. Pottmeyer E, Vassar MJ, Holcroft JW. Coagulation, inflammation, and responses to injury. *Crit Care Med*. 1986; 2:683–703.
41. Rutledge R, Sheldon GF, Collins ML. Massive transfusion. *Crit Care Med*. 1986; 2:791–805.
42. Drew JH. Ileus in retroperitoneal hematoma. *Med J Aust*. 1973; 1:246–248.
43. Gue S. Obstruction of second part of duodenum by retroperitoneal hematoma due to blunt abdominal trauma: a report of two cases. *Injury*. 1972; 4(1):65–68.
44. Jacques T, Lee R. Improvement of renal function after relief of raised intraabdominal pressure due to traumatic retroperitoneal hematoma. *Anesth Inten Care*. 1988; 16(4):478–482.
45. Ho KJ. Diffuse fatal pulmonary microembolism of retroperitoneal extravascular origin. *Arch Pathol Lab Med*. 1989; 113(12):1401–1403.
46. MacSweeney ST. Spontaneous retroperitoneal hematoma presenting as femoral neuropathy. Case Report. *Acta Chir Scand*. 1989; 155(11–12):621–622.
47. Mastroianni PP, Roberts MP. Femoral neuropathy and retroperitoneal hemorrhage. *Neurosurgery*. 1983; 13(1):44–47.

Index

(Italics indicate a table or a figure)

Abbreviated injury score (AIS), 218
Abdominal aorta, 344, *348*, 351, 365
Abdominal arterial trauma, 341–369
    anatomy, 344–347
    assessment, 347–348
    atherosclerotic, 365
    complications, 366–368
    exposure of specific injuries, 351–355
    history, 341
    initial operative management, 349–351
    management of specific injuries, 356–360
    mechanism of injury, 343
    pathophysiology, 342–343
    postoperative management, 365–366
    preoperative management, 348–349
    results, 368–369
    techniques of repair, 360–365
Abdominal trauma
    "conservation (nonoperative) management," 63–64
    general assessment, 1–12
    peritoneal lavage, 32–42
    resuscitation, 13–28
    surgery for, 57–70
        conduct of, 65–70
        indications, 58–63
        preoperative preparation, 64–65
    see also Abdominal arterial trauma; Abdominal venous trauma; Blunt trauma; Penetrating trauma
Abdominal venous trauma, 371–395
    anatomy, 373–375
    assessment, 376
    complications, 395
    history, 371–372
    mechanism of injury and pathophysiology, 372–373
    operative exploration and exposure, 377–385
    operative treatment, 391–392

    postoperative care, 392–393
    preoperative preparation, 376–377
    results, 393–394
    technical considerations, 385, 387–389
Abdominal wall injuries, 72–82
    anatomy, 74–77
    assessment, 77–80
    complications, 82
    definitive treatment, 80–81
    history, 72
    indications for operation, 80
    mechanism and significance of, 73–74
Air dermatome, 301
Airway, 14–16
Amniocentesis, 333
Amniotic membranes, 337
Anastomosis
    and abdominal venous trauma, *379*, 385, 387, 388, 389
    of colon, 220
    large vessel, *364*
    of small bowel, 203–204, *205*, 207
    small vessel, *363*
Angiography, 50–52
Antibiotics, 64, 219, 365
Arterial contusions, 342
Arteries *see* Abdominal arterial trauma; specific arteries
Arteriography, 351, 404
Arteriovenous fistulae (AVF), 388–389, *390*
Ascending colon, *221, 222*
Atherosclerotic arterial trauma, 365
Atrial caval shunting, 177
Avulsion injury, 73, 80, 81, 299

Back side, 8
Bentley autotransfusion device, 381
Bilateral hemothoraces, *48*
Bile duct, 150–152, 167–168

Biliary tract injuries, 147–150
Bladder, 69
  anatomy, 288
  complications, 291
  injuries, 62, 288–291
    assessment of, 288–289
    evaluation and repair, 289–291
    history, 277
  postoperative care, 291
Bleeding
  abdominal arterial trauma, 366
  abdominal venous trauma, 372, *380*
  bladder, 291
  liver, 176
  overt, 7
  pelvic, 103
  small bowel, 200–201, 207
  splenic, 247
  vaginal, 316
Blood pressure, 330–331
Blood transfusions, 218, 237
Blunt trauma
  of abdominal arteries, 342, 343
  abdominal venous, 376
  abdominal wall, 73, 80
  of diaphragm, 83, 85, 86, 89
  of duodenum, 62, 120, 128–129
  of female genitals, 313–314
  history, 1–2
  indications for surgery, 61–63
  lab and x-ray exams, 11–12
  of liver, 169, 187–188
  pathophysiology and etiology, 2, 5
  and peritoneal lavage, 34
  in pregnancy, 328–329, 338
  primary survey, 5–8
  retroperitoneal hematoma, 401, 407, 409–410
  secondary survey, 8–10
  and testicular rupture, 296
Bouchacourt's sign, 80
Bowel *see* Small bowel; Large bowel
Breathing *see* Respiration
Buck's fascia, 279
Burns, 300, 330

Cardiac compressive shock, 16, 23–24
Cardiovascular system, 14, 326
Catheters, 37, *39*, 178, 379, 381, *383*
Celiac artery, 345
Celiac axis, *353*, 357, 364

Celiotomy, 215, 219
Central nervous system, 14, 328, 335
Cervix, 316
Cesarean section, 336
Chest
  injuries, 72–82
    during pregnancy, 335
  inspection of, 8
  x-ray, 11, 88, *89*, 90
Circulation, 6–7, 16–25
  cardiac compressive shock, 16, 23–24
  collateral, 345–347
  hemorrhagic shock, 16, 17, 18–23
  neurogenic shock, 16, 24–25
  pathophysiology, 17–18
Coagulation, 395
Coagulopathy, 366, 411
Colles' fascia, 299
Colon, 200, *354*, 386
  anatomy and physiology, 211–212
  arterial supply, *213*
  ascending, *221*, *222*
  blood transfusions, 218
  complications, 226–227
  descending, *353*
  Flint severity score, 219
  methods of repair, 219–224
  operative exposure and evaluation, 215–216
  postoperative care, 225–226
  primary repair, 219–224
  sigmoid, *356*
  trauma to,
    adjunctive antibiotics, 219
    assessment of severity, 218–219
    associated risk factors, 216–218
    etiology and incidence, 210–211
    history, 209–210
    initial assessment, 213–214
    local wound exploration, 214
    pathophysiology, 212–213
    wound management, 225
Colostomy, 103–104, 220–223, *225*, 226
Computerized tomography, 42–49, 63
  for colon and rectum, 215
  for esophageal, gastric, and omental injuries, 112–113
  history, 42
  for liver injuries, 170–171
  versus peritoneal lavage, 49–50
  during pregnancy, 334

rationale and indications/contraindications, 42–43
for renal trauma, 256, *259*, *405*
results, 45
for retroperitoneal hematoma, 402–404, *405*
for small bowel injuries, 197
for spleen, *236*
technique, 43–45
for ureteral injury, 267, *269*
Constrictive bands, penile, 300
Contour, of abdomen, 9
Corpus cavernosum, 296
CT *see* Computerized tomography
Cystogram, 280, *282*, *285*, 288–289, *290*, 404

Decompensated shock, 17
Descending colon, *353*
Diagnostic peritoneal lavage (DPL), 214–215
Diametric fractures, 96–97, *98*
Diaphragm
anatomy, 83–85
average location, *10*
injuries, *61*
assessment of and preoperative work-up, 87–90
general mechanism, 85–86
pattern of, 86–87
treatment, 91–92
see also rupture *below*
postoperative management, 92
preoperative preparation, 90–91
rupture, 24, 62, 83–92
complications, 92
history, 83
tears, 91–92
Disseminated intravascular coagulation (DIC), 337, 338
Distal aortogram, *406*
Distal pancreatic resection, 139
Diverticulization procedure, 144, 146–147
Duodenojejunostomy, 141, *143*, 144, *145*
Duodenum, *354*, *386*
anatomy, 123, 125–128
blood vessels, 126
blunt trauma, 62, 120, 128–129
injuries, 120, 123, 124–125, 141
assessment of, 128–131
associated, 141
and biliary tract injuries, 147–150

classification of, 135–136
combined with bile duct and major pancreatic ductal injuries, 150–152
complications, 153–156
evaluation of, 134–135
isolated in absence of injury to pancreas or bile duct, 141–144
laceration, 144–147
mortality, 141
operative exploration and evaluation, 132–134
preoperative preparation, 131–132
rationale for choice of operation, 136–137

Endotracheal intubation, 15, 64, *383*
Esophageal, gastric, and omental injuries, 110–117
anatomy, 111–112
assessment, 112–113
blunt trauma, 62
complications and results, 116–117
definitive operative treatment, 115–116
history, 110
initial operative exposure and treatment, 113–115
postoperative management, 116
preoperative care, 113
Ethanol and resuscitation, 19
External sphincter, 280
Extrahepatic biliary tree, 185
Extremities, 10

Face, 7, 8
Fallopian tubes, 316
False aneurysms, 342
Fecal contamination, 217–218
Female genitals
anatomy, 311–313
assessment and management of injuries, 315–317
blunt trauma, 313–314
mechanism of injury, 313–315
penetrating trauma, 314–315
sports injuries, 314
Femoral vein, *384*
Fetus, 331–333, 337, 338–339
Fistulas, 153–154, 221, 223, *225*, 388–389
Fractures
diametric, 96–97, *98*
isolated, 98
pelvic, 51–52, 94–108, 280, 283, 317–319, 329

rib, 14
splenic, 241
stable, 98, *99*, 103
unstable, 96, 103
French catheter, *178*

Gastric blood supply, *112*
Gastric injuries *see* Esophageal, gastric, and omental injuries
Gastrointestinal system, 327
Genitals, female *see* Female genitals
Genital skin loss, 299–300
Gerota's capsule, 216
Gerota's fascia, 252, 253, 352
Glasgow Coma Scale, 26
Grafts
  for abdominal arterial trauma, 361, 364
  for abdominal venous trauma, 385, *389*, *390*
  penile, 301–303
  scrotal, 305–307
Gunshot wounds
  and abdominal trauma, 3–4
  abdominal wall, 73
  of female genitals, 314
  indications for surgery, 59
  laparotomy for, 1
  pelvic, 107
  during pregnancy, 337
  of prostatic urethra, *283*
  rectal and colonic, 212–213
  retroperitoneal hematoma, 401–402, 407, 410
  of small bowel, 193
  see also Shotgun injuries

Head injury, 25–27
Hematologic system, 326–327
Hematoma
  abdominal wall, 81
  mesenteric, 199, 200–201
  pelvic, 282
  perineal, 315
  rectus, 78
  see also Retroperitoneal hematoma
Hemopericardium, 24
Hemorrhage *see* Bleeding
Hemorrhagic shock, 16, 17, 18–23, 25
Hemothorax, 82
Hepatic artery, 164–166, 185, 352
Hepatic parenchyma, *170*
Hepatic resection, 178, 180–184

Hepatic trauma *see* Liver
Hepatic veins, 167
Hepatotomy, 175
Hernia, 83
Hilar injury, 241, *246*
Hollow viscus injury, 58, 61–62
Hyperventilation, 26
Hypotension, 64, 365
Hypovolemia, 19, 26, 202, 241, 330
Hysterectomy, 316

Ileostomy, 220
Ileum, 192, *193*, *194*
Iliac arteries, 352, 353, *355*, 359, *360*, *361*, *362*, 364, 379, *406*
Iliac veins, 373, 378, *379*, *384*, 391
Iliolumbar ligament, 96
Imaging
  for pelvic fractures, 100–102
  see also specific methods
In extremis management, 27–28
Infection, 106, 226, 299, 367
Inferior epigastric artery, 76
Inferior mesenteric artery, 346–347, 352, 359, 364
Inferior vena cava, *354*, 373, *384*, *390*, 394
Infrarenal aorta, 352, 359
Infrarenal vena cava, 391
Injury severity scale (ISS), 218
Intercostal nerves, 76
Internal sphincter, 279–280
Intraabdominal abscess, 367–368
Intravenous urogram (IVU), 256, 257, 267, *268*
Intubation, endotracheal *see* Endotracheal intubation
Ischemia, of bowel, 207–208
IVU *see* Intravenous urogram

Jaundice, 187
Jejunum, 192, *193*, *194*

Kidney, *48*, *51*, *353*
  anatomy, 252–254
  see also Renal trauma
Kleihauer-Betke test, 337
Kocher maneuver, 184, *354*, 378
Kussmaul's sign, 23

Laparotomy, 1, 59, 64–65, 91, 131–132, 190, 198
Large bowel, *212*

Left atrial segmentectomy, 181
Left gastric artery, 357
Left hepatic lobectomy, 181, *182*
Lithotomy, 277
Liver, 382, *384*
    anatomy, 161
        segmental, 161–164
    bile ducts, 167–168
    complications, 186–187
    drainage, 183, *184*
    Heaney maneuver, 177
    hepatic artery, 164–166
    hepatic veins, 167
    injuries, 160–188
        "Bear claw," 168, *169*
        classification, 172
        diagnosis and preoperative management, 169–171
        history, 160–161
        laceration, *46*
        minor, 74, *173*
        patterns of, 168–169
        results, 187–188
        treatment, 171–178
    portal vein, 166–167
    postoperative management, 186
    transplantation, 183
Lower urinary tract injury, 278

Magnetic resonance imaging, 53
Medical history, 10–11
Mesenteric artery, *201*
Mesenteric vein, *201*, 391, 394
Mesenteric vessels, 200
Meshed split thickness grafts, 302, *306*
Microvascular endothelial membrane, 18
Midline abdominal incision, 65, *66*, 132, 258, 290
Midline longitudinal abdominal wall incision, 77
Molestation, 319
Motor vehicle accidents *see* Traffic accidents
MRI *see* Magnetic resonance imaging
Mucous fistula, 221, 223, *225*
Musculoskeletal system, 328

Neck, 8
Nephrectomy, 251, 261, 262, 264
Neurogenic shock, 16, 24–25
Neurologic disability, 7
Nutrition, 411

Omental injuries *see* Esophageal, gastric, and omental injuries
Operations *see* Surgery; specific techniques and body parts
Organogenesis, 333
Ovaries, 316–317

Pain, 80
Pancreas, 69, *354*, *386*
    anatomy, 123, 125–128
    blood vessels, 126, *127*
    contusion of head, *47*
    injury to, 121–122, *405*
        assessment of, 128–131
        classification of, 135–136
        combined with duodenal and common bile duct injuries, 150–152
        complications, 153–156
        evaluation of, 134–135
        history, 118–120
        major ductal disruptions in head with associated duodenal laceration, 144–147
        and splenic injury, 246
        types of trauma, 137–140
    operative exploration and evaluation, 132–134
    postoperative care, 152–153
    preoperative preparation, 131–32
    preservation of tail, *140*
    rationale for choice of operation, 136–137
Pancreatic duct, 126, *130*
Pancreatitis, 154–155
Paracentesis, 32–33
Parietal peritoneum, 77
Pelvic abscess, *50*
Pelvic fractures, *49*, 94–108, 280, 283
    anatomy, 95–96
    assessment, 99–100
    complications, 106–107
    history, 94
    imaging, 100–102
    open, 317–319
    operative preparation and indication, 102
    postoperative management, 105–106
    in pregnancy, 329
    results, 107–108
    traumatic hemipelvectomy, 104–105
    treatment, 102–104
    types, 96–98
Pelvis, arterial anatomy, *403*

Penetrating abdominal trauma index (PATI), 218
Penetrating trauma
  of abdominal arteries, 343
  of diaphragm, 85, 86, 87–89, 91
  of female genitals, 314–315
  history, 1–2
  indications for operation, 58–61
  lab and x-ray exams, 11–12
  pathophysiology and etiology, 2–4
  in pregnancy, 330
  primary survey, 5–8
  retroperitoneal hematoma, 401, 407–408, 410
  secondary survey, 8–10
  thoracic, 14
Penile flaps, 303
Penile rupture, 293–296
  clinical findings, 294
  diagnosis, 294–295
  mechanism of, 294
  therapy, 295–296
Penile skin loss, 300–303
Perineal laceration, 103
Perineal region, female, 311–312, 315
Perirenal anatomy, 252–254
Perirenal aorta, 358–359
Peritoneal dialysis catheter, 37, *39*
Peritoneal irritation, 78
Peritoneal lavage, 32–42, 63, 64
  complications, 42
  versus computerized tomography, 49–50
  contraindications, 35–36
  diagnostic, 214–215
  history, 32–33
  interpretation, 40–41
  rapidity, 34
  rationale and indications, 33–35
  results, 41–42
  retroperitoneal injuries, 407
  technique, 36–40
Periurethral area, 315
Phrenic nerves, 84, *85*
Placenta, 325, 328, 336–337
Porta hepatis, 184–186
Portal triad, 175, 392
Portal vein, 127–128, 166–167, 184, 375, *381*, *386*, 392, 394
Portal venous system, 374–375, 395
Posterior peritoneum, *381*
Posterolateral aorta, *353*

Pregnancy, 324–339
  abdominal injuries and operative management, 335
  anatomy of, 324–325
    cardiovascular system, 326
    gastrointestinal system, 327
    hematologic system, 326–327
    musculoskeletal system, 328
    respiratory system, 327
    urinary system, 327–328
  blunt trauma in, 328–329, 338
  burns, 330
  central nervous system, 328, 335
  complications and postoperative care, 338
  diagnostic procedures, 333–334
  direct fetal injury, 336
  initial assessment and treatment of injury, 330–334
  injuries to uterus and placenta, 336–337
  management of maternal injuries, 335–337
  mechanism of injury, 328–330
  penetrating trauma in, 330
  physiology of, 325–328
  primary assessment of fetus, 331–333
  primary assessment of mother, 331
  resuscitation, 330–331
Premature labor, 338
Pringle maneuver, 172, 175, 176, 177
Prograde colonic lavage, 222
Prostamembranous disruptions, 286
Prostate, 287
Proximal fecal diversion, 223
Proximal right renal vein, *354*
Psoas hitch, *273*, 274
Pubic rami, 98
Pulsus paradoxus, 23

Rape *see* Sexual assault
Rectum
  anatomy and physiology, 211–212
  complications, 226–227
  exam as part of secondary survey, 9–10
  postoperative care, 225–226
  trauma to, 223–224
    associated risk factors, 216–218
    etiology and incidence, 210–211
    history, 209–210
    initial assessment, 213–214
    local wound exploration, 214
    pathophysiology, 212–213
  wound management, 225

Rectus hematoma, 78, 79–80, 81
Rectus muscles, 75, 76
Red blood cells, 40–41
Renal artery, 259, 350, 352, *353*, 358–359, 367
Renal failure, 367, 411
Renal function, 385
Renal parenchyma, 252, 261, *263*
Renal trauma, 252–266, *405*
  anatomy, 252–254
  classification, 252, *253*
  complications, 266
  detection and staging, 254–255
  history, 250–251
  postoperative care, 266
  radiographic staging, 255–257
  reconstructive techniques, 258–261
  scale, 255
  surgical staging and exploration, 257–258
Renal veins, 373, 391
Renorrhapy, 261
Reperfusion injury, 367
Respiration, 6
Respiratory distress syndrome (RDS), 17–18
Respiratory system, 327
Resuscitation, 13–28
  airway, 14–16
  circulation, 16–25
  history, 13–14
  in extremis management, 27–28
  of patients with concurrent head injury, 25–27
  in pregnancy, 330–331
  priorities and goals, 14
  shock, 20–23
Retroperitoneal hematoma, 350, 398–412
  anatomy, 399–401
  complications, 411
  diagnosis and evaluation, 402–407
  history, 398–399
  management, 407–410
  outcome, 411–412
  pathophysiology, 401–402
Retroperitoneum, *260*, *355*
Ribs
  fractures, 14
  lower six, 74, 77
Right hepatic lobectomy, 181, *183*
Right renal vein, 373
Roux-en-Y duodenojejunostomy, 141, *143*, 144, *145*

Roux-en-Y limb, 139, 146, 147, 148, *149*
Sacroiliac ligament, 95
Saphenous vein, *21*, 348, *390*
Scalp, 7, 8
Sciatic nerve, 100
Scrotal injuries, 303–309
  flaps in replacement, 308
  grafts, 305–307
  partial loss, 303–304
  testicular function after reconstruction, 308–309
  total loss, 304–308
Seat belts, 74, 195–196
Sepsis, 187, 207
Sexual assault, 319–322
  consent for information and exam, 319–320
  follow-up, 322
  history of assault, 320
  lab specimens, 321
  physical exam, 320–321
  support services, 319
  treatment, 321–322
Shock, 14, 16
  cardiac compressive, 16, 23–24
  colonic, 217
  decompensated, 17
  hemorrhagic, 16, 17, 18–23, 25
  neurogenic, 16, 24–25
  resuscitation, 20–23
Shotgun injuries, 4, 81
Sigmoid colon, *356*
Sigmoidoscopy, 407
Skin grafts *see* Grafts
Small bowel, 61, 190–208, 350, *386*
  anatomy, 192
  assessment, 196–197
  complications, 206–208
  history of repair, 190–192
  injuries, mechanism of, 193–196
  necrosis, *206*
  operative exploration, 198–199
  operative treatment, 199–204
  postoperative care, 204, 206
  preoperative preparation, 197–198
Small intestine, *355*
Sonourethrogram, *285*
Spasm, 343
Spermatic cords, 304
Sphincter, 279–280

Spleen, *353*, 357
  anatomy, 231
  arterial supply, *232*
  complications, 246–247
  function, 231–233
  injuries, 35, 230–247
    assessment of, 234–235
    history, 230
    lacerations, *245*, *246*
    mechanism of, 233–234
    nonoperative management, 236–238
    ruptured, *46*, *47*
    operative exploration and evaluation, 238–241
    and pancreatic injury, 138
    postoperative care, 243–246
    preoperative care, 235–236
Splenectomy, 241–243, 246, 247
Splenic artery, 231, 357
Splenic flexure, 215
Splenic vein, 127, 374–375, 385, 391
Splenorrhaphy, 243, 246
Split thickness grafts, 302, *306*
Sports injuries, 314
Stab wounds
  and abdominal trauma, 3
  abdominal wall, 73, 80
  indications for surgery, 59–60
  rectal and colonic, 212–213, 214
  and retroperitoneal hematoma, 408, 410
Stomach injuries *see* Esophageal, gastric, and omental injuries
Straddle injury, *284*, *285*
Superior epigastric artery, 76
Superior mesenteric artery, 192, 345–346, 352, *353*, 357–358
Superior mesenteric vein, 192, 385, 392
Supraceliac aorta, 352, 356
Suprarenal aorta, 352
Suprarenal vena cava, 373, 388, 391
Surgery
  for abdominal arterial trauma, 349–355, 360–365
  for abdominal trauma, 57–70
    conduct of, 65–70
    indications, 58–63
    preoperative preparation, 64–65
    priorities for associated injuries, 70
  for abdominal venous trauma, 376–393
  for esophageal, gastric, and omental injuries, 113–116
  hepatic resection, 178, 180–184
  for pancreatic and duodenal injury, 131–134, 136–137
  penile grafts, 301–303
  renal, 257–264
  small bowel, 197–206
  splenic, 238–243
  testicular, 298–299
  ureteral, 269–274
  urethral, 286–287
  see also specific techniques, body parts, and conditions

Tension pneumothorax, *9*, 24
Testes, *305*, 308
Testicles, 304, *306*, *307*, 308–309
Testicular rupture, 296–299
  approach to management, 297–298
  diagnosis, 297
  signs and symptoms, 296–297
  surgical reconstruction, 298–299
Thigh pouches, 304–305
Thoracic aorta, 352
Thoracic trauma, 9
Thoracotomy, 27–28, 352
Thrombosis, 259, 366–367, 395
Tissue elasticity, 168
Traffic accidents, 5, 328, 329
Transuretero-ureterostomy, 271
Transversus abdominis, 74
Traumatic hemipelvectomy, 104–105
Tripartite suture of Carrel, 387

Ultrasound, 52–53, 332
Underwater blast injuries, 194–195
Ureteral reimplantation, 271, *272*
Ureteral trauma, 266–274
  anatomy, 266
  complications, 274
  detection and staging, 267
  exploration and exposure, 269
  history, 251
  mechanism of, 267
  reconstructive techniques, 269–274
Urethra
  anatomy, 278–280
  complications, 288
  injuries, 277–288
    assessment of, 280–282
    evaluation and initial management for female, 283–284

evaluation and management of anterior, 284
evaluation and management of posterior, 284–286
initial management and operative exploration, 282–283
lacerations, 295
operative treatment, 286–287
postoperative care, 287
preoperative preparation, 282
Urethrogram, 280–281, *282*, *284*, *285*, 287, 288
Urinary system, 327–328
Urogram *see* Intravenous urogram
Uterus, 316, 324, 328, 331–332, 337

Vagina, 316, 320, 332
Vascular injury, 59, 261, 264–265
Vascular repair, *363*, 368
Vena cava, *354*, 373, *374*, 378–379, *380*, 381, *382*, *383*, 385, 391
Venous injury *see* Abdominal venous trauma
Veno-venous bypass, 177, *179*
Ventilatory system, 14
Vulva, 315

X-rays
for abdominal trauma, 11
chest, 11, 88, *89*, 90
during pregnancy, 333